CALCULATE
with Confidence

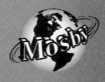

Visit our website at www.mosby.com

Third Edition

CALCULATE
with Confidence

Deborah Gray Morris, RN, BSN, MA, LNC

Professor of Nursing
Department of Nursing and Allied Health Sciences
Bronx Community College
Bronx, New York

With 614 Illustrations

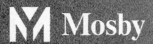 Mosby

An Affiliate of Elsevier Science

St. Louis   London   Philadelphia   Sydney   Toronto

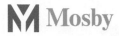

An Affiliate of Elsevier Science

Vice President and Publishing Director, Nursing: Sally Schrefer
Editor: Yvonne Alexopoulos
Developmental Editor: Kimberly A. Netterville
Project Manager: Catherine Jackson
Design Manager: Bill Drone

THIRD EDITION

NOTICE

Pharmacology is an ever-changing field. Standard safety precautions must be followed, but as new research and clinical experience broaden our knowledge, changes in treatment and drug therapy may become necessary or appropriate. Readers are advised to check the most current product information provided by the manufacturer of each drug to be administered to verify the recommended dose, the method and duration of administration, and contraindications. It is the responsibility of the treating physician, relying on experience and knowledge of the patient, to determine dosages and the best treatment for each individual patient. Neither the Publisher nor the editor assume any liability for any injury and/or damage to persons or property arising from this publication.

Mosby, Inc.
An Affiliate of Elsevier Science
11830 Westline Industrial Drive
St. Louis, Missouri 63146

Printed in the United States of America

Library of Congress Cataloging-in-Publication Data

Morris, Deborah Gray.
Calculate with confidence / Deborah Gray Morris.—3rd ed.
p. ; cm.
Includes bibliographical references and index.
ISBN 0-323-01349-X
1. Pharmaceutical arithmetic. 2. Nursing—Mathematics. I. Title.
[DNLM: 1. Pharmaceutical Preparations—administration & dosage—Nurses' Instruction. 2. Pharmaceutical Preparations—administration & dosage—Problems and Exercises. 3. Mathematics—Nurses' Instruction. 5. Mathematics—Problems and Exercises. QV 18.2 M875c 2002]
RS57 .M67 2002
615'.4—dc21

2001044609

02   03   04   05   GW/RDW   9   8   7   6   5   4   3   2

To my family, friends, nursing colleagues, and students past and present, but especially with love to my children, Cameron, Kimberly, Kanin, and Cory. You light up my life and have been proud of whatever I do.

To my mother, your guidance and nurturing has made me what I am today, thanks for always being there to support me.

To current practitioners of nursing and future nurses, I hope this book will be valuable in teaching the basic principles of medication administration and will ensure safe administration of medication to all clients regardless of the setting.

Reviewers

Milagros Y. Hall, BSN, RNC, CNA
Instructor
Nursing Department
Manhattan School–Practical Nursing Program
New York City Board of Education
New York, New York

Mary Welhaven, RN, PhD
Associate Professor
Nursing Department
Winona State University–Rochester Center
Rochester, Minnesota

Sandra C. Wardell, RN, BSN, MEd
Professor
Nursing Department
Orange County Community College
Middletown, New York

Preface

Calculate with Confidence is written to meet the needs of current and potential practitioners of nursing at any level. This book can be used for in-service education programs and as a reference for the inactive nurse returning to the work world. It is also suitable for courses of instruction whose content reflects the calculation of dosage and solutions for any health care professional whose responsibilities include safe administration of medications and solutions to clients in diverse clinical settings.

Despite the advent of what is called *unit dose* in some institutions, this procedure does not completely absolve health care professionals from the responsibility of calculation. With the increasing focus on providing health care outside the hospital, it becomes even more imperative that calculations be precise, done with thought, and done using critical thinking skills to ensure correct and safe administration of medications to clients. A working knowledge in the area of dosage calculation is necessary, regardless of the medication system used in an institution or in settings outside the institution.

Calculate with Confidence offers a simplified approach to the calculation and administration of drug doses. The book includes theoretical and mathematical concepts related to the administration of medications. An increased need for competency in basic math continues to be an essential prerequisite for dose calculation and demands a review of basic math skills, which each practitioner must be competent to do since it is the basis of all dose calculations. A step-by-step approach to dose calculation by the various rates of administration is also included.

Information related to systems of measurement and conversion is discussed in detail. Numerous illustrations, including full-color drug labels, syringes, and equipment used in medication administration, have been included to enhance learning and application to the clinical setting. Practice problems have been offered in each section to test the mastery of the content presented. In the area of basic math, a pretest and posttest have been included. The pretest will allow students to identify areas that need or do not need review. "Objectives," "Points to Remember," "Critical Thinking," and "Marginal Notes" are featured to guide students in learning the material in each chapter. Shading of syringes has been used to allow for visualization of dosages. Rationale for answers to dosage calculation problems has been included to enhance understanding of principles and answers related to dosages. Formulas that are simplified and encourage understanding of the dynamics in calculation are also presented, as well as dimensional analysis as a method of converting and calculation. Alternative vocabulary has been used in certain areas to enhance the learning of some material presented.

Calculate with Confidence is acknowledged for its simplicity in presenting material relevant to dose calculation and for enhancing the needs of the learner at different curricular levels. The book is also known for making content relevant to the needs of the student and for its use of realistic problems to enhance learning and to make material clinically applicable.

The third edition of *Calculate with Confidence* has maintained a style similar to the first. Revision of this edition is based on feedback from reviewers and on instructors' suggestions. It has been made more current to reflect the increasing responsibility of the nurse in medication administration and presents material necessary to reflect the current scope of practice. In addition to the revisions mentioned, the third edition, like the previous editions, is organized in a progression of basic to more complex information.

New features in the third edition include:

- Addition of new drug labels and discussion of equipment used in medication administration, including the computer-controlled dispensing system.
- Content about issues related to medication administration in home-care settings.
- Full color throughout the book to highlight and visually enhance material presented.
- New workbook-style format designed to allow notes and problems to be worked out in margins.
- Marginal Notes are featured throughout to highlight key information to remember for clinical practice.
- Chapter 9 on conversion in the heath care setting includes temperature conversions.
- Presentation of dimensional analysis in Chapter 24 as a method of converting and calculation.
- Many new practice problems to help students apply and evaluate learning in different types of calculations.
- An explanation of SI units and their use consistently throughout the book.
- Expanded content in the areas of I.V. calculation and pediatric doses, using the body-surface area (BSA) method and formula method; I.V. calculation chapter expanded to include methods of administering I.V. medications specific to the child, and easier formula for calculation of IV flow rates, including the shortcut method.
- Additional problems added to the comprehensive posttest at the end of the book, giving and serving as an overall evaluation of learning.

It is my hope that use of this book will help nurses and potential nurses calculate dosages accurately and with confidence, ensuring administration of medications safely to all clients in all settings, which is the primary responsibility of the nurse.

Deborah C. Gray Morris

Acknowledgments

I wish to extend sincere gratitude and appreciation to my family, friends, and colleagues for their support and encouragement during the writing of this third edition. I am indebted to the Nursing Department at Bronx Community College, who listened to me, made pertinent suggestions, helped with validation of content used in the text, and brought me problems from the clinical setting. Sincere thanks to Professor Lois Augustus, Chairperson of the Department of Nursing and Allied Health Sciences, for all your pep talks, encouragement, and understanding when I needed time to work on this edition. Special thanks to the reviewers of this text; their comments and suggestions were invaluable. Particular thanks to the math reviewers, Shirley S. Powell, BS, BSN, MSN, and Ann Dillon, MSN. Thanks to students past and present at Bronx Community College who brought practice problems from the clinical area, and helped me to have an appreciation for the problems that students encounter with basic math and calculation of drug doses. Thanks for your valuable feedback which helped with revisions.

I am sincerely grateful to the following people: Arlene Levey, a former and late colleague, who told me "I could fly" and whose encouragement helped me to "soar like an eagle." Professor Marie-Louise Nickerson of the English Department at Bronx Community College, who nurtured and encouraged me to first consider publication and worked closely with me on a project that resulted in the development of the text for publication. I am so grateful for your guidance; who would have thought it would now be in its third edition. Thank you, Professor Germana Glier, Chairperson of Mathematics and Computer Science at Bronx Community College; your help with the aspects of solving for the unknown in the I.V. chapter and validating mathematical answers was invaluable. And the late Dr. Gerald S. Lieblich, former Chairperson of the Department of Mathematics at Bronx Community College, who took the time to review and validate content, as well as to make pertinent suggestions for the unit on basic math. To my friend, the late Frank C. Rucker, your encouragement, inspiring words, and admiration for me as an author will always remain with me.

Thanks to the following hospitals for permission to reproduce records used in this text: St. Barnabas Hospital (Bronx, New York) and Jack D. Weiler Hospital of the Albert Einstein College of Medicine, a division of Montefiore Medical Center (Bronx, New York).

Thanks to the Research Foundation of New York for giving permission to use the I.V. formula and formula for dose calculations from the computer-assisted programs in pharmacology, which are copyrighted by the foundation.

I am especially grateful to the staff at Mosby for their support and help in planning writing, and producing the first edition of this text. A special thanks to Kimberly A. Netterville for her time, support, patience, and understanding with the revisions of the third edition. Thanks for your encouragement and sincere concerns at times when I needed it most.

To Reginald B. Morris, my husband, thanks for your help, encouragement, support, and understanding while I revised this text. Thanks for your support, confidence in me, and encouragement during those times when I had doubts that I would meet the deadline for this text. Thanks for the long hours you spent at the computer inputting the revisions and doing whatever to help complete the project. Without your continual support and assistance, this edition could not have been finished.

Anna, my dearest friend, and like a sister, thanks for all of your support, encouragement, and expressions of confidence in me during the times I needed it most, especially your statement to me: you'll get it done, I'm not even worried.

Finally I wish to thank all the pharmaceutical companies that allowed me to reproduce their medication labels in the book to provide a more realistic picture for the student.

Rhone-Paulenc Rorer Pharmaceuticals, Inc.
Hoechst Marion Roussel
Burroughs Wellcome Co.
Glaxo Wellcome, Inc.
Merck & Co., Inc.
Bayer Corporation
SmithKline Beecham
Bristol Meyers Squibb
Apothecon–a Bristol Meyer Squibb Company
The UpJohn Company
Dista–a divisionof Eli Lilly Corparation
Squibb
Astra USA, Inc.
Parke-Davis Divison of Warner Lambert
Eli Lilly and Company

Introduction to the Student

The nursing profession is undergoing profound changes. Today's nurses face many technological advances, not only in the hospital setting, but in settings outside of the hospital in the community and home. The nurse has to be competent and able to use critical thinking skills because application of dose calculations appears in a variety of settings. The accurate calculation of drug doses is a critical and necessary skill in health care. Serious harm can come to clients from mathematical errors in calculating a drug dose. Therefore it is a major responsibility of those administering drugs to ensure safe administration of medications by having the ability to accurately calculate a dose. Remember to always consult appropriate resources when necessary before administering any medication. This text is intended to provide you with the skills to calculate a dose with accuracy. Errors can be avoided if dose calculation is approached in a logical fashion, and consideration is given to the reasonableness of the answer based on the principles presented. It is hoped that this text will help to emphasize the importance of accurate medication administration to clients and will assist nurses to feel more confident in mastering the skill of dose calculation.

Deborah C. Gray Morris

Contents

UNIT ONE   Math Review, 1

   Pretest, 3

 1 *Roman Numerals*, 7

 2 *Fractions*, 11

 3 *Decimals*, 23

 4 *Ratio and Proportion*, 37

 5 *Percentages*, 45

   Posttest, 53

UNIT TWO   Systems of Measurement, 57

 6 *Metric System*, 59

 7 *Apothecaries' and Household Systems*, 69

 8 *Converting Within and Between Systems*, 77

 9 *Additional Conversions Useful in the Health Care Setting*, 93

UNIT THREE   Methods of Administration and Calculation, 101

10 *Medication Administration*, 103

11 *Understanding Medication Orders*, 119

12 *Medication Administration Records*, 131

13 *Reading Medication Labels*, 147

14 *Calculating Doses Using Ratio-Proportion*, 165

15 *Dose Calculation Using the Formula Method*, 187

UNIT FOUR   Oral and Parenteral Dose Forms, Insulin, and Pediatric Dose Calculations, 205

16 *Calculation of Oral Medications*, 207

17 *Parenteral Medications*, 247

18 *Powdered Drugs*, 291

19 Insulin, *317*

20 Pediatric Dose Calculation, *343*

UNIT FIVE   Basic I.V., Heparin, and Critical Care Calculations, *375*

21 Basic I.V. Calculations, *377*

22 Heparin Calculations, *439*

23 Critical Care Calculations, *455*

24 Dimensional Analysis, *467*

Comprehensive Posttest, *479*

Answer Key, *489*

Detailed Contents

UNIT ONE   Math Review, 1

Pretest, *3*

1 ***Roman Numerals***, *7*
Practice Problems, *9*
Chapter Review, *9*

2 ***Fractions***, *11*
Types of Fractions, *12*
Practice Problems, *14*
Reducing Fractions, *15*
Adding Fractions, *16*
Subtracting Fractions, *17*
Multiplying Fractions, *18*
Dividing Fractions, *19*
Practice Problems, *19*
Chapter Review, *21*

3 ***Decimals***, *23*
Reading and Writing Decimals, *24*
Practice Problems, *25*
Comparing the Value of Decimals, *25*
Practice Problems, *26*
Addition and Subtraction of Decimals, *26*
Practice Problems, *27*
Multiplying Decimals, *27*
Practice Problems, *29*
Division of Decimals, *29*
Rounding Off Decimals, *31*
Practice Problems, *31*
Changing Fractions to Decimals, *32*
Changing Decimals to Fractions, *32*
Practice Problems, *33*
Chapter Review, *33*

4 ***Ratio and Proportion***, *37*
Ratios, *37*
Proportions, *38*
Solving for *x* in Ratio-Proportion, *39*
Applying Ratio-Proportion to Dosage Calculation, *41*
Practice Problems, *42*
Chapter Review, *43*

5 *Percentages,* 45
    Practice Problems, 46
    Changing Percentages to Fractions, Decimals, and Ratios, 47
    Practice Problems, 47
    Changing Fractions, Decimals, and Ratios to Percentages, 48
    Practice Problems, 49
    Determining the Percent of a Quantity, 50
    Determining What Percent One Number Is of Another, 50
    Practice Problems, 51
    Chapter Review, 51
    Posttest, 53

UNIT TWO   Systems of Measurement, 57

6 *Metric System,* 59
    Particulars of the Metric System, 59
    Rules of Metric System, 61
    Units of Measure, 62
    Conversions Between Metric Units, 63
    Practice Problems, 63
    Chapter Review, 64

7 *Apothecaries' and Household Systems,* 69
    Apothecaries' System, 69
    Household System, 72
    Practice Problems, 75
    Chapter Review, 75

8 *Converting Within and Between Systems,* 77
    Equivalents Among Metric, Apothecaries', and Household Systems, 77
    Converting, 77
    Methods of Converting, 78
    Practice Problems, 79
    Converting Within the Same System, 81
    Practice Problems, 82
    Converting Between Systems, 83
    Calculating Intake and Output, 84
    Practice Problems, 89
    Chapter Review, 90

9 *Additional Conversions Useful in the Health Care Setting,* 93
    Converting Between Celsius and Fahrenheit, 93
    Formulas for Converting Between Fahrenheit and Celsius Scales, 95
    Practice Problems, 95
    Metric Measures Relating to Length, 96
    Practice Problems, 97
    Conversions Relating to Weight, 97
    Practice Problems, 98
    Chapter Review, 99

UNIT THREE   Methods of Administration and Calculation, 101

10 *Medication Administration,* 103
    Critical Thinking and Medication Administration, 104
    Factors That Influence Drug Doses and Action, 104
    Special Considerations for the Elderly, 105
    The Six Rights of Medication Administration, 106

Teaching the Client, *108*
Home Care Considerations, *109*
Routes of Medication Administration, *109*
Equipment Used for Dose Calculation, *111*
Equipment for Administering Oral Medications to a Child, *112*
Practice Problems, *115*
Chapter Review, *116*

11 *Understanding Medication Orders,* 119
Writing a Medication Order, *120*
Components of a Medication Order, *120*
Interpreting a Medication Order, *124*
Practice Problems, *126*
Chapter Review, *127*

12 *Medication Administration Records,* 131
Essential Information on a Medication Record, *132*
Documentation of Medications Administered, *132*
Explanation of Medication Administration Records, *135*
Computerized Medication Records, *137*
Unit Dose System, *137*
Scheduling Medication Times, *138*
Military Time, *139*
Practice Problems, *142*
Chapter Review, *143*

13 *Reading Medication Labels,* 147
Reading Medication Labels, *147*
Medication Labels for Combined Drugs, *153*
Practice Problems, *156*
Chapter Review, *158*

14 *Calculating Doses Using Ratio-Proportion,* 165
Use of Ratio-Proportion in Dose Calculation, *165*
Practice Problems, *168*
Chapter Review, *171*

15 *Dose Calculation Using the Formula Method,* 187
Formulas for Calculating Doses, *187*
Steps for Use of the Formulas, *188*
Practice Problems, *191*
Chapter Review, *193*

UNIT FOUR   Oral and Parenteral Dose Forms, Insulin,
and Pediatric Dose Calculations, 205

16 *Calculation of Oral Medications,* 207
Forms of Solid Medications, *207*
Calculating Doses Involving Tablets and Capsules, *210*
Practice Problems, *219*
Calculating Oral Liquids, *230*
Measuring Oral Liquids, *230*
Practice Problems, *242*
Chapter Review, *245*

17 *Parenteral Medications,* 247
Packaging of Parenteral Medications, *247*
Syringes, *251*
Practice Problems, *256*

Reading Parenteral Labels, *261*
Drugs Labeled in Percentage Strengths, *263*
Solutions Expressed in Ratio Strength, *264*
Parenteral Medications Measured in Units, *264*
Parenteral Medications in Milliequivalents, *265*
Practice Problems, *263*
Calculating Parenteral Dosages, *267*
Calculating Injectable Medications According to the Syringe, *267*
Calculating Doses for Medications in Units, *272*
Practice Problems, *274*
Chapter Review, *278*

18 *Powdered Drugs*, *291*
Basic Principles for Reconstitution, *291*
Practice Problems, *294*
Reconstituting Medications with More than One Direction
    for Mixing, *298*
Practice Problems, *300*
Reconstitution from Package Insert Directions, *301*
Calculations of Doses, *302*
Chapter Review, *305*

19 *Insulin*, *317*
Types of Insulin, *317*
Practice Problems, *318*
Appearance of Insulin, *320*
Fixed Combination Insulins, *320*
U-100 Syringe, *321*
Practice Problems, *323*
Insulin Orders, *326*
Preparing a Single Dose of Insulin in an Insulin Syringe, *329*
Measuring Two Types of Insulin in the Same Syringe, *329*
Chapter Review, *333*

20 *Pediatric Dose Calculation*, *343*
Principles Relating to Basic Calculations, *344*
Calculation of Doses Based on Body Weight, *344*
Converting lb to kg, *344*
Practice Problems, *345*
Converting kg to lb, *346*
Practice Problems, *346*
Calculation of Pediatric Doses Using Body Surface
    Area (BSA), *356*
Reading the West Nomogram Chart, *357*
Practice Problems, *358*
Dose Calculation Based on BSA, *359*
Calculating Using the Formula, *359*
Practice Problems, *360*
Calculating BSA with the Use of a Formula, *361*
Practice Problems, *363*
Pediatric Oral and Parenteral Medications, *364*
Chapter Review, *365*

UNIT FIVE Basic I.V., Heparin, and Critical Care Calculations, 375

21 *Basic I.V. Calculations*, 377
Methods of Infusion, *378*
I.V. Fluids, *387*
Practice Problems, *393*
I.V. Flow Rate Calculation, *394*
I.V. Tubing, *396*
Practice Problems, *398*
Calculating I.V. Flow Rates in gtt/min, *399*
Practice Problems, *399*
Formula Method for Calculating I.V. Flow Rate, *400*
Practice Problems, *403*
Calculating I.V. Flow Rates when Several Solutions
    Are Ordered, *407*
Practice Problems, *408*
I.V. Medications, *408*
Practice Problems, *409*
Determining the Amount of Drug in a Specific Amount
    of Solution, *410*
Practice Problems, *412*
Determining Infusion Times and Volumes, *412*
Steps to Calculating a Problem with an Unknown, *413*
Practice Problems, *414*
Recalculating an I.V. Flow Rate, *414*
Practice Problems, *416*
Calculating Total Infusion Times, *417*
Charting I.V. Therapy, *418*
Practice Problems, *416*
Calculating Infusion Time When mL/hr Is Not Indicated, *419*
Practice Problems, *420*
Labeling Solution Bags, *421*
I.V. Therapy and Children, *422*
Calculating I.V. Medications by Burette, *422*
Practice Problems, *425*
Enteral Feedings, *426*
Practice Problems, *428*
Chapter Review, *431*

22 *Heparin Calculations*, 439
Calculation of s.c. Doses, *440*
Calculation of I.V. Heparin Solutions, *441*
Determining If a Dose Is Within the Safe Heparinizing Range, *443*
Practice Problems, *444*
Chapter Review, *446*

23 *Critical Care Calculations*, 455
Calculating mL/hr Rate, *456*
Calculating Critical Care Doses Per Hour Or Per Minute, *456*
Drugs Ordered in Milligrams Per Minute, *457*
Calculating Doses Based on mcg/kg/min, *457*
Titration of Infusions, *458*
Practice Problems, *459*
Chapter Review, *460*

24 Dimensional Analysis, *467*
Understanding Dimensional Analysis, *467*
Understanding the Basics of Dimensional Analysis, *467*
Practice Problems, *469*
Dose Calculation Using Dimensional Analysis, *470*
Practice Problems, *473*
Using Dimensional Analysis to Calculate I.V. Flow Rates, *474*
Practice Problems, *476*
Chapter Review, *477*

Comprehensive Posttest, *479*

Answer Key, *489*

Index, *593*

UNIT ONE

Math Review

This unit contains a review of basic math skills essential for the calculation of doses and solutions, regardless of the problem-solving method used in calculation. Knowledge of basic math is a necessary component of dose calculation that nurses need to know to prevent medication errors and ensure the safe administration of medications. Although calculators are accessible for basic math operations, the nurse needs to be able to perform the processes involved in basic math. Controversy still exists among educators regarding the use of calculators in dose calculation. Calculators may indeed be recommended for complex calculations to ensure accuracy and save time; the types of calculations requiring their use are presented later in this text. However, because the basic math required for less complex calculations is often simple and can be done without the use of a calculator, it is a realistic expectation that each practitioner should be competent in the performance of basic math operations without their use. Performing basic math operations enables the nurse to think logically and critically about the dose ordered and the dose calculated.

Chapter 1
Roman Numerals
Chapter 2
Fractions
Chapter 3
Decimals
Chapter 4
Ratio and Proportion
Chapter 5
Percentages

A pretest and a posttest have been included in this unit, offering an opportunity for students to assess their skills.

Pretest

This test is designed to test your ability in the basic math areas reviewed in Unit One. The test consists of 55 questions. If you are able to complete the pretest with 100% accuracy, you may want to bypass Unit One. Any problems answered incorrectly should be used as a basis for what you might need to review. The purpose of this test and the review that follows is to build your confidence in basic math skills, and to help you avoid careless mistakes when you begin to perform dose calculations.

Express the following in Roman numerals.

1. 9 _____

2. 16 _____

3. 23 _____

4. $10\frac{1}{2}$ _____

5. 22 _____

Express the following in Arabic numbers.

6. $\overline{\text{xiss}}$ _____

7. $\overline{\text{xii}}$ _____

8. $\overline{\text{xviii}}$ _____

9. $\overline{\text{xxiv}}$ _____

10. $\overline{\text{vi}}$ _____

Reduce the following fractions to lowest terms.

11. $\dfrac{14}{21}$ _____

12. $\dfrac{25}{100}$ _____

13. $\dfrac{2}{150}$ _____

14. $\dfrac{24}{30}$ _____

15. $\dfrac{24}{36}$ _____

Perform the indicated operations; reduce to lowest terms where necessary.

16. $\dfrac{2}{3} \div \dfrac{3}{9}$ _____

17. $4 \div \dfrac{3}{4}$ _____

18. $\dfrac{2}{5} + \dfrac{1}{9} =$ _____

19. $7\dfrac{1}{7} - 2\dfrac{5}{6} =$ _____

20. $4\dfrac{2}{3} \times 4 =$ _____

Change the following fractions to decimals; express your answer to the nearest tenth.

21. $\dfrac{6}{7}$ _____   23. $\dfrac{2}{3}$ _____

22. $\dfrac{6}{20}$ _____   24. $\dfrac{7}{8}$ _____

Indicate the largest fraction in each group.

25. $\dfrac{3}{4}, \dfrac{4}{5}, \dfrac{7}{8}$ _____   26. $\dfrac{7}{12}, \dfrac{11}{12}, \dfrac{4}{12}$ _____

Perform the indicated operations with decimals.

27. $20.1 + 67.35 =$ _____   29. $4.6 \times 8.72 =$ _____

28. $0.008 + 5.0 =$ _____   30. $56.47 - 8.7 =$ _____

Divide the following decimals; express your answer to the nearest tenth.

31. $7.5 \div 0.004 =$ _____   33. $84.7 \div 2.3$ _____

32. $45 \div 1.9 =$ _____

Indicate the largest decimal in each group.

34. $0.674, 0.659$ _____   36. $0.25, 0.6, 0.175$ _____

35. $0.375, 0.37, 0.038$ _____

Solve for x, the unknown value.

37. $8 : 2 = 48 : x$ _____   39. $\dfrac{1}{10} : x = \dfrac{1}{2} : 15$ _____

38. $x : 300 = 1 : 150$ _____   40. $0.4 : 1 = 0.2 : x$ _____

Round off to the nearest tenth.

41. $0.43 =$ _____   43. $1.47 =$ _____

42. $0.66 =$ _____

Round off to the nearest hundredth.

44. $0.735 =$ _____   46. $1.227 =$ _____

45. $0.834 =$ _____

Complete the table below, expressing the measures in their equivalents where indicated. Reduce to lowest terms where necessary.

	Percent	Decimal	Ratio	Fraction
47.	6%	_____	_____	_____
48.	_____	_____	7:20	_____
49.	_____	_____	_____	$5\frac{1}{4}$
50.	_____	0.015	_____	_____

Find the following percentages.

51. 5% of 95 _____

52. $\frac{1}{4}$% of 2,000 _____

53. 2 is what % of 600 _____

54. 20 is what % of 100 _____

55. 30 is what % of 164 _____

Answers on p. 489

Roman Numerals

The Roman numeral system dates back to ancient Roman times and uses letters to designate amounts. Roman numerals may sometimes be used, especially in the **apothecaries' system** of measurement, with apothecary weights and measure.

Example:

                                grx

  Apothecary measure   Roman numeral
  unit of weight   (Arabic equivalent 10)

Roman numerals are also still used on objects that indicate time (i.e., watches, clocks).

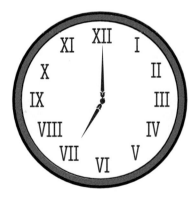

In the Arabic system, numbers, not letters, are used to express amounts. The Arabic system also uses fractions (1/2) and decimals (0.5).

To calculate drug doses the nurse needs to know both Roman numerals and Arabic numbers. Lower case letters are usually used to express Roman numerals in relation to medications. The Roman numerals you will see most often in the calculation of doses are built on the basic symbols i, v, and x. To prevent errors in interpretation a line is sometimes drawn over the symbol. If this line is used, the lower case "i" is dotted above the line, not below.

Example 1:   10 grains = gr$\overline{\text{x}}$

Example 2:   Two = ïi

When the symbol for 1/2 is used in conjunction with Roman numerals, the symbol (ss) is placed at the end.

Example 1: $3\frac{1}{2}$ = iiiss = iii$\overline{ss}$

Example 2: $1\frac{1}{2}$ grains = griss = gri$\overline{ss}$

Box 1-1 lists the common Arabic equivalents for Roman numerals (review them if necessary). They are often expressed with small case letters. Review this list before proceeding to the rules pertaining to Roman numbers in Box 1-2. You will most commonly see Roman numerals up to the value of 30 when used in relation to medications.

BOX 1-1	Arabic Equivalents for Roman Numerals
ARABIC NUMBER	**ROMAN NUMERAL**
$\frac{1}{2}$	ss or $\overline{ss}$
1	i or i̇, I
2	ii or i̇i, II
3	iii or i̇ii, III
4	iv or i̇v, IV
5	v or v̄, V
6	vi or v̄i, VI
7	vii or v̄ii, VII
8	viii or v̄iii, VIII
9	ix or i̇x, IX
10	x or x̄, X
15	xv or x̄v, XV
20	xx or x̄x, XX
30	xxx or x̄xx, XXX

Note:

Larger Roman numerals, such as L = 50, C = 100, and larger, are usually not used in relation to medications.

BOX 1-2	Rules Relating to the Roman System of Notation

When a Roman numeral is repeated twice it doubles the value; when repeated three times it triples the value. Example: x = 10, xx = 20, and xxx = 30.
1. The same numeral is never repeated more than three times.
2. When a Roman numeral of a lesser value is placed after one of greater value, the numeral of lesser value is added to the one of greater value.

Example: 25 = $\overline{xxv}$ $\overline{xx}$ = 20, v = 5 (10 + 10 + 5 = 25)

16 = $\overline{xvi}$ $\overline{x}$ = 10, v = 5, i = 1 (10 + 5 + 1 = 16)

3. When a Roman numeral of lesser value is placed **before** a numeral of greater value, the numeral of lesser value is subtracted from the one of greater value.

Example: i̇x = 9   x = 10, i = 1.

i being placed **before** the x is 10 − 1 = 9.

$\overline{xxi̇v}$ = 24

$\overline{xx}$ = 20, i̇v = 4

10 + 10 = 20, v being placed **after** i is 5 − 1 or 4.

20 + (5 − 1) = 20 + 4 = 24

PRACTICE PROBLEMS

Write the following as Roman numerals.

1. 15 _____   6. 14 _____

2. 13 _____   7. 29 _____

3. 28 _____   8. 4 _____

4. 11 _____   9. 19 _____

5. 17 _____   10. 34 _____

Answers on p. 490

CHAPTER REVIEW

Write the following Arabic numbers as Roman numerals.

1. 6 _____   6. 18 _____

2. 30 _____   7. 20 _____

3. $1\frac{1}{2}$ _____   8. 3 _____

4. 27 _____   9. 21 _____

5. 12 _____   10. 26 _____

Answers on p. 490

Write the following Roman numerals as Arabic numbers.

11. $\overline{\text{viiss}}$ _____   16. $\overline{\text{iii}}$ _____

12. $\overline{\text{xix}}$ _____   17. $\overline{\text{xxii}}$ _____

13. $\overline{\text{xv}}$ _____   18. $\overline{\text{xvi}}$ _____

14. $\overline{\text{xxx}}$ _____   19. $\overline{\text{v}}$ _____

15. $\overline{\text{ss}}$ _____   20. $\overline{\text{xxvii}}$ _____

Answers on p. 490

Fractions

Understanding fractions is necessary because the nurse often encounters fractions when dealing with apothecaries' measurements in dosage calculation.

A fraction is a part of a whole number (Figure 2-1). It is a division of a whole into units or parts (Figure 2-2).

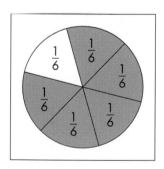

Figure 2-1 Diagram representing fractions of a whole. Five parts shaded out of six parts represents:

$$\frac{5}{6} \quad \frac{\text{Numerator}}{\text{Denominator}}$$

Example: $\frac{1}{2}$ is a whole divided into two parts.

Fractions are composed of two parts: a **numerator,** which is the top number, and a **denominator,** which is the bottom number.

$$\frac{\text{Numerator}}{\text{Denominator}} : \frac{\substack{\text{how many parts of the} \\ \text{whole you are taking}}}{\substack{\text{how many equal parts} \\ \text{the whole is divided into}}}$$

Example: In the fraction $\frac{5}{6}$, 5 is the numerator, and 6 is the denominator.

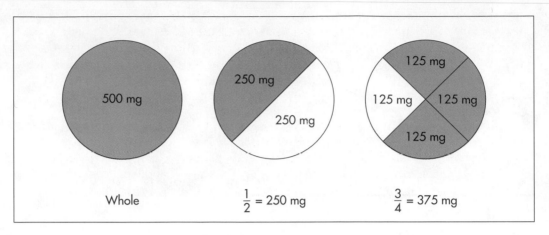

Figure 2-2   Fraction pie charts.

TYPES OF FRACTIONS

Proper Fraction: Numerator is less than the denominator.

Examples: $\dfrac{1}{8}, \dfrac{5}{6}, \dfrac{7}{8}, \dfrac{1}{150}$

Improper Fraction: Numerator is larger than, or equal to, the denominator.

Examples: $\dfrac{3}{2}, \dfrac{7}{5}, \dfrac{300}{150}, \dfrac{4}{4}$

Mixed Number: Whole number and a fraction.

Examples: $3\dfrac{1}{3}, 5\dfrac{1}{8}, 9\dfrac{1}{6}, 25\dfrac{7}{8}$

Complex Fraction: Numerator, denominator, or both, are fractions.

Examples: $\dfrac{3\frac{1}{2}}{2}, \dfrac{\frac{1}{3}}{\frac{1}{2}}, \dfrac{2}{\quad}, \dfrac{2}{\frac{1}{150}}$

Whole Numbers: Have an unexpressed denominator of one (1).

Examples: $1 = \dfrac{1}{1}, 3 = \dfrac{3}{1}, 6 = \dfrac{6}{1}, 100 = \dfrac{100}{1}$

An improper fraction can be changed to a mixed number or whole number by dividing the numerator by the denominator.

Examples: $\dfrac{6}{5} = 6 \div 5 = 1\dfrac{1}{5}, \dfrac{100}{25} = 100 \div 25 = 4$

A mixed number can be changed to an improper fraction by multiplying the whole number by the denominator, adding it to the numerator, and placing the sum over the denominator.

Example: $5\dfrac{1}{8} = \dfrac{(5 \times 8) + 1}{8} = \dfrac{41}{8}$

Two or more fractions with different denominators can be compared by changing both fractions to fractions with the same denominator (Box 2-1). This is done by finding the lowest common denominator (LCD), or the lowest number evenly divisible by the denominators of the fractions being compared.

Example: Which is larger, $\frac{3}{4}$ or $\frac{4}{5}$?

Solution: The lowest common denominator is 20, because it is the smallest number that can be divided by both denominators evenly. Change each fraction to the same terms by dividing the lowest common denominator by the denominator and multiplying that answer by the numerator. The answer obtained from this is the new numerator. The numerators are then placed over the lowest common denominator.

For the fraction $\frac{3}{4}$: $20 \div 4 = 5; 5 \times 3 = 15;$

therefore $\frac{3}{4}$ becomes $\frac{15}{20}$.

For the fraction $\frac{4}{5}$: $20 \div 5 = 4; 4 \times 4 = 16;$

therefore $\frac{4}{5}$ becomes $\frac{16}{20}$.

Therefore $\frac{4}{5}\left(\frac{16}{20}\right)$ is larger than $\frac{3}{4}\left(\frac{15}{20}\right)$.

Note:

LCD = 20

Box 2-2 presents fundamental rules of fractions.

BOX 2-1 Rules for Comparing Size of Fractions

Comparing the size of fractions is important in the administration of medications, it helps the new practitioner learn early the value of medication doses. Here are some basic rules to keep in mind when comparing fractions.

1. If the numerators are the same, the fraction with the smaller denominator has the larger value.

Example 1: $\frac{1}{2}$ is larger than $\frac{1}{3}$

Example 2: $\frac{1}{150}$ is larger than $\frac{1}{300}$

2. If the denominators are the same, the fraction with the larger numerator has the larger value.

Example 1: $\frac{3}{4}$ is larger than $\frac{1}{4}$

Example 2: $\frac{3}{100}$ is larger than $\frac{1}{100}$

Notes

BOX 2-2   Fundamental Rules of Fractions

In working with fractions, there are some fundamental rules we need to remember.

1. When the numerator and denominator of a fraction are both multiplied or divided by the same number, the value of the fraction remains unchanged.

Examples:

$$\frac{1}{2} = \frac{1 \times (2)}{2 \times (2)} = \frac{2}{4} = \frac{2 \times (25)}{4 \times (25)} = \frac{50}{100} \text{, etc.,}$$

$$\frac{50}{100} = \frac{50 \div (10)}{100 \div (10)} = \frac{5}{10} = \frac{5 \div (5)}{10 \div (5)} = \frac{1}{2} \text{, etc.}$$

As shown in the examples, common fractions can be written in varied forms, provided always that the numerator, divided by the denominator, yields the same number (quotient). The particular form of a fraction that has the smallest possible whole number for its numerator and denominator is called the *fraction in its lowest terms*. In the example, therefore, 50/100, or 5/10, or 2/4, is 1/2 in its lowest terms.

2. To change a fraction to its lowest terms, divide its numerator and its denominator by the largest whole number that will divide both evenly.

Example: Reduce 128/288 to lowest terms.

$$\frac{128}{288} = \frac{128 \div 32}{288 \div 32} = \frac{4}{9}$$

Note: When you do not see at once the largest number that can be divided evenly, the fraction may have to be reduced using repeated steps.

Example: $$\frac{128}{288} = \frac{128 \div 4}{288 \div 4} = \frac{32}{72} = \frac{32 \div 8}{72 \div 8} = \frac{4}{9}$$

Note: If both the numerator and denominator cannot be divided evenly by a whole number, the fraction is in lowest terms. Fractions should always be expressed in their lowest terms.

3. LCD (lowest common denominator) is the smallest whole number that can be divided evenly by all of the denominators within the problem.

Example: 1/3 and 5/12—12 is evenly divisible by 3; therefore 12 is the LCD. 3/7, 2/14, and 2/28—28 is evenly divisible by 7 and 14, therefore 28 is the LCD.

PRACTICE PROBLEMS

Circle the fraction with the lesser value in each of the following sets.

1. $\frac{6}{30}$, $\quad \frac{4}{5}$

2. $\frac{5}{4}$, $\quad \frac{6}{8}$

3. $\frac{1}{75}$, $\quad \frac{1}{100}$, $\quad \frac{1}{150}$

4. $\frac{6}{18}$, $\quad \frac{7}{18}$, $\quad \frac{8}{18}$

5. $\frac{4}{5}$, $\quad \frac{7}{5}$, $\quad \frac{3}{5}$

6. $\frac{4}{8}$, $\quad \frac{1}{8}$, $\quad \frac{3}{8}$

7. $\frac{1}{40}$, $\quad \frac{1}{10}$, $\quad \frac{1}{5}$

8. $\frac{1}{300}$, $\quad \frac{1}{200}$, $\quad \frac{1}{175}$

9. $\frac{4}{24}$, $\quad \frac{5}{24}$, $\quad \frac{10}{24}$

10. $\frac{4}{3}$, $\quad \frac{1}{2}$, $\quad \frac{1}{6}$

Notes

Circle the fraction with the higher value in each of the following sets.

11. $\dfrac{6}{8}$, $\quad \dfrac{5}{9}$

16. $\dfrac{2}{5}$, $\quad \dfrac{6}{5}$, $\quad \dfrac{3}{5}$

12. $\dfrac{7}{6}$, $\quad \dfrac{2}{3}$

17. $\dfrac{1}{8}$, $\quad \dfrac{4}{6}$, $\quad \dfrac{1}{4}$

13. $\dfrac{1}{72}$, $\quad \dfrac{6}{12}$, $\quad \dfrac{1}{24}$

18. $\dfrac{7}{9}$, $\quad \dfrac{5}{9}$, $\quad \dfrac{8}{9}$

14. $\dfrac{1}{10}$, $\quad \dfrac{1}{6}$, $\quad \dfrac{1}{8}$

19. $\dfrac{1}{10}$, $\quad \dfrac{1}{50}$, $\quad \dfrac{1}{150}$

15. $\dfrac{1}{75}$, $\quad \dfrac{1}{125}$, $\quad \dfrac{1}{225}$

20. $\dfrac{2}{15}$, $\quad \dfrac{1}{15}$, $\quad \dfrac{6}{15}$

Answers on pp. 490-491

REDUCING FRACTIONS

Fractions should always be reduced to their lowest terms.

> To reduce a fraction to its lowest terms, the numerator and denominator are each divided by the largest number by which they are both evenly divisible.

Example 1:   Reduce the fraction $\dfrac{6}{20}$

Solution: Both numerator and denominator are evenly divisible by 2.

$6 \div 2 = 3; 20 \div 2 = 10$

$\dfrac{6}{20} = \dfrac{3}{10}$

Example 2:   Reduce the fraction $\dfrac{75}{100}$

Solution: Both numerator and denominator are evenly divisible by 25.

$75 \div 25 = 3; 100 \div 25 = 4$

$\dfrac{75}{100} = \dfrac{3}{4}$

 PRACTICE PROBLEMS

Reduce the following fractions to their lowest terms.

21. $\dfrac{10}{15} = $ _____

25. $\dfrac{20}{28} = $ _____

22. $\dfrac{7}{49} = $ _____

26. $\dfrac{14}{98} = $ _____

23. $\dfrac{64}{128} = $ _____

27. $\dfrac{10}{18} = $ _____

24. $\dfrac{100}{150} = $ _____

28. $\dfrac{24}{36} = $ _____

29. $\dfrac{10}{50} =$ _____

30. $\dfrac{9}{27} =$ _____

31. $\dfrac{9}{9} =$ _____

32. $\dfrac{15}{45} =$ _____

33. $\dfrac{124}{155} =$ _____

34. $\dfrac{12}{18} =$ _____

35. $\dfrac{36}{64} =$ _____

Answers on p. 491

ADDING FRACTIONS

To add fractions with the same denominator, add the numerators, place the sum over the denominator, and reduce to lowest terms.

Example 1: $\dfrac{1}{6} + \dfrac{4}{6} = \dfrac{5}{6}$

Example 2: $\dfrac{1}{6} + \dfrac{3}{6} + \dfrac{4}{6} = \dfrac{8}{6}$

$\dfrac{8}{6} = \dfrac{4}{3} = 1\dfrac{1}{3}$

Note:

In addition to reducing to lowest terms in example 2, the improper fraction was changed to a mixed number.

To add fractions with different denominators, change fractions to their equivalent fraction with the lowest common denominator, add the numerators, write the sum over the common denominator, and reduce if necessary.

Example 1: $\dfrac{1}{4} + \dfrac{1}{3}$

Solution: The lowest common denominator is 12. Change to equivalent fractions.

$$\dfrac{1}{4} = \dfrac{3}{12}$$

$$+ \dfrac{1}{3} = \dfrac{4}{12}$$

$$\dfrac{7}{12}$$

Example 2: $\dfrac{1}{2} + 1\dfrac{1}{3} + \dfrac{2}{4}$

Solution: Change the mixed number 1 1/3 to 4/3. Find the lowest common denominator, change fractions to equivalent fractions, add, and reduce if necessary. The lowest common denominator is 12.

$$\frac{1}{2} = \frac{6}{12}$$

$$\frac{4}{3} = \frac{16}{12}$$

$$+\frac{2}{4} = \frac{6}{12}$$

$$\frac{28}{12} = 2\frac{4}{12} = 2\frac{1}{3}$$

Notes

SUBTRACTING FRACTIONS

To subtract fractions with the same denominator, subtract the numerators, and place this amount over the denominator. Reduce to lowest terms, if necessary.

Example 1: $\qquad \frac{5}{4} - \frac{3}{4} = \frac{2}{4} = \frac{1}{2}$

Example 2: $\qquad 2\frac{1}{6} - \frac{5}{6}$

Solution: Change the mixed number 2 1/6 to 13/6

$$\frac{13}{6} - \frac{5}{6} = \frac{8}{6} = \frac{4}{3} = 1\frac{1}{3}$$

To subtract fractions with different denominators, find the lowest common denominator, change to equivalent fractions, subtract the numerators, and place the sum over the common denominator. Reduce to lowest terms, if necessary.

Example 3: $\qquad \frac{15}{6} - \frac{3}{5}$

Solution: The lowest common denominator is 30. Change to equivalent fractions and subtract.

$$\frac{15}{6} = \frac{75}{30}$$

$$-\frac{3}{5} = \frac{18}{30}$$

$$\frac{57}{30} = 1\frac{27}{30} = 1\frac{9}{10}$$

Example 4: $\qquad 2\frac{1}{5} - \frac{4}{3}$

Solution: Change the mixed number $2\frac{1}{5}$ to $1\frac{1}{5}$. Find the lowest

common denominator, change to equivalent fractions, subtract, and reduce if necessary. The lowest common denominator is 15.

$$\frac{11}{5} = \frac{33}{15}$$

$$-\frac{4}{3} = \frac{20}{15}$$

$$\frac{13}{15}$$

MULTIPLYING FRACTIONS

To multiply fractions, multiply the numerators, multiply the denominators, and reduce, if necessary.

Note:

If fractions are not in lowest terms, reduction can be done before multiplication.

Example 1: $\dfrac{3}{4} \times \dfrac{2}{5} = \dfrac{6}{20} = \dfrac{3}{10}$

Example 2: $\dfrac{2}{4} \times \dfrac{3}{4}$

reduce $\dfrac{2}{4}$ to $\dfrac{1}{2}$ then multiply.

$$\frac{1}{2} \times \frac{3}{4} = \frac{3}{8}$$

Example 3: $6 \times \dfrac{5}{6}$

$$\frac{6}{1} \times \frac{5}{6} = \frac{30}{6} = 5$$

Note:

The whole number 6 is expressed as a fraction here, by placing 1 as the denominator.

or

$$\frac{6 \times 5}{6} = \frac{30}{6} = 5$$

Example 4: $3\dfrac{1}{3} \times 2\dfrac{1}{2}$

Solution: Change the mixed numbers to improper fractions. Proceed with multiplication.

$$3\frac{1}{3} = \frac{10}{3} ; 2\frac{1}{2} = \frac{5}{2}$$

$$\frac{10}{3} \times \frac{5}{2} = \frac{50}{6} = 8\frac{2}{6} = 8\frac{1}{3}$$

DIVIDING FRACTIONS

Notes

To divide fractions, invert (turn upside down) the second fraction (divisor), and multiply. Reduce where necessary.

Example 1:
$$\frac{3}{4} \div \frac{2}{3}$$

Solution:
$$\frac{3}{4} \times \frac{3}{2} = \frac{9}{8} = 1\frac{1}{8}$$

Example 2:
$$1\frac{3}{5} \div 2\frac{1}{10}$$

Solution: Change mixed numbers to improper fractions. Proceed with steps of division.

$$1\frac{3}{5} = \frac{8}{5}; 2\frac{1}{10} = \frac{21}{10}$$

$$\frac{8}{5} \times \frac{10}{21} = \frac{80}{105} = \frac{16}{21}$$

Example 3:
$$5 \div \frac{1}{2}$$

Solution:
$$5 \times \frac{2}{1} = \frac{10}{1} = 10$$

or

$$\frac{5}{1} \times \frac{2}{1} = \frac{10}{1} = 10$$

(*Note:* When doing dosage calculations that involve division, the fractions may be written as follows: $\dfrac{\frac{1}{4}}{\frac{1}{2}}$. In this case $\frac{1}{4}$ is the numerator, and $\frac{1}{2}$ is the denominator. Therefore the problem is set up as: $\frac{1}{4} \div \frac{1}{2}$, which becomes $\frac{1}{4} \times \frac{2}{1} = \frac{2}{4} = \frac{1}{2}$.)

 PRACTICE PROBLEMS

Change the following improper fractions to mixed numbers and reduce to lowest terms.

36. $\dfrac{18}{5} =$ _____

37. $\dfrac{60}{14} =$ _____

38. $\dfrac{13}{8} =$ _____

39. $\dfrac{35}{12} =$ _____

40. $\dfrac{112}{100} =$ _____

Change the following mixed numbers to improper fractions.

41. $1\dfrac{4}{25}$ = _____   44. $3\dfrac{3}{8}$ = _____

42. $4\dfrac{2}{8}$ = _____   45. $15\dfrac{4}{5}$ = _____

43. $4\dfrac{1}{2}$ = _____

Add the following fractions and mixed numbers and reduce fractions to lowest terms.

46. $\dfrac{2}{3} + \dfrac{5}{6}$ = _____   49. $7\dfrac{2}{5} + \dfrac{2}{3}$ = _____

47. $2\dfrac{1}{8} + \dfrac{2}{3}$ = _____   50. $12\dfrac{1}{2} + 10\dfrac{1}{3}$ = _____

48. $2\dfrac{3}{10} + 4\dfrac{1}{5} + \dfrac{2}{3}$ = _____

Subtract and reduce fractions to lowest terms.

51. $\dfrac{4}{3} - \dfrac{3}{7}$ = _____   54. $2\dfrac{5}{6} - 2\dfrac{3}{4}$ = _____

52. $3\dfrac{3}{8} - 1\dfrac{3}{5}$ = _____   55. $\dfrac{1}{8} - \dfrac{1}{12}$ = _____

53. $\dfrac{15}{16} - \dfrac{1}{4}$ = _____

Multiply the following fractions and mixed numbers and reduce to lowest terms.

56. $\dfrac{2}{3} \times \dfrac{4}{5}$ = _____   59. $2\dfrac{5}{8} \times 2\dfrac{3}{4}$ = _____

57. $\dfrac{6}{25} \times \dfrac{3}{5}$ = _____   60. $\dfrac{5}{12} \times \dfrac{4}{9}$ = _____

58. $\dfrac{1}{50} \times 3$ = _____

Divide the following fractions and mixed numbers and reduce to lowest terms.

61. $2\dfrac{6}{8} \div 1\dfrac{2}{3}$ = _____   64. $\dfrac{7}{8} \div \dfrac{7}{8}$ = _____

62. $\dfrac{1}{60} \div \dfrac{1}{2}$ = _____   65. $3\dfrac{1}{3} \div 1\dfrac{7}{12}$ = _____

63. $6 \div \dfrac{2}{5}$ = _____

Answers on p. 491

CHAPTER REVIEW

Notes

Change the following improper fractions to mixed numbers and reduce to lowest terms.

1. $\dfrac{10}{8} =$ _____

2. $\dfrac{30}{4} =$ _____

3. $\dfrac{22}{6} =$ _____

4. $\dfrac{11}{4} =$ _____

5. $\dfrac{59}{14} =$ _____

6. $\dfrac{67}{10} -$ _____

7. $\dfrac{9}{2} =$ _____

8. $\dfrac{11}{5} =$ _____

9. $\dfrac{64}{15} =$ _____

10. $\dfrac{100}{13} =$ _____

Change the following mixed numbers to improper fractions.

11. $2\dfrac{1}{2} =$ _____

12. $7\dfrac{3}{8} =$ _____

13. $8\dfrac{3}{5} =$ _____

14. $16\dfrac{1}{4} =$ _____

15. $3\dfrac{1}{5} =$ _____

16. $2\dfrac{3}{5} =$ _____

17. $8\dfrac{4}{10} =$ _____

18. $9\dfrac{1}{4} =$ _____

19. $12\dfrac{3}{4} =$ _____

20. $6\dfrac{5}{7} -$ _____

Add the following fractions and mixed numbers. Reduce to lowest terms.

21. $\dfrac{2}{5} + \dfrac{1}{3} + \dfrac{7}{10} =$ _____

22. $\dfrac{1}{4} + \dfrac{1}{6} + \dfrac{1}{8} =$ _____

23. $20\dfrac{1}{2} + \dfrac{1}{4} + \dfrac{5}{4} =$ _____

24. $\dfrac{1}{2} + \dfrac{1}{5} =$ _____

25. $6\dfrac{1}{4} + \dfrac{2}{9} + \dfrac{1}{36} =$ _____

Subtract the following fractions and mixed numbers. Reduce to lowest terms.

26. $\dfrac{4}{9} - \dfrac{3}{9} =$ _____

27. $2\dfrac{1}{4} - 1\dfrac{1}{2} =$ _____

28. $2\dfrac{3}{4} - \dfrac{1}{4} =$ _____

29. $\dfrac{4}{5} - \dfrac{1}{6} =$ _____

30. $\dfrac{6}{4} - \dfrac{1}{2} =$ _____

31. $\dfrac{4}{5} - \dfrac{1}{4} =$ _____

32. $\dfrac{4}{6} - \dfrac{3}{8} =$ _____

33. $4\dfrac{1}{6} - 1\dfrac{1}{3} =$ _____

34. $\dfrac{8}{5} - \dfrac{1}{3} =$ _____

35. $\dfrac{4}{7} - \dfrac{1}{3} =$ _____

Notes

Multiply the following fractions and mixed numbers. Reduce to lowest terms.

36. $\dfrac{1}{3} \times \dfrac{4}{12} =$ _____

37. $2\dfrac{7}{8} \times 3\dfrac{1}{4} =$ _____

38. $8 \times 1\dfrac{3}{4} =$ _____

39. $15 \times \dfrac{2}{3} =$ _____

40. $36 \times \dfrac{3}{4} =$ _____

41. $\dfrac{5}{4} \times \dfrac{2}{4} =$ _____

42. $\dfrac{2}{5} \times \dfrac{1}{6} =$ _____

43. $\dfrac{3}{10} \times \dfrac{4}{12} =$ _____

44. $\dfrac{1}{9} \times \dfrac{7}{3} =$ _____

45. $\dfrac{10}{25} \times \dfrac{5}{3} =$ _____

Divide the following fractions and mixed numbers. Reduce to lowest terms.

46. $2\dfrac{1}{3} \div 4\dfrac{1}{6} =$ _____

47. $\dfrac{1}{3} \div \dfrac{1}{2} =$ _____

48. $25 \div 12\dfrac{1}{2} =$ _____

49. $\dfrac{7}{8} \div 2\dfrac{1}{4} =$ _____

50. $\dfrac{6}{2} \div \dfrac{3}{4} =$ _____

51. $\dfrac{4}{6} \div \dfrac{1}{2} =$ _____

52. $\dfrac{3}{10} \div \dfrac{5}{25} =$ _____

53. $3 \div \dfrac{2}{5} =$ _____

54. $\dfrac{15}{30} \div 10 =$ _____

55. $\dfrac{8}{3} \div \dfrac{8}{3} =$ _____

Answers on p. 492

Decimals

An understanding of decimals is crucial to the calculation of doses. Most medications are ordered in metric measures that use decimals.

Example 1:   Digoxin 0.125 mg

Example 2:   Capoten 6.25 mg

A decimal is a fraction that has a denominator that is a multiple of 10. A decimal fraction is written as a decimal by the use of a decimal point (.). The decimal point is used to indicate place value. Some examples are as follows:

Fraction	Decimal number
$\dfrac{3}{10}$	0.3
$\dfrac{18}{100}$	0.18
$\dfrac{175}{1000}$	0.175

The decimal point represents the center. Notice that the numbers written to the right of the decimal point are decimal fractions with a denominator of 10 or a multiple of 10, and represent a value that is less than one (1) or part of one (1). Num-

Notes

bers written to the left of the decimal point are whole numbers, or have a value of one (1) or greater.

The easiest way to understand decimals is to memorize the place values (see Box 3-1).

BOX 3-1   Decimal Place Values

The decimal value is determined by its position to the right of the decimal point.

(100,000)	(10,000)	(1,000)	(100)	(10)	(1)	Decimal point	(.1)	(.01)	(.001)	(.0001)	(.00001)
Hundred-thousands	Ten-thousands	Thousands	Hundreds	Tens	Ones (Units)	↓	Tenths	Hundredths	Thousandths	Ten-thousandths	Hundred-thousandths
6	5	4	3	2	1	.	1	2	3	4	5

WHOLE NUMBERS TO THE LEFT   **DECIMAL NUMBERS TO THE RIGHT**

The **first** place to the right of the decimal is tenths.

The **second** place to the right of the decimal is hundredths.

The **third** place to the right of the decimal is thousandths.

The **fourth** place to the right of the decimal is ten-thousandths.

In the calculation of medication dosages it is necessary to **consider only three figures after the decimal point (thousandths) (e.g., 0.375 mg). When there is no whole number before it, it is important to place a zero (0) in front of the decimal point to indicate that it is a fraction. This will emphasize its value and prevent errors in interpretation.** *The source for many medication errors is misplacement of a decimal point or incorrect interpretation of a decimal value.*

READING AND WRITING DECIMALS

Once you have an understanding of the place value of decimals, reading and writing them is simple.

To read the decimal numbers read:
1. The whole number,
2. the decimal point as "and," and
3. the decimal fraction.

Example 1:   The number 8.3 is read as "eight and three tenths."

Example 2:   The number 0.4 is read as "four tenths."

Example 3: The decimal 4.06 is read as "four and six hundredths."

When there is only a zero (0) to the left of the decimal, as in example 2, the zero is not read aloud.

An exception to this is in an emergency situation where a nurse has to take a verbal order over the phone from a doctor. When repeating back an order for a medication involving a decimal, the zero should be read aloud to prevent a medication error.

To write a decimal number, write the following:
  1. The whole number. (If there is no whole number, write zero [0].)
  2. The decimal point to indicate the place value of the rightmost number.
  3. The decimal portion of the number.

Example 1:   Written, seven and five tenths = 7.5

Example 2:   Written, one hundred twenty-five thousandths = 0.125

Example 3:   Written, five tenths = 0.5

 PRACTICE PROBLEMS

Write each of the following numbers in word form.

1. 8.35 _____

2. 11.001 _____

3. 4.57 _____

4. 5.0007 _____

5. 10.5 _____

6. 0.163 _____

Write each of the following in decimal form.

7. four tenths _____

8. eighty-four _____
   and seven hundredths

9. seven hundredths _____

10. two and twenty-three
    hundredths _____

11. five hundredths _____

12. nine thousandths _____

Answers on p. 493

COMPARING THE VALUE OF DECIMALS

Understanding which decimal is larger or smaller is important in the calculation of dosage problems. This avoids errors in dosage, and gives the nurse an understanding of the size of a dose (e.g., 0.5 mg, 0.05 mg). Understanding the value of decimals avoids errors in misinterpretation. There is an appreciable difference between 0.5 mg and 0.05 mg.

When decimal numbers contain whole numbers, the whole numbers are compared to determine which is greater.

Example 1:   4.8 is larger than 2.9

Example 2:   11.5 is larger than 7.5

Example 3:   7.37 is larger than 6.94

If the whole numbers being compared are the **same** (e.g., 5.6 and 5.2) or if there is **no whole number** (e.g., 0.45 and 0.37), then the number in the **tenths** place determines which decimal is larger.

Example 1:   0.45 is larger than 0.37

Example 2:   1.75 is larger than 1.25

If the whole numbers are the same or zero and the numbers in the **tenths place** are the **same,** then the decimal with the higher number in the **hundredths place** has the larger value, and so forth.

Note:

The addition of zeros at the end of a decimal does not alter its value; they are therefore un-necessary and could result in a calculation error.

Example 1:   0.67 is larger than 0.66

Example 2:   0.17 is larger than 0.14

Example 1:   0.2 is the same as 0.2000, 0.20

Example 2:   4.4 is the same as 4.40, 4.400

 PRACTICE PROBLEMS

Circle the decimal with the largest value in the following:

13. 0.5,   0.15,   0.05   16. 0.175,   0.1,   0.05

14. 2.66,   2.36,   2.87   17. 7.02,   7.15,   7.35

15. 0.125,   0.375,   0.25   18. 0.067,   0.087,   0.077

Answers on p. 493

ADDITION AND SUBTRACTION OF DECIMALS

To add or subtract decimals, place the numbers in columns so that the decimal points are lined up directly under one another and add or subtract from right to left.

Example 1: Add 16.4 + 21.8 + 13.2

$$\begin{array}{r} 16.4 \\ 21.8 \\ + \ 13.2 \\ \hline 51.4 \end{array}$$

Example 2: Add 11.2 + 16

$$\begin{array}{r} 11.2 \\ + \ 16.0 \\ \hline 27.2 \end{array}$$

Note:

The addition of a zero to make the columns the same length.

Example 3: Subtract 3.78 from 12.84

$$\begin{array}{r} 12.84 \\ - \ 3.78 \\ \hline 9.06 \end{array}$$

Example 4: Subtract 0.007 from 0.05

$$\begin{array}{r} 0.050 \\ - \ 0.007 \\ \hline 0.043 \end{array}$$

Note:

The addition of a zero to make the columns the same length.

 PRACTICE PROBLEMS

Add the following decimals.

19. 4.7 + 5.3 + 8.4 = _____

20. 38.52 + 0.029 + 1.90 = _____

21. 0.7 + 3.25 = _____

22. 2.2 + 1.67 = _____

Subtract the following decimals.

23. 3.67 − 0.75 = _____

24. 64.3 − 21.2 = _____

25. 0.08 − 0.045 = _____

26. 6.75 − 0.87 = _____

Answers on p. 493

MULTIPLYING DECIMALS

When multiplying decimals, be sure the decimal is placed in the correct position in the answer (product).

To multiply decimals, multiply as with whole numbers. In the answer (product), count off from right to left as many decimal places as there are in the numbers being multiplied.

Notes

Example 1:

$$1.2 \times 3.2$$

$$
\begin{array}{r}
1.2 \\
\times\ 3.2 \\
\hline
24 \\
36 \\
\hline
384. \\
\end{array}
$$

Answer: 3.84

In example 1, 1.2 has one number after the decimal, and 3.2 also has one. Therefore you will need to place the decimal point 2 places to the left in the answer (product).

When there are insufficient numbers in the answer for correct placement of the decimal point, add as many zeros as needed to the left of the answer.

Example 2:

$$1.35 \times 0.65$$

$$
\begin{array}{r}
1.35 \\
\times\ 0.65 \\
\hline
675 \\
810 \\
\hline
8775. \\
\end{array}
$$

Answer: 0.8775

In example 2, 1.35 has two numbers after the decimal, and 0.65 also has two. Therefore you will need to place the decimal point 4 places to the left in the answer (product), and add a zero in front.

Example 3:

$$0.11 \times 0.33$$

$$
\begin{array}{r}
0.11 \\
\times\ 0.33 \\
\hline
33 \\
33 \\
\hline
0363. \\
\end{array}
$$

Answer: 0.0363

In example 3, there are four decimal places needed (two numbers after each decimal in 0.11 and 0.33), but there are only three numbers in the product. A zero must be placed to the left of these numbers for correct placement of the decimal point.

Multiplication by Decimal Movement

This method may be preferred when doing metric conversions because it is based on the decimal system. Multiplying by 10, 100, 1,000, and so forth can be done by moving the decimal point to the right the same number of places as there are zeros in the number by which you are multiplying.

Notes

Example: When multiplying by 10, move the decimal one place to the right; by 100, two places to the right; by 1,000, three places to the right, and so forth.

Example 1: 1.6 × 10 = 16 (decimal moved one place to the right)

Example 2: 5.2 × 100 = 520 (decimal moved two places to the right)

Example 3: 0.463 × 1,000 = 463 (decimal moved three places to the right)

Example 4: 6.64 × 10 = 66.4 (decimal moved one place to right)

 PRACTICE PROBLEMS

Multiply the following decimals.

27. 3.15 × 0.015 = _____

28. 3.65 × 0.25 = _____

29. 9.65 × 1,000 = _____

30. 8.9 × 0.2 = _____

31. 14.001 × 7.2 = _____

Answers on p. 493

DIVISION OF DECIMALS

The division of decimals is done in the same manner as dividing whole numbers except for placement of the decimal point. Incorrect placement of the decimal point changes the numerical value and can cause error in calculation. Errors made in the division of decimals are commonly due to improper placement of the decimal point, incorrect placement of numbers in the quotient, and omission of necessary zeros in the quotient.

The parts of a division problem are as follows:

$$\text{Divisor)}\overline{\text{Dividend}}^{\text{Quotient}}$$

The number being divided is called the **dividend,** the number used for the division is the **divisor,** and the answer is the **quotient.**

Symbols used to indicate division are as follows:

1. $\overline{)}$

Example: $9\overline{)27}$

2. ÷

Example: 27 ÷ 9

3. The horizontal bar with the dividend on the top and the divisor on the bottom.

Example: $\dfrac{27}{9}$

4. The slanted bar with the dividend to the left and the divisor to the right.

Example: 27/9

Notes

Dividing a Decimal by a Whole Number

> To divide a decimal by a whole number, place the decimal point in the quotient directly above the decimal point in the dividend. Proceed to divide as with whole numbers.

Example: Divide 17.5 by 5

$$
\begin{array}{r}
3.5 \\
5\overline{)17.5} \\
-15 \\
\hline
25 \\
-25 \\
\hline
0
\end{array}
$$

Dividing a Decimal or a Whole Number by a Decimal

> To divide by a decimal, the decimal point in the divisor is moved to the right until the number is a whole number. The decimal point in the dividend is moved the same number of places to the right, and zeros are added as necessary. Proceed to divide as with whole numbers.

Example: Divide 6.96 by 0.3

$$6.96 \div 0.3 = 0.3\overline{)6.96}$$

Step 1: $3\overline{)69.6}$ (After moving decimals in the divisor the same number of places as the dividend.)

Step 2:

$$
\begin{array}{r}
23.2 \\
3\overline{)69.6} \\
-6 \\
\hline
9 \\
-9 \\
\hline
6 \\
-6 \\
\hline
0
\end{array}
$$

Division by Decimal Movement

> To divide a decimal by 10, 100, or 1000, move the decimal point to the **left** the same number of places as there are zeros in the divisor.

Example 1: $0.46 \div 10 = 0.046$ (The decimal is moved one place to the left.)

Example 2: $0.07 \div 100 = 0.0007$ (The decimal is moved two places to the left.)

Example 3: $0.75 \div 1{,}000 = 0.00075$ (The decimal is moved three places to the left.)

Notes

ROUNDING OFF DECIMALS

The determination of how many places to carry your division when calculating dosages is based on the materials being used. Some syringes are marked in **tenths,** some in **hundredths.** As you become familiar with the materials used in dosage calculation, you will learn how far to carry your division and when to round off. To ensure accuracy, most calculation problems require that you carry your division at least **two decimal places (hundredths place)** and **round off to the nearest tenth.**

To express an answer to the nearest tenth, carry the division to the hundredths place (two places after the decimal). If the number in the hundredths place **is 5 or greater**, **add** one to the tenths place. If the number **is less than 5**, **drop** the number to the right of the desired decimal place.

Example 1:   Express 4.15 to the nearest tenth.

Answer: 4.2 (The number in the hundredths place is 5, so the number in the tenths place is **increased by one.** 4.1 becomes 4.2.)

Example 2:   Express 1.24 to the nearest tenth.

Answer: 1.2 (The number in the hundredths place is less than 5, so the number in the **tenths place does not change.**)

To express an answer to the nearest hundredth, carry the division to the thousandths place (three places after the decimal). If the number in the thousandths place is 5 or greater, add one to the hundredths place. If the number is less than 5, drop the number to the right of the desired decimal place.

Example 1:   Express 0.176 to the nearest hundredth.

Answer: 0.18 (The number in the thousandths place is 6, so the number in the hundredths place is increased by one. 0.17 becomes 0.18.)

Example 2:   Express 0.554 to the nearest hundredth.

Answer: 0.55 (The number in the thousandths place is less than 5, so the number in the hundredths place does not change.)

 ## PRACTICE PROBLEMS

Divide the following decimals. Carry division to the hundredths place where necessary. Do not round off.

32. 2 ÷ 0.5 = _____   35. 39.6 ÷ 1.3 = _____

33. 1.4 ÷ 1.2 = _____   36. 1.9 ÷ 3.2 = _____

34. 63.8 ÷ 0.9 = _____

Express the following decimals to the nearest tenth.

37. 3.57 _____   39. 1.98 _____

38. 0.95 _____

Express the following decimals to the nearest hundredth.

40. 3.550 _____   42. 0.738 _____

41. 0.607 _____

Divide the following decimals.

43. 0.005 ÷ 10 = _____   44. 0.004 ÷ 100 _____

Multiply the following decimals.

45. 58.4 × 10 = _____   46. 0.5 × 1,000 = _____

Answers on p. 493

CHANGING FRACTIONS TO DECIMALS

To change a fraction to a decimal, divide the numerator by the denominator and add zeros as needed. If the numerator doesn't divide evenly into the denominator, carry division three places.

Example 1: $\dfrac{2}{5} = 5\overline{)2} = 5\overline{)2.0}\;\;^{0.4}$

Example 2: $\dfrac{3}{8} = 8\overline{)3} = 8\overline{)3.000}\;\;^{0.375}$

Changing fractions to decimals can also be a method of comparing fraction size. The fractions being compared are changed to decimals, and the rules relating to comparing decimals are then applied. (See Comparing the Value of Decimals, p. 25.)

Example: Which fraction is larger, $\dfrac{1}{3}$ or $\dfrac{1}{6}$?

Solution: $\dfrac{1}{3} = 0.333$ as a decimal

$\dfrac{1}{6} = 0.166$

$\dfrac{1}{3}$ is therefore the larger fraction.

CHANGING DECIMALS TO FRACTIONS

To change a decimal to a fraction, simply read the decimal as a fraction and write it as it is read. Reduce if necessary. (*Note:* See Reading and Writing Decimals, p. 24.)

Notes

Example 1:   0.4 is read "four tenths" and written $\frac{4}{10}$, which $= \frac{2}{5}$ when reduced.

Example 2:   0.65 is read "sixty-five hundredths" and written $\frac{65}{100}$, which $= \frac{13}{20}$ when reduced.

PRACTICE PROBLEMS

Change the following fractions to decimals and carry the division three places as indicated. Do not round off.

47. $\frac{3}{4}$ _____

49. $\frac{1}{2}$ _____

48. $\frac{5}{9}$ _____

Change the following decimals to fractions and reduce to lowest terms.

50. 0.75 _____

52. 0.04 _____

51. 0.0005 _____

Answers on p. 493

POINTS TO REMEMBER

- Read decimals carefully.

- When the decimal fraction is **not** preceded by a whole number (e.g., 12), **always place a "0"** to the left of the decimal (0.12) to avoid interpretation errors.

- Never follow a whole number with a decimal point and zero. This could result in medication error due to misinterpretation (e.g., 3, not 3.0).

- Add zeros to the right as needed for making decimals of equal spacing for addition and subtraction. These zeros do not change the value.

- Adding zeros at the end of a decimal (except when called for to create decimals of equal length for addition or subtraction) can result in error (e.g., 1.5, not 1.50).

- Double-check work to avoid errors.

CHAPTER REVIEW

Identify the decimal with the largest value in the following sets.

1. 0.4, 0.44, 0.444 _____

4. 0.1, 0.05, 0.2 _____

2. 0.8, 0.7, 0.12 _____

5. 0.725, 0.357, 0.125 _____

3. 1.32, 1.12, 1.5 _____

Perform the indicated operations.

6. $3.005 + 4.308 + 2.47 =$ _____

7. $20.3 + 8.57 + 0.03 =$ _____

8. $5.886 - 3.143 =$ _____

9. $8.17 - 3.05 =$ _____

10. $3.8 - 1.3 =$ _____

Solve the following. Carry division to the hundredths place where necessary.

11. $5.7 \div 0.9 =$ _____

12. $3.75 \div 2.5 =$ _____

13. $1.125 \div 0.75 =$ _____

14. $0.15 \times 100 =$ _____

15. $15 \times 2.08 =$ _____

16. $472.4 \times 0.002 =$ _____

Express the following decimals to the nearest tenth.

17. 1.75 _____

18. 0.13 _____

Express the following decimals to the nearest hundredth.

19. 1.427 _____

20. 0.147 _____

Change the following fractions to decimals. Carry division three decimal places as necessary.

21. $\dfrac{8}{64}$ _____

22. $\dfrac{3}{50}$ _____

23. $6\dfrac{1}{2}$ _____

Change the following decimals to fractions and reduce to lowest terms.

24. 1.01 _____

25. 0.065 _____

Add the following decimals.

26. You are to give a client one tablet labeled 0.15 mg, and one labeled 0.025 mg. What is the total dose of these two tablets? _____

27. If you administer two tablets labeled 0.04 mg, what total dose will you administer? _____

28. You have two tablets, one labeled 0.025 mg and the other 0.1 mg. What is the total dose of these two tablets? _____

29. You have just administered 3 tablets with dose strength of 1.5 mg. What was the total dose ordered? _____

30. If you administer two tablets labeled 0.6 mg, what total dose will you administer? _____

Multiply the following numbers by moving the decimal.

31. $0.08 \times 10 =$ _____

32. $5.65 \times 100 =$ _____

33. $0.849 \times 1{,}000 =$ _____

34. $2.34 \times 10 =$ _____

35. $0.002 \times 100 =$ _____

Divide the following numbers and round to the nearest hundredth.

36. $6.45 \div 10 =$ _____

37. $37.5 \div 100 =$ _____

38. $0.13 \div 0.25 =$ _____

39. $4 \div 4.1 =$ _____

40. $5 \div 14.3 =$ _____

Round the following decimals to the nearest thousandth.

41. 4.2475 _____

42. 0.5673 _____

43. 2.3249 _____

44. 7.8393 _____

45. 5.8333 _____

Answers on p. 493

Ratio and Proportion

Ratio and proportion is one logical method for calculating medications. It can be used to calculate all types of medication problems. Nurses use ratios to check doses and to calculate medication doses. There are some medications that express the strength of the solution using a ratio. Example: epinephrine label may state 1:1,000. Ratios are used in hospitals to determine the client to nurse ratio. Example: If there are 28 clients and 4 nurses on a unit, the ratio of clients to nurses is 28:4, or "28 to 4." Like a fraction, which indicates the division of two numbers, a ratio indicates the division of two quantities. Ratio proportion is a logical approach to calculating dosages.

RATIOS

A ratio is used to indicate a relationship between two numbers. These numbers are separated by a colon (:).

Example: 3 : 4

The colon indicates division; therefore a ratio is a fraction and the numbers or terms of the ratio are the numerator and denominator. The numerator is always to the left of the colon, and the denominator is always to the right of the colon.

Example: 3 : 4 (3 is the numerator, 4 is the denominator, and the expression

can be written as $\frac{3}{4}$.)

PROPORTIONS

A proportion is an equation of two ratios of equal value. The terms of the first ratio have a relationship to the terms of the second ratio. A proportion can be written in any of the following formats:

Example 1: $3 : 4 = 6 : 8$ (separated with an equal sign)

Example 2: $3 : 4 :: 6 : 8$ (separated with a double colon)

Example 3: $\dfrac{3}{4} = \dfrac{6}{8}$ (written as a fraction)

Read as follows: 3 is to 4 equals 6 is to 8; 3 is to 4 as 6 is to 8; or, as a fraction, three fourths equals six eighths.

Proving that ratios are equal and that the proportion is true can be done mathematically.

Example: $5 : 25 = 10 : 50$

or

$5 : 25 :: 10 : 50$

The terms in a proportion are called the *means* and *extremes*. Confusion of these terms can result in an incorrect answer. To avoid confusion of terms in proportions, remember **m** for middle terms **(means)** and **e** for the end terms **(extremes)** of the proportion. Let's refer to our example to identify these terms.

The extremes are the outer or end numbers (previous example 5, 50), and the means are the inner or middle numbers (previous example 25, 10).

Example:

means
⌐‾‾‾⌐
$5 : 25 = 10 : 50$
⌐_____ extremes _____⌐

| In a proportion the product of the means equals the product of the extremes.

In other words, the answers obtained when you multiply the means and extremes are equal.

Example: $5 : 25 = 10 : 50$

$25 \times 10 = 50 \times 5$
⌐___⌐   ⌐___⌐
means   extremes

$250 = 250$

Note:

The product of the means, 250, equals the product of the extremes, 250, proving the ratios are equal and the proportion is true.

To verify that the two ratios in a proportion expressed as a fraction are equal and that it is a true proportion, multiply the numerator of each ratio by its opposite denominator. The sum of the products are equal. The numerator of the first fraction and the denominator of the second fraction are the extremes. The numerator of the second fraction and denominator of the first fraction are the means.

Example:

$$5 : 25 = 10 : 50$$

$$\frac{5}{25} = \frac{10}{50} \text{ (proportion written as a fraction)}$$

$$\frac{5 \text{ (extreme)}}{25 \text{ (mean)}} = \frac{10 \text{ (mean)}}{50 \text{ (extreme)}}$$

Note:

When stated as a fraction, the proportion is solved by cross multiplication.

$$5 \times 50 = 25 \times 10$$
$$250 = 250$$

SOLVING FOR *x* IN RATIO-PROPORTION

Because the product of the means is always equal to the product of the extremes, if three numbers of the two ratios are known the fourth number can be found. In a proportion problem, the unknown quantity is represented by *x*.

Example: $12 : 9 = 8 : x$

Steps: $72 = 12x$ 1. Multiply the means and extremes.

$$\frac{72}{12} = \frac{12x}{12}$$

2. Divide both sides of the equation by the number in front of *x* to obtain the value for *x*.

$$x = 6$$

Proof: Place the answer obtained for *x* in the equation and multiply to be certain that the product of the means equals the product of the extremes.

$$12 : 9 = 8 : 6$$
$$9 \times 8 = 12 \times 6$$
$$72 - 72$$

Solving for *x* with a proportion in a fraction format can be done by cross multiplication to determine the value of *x*.

Example 1: $\dfrac{4}{3} = \dfrac{12}{x}$

Steps: $4x = 36$ 1. Cross multiply to obtain the product of the means and extremes.

$$\frac{4x}{4} = \frac{36}{4}$$

2. Divide by the number in front of *x* to obtain the value for *x*.

$$x = 9$$

Proof: Place the value obtained for *x* in the equation; the cross products should be equal.

Notes

$$\frac{4}{3} = \frac{12}{9}$$

$$4 \times 9 = 12 \times 3$$

$$36 = 36$$

Solving for x in proportions that involve decimals in the equation can be done by the same process.

Example: $25 : 5 = 1.5 : x$

Steps: $5 \times 1.5 = 25x$ 1. Multiply the means and extremes.

$$\frac{7.5}{25} = \frac{25x}{25}$$ 2. Divide by the number in front of x to solve for x.

$$x = 0.3$$

Proof: $25 : 5 = 1.5 : 0.3$

$$5 \times 1.5 = 25 \times 0.3$$

$$7.5 = 7.5$$

Proportions with unknowns that also involve fractions may be solved by the same method.

Example: $\frac{1}{5} : 1 = \frac{1}{2} : x$

Steps: $\frac{1}{2} \times 1 = \frac{1}{5} \times x$ 1. Multiply the means and extremes.

$$\frac{1}{2} = \frac{1}{5} x$$

$$x = \frac{1}{2} \div \frac{1}{5}$$ 2. Divide both sides by the number in front of x. Division of two fractions becomes multiplication, and the second fraction is inverted. Multiply numerators and denominators.

$$x = \frac{1}{2} \times \frac{5}{1}$$

$$x = \frac{5}{2} = 2.5 \text{ or } 2\frac{1}{2}$$ 3. Divide the final fraction to solve for x.

Proof: $\frac{1}{5} : 1 = \frac{1}{2} : 2\frac{1}{2}$

$$1 \times \frac{1}{2} = \frac{1}{5} \times 2\frac{1}{2} = \frac{1}{5} \times \frac{5}{2}$$

$$\frac{1}{2} = \frac{5}{10} = \frac{1}{2}$$

$$\frac{1}{2} = \frac{1}{2}$$

Note: If the answer is expressed in fraction format for *x*, it must be reduced to **lowest terms.** Division should be carried **two decimal places** when an answer does not work out evenly and may have to be **rounded to the nearest tenth** to prove the answer correct.

APPLYING RATIO-PROPORTION TO DOSE CALCULATION

Now that we have reviewed the basic definitions and concepts relating to ratio and proportion, let's look at how this might be applied in dose calculation.

In dose calculation, ratio proportion may be used to represent **the weight of a drug that is in tablet or capsule form.**

Example 1:
$$1 \text{ tab} : 0.125 \text{ mg or } \frac{1 \text{ tab}}{0.125 \text{ mg}}$$

This may also be expressed stating the weight of the drug first:

$$0.125 \text{ mg} : 1 \text{ tab or } \frac{0.125 \text{ mg}}{1 \text{ tab}}$$

This means that 1 tablet contains 0.125 mg or is equal to 0.125 mg of drug.

Example 2: If a capsule contains a dosage of 500 mg, this could be represented by a ratio as follows:

$$1 \text{ cap} : 500 \text{ mg or } \frac{1 \text{ cap}}{500 \text{ mg}}$$

This may also be expressed stating the weight of the drug first:

$$500 \text{ mg} : 1 \text{ cap or } \frac{500 \text{ mg}}{1 \text{ cap}}$$

Another use of ratio and proportion in dose calculation is to express liquid medications used for oral administration and for injection. When stating a dose of a liquid medication, a ratio expresses the **weight (strength) of a drug in a certain volume of solution.**

Example 3: A solution that contains 250 mg of drug in each **1 mL** could be written as:

$$\textbf{250 mg} : 1 \text{ mL or } \frac{250 \text{ mg}}{\textbf{1 mL}}$$

1 mL contains 250 mg of drug

Example 4: A solution that contains 80 mg of drug in each **2 mL** would be written as:

$$80 \text{ mg} : \textbf{2 mL or } \frac{80 \text{ mg}}{\textbf{2 mL}}$$

2 mL contains 80 mg of drug

Proving mathematically that ratios are equal and the proportion is true is important with medications. This can be illustrated by using our previous drug strength examples.

Notes

Example 1:   1 cap : 500 mg = 2 cap : 1,000 mg

If 1 cap contains 500 mg, 2 cap will contain 1,000 mg

→ extremes ←

1 cap : 500 mg = 2 cap : 1,000 mg

→ means ←

$$500 \times 2 = 1,000 \times 1$$

$$1,000 = 1,000$$

(In true proportion, the product of means equals product of extremes.)

Example 2:   2 mL : 80 mg = 1 mL : 40 mg

$$80 \times 1 = 2 \times 40$$

$$80 = 80$$

(In true proportion, the product of means equals product of extremes.)

POINTS TO REMEMBER

- Proportions represent two ratios that are equal and have a relationship to each other.
- When 3 values are known, the fourth can be easily calculated.
- Proportions can be stated using an (=) sign, a double colon (::), or a fraction format.
- Ratio can be used to state the amount of drug contained in a volume of solution, tablet, or capsule.
- Proportions are solved by multiplying the means and extremes.
- Ratios are always stated in their lowest terms.
- Double-check work.

PRACTICE PROBLEMS

1. Assume that the ratio of clients to nurses is 15 to 2. Express the ratio in

   fraction and colon form. _____

Express the following doses as ratios. Include the units of weight and the numerical value.

2. An injectable liquid that contains 100 mg in each 0.5 mL. _____

3. A tablet that contains 0.2 mg of the drug. _____

4. An oral liquid that contains 1 g in each 10 mL. _____

5. A capsule that contains 500 mg of the drug. _____

Determine the value for x in the following problems. Express your answer to the nearest tenth as indicated.

6. $12.5 : 5 = 24 : x$ _____

9. $1/300 : 3 = 1/120 : x$ _____

7. $1.5 : 1 = 4.5 : x$ _____

10. $x : 12 = 9 : 6$ _____

8. $750/3 = 600/x$ _____

Answers on p. 494

 CHAPTER REVIEW

Express the following fractions as ratios. Reduce to lowest terms.

1. $\dfrac{2}{3}$ _____

4. $\dfrac{1}{5}$ _____

2. $\dfrac{1}{9}$ _____

5. $\dfrac{5}{10}$ _____

3. $\dfrac{6}{8}$ _____

6. $\dfrac{2}{10}$ _____

Express the following ratios as fractions. Reduce to lowest terms.

7. $3 : 7$ _____

10. $8 : 6$ _____

8. $4 : 6$ _____

11. $3 : 4$ _____

9. $1 : 7$ _____

Solve for x in the following proportions. Carry division two decimal places as necessary.

12. $20 : 40 = x : 10$ _____

17. $\dfrac{1}{4} : 1.6 = \dfrac{1}{8} : x$ _____

13. $\dfrac{1}{4} : \dfrac{1}{2} = 1 : x$ _____

18. $\dfrac{1}{2} : 2 = \dfrac{1}{3} : x$ _____

14. $0.12 : 0.8 = 0.6 : x$ _____

19. $125 : 0.4 = 50 : x$ _____

15. $\dfrac{1}{250} : 2 = \dfrac{1}{150} : x$ _____

20. $x : 1 = 0.5 : 5$ _____

16. $x : 9 = 5 : 10$ _____

Express the following doses as ratios. Be sure to include the units of measure and numerical value.

21. An injectable solution that contains 1,000 units (U) in each mL. _____

22. A tablet that contains 0.2 mg of drug. _____

Notes

23. A capsule that contains 250 mg of drug. _____

24. An oral solution that contains 125 mg in each 5 mL. _____

25. An injectable solution that contains 40 mg in each mL. _____

Answers on p. 494

Percentages

Percentage is a commonly used word. Sale taxes are a *percentage* of the sale price; a final examination is a certain *percentage* of the final grade; interest on a home mortgage represents a percentage of the balance owed; interest on a savings account is expressed as a *percentage*. **Health care professionals see percentages written with medications** (e.g., magnesium sulfate 50%). In addition to using percentage with medications, it is also used in the assessment of burns. The size of a burn (percentage of injured skin) is determined using the rule of nines in an adult (Figure 5-1). The basis of the rule is that the body is divided into anatomic sections, each of which represents 9% or a multiple of 9% of the total body surface area. The total body surface area is represented by 100%. Another method used is the age-specific burn diagram or chart. Burn size is expressed as a percentage of the total body surface area (BSA). In children, age-related charts are used because their body proportions are different from those of an adult and the rules of nine cannot be applied.

Many health care providers use solutions that are expressed in percentages for external as well as internal use (e.g., hydrocortisone cream, Dakin's solution, and intravenous solutions).

In current practice, percentage solutions are prepared by the pharmacy and people can purchase solutions or components of the solutions over the counter. There are institutions that require nurses to prepare solutions in many institutions as well as in home care for clients being cared for at home. Understanding percentages provides the foundation for preparing and calculating doses for medication that are ordered in percentages.

The term *percent* (%) means hundredth. A percentage is the same as a fraction in which the denominator is 100, and the numerator indicates the part of 100 that is being considered.

Example:
$$4\% = \frac{4}{100}$$

Notes

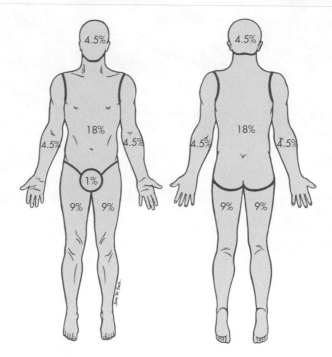

Figure 5-1   "Rule of Nines." Rule of nines is one method to estimate amount of skin surface burned in an adult. (From Thibodeau GA, Patten KT: *Anatomy & physiology*, ed 4, St Louis, 1999, Mosby.)

Intravenous solutions are ordered in percentage strengths, and nurses need to be familiar with their meaning (e.g., 1000 mL/cc 5% dextrose and water). **Percentage solution means the number of grams of solute per 100 mL/cc of diluent.**

Example 1:   1,000 mL IV of 5% dextrose and water contains 50 g (grams) of dextrose

Example 2:   250 mL IV of 10% dextrose contains 25 g (grams) of dextrose

A point to remember with percentage solutions such as intravenous fluids is the higher the percentage strength the more drug/solute it contains, and the more potent the solution will be.

Example: 10% I.V. solution is more potent than 5%. **Always check the percentage of I.V. solution prescribed.**

 PRACTICE PROBLEMS

1. How many grams of drug will 500 mL of a 10% solution contain?

   _____

2. How many grams of dextrose will 1,000 mL of a 10% solution contain?

   _____

3. How many grams of dextrose will 250 mL of a 5% solution contain?

_____

4. How many grams of drug will 100 mL of a 50% solution contain?

_____

5. How many grams of dextrose will 150 mL of 5% solution contain?

_____

Answers on p. 494

CHANGING PERCENTAGES TO FRACTIONS, DECIMALS, AND RATIOS

The percent symbol may be used with a whole number (15%), a fraction (1/2%), a mixed number (14 1/2%), or a decimal (0.6%).

> To change a percent to a fraction, drop the % sign, place the number over 100, and reduce to lowest terms.

Example 1: $8\% = \dfrac{8}{100}$, reduced is $\dfrac{2}{25}$

Example 2: $\dfrac{1}{4}\% = \dfrac{1}{4} \div 100 = \dfrac{1}{4} \times \dfrac{1}{100} = \dfrac{1}{400}$

 PRACTICE PROBLEMS

Change the following percents to fractions and reduce to lowest terms.

6. 1% _____

7. 2% _____

8. 50% _____

9. 80% _____

10. 3% _____

Answers on p. 494

> To change a percent to a decimal, drop the % sign, and move the decimal point two places to the left (add zeros as needed).

Example 1: $25\% = 0.25$

Example 2: $1.4\% = 0.014$

Example 3: $75\% = \dfrac{75}{100} = \dfrac{3}{4}$ (lowest terms). Divide the numerator of the fraction (3) by the denominator (4).

$$4\overline{)3.00} = 0.75$$

Note:

Example 3 is an alternative method is to drop the % sign, express the percent as a fraction in its lowest terms, and divide the numerator by the denominator to obtain a decimal.

Notes

 PRACTICE PROBLEMS

Change the following percents to decimals.

11. 10% _____   14. 14.2% _____

12. 35% _____   15. $\frac{1}{4}$% _____

13. 50% _____   Answers on pp. 494-495

> To change a percent to a ratio, change it to a fraction and reduce to the lowest terms, then place the numerator as the first term of the ratio and the denominator as the second term. Separate the two terms with a colon (:).

Example: $10\% = \dfrac{10}{100} = \dfrac{1}{10} = 1 : 10$

 PRACTICE PROBLEMS

Change the following percents to a ratio. Express in lowest terms:

16. 25% _____   19. 4.5% _____

17. 11% _____   20. $\frac{2}{5}$% _____

18. 75% _____   Answers on p. 495

CHANGING FRACTIONS, DECIMALS, AND RATIOS TO PERCENTAGES

> To change a fraction to a percent, multiply the fraction by 100, reduce if necessary, and add the percent sign.

Example 1: $\frac{3}{4}$ changed to a percent is

$$\frac{3}{4} \times \frac{100}{1} = \frac{300}{4} = \frac{75}{1} = 75$$

Add symbol for percent: 75%

Example 2: $5\frac{1}{2}$ changed to a percent is

$5\frac{1}{2}$: change to an improper fraction $\frac{11}{2}$

$$\frac{11}{2} \times \frac{100}{1} = \frac{1,100}{2} = \frac{550}{1} = 550$$

Add symbol for percent: 550%

PRACTICE PROBLEMS

Change the following fractions to percents.

21. $\dfrac{2}{5}$ _____

24. $\dfrac{1}{4}$ _____

22. $\dfrac{11}{4}$ _____

25. $\dfrac{7}{10}$ _____

23. $\dfrac{1}{2}$ _____

Answers on p. 495

To change a decimal to a percent, move the decimal point two places to the right (multiply), add zeros if necessary, and add the percent symbol.

Example 1: Change 0.45 to %

Move the decimal point two places to the right.

Add the symbol for percent: 45%

Example 2: Change 2.35 to %

Move the decimal point two places to the right.

Add the symbol for percent: 235%

A decimal may also be changed to a percent by changing the decimal to a fraction and following the steps to change a fraction to a percent. If the percentage does not end in a whole number, express the percentage with the remainder as a fraction, to the nearest whole percent, or to the nearest tenth of a percent.

Example: $0.625 = \dfrac{625}{1000} = \dfrac{5}{8} = 62\dfrac{1}{2}\%$, 63%, or 62.5%.

$$\dfrac{625}{1,000} = \dfrac{5}{8}; \ \dfrac{5}{8} \times \dfrac{100}{1} = \dfrac{500}{8} = 62.5\%$$

To change a ratio to percent, change the ratio to a fraction, and proceed with steps for changing a fraction to percent.

Example: $1:4 = \dfrac{1}{4}, \ \dfrac{1}{4} \times \dfrac{100}{1} = 25$

Add the symbol for percent: 25%

PRACTICE PROBLEMS

Change the following ratios to percent.

26. 1 : 25 _____

29. 1 : 100 _____

27. 3 : 4 _____

30. 1 : 2 _____

28. 1 : 10 _____

Answers on p. 495

Notes

DETERMINING THE PERCENT OF A QUANTITY

Nurses may find it necessary to determine a given percentage or part of a quantity.

When determining a given percent of a number, first change the percent to a decimal or fraction, then multiply the decimal or fraction by the number.

Example 1:   A client reports that he drank 25% of his 8 ounce cup of tea. Determine what amount 25% is of 8 ounces.

Solution: Change the percent to a decimal:

$$25\% = \frac{25}{100} = .25 = 0.25$$

Multiply the decimal by the number:

$$0.25 \times 8 = 2 \text{ ounces}$$

Therefore, 25% of 8 ounces is 2 ounces.

Example 2:   40% of 90

$$40\% = \frac{40}{100} = .40 = 0.40$$

$$0.40 \times 90 = 36$$

Therefore, 40% of 90 = 36

DETERMINING WHAT PERCENT ONE NUMBER IS OF ANOTHER

To determine what percent one number is of another it is necessary to make a fraction using the numbers. The denominator of the fraction is the number following the word "of" in the problem and the other number is the numerator of the fraction. Convert the fraction to a decimal, then convert to a percent.

Example 1:   12 is what % of 60? Or what % of 60 is 12?

Solution: Make a fraction using the two numbers.

$$\frac{12}{60}$$

Convert the fraction to a decimal.

$$60\overline{)12.0}^{\;0.2}$$

Convert the decimal to a percent:

$$0.2 = 20\%$$

Therefore, 12 is 20% of 60 or 20% of 60 = 12.

PRACTICE PROBLEMS

Perform the indicated operations.

31. 60% of 30 _____

32. 20% of 75 _____

33. 2 is what % of 200 _____

34. 50 is what % of 500 _____

35. 40 is what % of 1,000 _____

Answers on p. 495

CHAPTER REVIEW

Complete the table below. Express each of the following measures in their equivalents where indicated. Reduce to lowest terms where necessary.

	Percent	Ratio	Fraction	Decimal
1.	0.25%	_____	_____	_____
2.	71%	_____	_____	_____
3.	_____	_____	$\frac{7}{100}$	_____
4.	_____	1 : 50	_____	_____
5.	_____	_____	_____	0.06
6.	_____	_____	$\frac{1}{30}$	_____
7.	_____	_____	$\frac{61}{100}$	_____
8.	_____	7 : 1000	_____	_____
9.	5%	_____	_____	_____
10.	2.5%	_____	_____	_____

Perform the indicated operations.

11. A client reports that he drank 40% of his 12 ounce can of gingerale. How many ounces did the client drink? _____

12. 40% of 140 _____

13. $\frac{1}{2}$ is what % of 60? _____

14. 100 is what % of 750? _____

15. 15% of 250 _____

Answers on p. 495

Posttest

After completing Unit One of this text, you should be able to complete this test. The test consists of a total of 50 questions. If you miss three or more questions in any section, review the chapter relating to that content.

Express the following in Roman numerals.

1. 5 _____

2. 17 _____

3. 27 _____

4. 29 _____

5. 30 _____

Express the following in Arabic numbers.

6. $\overline{\text{viss}}$ _____

7. $\overline{\text{xxiv}}$ _____

8. $\overline{\text{xix}}$ _____

9. $\overline{\text{xxv}}$ _____

10. $\overline{\text{xv}}$ _____

Reduce the following fractions to lowest terms.

11. $\dfrac{8}{6}$ _____

12. $\dfrac{22}{33}$ _____

13. $\dfrac{27}{63}$ _____

14. $\dfrac{10}{15}$ _____

15. $\dfrac{16}{10}$ _____

Perform the indicated operations with fractions; reduce to lowest terms where needed.

16. $\dfrac{5}{6} \div \dfrac{7}{10} =$ _____

17. $5\dfrac{1}{2} \div 4\dfrac{1}{2} =$ _____

18. $6\dfrac{1}{3} \times 4 =$ _____

19. $5\dfrac{1}{5} - 3\dfrac{4}{7} =$ _____

20. $\dfrac{5}{4} + \dfrac{2}{9} =$ _____

Notes

Change the following fractions to decimals; express your answer to the nearest tenth.

21. $\dfrac{8}{7}$ _____

23. $\dfrac{1}{15}$ _____

22. $\dfrac{1}{8}$ _____

24. $\dfrac{12}{13}$ _____

Indicate the largest fraction in each group.

25. $\dfrac{1}{2}, \dfrac{2}{3}, \dfrac{5}{9}$ _____

26. $\dfrac{3}{4}, \dfrac{7}{10}, \dfrac{5}{8}$ _____

Perform the indicated operation with decimals.

27. $16.7 + 21.0 =$ _____

29. $10.57 \times 10 =$ _____

28. $0.007 + 17.4 =$ _____

30. $36.8 - 3.86 =$ _____

Divide the following decimals; express your answer to the nearest tenth.

31. $67.8 \div 0.8 =$ _____

33. $5.01 \div 10 =$ _____

32. $9 \div 0.4 =$ _____

Indicate the largest decimal in each group.

34. $0.850, 0.085$ _____

36. $0.478, 0.445, 0.493$ _____

35. $3.002, 0.390, 0.399$ _____

Solve for x, the unknown value.

37. $10 : 20 = x : 8$ _____

39. $0.3 : x = 1.8 : 0.6$ _____

38. $500 : x = 200 : 1$ _____

40. $\dfrac{1}{4} : x = \dfrac{1}{8} : 2$ _____

Round off to the nearest tenth.

41. 0.57 _____

43. 1.42 _____

42. 0.99 _____

Round off to the nearest hundredth.

44. 0.677 _____

46. 1.222 _____

45. 0.832 _____

Complete the table below. Express each of the measures in their equivalents where indicated. Reduce to lowest terms where necessary or round off to nearest hundredth.

	Percent	**Decimal**	**Ratio**	**Fraction**
47.	_____	_____	1 : 10	_____
48.	60%	_____	_____	_____
49.	$66\frac{2}{3}\%$	_____	_____	_____
50.	25%	_____	_____	_____

Find the percentage.

51. 9% of 200 _____   54. 5 is what % of 2,000 _____

52. 2.5% of 750 _____   55. 25 is what % of 65 _____

53. 30 is what % of 45 _____   Answers on pp. 495-496

UNIT TWO

Systems of Measurement

Three systems of measurement are used to compute medication doses: metric, apothecaries', and household. To be competent in the administration of medications, it is essential that the nurse be familiar with all three systems.

Chapter 6
Metric System

Chapter 7
Apothecaries' and Household Systems

Chapter 8
Converting Within and Between Systems

Chapter 9
Additional Conversions Useful in the Health Care Setting

Chapter 6

Metric System

Objectives

After reviewing this chapter, you should be able to:

1. **Express metric measures correctly using rules of the metric system**
2. **State common equivalents in the metric system**
3. **Convert measures within the metric system**

The metric system is an international decimal system of weights and measures that was introduced in France in the late 17th and 18th centuries. The system is also referred to as the International System of Units (SI). SI is the abbreviation for the French *Système International d'Unités*. Although the system was rooted in the late 17th and 18th centuries, the standard system of abbreviations was not adopted until 1960. The metric system is more precise than the apothecaries' and household systems. Apothecaries' and household measures are gradually being replaced with the metric system. More and more in everyday situations we are encountering the use of metric measures. For example, soft drinks come in bottles labeled in liters; engine sizes are also expressed in liters.

Most medications and measurements used in health care are calibrated and calculated using the metric system. For example, newborn weights are recorded in grams and kilograms, and adult weights are expressed in kilograms, as opposed to pounds and ounces. In obstetrics we express fundal height (upper portion of the uterus) in centimeters. Although some medications are still prescribed in apothecaries' and household terms, the nurse will find the majority of medication calculation and administration skills involve **accurate** use of the metric system.

PARTICULARS OF THE METRIC SYSTEM

1. The metric system is based on the decimal system, in which divisions and multiples of ten are used. Therefore a lot of math can be done by decimal point movement.
2. Three basic units of measure are used:
   a) **Gram**—the basic unit for weight
   b) **Liter**—the basic unit for volume
   c) **Meter**—the basic unit for length

   Doses are calculated using metric measurements that relate to weight and volume. Meter, which is used for linear (length) measurement, is not used in the calculation of doses. Linear measurements (meter, centimeter) are commonly used to measure the height of an individual and to determine growth patterns.

3. Common prefixes in this system denote the numeric value of the unit being discussed. Memorization of these prefixes is necessary for quick and accurate calculations. The prefixes in bold in Table 6-1 are the ones used most often in health care for dosage calculations. However, some of the prefixes may be seen to express other values, such as laboratory values. *Kilo* is a common prefix used to identify a measure larger than the basic unit. The other common prefixes used in medication administration are smaller units, such as *centi, milli,* and *micro.*

Let's look at the following example to see how the prefixes may be used.

Example: 67 milligrams

Prefix—*milli*—means measure in thousandths of a unit.
Gram is a unit of weight.
Therefore 67 milligrams = 67 thousandths of a gram.

4. Regardless of the size of the unit, the name of the basic unit is incorporated into the measure. This allows easy recognition of the unit of measure.

Example 1: milli**liter**—the word *liter* indicates you are measuring volume (*milli* indicates 1/1,000 of that volume).

Example 2: kilo**gram**—the word *gram* indicates you are measuring weight (*kilo* indicates 1,000 of that weight; 1 kilogram = 1,000 grams).

Example 3: kilo**liter**—the word *liter* indicates you are measuring volume (*kilo* indicates 1,000 of that volume; 1 kiloliter = 1,000 liters).

Example 4: deci**liter**—the word *liter* indicates that you are measuring volume (*deci* indicates 0.1 of that volume (liter), or 100 milliliters). The note, "Female's normal hemoglobin is 12-16g/dL," for example, therefore means there is 12-16 grams of hemoglobin contained in 100 milliliters of blood.

Example 5: cubic milli**meter** (mm)—cubic millimeter is a unit of volume of three-dimensional space (length $\times$ width $\times$ height). In a normal individual the white blood cell count ranges between 5,000 and 10,000 cells per cubic millimeters of blood. Therefore 1 mm of blood contains between 5,000 and 10,000 white blood cells (5,000/mm and 10,000/mm).

5. The abbreviation for a unit of measure in the metric system is often the first letter of the word. Lower case letters are used more often than capital letters.

TABLE 6-1 Common Prefixes Used in Health Care

Prefix	Numeric value	Meaning
Kilo	**1,000**	**one thousand times**
Centi	**0.01**	**one hundredth part of**
Milli	**0.001**	**one thousandth part of**
Micro	**0.000001**	**one millionth part of**
Hecto	100	one hundred times
Deka	10	ten times
Deci	0.1	one tenth

Notes

Example 1: g = gram

Example 2: mg = milligram

The exception to this rule is liter, which uses a capital letter.

Example 3: liter = L

6. When prefixes are used in combination with the basic unit, the first letter of the prefix and the first letter of the unit of measure are written together in lower case letters.

Example 1: milligram—Abbreviated as **mg.** The *m* is taken from the prefix *milli* and the *g* from *gram,* the unit of weight.

Example 2: Microgram—Abbreviated as **mcg.** Microgram is also written using the symbol μ in combination with the letter *g* from the basic unit *gram* (μg). **However, using the symbol μg should be avoided when transcribing orders, because it might be interpreted as mg.**

Example 3: Milliliter—Abbreviated as **mL.** Note that when *L (liter)* is used in combination with a prefix, it **remains capitalized.**

You may see gram abbreviated as Gm or gm, liter as lowercase l, or milliliter as ml. These abbreviations are outdated and can lead to misinterpretation. Use only the standardized SI abbreviations. See Box 6-1 for common metric abbreviations.

RULES OF METRIC SYSTEM

Certain rules specific to the metric system are important to remember. See Box 6-2.

A zero should always be placed in front of the decimal when the quantity is not a whole number. When the quantity expressed is preceded by a whole number, a zero is not necessary.

Example 1: .52 mL is written as 0.52 mL to **reinforce the decimal** and avoid being misread as 52 mL.

Example 2: 2.5 mL is written as 2.5 mL, not 2.50 mL. **Addition of unnecessary zeros can lead to errors in reading;** 2.50 mL may be misread as 250 mL instead of 2.5 mL.

B O X 6-1 Common Metric Abbreviations

gram = g
microgram = mcg
milligram = mg
kilogram = kg
liter = L
milliliter = mL

Notes

BOX 6-2   **Metric System Rules**

1. Arabic numbers are used to express quantities in this system.

   Example: 1; 1,000; 0.5

2. Parts of a unit or fractions of a unit are expressed as decimals.

   Example: 0.4 g, 0.5 L $\left(\text{not } \frac{2}{5} \text{ g}, \frac{1}{2} \text{ L}\right)$

3. The quantity, whether in whole numbers or in decimals, is always written before the abbreviation or symbol for a unit of measure.

   Example: 1,000 mg, 0.75 mL (not mg 1,000, mL 0.75)

UNITS OF MEASURE

Weight

The gram is the basic unit of weight. Medications may be ordered in grams or fractions of a gram, such as milligram or microgram.

1. The milligram is 1,000 times smaller than a gram;

$$1,000 \text{ mg} = 1 \text{ g}$$

2. The microgram is 1,000 times smaller than a milligram and 1 million times smaller than a gram. The word *micro* also means tiny or small. Micrograms are tiny parts of a gram: 1,000 mcg = 1 mg. A milligram is 1,000 times larger than a microgram. It takes 1 million mcg to make 1 g.

3. The kilogram is very large and is not used for measuring medications. A kilogram is 1,000 times larger than a gram: 1 kg = 1,000 g. This measure is often used to denote weights of clients, upon which medication doses are based. This is the only unit you will see used to identify a unit larger than the basic unit.

Box 6-3 presents units of weight to memorize.

Volume

1. The **liter** is the basic unit.

$$1,000 \text{ mL} = 1 \text{ L}$$

2. The **milliliter** is 1000 times smaller than a liter. It is abbreviated as mL.

$$1 \text{ mL} = 0.001 \text{ L}$$

3. The **cubic centimeter** is the amount of space that 1 mL of liquid occupies. It is abbreviated as cc.

$$1 \text{ mL} = 0.001 \text{ L}$$

$$1 \text{ L} = 1,000 \text{ mL}$$

Note:

Although cc and mL have been used interchangeably, mL is the correct term for volume.

Cubic centimeter (cc) and milliliter (mL) are considered to be the **same** and are used **interchangeably.** However mL is the correct term that should be used in relation to volume, not cc. (Figure 6-1 illustrates metric measures that may be seen on a medication cup.)

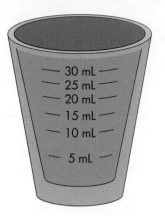

Figure 6-1   Medicine cup showing volume measure in milliliters (mL).

BOX 6-3   **Units of Weight to Memorize**

1 kilogram (kg) = 1,000 grams (g)
1 gram (g) = 1,000 milligrams (mg)
1 milligram (mg) = 1,000 micrograms (mcg)

Unit of Volume to Memorize
1 liter = 1,000 milliliters (mL)

Although pint and quart are not metric measures, they have metric equivalents. For example, a quart is approximately the size of a liter: 1 quart = 1,000 mL and 1 pint = 500 mL. Although pint and quart are not measures used in medication administration, you may need them to calculate a solution, especially in homecare.

CONVERSIONS BETWEEN METRIC UNITS

Because the metric system is based on the decimal system, conversions between one metric system unit and another can be done by moving the decimal point. The number of places to move the decimal point depends on the equivalent. In health care, each unit of measure in common use for purposes of medication administration differs by 1,000. In the metric system the most common terms used are the gram, liter, microgram, milligram, milliliter, centimeter, and kilogram. To **convert** or make a **conversion** means to change from one form to another. This converting can be simply changing a measure to its equivalent in the same system. Changing from grams to milligrams illustrates a metric measure changed to another metric measure. Each metric unit in common use differs from the next by a factor of 1,000. Metric conversions can therefore be made by dividing or multiplying by **1,000.** Knowledge concerning the size of a unit is important when converting by moving the decimal, because this determines whether division or multiplication is necessary to make the conversion.

Nurses often make conversions within the metric system when administering medications; for example, g to mg.

To make conversions within the metric system, remember the common conversion factors (1 kg = 1,000 g, 1 g = 1,000 mg; 1 mg = 1,000 mcg, and 1 L = 1,000 mL) and the following rules:

1. To convert a **smaller** unit to a **larger** one, **divide** by moving the decimal point **three places to the left.**

Example 1:   100 mL = ___ L   (conversion factor
                    (smaller)   (larger)   1,000 mL = 1 L)

100 mL = .100 = 0.1 L (Placing zero in front of the decimal is important.)

Example 2:   50 mg = ___ g   (conversion factor
                    (smaller)   (larger)   1,000 mg = 1 g)

50 mg = .050 = 0.05 g (Placing zero in front of the decimal is important.)

2. To convert a **larger** unit to a **smaller** one, **multiply** by moving the decimal **three places to the right.**

Example 1:   0.75 g = ___ mg   (conversion factor
                     (larger)   (smaller)   1 g = 1,000 mg)

0.75 g = 0.750 = 750 mg

Note:

Answers to conversions should be labeled with the unit of measure. A comma should be placed in values greater than 1,000.

Example 2:   0. 04 kg = ___ g   (conversion factor
                     (larger)   (smaller)   1 kg = 1,000 g)

0.04 kg = 0.040 = 40 g

 PRACTICE PROBLEMS

Convert the following metric measures by moving the decimal.

1. 300 mg = _____ g   11. 529 mg = _____ g

2. 6 mg = _____ mcg   12. 645 mcg = _____ mg

3. 0.7 L = _____ mL   13. 347 L = _____ mL

4. 180 mcg = _____ mg   14. 238 g = _____ mcg

5. 0.02 mg = _____ mcg   15. 3,500 mL = _____ L

6. 4.5 L = _____ mL   16. 0.04 kg = _____ g

7. 4.2 g = _____ mg   17. 658 kg = _____ g

8. 0.9 g = _____ mg   18. 51 mL = _____ L

9. 3,250 mL = _____ L   19. 1.6 mg = _____ mcg

10. 42 g = _____ kg   20. 28 mL = _____ L

Answers on p. 496

Notes

POINTS TO REMEMBER

- The liter and the gram are the basic units used for medication administration.

- Conversion factors must be memorized to do conversions. The common conversion factors in the metric system are 1 kg = 1,000 g, 1 g = 1,000 mg, 1 mg = 1,000 mcg, and 1 L = 1,000 mL (mL is the correct term to use in relation to volume, instead of cc).

- Express answers using the following rules of the metric system:
    1. Fractional parts are expressed as a decimal.
    2. Place a zero in front of the decimal point when it is not preceded by a whole number.
    3. Omit unnecessary zeros to avoid misreading of a value.
    4. The abbreviation for a measure is placed after the quantity.

- Converting common metric units used in medication administration from one unit to another is done by moving the decimal point three places.

- Answers should be stated with the unit of measure as the label.

- Values greater than 1,000 should be written with a comma.

 ## CHAPTER REVIEW

1. List the three units of measurement used in the metric system.

    a) _____

    b) _____

    c) _____

2. Which is larger, kilogram or milligram? _____

3. 1 mL = _____ L

4. What units of measure are used in the metric system for:

    a. liquid capacity? _____

    b. weight? _____

5. 1,000 mg = _____ g

6. 1 L = _____ mL

7. 1,000 mcg = _____ mg

8. 1,000 mL = _____ L

Notes

9. The abbreviation for liter is _____

10. The abbreviation for microgram is _____

11. The abbreviation for milliliter is _____

12. The abbreviation for gram is _____

13. The abbreviation for kilogram is _____

14. The prefix *kilo* means _____

15. The prefix *milli* means _____

Using abbreviations and the rules of the metric system, express the following quantities correctly.

16. Six tenths of a gram _____

17. Fifty kilograms _____

18. Four tenths of a milligram _____

19. Four hundredths of a liter _____

20. Four and two tenths micrograms _____

21. Five thousandths of a gram _____

22. Six hundredths of a gram _____

23. Two and six tenths milliliters _____

24. One hundred milliliters _____

25. Three hundredths of a milliliter _____

Convert the following metric measures by moving the decimal.

26. 950 mcg = _____ mg

27. 58.5 L = _____ mL

28. 130 mL = _____ L

29. 276 g = _____ mg

30. 550 mL = _____ L

31. 56.5 L = _____ mL

32. 205 g = _____ kg

33. 0.025 kg = _____ g

34. 1 L = _____ mL

35. 0.015 g = _____ mg

36. 250 mcg = _____ mg

37. 8 kg = _____ g

38. 2 kL = _____ L

39. 5 L = _____ mL

40. 0.75 L = _____ mL

41. 0.33 g = _____ mg

42. 750 mg = _____ g

43. 6.28 kg = _____ g

44. 36.5 mg = _____ g

45. 2.2 mg = _____ g

46. 400 g = _____ kg

47. 0.024 L = _____ mL

48. 100 mg = _____ g

49. 150 g = _____ mg

50. 85 mcg = _____ mg

Answers on p. 496

Notes

Apothecaries' and Household Systems

APOTHECARIES' SYSTEM

The apothecaries' system is one of the oldest systems of measure. Historically it was brought to this country from England during the colonial period. In Europe, the apothecaries' system has been totally replaced by the metric system. This transition in the United States has been a gradual and slow process; however, it is quite possible that within the next few years the metric system will totally replace the apothecaries' and be used exclusively in the calculation of dosages. Although the apothecary measures are seldom used today, it is important for health care providers to be aware of them.

Apothecaries' measures are seen on medication labels that have been in use for many years (e.g., morphine, atropine, and aspirin). Health care providers may write orders using some apothecaries' measures (e.g., "aspirin grains ten"). Pharmaceutical companies may label drugs using both apothecary and metric measures on the label. For example, if we look at the label on a bottle of nitroglycerin (Nitrostat) tablets, we see that the tablets are labeled in milligrams, which is a metric measure, and also grains (in parenthesis), which is an apothecaries' measure. Figure 7-1 illustrates the use of metric and apothecaries' measures on a drug labels.

Apothecaries' measures are also still on syringes (minim) and medication cups (dram); it is important to note, however, use of these measures has been discouraged. In some institutions, due to the inaccuracy of minims, syringes that are purchased do not have minims on them. Because the apothecaries' system is still in use, even minimally, it is necessary for those involved in the administration of medications to be familiar with it.

Notes

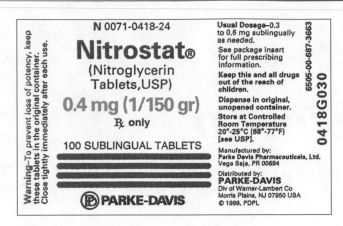

Figure 7-1 Drug label showing apothecaries' and metric measures (*mg*, metric; *gr*, apothecaries').

Particulars of the Apothecaries' System

1. The measures used in this system are approximations, not exact as the metric system, and caution should be exercised when using this system; you could place a client at risk. When orders are written using apothecaries' measures they should be converted to metric measures by referring to an equivalents table, which are often posted in the medication room. It is wise to check a reference whenever an uncommon measure is used.
2. Roman numerals, as well as Arabic numbers, are often used in this system. When Roman numerals are written in the apothecaries' system they are written using lower case letters to express numbers (e.g., gr v).
3. Fractions are used to express quantities that are less than one, as opposed to the use of decimals in the metric system.
4. The symbol *ss* is used for the fraction 1/2. When used it can be written ss or $\overline{ss}$.

Example: half of a grain in abbreviated form would be gr ss or gr $\overline{ss}$.

The symbol *ss* can also be used with Roman numerals. When used with Roman numerals, it is placed at the end.

Example: seven and a half grains = gr $\overline{viiss}$.

5. Unlike the metric system, in the apothecaries' system the abbreviation or symbol for a unit of measure is written **before** the amount or quantity. Small case letters are used for abbreviations.

Example: six grains. The symbol for grains is gr. Therefore six grains would be written as 6 grvi, gr6, or gr$\overline{vi}$.

6. A combination of Arabic numerals and fractions can also be used in this system to express units of measure.

Example: $gr\ 7\frac{1}{2}$

gr	7	$\frac{1}{2}$
↓	↓	↓
abbreviation	Arabic	fraction

The notations for the apothecaries' system are unusual, and often time inconsistent. The specifics previously mentioned relating to notations within this system may be seen and a few may be followed.

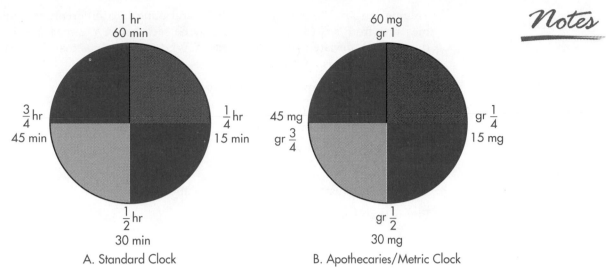

Notes

Figure 7-2 **A,** 60 minutes = 1 hour, and fractions of an hour are shown in minutes. **B,** Because 60 mg = grl and there are 60 minutes in one hour, you can visualize milligrams as representing minutes on a clock, and the fractions of an hour as grains.

Apothecaries' Units of Measure

The units of measure used for medication administration are few.

Weight

The basic unit for weight is the **grain.**

1. Grain is abbreviated in lower case letters as gr. The abbreviations for grain and gram are often confused. Remember **grain** is abbreviated as **gr,** and **gram** is abbreviated as **g.** Grain, which is an apothecaries' measure for weight, has some metric equivalents. Two important conversions to remember are **gr 15 − 1 g** and **60 mg = gr 1.** Another way to remember common apothecaries' and metric conversions is to remember the **conversion clock.** First let's visualize the relationship of a standard clock to a clock illustrating metric and apothecary conversion (Figure 7-2).

2. Dram is also a unit of weight; however, dry medications are not measured in drams anymore. The symbol for dram is a **single-headed** z with a tail (ʒ). Dram is also abbreviated as dr. Drams are often seen on medication cups; however, like minims, their use is discouraged.

3. Ounce—the symbol for ounce is a **double-headed** z with a tail (℥). Note: The extra loop on the z differentiates it from the symbol for dram. It is important not to confuse the symbols for dram and ounce because of the large difference in measures. A way to avoid confusion is to remember that an ounce is larger than a dram, thus the symbol is bigger. Another differentiating cue is to remember that the **"ounce (symbol) has the extra bounce."** Ounce is also abbreviated as oz.

Volume

The smallest unit for volume is the **minim.**

1. The most current abbreviation for minim is a lower case m. A minim is extremely small (the size of one drop), and minims are therefore always expressed as whole numbers. A way to remember the size of a minim is to think about the beginning three letters of the word (min) and think of words such as minute and minimal. Syringes still have a minim scale on them; however, their use is discouraged due to their inaccuracy.

2. Volume can also be measured by dram and ounce. To differentiate liquid measures from solid measures, an f may be seen before the measure. F = fluid; it is abbreviated with a lower case f. When it is obvious that the measure is a liquid, it is omitted.

Example: f3 = fluid dram; f3̄ = fluid ounce

1 fluid dram = 60 minims
(f3i = m 60), or f3i = mlx

1 fluid ounce = 8 fluid drams
(f3̄i = f3viii)

3. The pint and quart are also apothecaries' measures.

Pint is abbreviated as pt

1 pint = 16 fluid ounces

Quart is abbreviated as qt

1 quart = 32 fluid ounces or 2 pints

4. Some apothecaries' measures have equivalents in the metric system that must be memorized:

1 dram = 4 mL

1 ounce = 30 mL

1 pint = 500 mL

1 quart = 1,000 mL

Discrepancies in Apothecaries' Equivalents

Discrepancies in the apothecaries' system exist because of the inaccuracy and approximation within this system. Tables of equivalents may state that **gr 1 equals 60-65 mg.** The equivalent recognized and used in drug orders is gr 1 = 60 mg (for example, aspirin 300 mg = gr 5). In some instances labels may indicate gr 5 is equivalent to 325 mg or 324 mg. It is important for the nurse to realize discrepancies do exist.

For medication administration it is necessary to be familiar with the apothecaries' system units shown in Box 7-1.

BOX 7-1 **Units of the Apothecaries' System**

Weight: grain (gr)
 Volume: minim (m)
       dram (dr) (3)
       ounce (oz) (3̄)

HOUSEHOLD SYSTEM

Like the apothecaries' system, the household system is an old system. It is a modified system designed for everyday use at the home. The household system is still in use for doses given primarily at home, as indicated by the name. The nurse needs to be familiar with household measures, because clients often use utensils in the home to take prescribed medications. The household system is the **least accurate** of the three systems of measure. Capacities of utensils such as teaspoon, tablespoon, and cup vary from one house to another; therefore liquid measures are approximate. With the increase in nursing provided at home (home care, visiting nurse), it is imperative that nurses become adept in converting from one system to another. When calculating doses or interpreting the health care provider's instructions for the client at home, the nurse must remember that household measures are used. Consequently the nurse must be able to calculate equivalents for adaptation in the home, even though medication administration spoons, droppers, and medication measuring cups (Figure 7-3) are available.

Common household measures to memorize are the following:

1 teaspoon (tsp) = 5 mL (cc)

1 tablespoon (tbs) = 15 mL (cc)

1 measuring cup = 8 oz

Note:

Anything less than a teaspoon should be measured in a syringe-type device and not a measuring cup.

Particulars of the Household System

1. Some of the units for liquid measures are the same as those in the apothecaries' system; for example, pint and quart.
2. There are no standard rules for expressing household measures, which accounts for variations in their use.
3. Standard cookbook abbreviations are used in this system.
4. Arabic numerals and fractions are used to express quantities.
5. The smallest unit of measure in the household system is the drop (gtt).
   Note: **Drops should never be used as a measure for medications because the size of drops varies and therefore can be inaccurate. When drops are used as a measure for medications, they should be calibrated or used only when associated with a dropper size, as in intravenous (I.V.) flow rates.**
6. Common household measures and conversions within this system are as follows. See also Box 7-2.

Drop (gtt)

Teaspoon (t, tsp)

Tablespoon (T, tbs) (3 tsp = 1 tbs)

Cup (C) (16 tbs = 1 C)

Pint (pt) (2 C = 1 pt)

Quart (qt) (2 pt = 1 qt)

1 glassful = 8 ounces

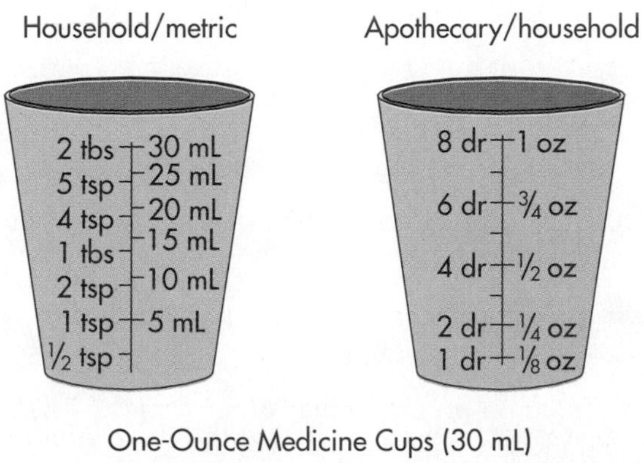

Household/metric   Apothecary/household

2 tbs	30 mL
5 tsp	25 mL
4 tsp	20 mL
1 tbs	15 mL
2 tsp	10 mL
1 tsp	5 mL
½ tsp	

8 dr	1 oz
6 dr	¾ oz
4 dr	½ oz
2 dr	¼ oz
1 dr	⅛ oz

One-Ounce Medicine Cups (30 mL)

Figure 7-3 Medicine cups showing household/metric and apothecaries'/household measurements.

Note:

The abbreviations mL and cc are used interchangeably; however, mL is more accurate and a measure of volume.

B O X 7-2 **Apothecaries'/Household/Metric Equivalents**

VOLUME (LIQUID)
1 ounce (oz, ℥) = 30 mL
1 dram (dr, ʒ) = 4 mL or 1 fluid dram
1 tablespoon (T or tbs) = 15 mL
1 teaspoon (t or tsp) = 5 mL
1 cup (standard measuring cup) = 240 mL (8 ounces)
1 pint (pt) = 500 mL (16 ounces)
1 quart (qt) = 1,000 mL (32 ounces)
15 or 16 minims (m) = 1 mL*

WEIGHT
15 grains (gr) = 1,000 mg = 1 gram (g)
1 grain (gr) = 60 mg
*Minims are inaccurate and not used

It is important for the nurse providing care in the home to remember that clients need specific instructions for measuring accurately at home. Sometimes solutions may have to be made at home using household measures. Below are some examples illustrating making solutions in the home using household devices.

  a) Normal saline (0.9%)—2 teaspoons of salt to 4 cups of water.
  b) Acetic acid solution (0.25%)—3 tablespoons of white vinegar to 4 cups of water for wound/dressing care and cleaning equipment.
  c) Dakins solution—1/3 cup household liquid bleach to 3 cups of water for wound/dressing care.

POINTS TO REMEMBER

- In the apothecaries' system, the abbreviation or symbol is placed before the quantity. There are inconsistencies in notation rules in the apothecaries' system.

- Apothecaries' measures are approximate measures.

- The apothecaries' system uses fractions, Roman numerals, and Arabic numerals.

- Teaspoon, tablespoon, and drop are common measures used in the household system.

- There are no rules for stating household measures.

- The household system uses fractions and Arabic numerals.

- Conversions between metric, apothecaries', and household are not equal measures.

- Doses less than a teaspoon should be measured with a syringe-type device.

- When possible, convert apothecaries' and household to metric measures

- When in doubt about an unfamiliar unit or one that is not used often, consult a reference or an equivalency table.

- mL and cc are used interchangeably; however, mL is a measure of volume and is more accurate.

PRACTICE PROBLEMS

Write the symbols and or abbreviations for the following measures.

1. minim _____

4. dram _____

2. ounce _____

5. pint _____

3. grain _____

Use Box 7-2 to determine the following equivalents.

6. oz $\frac{1}{2}$ = _____ mL

9. $\frac{1}{2}$ pt = oz _____

7. 2 tsp = _____ mL

10. 30 mL = oz _____

8. 10 mL = ℥ _____

Write the following amounts correctly. Make sure they are written using the notation rules of the apothecaries' system.

11. 10 ounces _____

12. one-half grain _____

13. 16 minims _____

14. What household measure might be used to give a $\frac{1}{2}$ ounce of cough syrup?

_____

15. The nurse encouraged a client with diarrhea to drink 40 oz of water per day. How many glassfuls does this represent? (1 glassful = 8 ounces)

_____   Answers on p. 497

 CHAPTER REVIEW

Using the rules of the apothecaries' system, write the following using the correct abbreviations or symbols.

1. Eight and one-half grains _____

2. Three minims _____

3. Five drams _____

4. Eight ounces _____

5. Quart _____

6. Pint _____

7. One hundred twenty-fifth of a grain _____

8. Six and a half fluid drams

_____

9. Two fluid ounces _____

10. Five ounces _____

Notes

Complete the following.

11. The volume
    of one drop equals _____

12. ℥ i = m _____

13. f℥ i = f℥ _____

14. 1 pt = f℥ _____

15. 1 qt = f℥ _____

16. 1 tbs = f℥ _____

17. The abbreviation for drop

    is _____.

18. T is the abbreviation for

    _____.

19. The abbreviation t is used for

    _____.

20. 1 t = _____ mL

21. ℥i = _____ mL

22. 1 cup = _____ ounces

23. 1 tbs = _____ mL

24. 1 pt = _____ ounces

25. 1 qt = _____ ounces

Answers on p. 497

Converting Within and Between Systems

EQUIVALENTS AMONG METRIC, APOTHECARIES', AND HOUSEHOLD SYSTEMS

As discussed in the previous chapters dealing with the systems of measure, some measures in one system have equivalents in another system; however, equivalents are not exact measures, and there are discrepancies. Several tables have been developed illustrating conversions/equivalents. Sometimes drug companies use different equivalents for a measure. As mentioned previously, a common discrepancy is with grains, which is an apothecaries' measure. Some sources indicate 60-65 mg = gr 1. However, remember that **60 mg = gr 1** is used in medication administration.

In the health care system it is imperative that nurses be proficient in converting between all three systems of measure (metric, apothecaries', and household). Nurses are becoming increasingly responsible for administration of medications to clients outside of the conventional hospital setting (for example, home care). Nurses have become more involved in discharge planning and are responsible for ensuring that the client can safely self-administer medications in the correct dose. Table 8-1 lists some of the equivalents between systems. Memorize these common equivalents!

CONVERTING

The term *convert* means to change from one form to another. Converting can mean changing a measure to its equivalent in the same system or changing a measurement from one system to another system, which is called *converting between systems*. The measurement obtained when converting between systems is approximate, not exact. Thus certain equivalents have been established to ensure continuity.

Notes

It is important that nurses be able to make conversions because they are often called upon to convert medication doses between metric, apothecaries', and household systems. The nurse therefore must understand the systems of measurement and be able to convert within the same system, and from one to another, with accuracy.

Before beginning the actual process of converting, the nurse should remember the following important points that can make converting simple.

Points for Converting

1. Memorization of the equivalents/conversions is essential.
2. Think of memorized equivalents/conversions as essential conversion factors.

   Example: 1,000 mg = 1 g is called a conversion factor.

3. Follow basic math principles regardless of the conversion method used.
4. Answers should be expressed applying specific rules that relate to the system to which you are converting.

   Example: The metric system uses decimals; the apothecaries' system uses fractions.

5. THINK CRITICALLY—select the appropriate equivalent to make conversions.

METHODS OF CONVERTING

Moving the Decimal Point

This method was discussed in Chapter 6. Because the metric system is based on the decimal system, conversions within the metric system can be done easily by moving the decimal point. This method cannot be applied in the apothecaries' or household system because decimal points are not used in either system. **Remember the two rules in moving decimal points:**

1. To convert a smaller unit to a larger one, divide or move the decimal point to the left.

Note:

Equivalents indicated in this table are those used most often. *mL* and *cc* are used interchangeably; however, mL is the accurate and preferred term for liquids.

TABLE 8-1 **Approximate Equivalents of Metric, Apothecaries', and Household Measures**

Household	Apothecaries'	Metric
	m 15 or 16★	1 mL
	dr 1 (ℨi)	4 mL
1t, 1tsp		5 mL
1T, 1tbs		15 mL
	gr 15	1 g (1,000 mg)
	gr i	60 mg
	1 oz (℥i)	30 mL
	1 pt (16 oz.)	500 mL
	1 qt (32 oz.)	1000 mL, 1L
	2.2 lb	1 kg (1,000 g)

★Minims is an inaccurate measure and should not be used.

Example: 350 mg = _____ g

                          (smaller) (larger)

Solution: After determining that mg is the smaller unit and you are converting to a larger unit (g), recall the conversion factor that allows you to change milligrams to grams: 1 g = 1,000 mg. Therefore 350 is divided by 1,000 by moving the decimal point three places to the left, indicating 350 mg = 0.35 g.

                          350. mg = 0.35 g

Note: The final answer is expressed in decimal format. Remember to always place a (0) in front of the decimal point to indicate a value that is less than one.

2. To convert a larger unit to a smaller one, multiply or move the decimal point to the right.

Example: 0.85 L = _____ mL

                          (larger)   (smaller)

Solution: After determining that L is the larger unit and you are converting to a smaller unit (mL), recall the conversion factor that allows you to change liters to milliliters: 1L = 1,000 mL. Therefore 0.85 is multiplied by 1,000 by moving the decimal point three places to the right, indicating 0.85 L = 850 mL.

                          0.850 L = 850 mL

Note the addition of a zero here to allow movement of the decimal point the correct number of places.

PRACTICE PROBLEMS CONVERTING WITHIN THE METRIC SYSTEM

For additional practice in converting by decimal movement, convert the following metric measures to the equivalent units indicated.

1. 600 cc = _____ L   11. 0.04 g = _____ mg

2. 0.016 g = _____ mg   12. 0.12 g = _____ kg

3. 4 kg = _____ g   13. 180 mg = _____ g

4. 3 mcg = _____ mg   14. 1,700 mL = _____ L

5. 0.3 mg = _____ g   15. 15 kg = _____ g

6. 0.01 kg = _____ g   16. 3.5 g = _____ mg

7. 1.9 L = _____ mL   17. 0.16 kg = _____ g

8. 0.5 g = _____ kg   18. 0.004 L = _____ mL

9. 0.07 mg = _____ mcg   19. 1 mL = _____ L

10. 650 mL = _____ L   20. 8 mg = _____ g

Answers on p. 497

Using Ratio-Proportion

This is one of the easiest ways to make conversions, whether within the same system or between systems. The basics on how to state ratio-proportions and how to solve them when looking for one unknown are presented in Chapter 4. To make conversions using ratio-proportion, a proportion must be set up that expresses a numerical relationship between the two systems. A proportion may be written in colon format or as a fraction when making conversions. Regardless of the format used, there are some basic rules to follow when using this method.

Rules for Ratio-Proportion

1. State the known equivalent first (memorized equivalent).
2. Add the incomplete ratio on the other side of the equal sign, making sure the units of measurement are written in the same sequence.

Example: mg : g = mg : g

3. Label all terms in the proportion, including x (These labels are ignored when multiplying or dividing.)
4. Solve the problem by using the principles for solving ratio-proportions. (The product of the means equals the product of the extremes.)
5. The final answer for x should be labeled with the appropriate unit of measure or desired unit.

When using the method of ratio-proportion to make conversions, as with any method used, the known equivalents must be memorized. Stating the proportion in the fraction format may be a way of avoiding confusion with the terms (means and extremes). However, regardless of the format used, the terms must correspond to each other in value and have a relationship. Division should always be carried at least two decimal places to ensure accuracy.

Example: 8 mg = _____ g

Solution: State the known equivalent first, then add the incomplete ratio, making sure the units are in the same sequence. Label all the terms in the proportion, including x.

$$1{,}000 \text{ mg} : 1 \text{ g} \quad = \quad 8 \text{ mg} : x \text{ g}$$

$$\text{(known equivalent)} \qquad \text{(unknown)}$$

Read as "1,000 mg is to 1 g as 8 mg is to x g"

Note:

The terms of the proportion are the same sequence, (mg : g = mg : g), and there is a correspondence in the ratio: small : large = small : large.

Once the proportion is stated, solve it by multiplying the means (inner terms) and the extremes (outer terms).

Result:

$$\overset{\ulcorner \text{means} \urcorner}{1{,}000 \text{ mg} : 1 \text{ g} = 8 \text{ mg} : x \text{ g}}$$
$$\underset{\llcorner\text{extremes}\lrcorner}{}$$

$$1 \times 8 = 1{,}000 \times x$$

$$\frac{8}{1{,}000} = \frac{1{,}000\,x}{1{,}000}$$

$$x = \frac{8}{1{,}000}$$

Because the measure you are converting to is metric, the fraction is changed to a decimal by dividing 8 by 1,000 to obtain an answer of 0.008 g. However, because the measures are metric in this example, perhaps moving the decimal point would be the preferred method as opposed to actual division.

Example:
$$8 \text{ mg} = \underline{\hspace{1cm}} \text{ g}$$

1. Note that conversion is going from smaller to larger, thus division or moving the decimal point to the left is indicated.
2. Note that the unit is going from mg to g, thus changing by a factor of 1,000.
3. The decimal point will be moved three places to the left to complete this conversion: 8 mg = 0.008 g.

An alternate way of stating the problem illustrated in the previous example would be stating it as a fraction and cross multiplying to solve for *x*.

$$\frac{1,000 \text{ mg}}{1 \text{ g}} = \frac{8 \text{ mg}}{x \text{ g}}$$

$$\frac{1,000 \, x}{1,000} = \frac{8}{1,000}$$

$$x = 0.008 \text{ g}$$

The remainder of this chapter will show examples of the methods used in converting within the same system and between systems.

CONVERTING WITHIN THE SAME SYSTEM

Converting within the same system is often seen with metric measures; however, it can be done using the other systems of measurement, such as one apothecaries' measure being converted to an equivalent within the apothecaries' system. Any one of the methods discussed can be used, but movement of decimal points is limited to the metric system. Ratio-proportion can be used for all systems.

Example 1:   (metric)   (metric)

$$0.6 \text{ mg} = \underline{\hspace{1cm}} \text{ mcg}$$

Solution: Equivalent: 1,000 mcg = 1 mg

A milligram is larger than a microgram; the answer is obtained by moving the decimal point three places to the right (multiply).

Answer: 600 mcg

Alternative: Set up as a proportion, a fraction, or using the colon.

Example 2:   (apothecaries')   (apothecaries')

$$f\mathfrak{Z} \text{ iv} \quad = \quad m \underline{\hspace{1cm}}$$

Solution: m 60 = f℥ i
A dram is larger than a minim; the answer is obtained by multiplying 4 by 60.

Answer: m 240

Alternative: Set up as a proportion using the colon format or as a fraction.

Note:

This is an illustration of converting within the same system; drams and minims are no longer used.

Notes

Because it may be confusing to write using apothecaries' symbols when stating the proportion, it can be written as follows:

1 fluid dram : 60 minims = 4 fluid dram : x minims

or

$$\frac{1 \text{ fluid dram}}{60 \text{ minims}} = \frac{4 \text{ fluid dram}}{x \text{ minims}}$$

The principles presented for solving ratio-proportion problems are used to solve for x, when presented in colon format or fraction.

Dimensional Analysis

Dimensional analysis is a conversion method that has been used in chemistry and other sciences, and will be discussed in more detail in a later chapter. Dimensional analysis involves manipulation of units to get the desired unit. This method can be used to convert for all systems. As with other methods discussed, you must know the conversion factor (equivalent).

Steps:

1. Identify the unit you are converting to.
2. Write the conversion factor so that the desired unit is in the denominator to allow you to cancel units.
3. Cancel the unwanted units.
4. Perform the mathematic process indicated.

Example: (metric)   (metric)

0.12 kg to g

Solution: You want to cancel the kg and obtain the equivalent amount in g. Because 1 kg = 1,000 g, the fraction that will allow you to cancel kg

is: $\dfrac{1{,}000 \text{ g}}{1 \text{ kg}}$

Note: The unit you want to cancel is always written in the denominator of the

fraction. Therefore 0.12 kg $\times \dfrac{1{,}000 \text{ g}}{1 \text{ kg}} = x$ g

Cancel the units 0.12 k̶g̶ $\times \dfrac{1{,}000 \text{ g}}{1 \text{ k̶g̶}} = x$ g

0.12 $\times$ 1,000 = 120 g. 0.12 kg is equivalent to 120 g.

Answer: 120 g.

 PRACTICE PROBLEMS

21. 500 mL = _____ L   27. 6.5 L = _____ mL

22. 4 kg = _____ g   28. 60 g = _____ kg

23. 1.4 L = _____ mL   29. 600 mg = _____ g

24. ℥ vi = ℥ _____   30. 0.736 mg = _____ mcg

25. 4.5 mg = _____ mcg   31. 1,600 mL = _____ L

26. ℥ ss = ℥_____   32. 0.015 L = _____ mL

33. 0.18 g = _____ mg   35. 5.2 g = _____ kg

34. 25 mcg = _____ mg   Answers on p. 497

CONVERTING BETWEEN SYSTEMS

The methods presented previously can be used to change a measure in one system to its equivalent in another.

Example 1:   (apothecaries')   (metric)

$$\text{gr } \frac{1}{100} \quad = \quad \underline{\quad} \text{ mg}$$

Solution: Equivalent: gr 1 = 60 mg

A grain is larger than a milligram.

Multiply 1/100 by 60 to obtain 60/100.

Because the final answer is a metric measure, 60/100 is changed to a decimal by dividing 100 into 60. The fraction could also be reduced first to its lowest term (3/5) then changed to a decimal by dividing 5 into 3.

Answer: 0.6 mg

Alternative: Express the conversion in proportion format and solve for *x*.

$$\text{gr } 1 : 60 \text{ mg} = \text{gr } \frac{1}{100} : x \text{ mg}$$

$$60 \times \frac{1}{100} = x$$

$$\frac{60}{100} = x$$

$$x = 0.6 \text{ mg}$$

OR

$$\frac{\text{gr } 1}{60} \text{ mg} = \text{gr } \frac{\text{gr } 1/100}{x} \text{ mg}$$

$$x = \frac{1}{100} \times 60$$

$$x = \frac{60}{100}$$

$$x = 0.6 \text{ mg}$$

Example 2:   (apothecaries')   (metric)

$$110 \text{ lb} \quad = \quad \underline{\quad} \text{ kg}$$

Solution: Equivalent: 1 kg = 2.2 lbs

A pound is smaller than a kilogram; 110 is divided by 2.2.

Answer: 50 kg

Example 3:   (apothecaries')   (metric)

$$\text{gr } 1/10 \quad = \quad \underline{\quad} \text{ mg}$$

Solution: Here you want to cancel gr to find the equivalent amount in mg. Because gr 1 = 60 mg, the fraction you desire so you can cancel gr is:

$$\frac{60 \text{ mg}}{\text{gr } 1}$$

$$\text{Therefore gr } \frac{1}{10} \times \frac{60 \text{ mg}}{\text{gr } 1} = x \text{ mg}$$

$$\frac{1}{10} \times 60 = \frac{60}{10} = 6$$

6 mg is equivalent to gr $\frac{1}{10}$.

Answer: 6 mg

CALCULATING INTAKE AND OUTPUT

The nurse often converts between systems to calculate a client's **intake and output.** Intake and output is abbreviated **I&O.** Intake refers to the monitoring of fluid a client takes orally (p.o.), by feeding tube, or parenterally. Oral intake includes fluids and solids that become liquid at body and room temperature, such as jello and popsicles. Intake also includes water, broth, and juice. Intake does not include solids such as bread, cereal, or meats. Liquid output refers to fluids that exit the body, such as diarrhea, vomitus, gastric suction, and urine. A client's intake and output are usually recorded on a special form called an intake and output sheet (Figure 8-1), which varies from institution to institution. A variety of clients require I&O monitoring, such as those whose fluids are restricted or who are receiving diuretic or I.V. therapy.

Intake and output are recorded using cubic centimeters or milliliters. Milliliters should, however, be used for volume. When measuring output, the nurse uses a graduated receptacle calibrated in metric measures (mL and cc), and conversions are not necessary. Oral intake usually must be converted from household measures to metric measures before it can be recorded. Some agencies have cups calibrated to facilitate easy measuring and accurate recording of intake and output. Each time a client takes oral liquids, even those administered with medications, the amount and time are recorded on the appropriate form. The total intake and output are recorded at the end of each shift and also totalled for a 24-hr period.

Conversion of a client's intake is usually required when recording measurements such as a bowl or coffee cup. Each agency usually has an I&O sheet with a ledger that indicates the standard measurement for the utensils used in its facility. For example, it may indicate a standard cup is 6 oz or a coffee cup is 180 mL. A client's oral intake is calculated in the same manner as other conversion problems. After each item is converted, the items are added together for the total intake.

Example: Calculate the client's intake for breakfast in milliliters. Assume the glass holds 6 oz and the cup 8 oz. The client had the following for breakfast at 8 AM:

Items	Conversion factors
1/3 glass of apple juice	1 oz = 30 mL
2 sausages	1 pint = 500 mL
1 boiled egg	1 cup = 8 oz
1/2 cup of coffee	1 glass = 6 oz
1/2 pint of milk	

Note:

2 sausages and 1 boiled egg are not part of fluid intake. Although many institutions use cc on I&O, mL will be used in this exercise.

Juice glass	– 180 mL	Jello cup	– 150 mL
Water glass	– 210 mL	Ice cream	– 120 mL
Coffee cup	– 240 mL	Creamer	– 30 mL
Soup bowl	– 180 mL		
Small water cup	– 120 mL		

Addressograph with Client Information

Date ___October 30, 2001___

	INTAKE						OUTPUT			OTHER	
	ORAL			IV							
TIME	TYPE	AMT	TIME	TYPE	AMOUNT ABSORBED	TIME	URINE	STOOL			
8A	Juice	60 mL									
	Coffee	120 mL									
	Milk	250 mL									

Figure 8-1 Sample I&O sheet.

Solution:

1. $\frac{1}{3}$ glass of apple juice

$$1 \text{ glass} = 6 \text{ oz}; \frac{1}{3} \text{ of } 6 \text{ oz} = 2 \text{ oz}$$

Therefore 1 oz = 30 mL, 2 oz × 30 mL = 60 mL

OR 1 oz : 30 mL = 2 oz : x mL, 60 mL = x

2. $\frac{1}{2}$ cup of coffee

$$1 \text{ cup} = 8 \text{ oz}; \frac{1}{2} \text{ of } 8 \text{ oz} = 4 \text{ oz}$$

Therefore 4 oz × 30 = 120 mL

OR 1 oz : 30 mL = 4 oz : x mL, 120 mL = x

3. 1 pint of milk

$$1 \text{ pint} = 500 \text{ mL}; \frac{1}{2} \text{ of } 500 \text{ mL} = 250 \text{ mL}$$

$$\text{Total mL} = 60 \text{ mL} + 120 \text{ mL} + 250 \text{ mL} = 430 \text{ mL}$$

Another solution could have been to total the number of ounces, which in this example is 6 ounces, convert that amount to milliliters, and add the half pint of milk (expressed in milliliters).

$$1 \text{ oz} : 30 \text{ mL} = 6 \text{ oz} : x \text{ mL}$$

$$180 \text{ mL} = x$$

$$180 \text{ mL} + 250 \text{ mL} \ (\frac{1}{2} \text{ pint}) = 430 \text{ mL}$$

The conversions are recorded on an I&O sheet next to time ingested. The I&O sheet in Figure 8-1 is filled out with the data for this sample problem.

8:00 AM   juice, 60 mL
              coffee, 120 mL
              milk, 250 mL

In addition to the oral intake, if a client is receiving intravenous (I.V.) therapy the amount of I.V. fluid given is also recorded on the I&O sheet. When an I.V. bottle or bag is hung or added, the nurse indicates the time and the type and amount of fluid in the appropriate column on the I&O sheet. When the I.V. fluid has infused or the I.V. is changed, the nurse records the actual amount of fluid **infused,** or **absorbed.**

In the situation where a bag or bottle of I.V. fluid is not completed by the end of the shift, it is communicated to the oncoming nurse how much fluid is left in the bag. The amount is also indicated on the I&O with the abbreviation LIB (left in bag or bottle).

Example: The nurse hangs a 1,000 mL bag of D_5W at 7 AM. At 3 PM 150 mL is left in the bag. The nurse records 850 mL was absorbed and indicates 150 mL is LIB. Refer to the sample I&O form in Figure 8-2 showing how this example is charted.

I&O sheets usually have a place for recording p.o. intake, I.V. intake, and a column or columns for output. Figure 8-3 shows a sample 24-hr I&O sheet illustrating the charting of intake.

As discussed, output is also recorded on the I&O form. The most commonly measured output is urine. After a client's output is recorded, sometimes the nurse needs to compute an average. The most important average nurses compute in most health care settings is the hourly urine output. The **hourly** urine output for an adult **should be** 30 mL or more. Usually the hourly amount is more significant than each voiding. To find the hourly average of urinary output, take the total and divide by the number of hours.

Juice glass – 180 mL Small water cup – 120 mL
Water glass – 210 mL Jello cup – 150 mL
Coffee cup – 240 mL Ice cream – 120 mL
Soup bowl – 180 mL Creamer – 30 mL

Date: May 21, 2001

Client information

INTAKE					OUTPUT				
Time	Type	Amt	Time	IV/ blood type	Amount absorbed	Time	Urine	Stool	Other
			7A	D5W 1000 mL	850 mL				
8 hr total									
			3P	D5W 150 mL LIB					

Figure 8-2 Charting IV fluids on an I&O sheet.

Example $$\frac{400\ \text{mL/urine}}{8\ \text{hr}} = 50\ \text{mL of urine/hr}$$

Each institution varies relating to I&O charting. Always check the policies to ensure compliance with a particular institution.

Note:

This amount is above the minimum hourly average (30 mL/hr) for adequate kidney functioning.

Juice glass – 180 mL Small water
Water glass – 210 mL   cup   – 120 mL
Coffee cup – 240 mL Jello cup – 150 mL
Soup bowl   – 180 mL Ice cream – 120 mL
                      Creamer   – 30 mL

Date: May 21, 2001

Client information

INTAKE					OUTPUT				
Time	Type	Amt	Time	IV/ blood type	Amount absorbed	Time	Urine	Stool	Other
8A	juice	240 mL	7A	D5W 1000 mL	850 mL	8A	300 mL		
	milk	120 mL				10A	200 mL		
	coffee	200 mL				1³⁰/P	425 mL		
9³⁰/A	water	60 mL							
12P	broth	180 mL							
	juice	120 mL							
1P	water	120 mL							
8 hr total		1,040 mL			850 mL		925 mL		
5P	tea	100 mL	3P	D5W 150 mL LIB	150 mL	4p	425 mL		
	broth	360 mL	5P	D5W 1000 mL	750 mL	7p	350 mL		
	ice-cream	120 mL				9³⁰/P	200 mL		
9 P	water	240 mL							
8 hr total		820 mL			900 mL		975 mL		
1A	water	120 mL	11P	D5W 250 mL LIB	250 mL				
5A	tea	200 mL	3A	D5W 1000 mL	600 mL	2A	350 mL		
						5A	150 mL		
8 hr total		320 mL			850 mL		500 mL		
24 hr total		2,180 mL			2,600 mL		2,400 mL		

Total intake 24 hr: (4,780 mL)   (2,180 mL + 2,600 mL)

Total output 24 hr: (2,400 mL)

Figure 8-3   I&O sheet (completed 24 hours).

PRACTICE PROBLEMS

Convert the following to the equivalent measures indicated.

36. 60 lb = _____ kg

37. 15 mg = gr _____

38. ℥ v = _____ mL

39. gr v = _____ mg

40. ℥ vii = _____ mL

41. 250 mL = _____ qt

42. 45 mL = _____ tbs

43. gr 45 = _____ g

44. gr 1¹/₂ = _____ mg

45. 20 mL = _____ tsp

46. gr 5¹/₂ = _____ mg

47. 4 qt = _____ mL

48. 72 kg = _____ lb

49. gr $\dfrac{1}{125}$ = _____ mg

50. 2.4 L = _____ mL

Compute how much I.V. fluid you would document on an I&O form as being absorbed from a 1,000 mL bag if the following amounts are left in a bag.

51. 300 mL _____

52. 450 mL _____

53. 100 mL _____

Compute the average hourly output in the following situations (round to nearest whole number).

54. 650 mL in 8 hr _____

55. 250 mL in 8 hr _____

56. 1,000 mL in 24 hr _____

Answers on p. 497

Notes

POINTS TO REMEMBER

- Regardless of the method used for converting, **memorizing equivalents** is a necessity.
- Answers stated in fraction format should be **reduced** as necessary.
- When more than one equivalent is learned for a unit, use the **most common equivalent** for the measure or use the number that divides equally without a remainder.
- The apothecaries' system does not convert exactly to metric.
- Division should be carried out **two decimal** places to ensure accuracy, and is not rounded.
- Decimal point movement as a method for converting is limited to the metric system; ratio-proportion and dimensional analysis can be used for all systems of measure.
- Oral intake is converted before placing data on an I&O sheet. The amount is usually recorded in cc at many institutions; however, mL is the correct unit for volume.
- The most common conversions used to calculate dosages are metric.
- Always check the policy of the institution regarding I&O and the charting of it.

CHAPTER REVIEW

Convert the following to the equivalent measures indicated.

1. 0.007 g = _____ mg

2. 1 mg = _____ g

3. 6,000 g = _____ kg

4. 5 mL = _____ L

5. 0.45 L = _____ mL

6. 60 mL = ℨ _____

7. gr $\dfrac{1}{300}$ = _____ mg

8. 1 mg = gr _____

9. 12 mL = ℨ _____

10. gr ⅱ = _____ mg

11. $1\dfrac{1}{2}$ qt = _____ mL

12. 30 mg = gr _____

13. 1.6 L = _____ mL

14. 47 kg = _____ lb

15. 3 mL = _____ L

16. 75 lb = _____ kg

17. 0.008 g = _____ mg

18. $4\dfrac{1}{2}$ pt = _____ mL

19. gr $\dfrac{1}{2}$ = _____ mg

20. gr $\dfrac{1}{150}$ = _____ mg

21. 6,172 g = _____ kg

22. 200 mL = _____ tsp

23. 102 lb = _____ kg

24. 204 g = _____ kg

25. 1.5 L = _____ mL

26. 200 mcg = _____ mg

27. 48.6 L = _____ mL

28. 0.7 L = _____ mL

29. ℥ vss = _____ mL

30. 4 tsp = _____ mL

31. gr iv = _____ mg

32. 2 tbs = _____ mL

33. ℥ ii = _____ mL

34. 45 mg = gr _____

35. gr 45 = _____ g

36. ℥ xx = _____ mL

37. gr iiss = _____ mg

38. gr $\dfrac{3}{8}$ = _____ mg

39. gr x = _____ mg

40. 4 kg = _____ lb

41. 3.25 mg = _____ mcg

42. 75 mL = ℥ _____

43. gr $\dfrac{1}{120}$ = _____ mg

44. 6.653 g = _____ mg

45. 4 g = _____ mg

46. 36 mg = _____ g

47. 0.8 g = _____ mg

48. 9 g = gr _____

49. 0.5 mg = gr _____

50. 2 qt = _____ L

Calculate the fluid intake in mL. (Assume a cup holds 8 oz and a glass holds 4 oz for the following problems. Calculate the number of milliliters.)

51. Client had the following at lunch:
    4 oz fruit cocktail, 1 tunafish sandwich, 1/2 cup of tea, 1/4 pt of milk.

    Total mL = _____

52. Calculate the following individual items and give the total number of cubic milliliters:
    3 popsicles (3 oz each), 1/2 qt iced tea,1 1/2 glasses water, 12 oz soft drink

    Total mL = _____

53. Client had the following:
    8 oz milk
    6 oz orange juice
    4 oz water with medication

    Total mL = _____

54. Client had the following:
    10 ounces of coffee
    8 ounces of water
    6 ounces of broth.

    Total mL = _____

Notes

55. Client had the following:
    3/4 glass of milk
    4 oz water
    2 oz beef broth.

    Total mL = _____

Convert the following amounts of fluid to milliliters.

56. $3\frac{1}{2}$ oz = _____ mL

57. $\frac{3}{4}$ C (8 oz cup) = _____ mL

Compute how much I.V. fluid you would document on an I&O form as being absorbed from a 1000 mL bag if the following amounts are left in the bag.

58. 275 mL _____

59. 550 mL _____

60. 75 mL _____

Compute the average hourly urinary output in each of the following situations (round to nearest whole number).

61. 500 mL in 8 hr _____

62. 640 mL in 24 hr _____

63. 700 mL in 8 hr _____

Compute how much I.V. fluid you would document on an I&O form as being absorbed from a 500 mL bag if the following amounts are left in the bag.

64. 125 mL _____

65. 225 mL _____

Answers on p. 498

Additional Conversions Useful in the Health Care Setting

CONVERTING BETWEEN CELSIUS AND FAHRENHEIT

Many health care facilities use electronic temperature-taking devices that instantly convert between the two scales; however, such devices don't eliminate the need for the nurse to understand the difference between Celsius and Fahrenheit. In addition, it may be necessary for the nurse to explain to clients or families how to convert from one to the other.

Another factor is the recognition that all persons involved in client care do not have a "universal" measurement for temperature; therefore, Fahrenheit or Celsius may be used. Let's look first at some general information that will help you understand the formulas used.

Differentiating Between Celsius and Fahrenheit

To differentiate which scale is being used (Fahrenheit or Celsius), the temperature reading is followed by an *F* or *C*. *F* indicates Fahrenheit, *C* Celsius. (*Note:* Celsius was formerly known as *centigrade*.)

Example: 98° F

   36° C

Notes

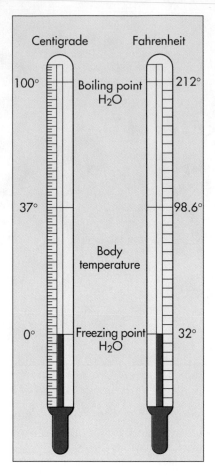

Figure 9-1 Celsius and Fahrenheit temperature scales. (From Clayton BD, Stock YN: *Basic pharmacology for nurses,* ed 12, St Louis, 2001, Mosby.)

The freezing point of water on the Fahrenheit scale is **32° F,** and the boiling point is **212° F.** The freezing point of water on the Celsius scale is **0° C,** and the boiling point is **100° C.**

The difference between the freezing and boiling points on the Fahrenheit scale is **180°,** whereas the difference between these points on the Celsius scale is **100°.**

The differences between Fahrenheit and Celsius in relation to the freezing and boiling points led to the development of appropriate conversion formulas. Figure 9-1 shows two thermometers reflecting the relationship of pertinent values between the two scales. Figure 9-2 shows medically important Celsius and Fahrenheit temperature ranges.

The **32° difference** between the freezing point on the scales is used for converting temperature from one scale to the other. There is a **180°** difference between the boiling and freezing points on the Fahrenheit thermometer and **100°** between the boiling and freezing points on the Celsius scale. These differences can be set as a ratio, 180:100. Therefore consider the following:

$$180{:}100 = \frac{180}{100} = \frac{9}{5}$$

The fraction 9/5 expressed as a decimal is 1.8; therefore, each Celsius degree **is 1.8 times** greater than each Fahrenheit degree.

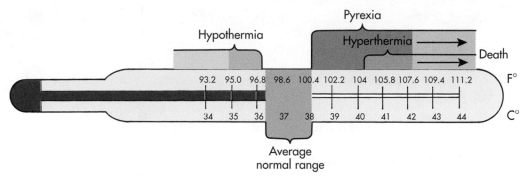

Figure 9-2 Celsius and Fahrenheit temperatures related to temperature ranges. Hypothermia—abnormal lowering of body temperature below 35° C (93° F). Pyrexia—abnormal elevation of the temperature of the body above 37° C (98.6° F); refers to fever also. Hyperthermia—Body temperature exceeds the set point. (From Elkin MK, Perry AG, and Potter PA: *Nursing interventions & clinical skills*, ed 2, St Louis, 2000, Mosby.)

FORMULAS FOR CONVERTING BETWEEN FAHRENHEIT AND CELSIUS SCALES:

▎ To convert from Celsius to Fahrenheit, multiply by 1.8 and add 32.

$$° F = 1.8(° C) + 32$$

or

$$° F = \frac{9}{5}(° C) + 32$$

Note:

Your preference between these formulas is based on whether you find it easier to work with decimals or fractions.

Example: Convert 37.5° C to ° F.

$$° F = (1.8) \times 37.5 + 32 \qquad\qquad ° F = \left(\frac{9}{5}\right) \times 37.5 + 32$$

$$° F = 67.5 + 32 \qquad \text{or} \qquad ° F = 67.5 + 32$$

$$° F = 99.5° \qquad\qquad\qquad ° F = 99.5°$$

▎ To convert from Fahrenheit to Celsius, subtract 32 and divide by 1.8.

$$° C = \frac{° F - 32}{1.8} \qquad \text{or} \qquad ° C = (° F - 32) \div \frac{9}{5}$$

Example: Convert 68° F to ° C.

$$° C = \frac{68 - 32}{1.8} \qquad\qquad ° C = (68 - 32) \div \frac{9}{5}$$

$$° C = \frac{36}{1.8} \qquad \text{or} \qquad ° C = 36 \div \frac{9}{5}$$

$$° C = (36) \times \frac{5}{9}$$

$$° C = 20° \qquad\qquad\qquad ° C = 20°$$

Note:

When converting between Fahrenheit and Celsius, if necessary carry the math process to hundredths and round to tenths.

PRACTICE PROBLEMS

Convert the following temperatures as indicated (round your answer to tenths).

1. 4° C = _____ ° F   2. 101° F = _____ ° C

Notes

3. 38.1° C = _____ ° F   5. 37.5° C = _____ ° F

4. 101.3° F = _____ ° C

Change the given temperature in the following statements to their corresponding equivalent in ° C or ° F.

6. Store medication at room temperature 20 to 25 C°. _____ ° F

7. Notify MD for temperature > (greater than) 101° F. _____ ° C

8. Store vaccine serum at 7° F. _____ ° C

9. Normal body temperature is 37° C. _____ ° F

10. Do not store IV solutions < (less than) 46° F. _____ ° C

Answers on p. 498

In addition to temperature conversions, other measures that may be encountered in the health care setting relate to linear measurement. Like temperature conversion, even though there are devices that instantly convert these measures, nurses need to understand the process. For the purpose of this chapter, we will focus on millimeters (mm) and centimeters (cm).

METRIC MEASURES RELATING TO LENGTH

In health care settings metric measures relating to length are used. Diameter of pupils of the eye may be described in mm (millimeters); the normal diameter of pupils is 3 to 7 mm. Charts may show pupillary size in mm (millimeters). Accommodation of pupils is tested by asking a client to gaze at a distant object (e.g., a far wall), and then at a test object (e.g., a finger or pencil) held by the examiner approximately 10 cm (4 in) from the bridge of the client's nose.

A baby's head and chest circumference are expressed in cm (centimeters). Gauze for dressings is available in different size squares.

Example: 10 × 10 cm (4 × 4 in). 5 × 5 cm (2 × 2 in).

Also, incisions may be expressed using measures such as cm (Box 9-1).

Now let's try some conversions using these equivalents.

Example 1: A client's incision measures 25 millimeters. How many centimeters is this?

Conversion factor: 1 cm = 10 mm

Solution: Think: mm is smaller and cm is larger. Divide by 10 or move the decimal point one place to the left.

$$25 \text{ mm} = 25 \div 10 = 2.5 \text{ cm or } 2.5 = 2.5 \text{ cm}$$

Answer: 2.5 cm

BOX 9-1 Conversions Relating to Length

1 cm = 10 mm
1 in = 2.54 cm

★The approximate conversion of 1 in = 2.5 cm is used for conversions.

Example 2:   Convert 30 centimeters to inches.
Conversion factor: 1 inch = 2.5 cm
Solution: Think smaller to larger (divide).

$$30 \text{ cm} = 30 \div 2.5 = 12 \text{ inches}$$

Answer: 12 inches

Example 3:   An infant's head circumference is 35.5 centimeters. How many millimeters is this?
Conversion factor: 1 cm = 10 mm.
Solution: Think larger to smaller (multiply). Multiply by 10 or move the decimal point one place to the right.

$$35.5 \text{ cm} = 35.5 \times 10 = 355 \text{ mm or } 35.5 = 355 \text{ mm}$$

Answer: 355 mm

 PRACTICE PROBLEMS

Convert the following to the equivalent indicated.

11. A gauze pad for a dressing is

     10 cm. _____ inches

12. A client's incision measures 45

     mm. _____ cm

13. An infant's head circumference is

     37.5 cm. _____ mm

14. A newborn is $20\frac{1}{2}$ inches long.

     _____ cm

15. 14.8 inches = _____ cm

16. 6.5 cm = _____ inches

17. 100 inches = _____ cm

18. An infant's chest circumference is

     32 cm. _____ inches

19. An infant's head circumference is

     38 cm. _____ inches

20. A newborn is 20 inches long.

     _____ cm

Answers on p. 498

Note:

In Example 2, you cannot get this answer by decimal movement. You are converting to inches, which is a household measure.

Note:

Any of the methods presented in previous chapters may be used for conversion. Remember, however, decimal movement is limited to conversions from one metric measure to another, and the number of places the decimal is moved is based on the conversion factor. If necessary, review previous chapters relating to converting.

CONVERSIONS RELATING TO WEIGHT

Body weight is essential for calculating dosages in adults, children, and, because of the immaturity of their systems, even more so in infants and neonates. This chapter will focus on converting weights for adults and children. Because medication doses in drug references are usually based on kg, it is essential to be able to convert from lb to kg. However, the nurse also needs to know how to do the opposite (kg to lb) for general knowledge, to explain it to others, and to decide if the amount of medication makes sense based on weight.

Converting lb to kg

Equivalent: 2.2 lb = 1 kg
To convert lb to kg divide by 2.2 (think smaller to larger).
The answer is rounded to the nearest tenth.

Example 1:   A child weighs 65 lb. Convert to kg.

$$65 \text{ lb} = 65 \div 2.2 = 29.54 = 29.5 \text{ kg}$$

Example 2:   An adult weighs 135 lb. Convert to kg.

$$135 \text{ lb} = 135 \div 2.2 = 61.36 = 61.4 \text{ kg}$$

 PRACTICE PROBLEMS

Convert the following weights in lb to kg (round to the nearest tenth where indicated).

21. 20 lb = _____ kg   24. 121 lb = _____ kg

22. 64 lb = _____ kg   25. 85 lb = _____ kg

23. 22 lb = _____ kg   Answers on p. 498

Converting kg to lb

Equivalent: 2.2 lb = 1 kg
To convert kg to lb, multiply by 2.2. (Think: larger to smaller.)
Answer is expressed to nearest lb.

Example 1:   A child weighs 24.1 kg. Convert to lb.

$$24.1 \text{ kg} = (24.1) \times 2.2 = 53.02 = 53 \text{ lb}$$

Example 2:   An adult weighs 72.2 kg. Convert to lb.

$$72.2 \text{ kg} = (72.2) \times 2.2 = 158.84 = 159 \text{ lb}$$

 PRACTICE PROBLEMS

Note:

Although lb is an apothecaries' measure, a decimal may be used to express weights.

Convert the following weights in kg to lb (round to the nearest lb).

26. 20 kg = _____ lb   29. 10.4 kg = _____ lb

27. 46 kg = _____ lb   30. 34.9 kg = _____ lb

28. 98.2 kg = _____ lb   Answers on p. 498

 Think Critically to Avoid Drug Calculation Errors

Although there are charts that provide instant conversions, critical thinking involves asking why or how something is derived at.

POINTS TO REMEMBER + − > =

Use these formulas to convert between Fahrenheit and Celsius temperature.

- To convert from ° C to ° F: ° F = 1.8 (° C) + 32, or $\dfrac{9}{5}$ (° C) + 32.

- To convert from ° F to ° C: ° C = $\dfrac{° F - 32}{1.8}$, or (F − 32) ÷ $\dfrac{9}{5}$.

- When converting between Fahrenheit and Celsius, carry math to hundredths and round to tenths.

Conversions Relating to Length

- Conversions can be made using any of the methods presented in the chapter on conversions; however, moving of decimals is limited to converting between metric measures.

$$1 \text{ cm} = 10 \text{ mm}$$

$$1 \text{ inch} = 2.5 \text{ cm}$$

Conversions Relating to Weight

- Weight conversion of lb to kg is done most often because many medications are based on kg of body weight.

- Body weight is **essential** for determining doses in infants and neonates.

- To convert lb to kg, divide by 2.2. Round answer to the nearest tenth.

- To convert kg to lb, multiply by 2.2. Round answer to the nearest lb.

 CHAPTER REVIEW

For each of the following statements, change the given temperature to their corresponding equivalent in ° C or ° F. (round to nearest tenth).

1. Notify physician for temperature > (greater than) 101.4° F. _____ ° C

2. Store medication at room temperature, 77° F. _____ ° C

3. Store medication within temperature range of 15° C to 30° C. _____ ° F

4. An infant has a body temperature of 36.5° C. _____ ° F

5. Store vaccine at 6° C. _____ ° F

Convert temperatures as indicated. Round your answer to the nearest tenth.

6. −10° C = _____ ° F   8. 102.8° F = _____ ° C

7. 0° F = _____ ° C   9. 29° C = _____ ° F

Notes

10. 106° C = _____ ° F   12. 39.6° C = _____ ° F

11. 70° F = _____ ° C   13. 64.4° F = _____ ° C

Convert the following to the equivalent indicated.

14. 18 inches = _____ cm   18. 3 cm = _____ mm

15. 31 cm = _____ inches   19. 7.9 cm = _____ mm

16. 44.5 cm = _____ mm   20. 4 inches = _____ cm

17. 32 inches = _____ cm

Convert the following weights in lb to kg (round to the nearest tenth where indicated).

21. 63 lb = _____ kg   24. 81 lb = _____ kg

22. 150 lb = _____ kg   25. 27 lb = _____ kg

23. 78 lb = _____ kg

Convert the following weights in kg to lb (round to the nearest lb).

26. 77.3 kg = _____ lb   29. 9 kg = _____ lb

27. 7 kg = _____ lb   30. 56.1 kg = _____ lb

28. 4.5 kg = _____ lb   Answers on pp. 498-499

UNIT THREE

Methods of Administration and Calculation

The safe and accurate administration of medications to a client is an important and primary responsibility of a nurse. Being able to read and calculate medication orders is necessary for accurate administration.

Chapter 10

Medication Administration

Chapter 11

Understanding Medication Orders

Chapter 12

Medication Administration Records

Chapter 13

Reading Medication Labels

Chapter 14

Calculating Doses Using Ratio-Proportion

Chapter 15

Dose Calculation Using the Formula Method

Medication Administration

Objectives

After reviewing this chapter, you should be able to:

1. State the six "rights" of safe medication administration
2. Identify factors that influence medication doses
3. Identify the common routes for medication administration
4. Define *critical thinking*
5. Explain the importance of critical thinking in medication administration
6. Identify important critical thinking skills necessary in medication administration
7. Discuss the importance of client teaching
8. Identify special considerations relating to the elderly and medication administration
9. Identify home care considerations in relation to medication administration

Medications are therapeutic measures for a client; however, when administered haphazardly they can cause harmful effects. When a medication error is made, it is often caused by multiple factors. Some causes of medication errors are as follows:

1. The way in which a drug is ordered
2. Errors in the mathematical calculation of doses
3. Incorrect reading of labels on medications
4. Poor labeling and/or packaging of drugs by the pharmaceutical companies (e.g., look-alike packaging, generic names that are strikingly similar)
5. Lack of knowledge concerning the medication to be administered
6. Use of improper abbreviations, incorrect expression of drug doses, or illegible and incorrect preparation of medication records
7. Failure to properly identify a client before administering medications or failure to listen to a client and to double-check when a client raises questions regarding a medication
8. Failure to educate clients properly about medications they are taking
9. Administration of medications without any thought
10. Failure to comply with required policy or procedure
11. Failure in communication, which includes incorrect reading, hearing, and documenting

The reasons for medication errors are not limited to those listed and are not nursing errors alone. The best solution for medication errors is prevention. To prevent medication errors, personnel involved in the administration of medications must perform the task properly, paying close attention to detail.

The administration of medications is more than just giving the medication ordered merely because it is what the health care provider ordered. The health care provider orders the medication, but the nurse should know the action, uses, side effects, expected response, and the range of dosage for the medication being administered. Nurses are accountable when administering medications, and must understand the activity, indications, and contraindications of the full range of medications they may be called on to administer.

Medication administration involves using the nursing process, which includes assessment, nursing diagnosis, planning, intervention, evaluation, and teaching clients about safe administration.

Note:

Failure to think about what you are doing and why you are doing it and failure to assess a client can result in errors.

CRITICAL THINKING AND MEDICATION ADMINISTRATION

There are numerous definitions for *critical thinking*. The best way to define critical thinking is as a process of thinking that includes being reasonable and rational. Thinking is based on reason. Critical thinking is important to all phases of nursing, but is particularly relevant in the discussion of medication administration.

Critical thinking encompasses several skills relevant to medication administration. One such skill is the ability to identify an organized approach to the task at hand. An example of this in medication administration involves calculating doses in an organized, systematic manner (formula, ratio-proportion) to decrease the likelihood of errors.

A second skill characteristic of critical thinking is the ability to be an autonomous thinker—for example, challenging a medication order that is written incorrectly rather than passively accepting the order. Critical thinking also involves the ability to distinguish irrelevant data from that which is relevant. For example, when reading a medication label, the nurse is able to decipher from the label the information necessary for calculating the correct dose. Critical thinking involves reasoning and the application of concepts—for example, choosing the correct type of syringe to administer a dose, and using concepts learned to decide the appropriateness of a dose. Critical thinking also involves asking for clarification of what you don't understand and not making assumptions. Clarifying a medication order and dosage indicates critical thinking. Checking the accuracy and reliability of information decreases the chance of medication errors. The ability to validate information requires a high level of thinking and decreases the chance of medication errors that could be harmful to the client.

Critical thinking is essential to the safe administration of medications. This process allows a nurse to think before doing, translate knowledge into practice, and make appropriate judgments. To safely administer medication the nurse must base decisions on rational thinking and thorough knowledge of medication administration. A nurse who administers medications in a routine manner rather than with thought and reasoning is not using critical thinking skills.

FACTORS THAT INFLUENCE DRUG DOSES AND ACTION

Several factors influence drug doses and the way they act, including the following:
1. Route of administration
2. Time of administration
3. Age of the client

4. Nutritional status of the client
5. Absorption and excretion of the drug
6. Health status of the client
7. Sex of the client
8. Ethnicity and culture of the client
9. Genetics

All of these factors affect how clients react to a medication and the dose they receive, and all must be considered when medications are prescribed and administered. Due to differences in the actions and types of drugs, clients respond in various ways, and therefore doses must be individualized. No two clients will respond to a medication in the same manner. Nurses must bear these factors in mind when administering medications. These factors can account for individuals responding differently to the same medication.

SPECIAL CONSIDERATIONS FOR THE ELDERLY

Elderly individuals can be considered high-risk drug consumers. As a person grows older there is a tendency to consume more medications. According to an article entitled "The Effect of Medication on Older Adults" by Cervantes et al in *Caring Magazine,* March 1996, "People over 65 consume four times more health care products than those under 65, and take 25% of the medications." The article also indicated that older people account for taking 30% of prescribed and 40% to 50% of over-the-counter (OTC) medications. These numbers have increased since 1996. Persons over 85 have become the most rapidly increasing portion of the population in the United States.

People are now living longer, and older people tend to use health care services more often. As with children (see Chapter 20), special consideration should be given to the client who is over 65 years of age. With the aging process come physiological changes that have a direct effect on medications and their action in the elderly individual. Aging causes the slowing down of the body's functions. Other physiological changes include a decrease in circulation, slower absorption, slower metabolism, a decrease in excretory functions, and a decrease in the ability to respond to stress such as the stress of drugs on the system. Other changes with aging include a decrease in body weight, which can affect the dose of medications, and changes in mental status, possibly due to the effects of physical illness or physiological changes in the neurological system that can occur with aging. These physiological changes can cause unexpected drug reactions and cause the elderly person to be more sensitive to the effects of many drugs. Often the elderly client is taking more than one medication at a time (the average is four or more), which causes problems such as drug interactions, severe adverse reactions, drug and food interactions, and an increase in medication errors. Many elderly persons are hospitalized each year for problems caused by medications.

As a rule the elderly client will require smaller doses of medications (as dose size increases, the number of side effects and their severity increase), and the doses should be given farther apart to prevent accumulation of drugs and toxicity. With aging, visual and hearing problems may develop. Special attention must be given when teaching clients about their medications to avoid medication errors. Develop a relationship with the client; building rapport and trust is important for the elderly. Take time and talk to the elderly, listen to what they say, and never assume they don't know how much or what medications they are taking. Ascertain that all instructions are written as clearly as possible. Make sure the client has appropriate measuring devices (for example, a measurer with calibrated lines to indicate small doses [0.2 mg, 0.4 mg, etc.] such as a dropper or measuring cup to facilitate ease and accuracy when measuring). To lessen the chance of taking too much medication or forgetting

Notes

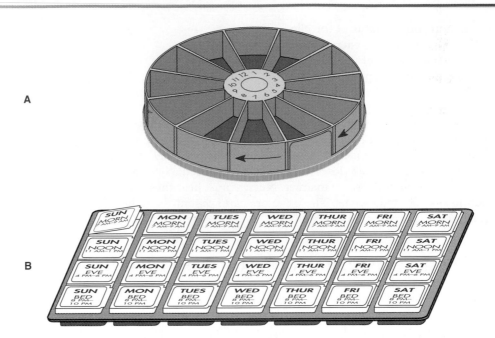

Figure 10-1 **A,** Example of a container that holds a day's medications, stored by hour of administration. **B,** Container that holds a week's medications. (**A,** Modified from Ogden SJ: *Radcliff & Ogden's calculation of drug dosages,* ed 6, St Louis, 1999, Mosby.)

a dose, try to establish specific times compatible with the client's routine for taking medications. Help the client to recognize pills by the name on the bottle, not by color. If the print on medications is too small for the client to read, encourage the use of a magnifying glass. Other measures might include a simple chart that outlines the medications to be taken, time they are to be taken, and special instructions if needed. These charts should be geared to the client's visual ability and comprehension level. Encourage the elderly client to request that childproof containers not be used; some will have difficulty opening child-resistant containers. Recommend medication aids for the client, such as special medication containers divided into separate compartments for storing daily or weekly drug doses. (Figure 10-1 shows examples of medication containers.)

In teaching elderly clients it is important to remember that the elderly are mature adults who are capable of learning; they may need and deserve additional time for learning to take place. Be patient, use simple language, and maintain the independence of the elderly as much as possible.

THE SIX RIGHTS OF MEDICATION ADMINISTRATION

When the nurse is administering medications to a client, the six rights of medication administration should serve as guidelines. Failure to achieve any of these "rights" constitutes a medication error. The six rights (Box 10-1) should be checked before administering any medication to avoid errors and to ensure client safety.

1. **The right drug**—When medications are ordered, the nurse should compare them with the written order. When administering medications, the nurse should check the label on the medication container against the Medication Administration Record (MAR) or medication ticket. Medications should be checked three times: before pouring, after pouring, and before replacing the container. With unit doses (each drug dose is prepared in the prescribed dose, packaged, labeled, and ready to use), the label should still be checked three times.

BOX 10-1

THE SIX RIGHTS
1. The right drug
2. The right dose
3. The right client
4. The right route
5. The right time
6. The right documentation

2. **The right dose**—Always perform and check calculations carefully, without ignoring decimal points. Have someone else double-check a dose that causes concern. In some agencies certain medication doses are always checked by another nurse (for example, insulin and heparin). After doses are calculated, they should be given using standard measuring devices such as calibrated medicine droppers and cups.

3. **The right client**—Always make sure you are administering medications to the right client. Ask for the client's name, and check the client's identification bracelet against the MAR. If a client does not have an identification bracelet, obtain one; secure the help of a staff member in establishing proper identification. Never go by room number or last name only.

4. **The right route**—Medications should be given by the correct route (for example, orally or by injection). The route of the medication should be stated on the order. Do not assume which route is appropriate.

5. **The right time**—Drugs should be given at the correct time of day and interval (for example, three times a day [t.i.d.] or every 6 hr [q6h]). Judgment should be used as to when medications should be given or not given. If several medications are ordered, set priorities and administer medications that must act at a certain time. For example, insulin should be given at an exact time before meals. The right time should also include the right time sequence! For example a client maybe on a diuretic b.i.d. and the institution may have b.i.d. as 9:00 AM and 9:00 PM. The nurse will need to know that the diuretic should be given in the late afternoon, so the individual is not up to the bathroom all night. This requires critical thinking. The nurse must know if a time schedule can be altered or requires judgment in determining the proper time to be administered.

6. **The right documentation**—Correct documentation is referred to as the sixth right of medication administration. Medications should be charted accurately as soon as they are given—on the right client's medication record, under the right date, and next to the right time. If a medication is refused, it should be documented as such with a notation on the medication record or in the nurse's notes. Never chart a medication as given before administering it or without documentation as to why it was not given. Follow the policy of the institution when documenting. All documentation should be legible.

In addition to the six rights of medications, a **client has the right to refuse medications.** When this occurs the nurse needs to document the refusal correctly and make appropriate persons aware of the refusal. The right to refuse may be denied to the client who has a mental illness. A client deemed to be dangerous to self or others can be taken to court and mandated to take medication. While the client does have the right to refuse medication or treatment, the law referred to as "Kendra's Law" in New York state may provide some exception to a client's right to refuse treatment (e.g., medication). Kendra's Law is legislation designed to protect the public and individuals living with mental illness by ensuring that potentially dangerous mentally ill outpatients are safely and effectively treated.

Notes

Kendra's Law is court-ordered assisted outpatient treatment (AOT). It authorizes the courts to issue orders that would require mentally ill persons, who are unlikely to survive safely in the community without supervision, to accept medications and other needed mental health services. In other words, if a client is in the community and noncompliant with the treatment regimen (e.g., medication), the client can be petitioned to court by an individual (e.g., spouse, parent, adult roommate). The judge can then mandate the client to take medication if he or she is of danger to self or others.

It is important to realize however that although there is a right to refuse, during an emergency situation, if danger is imminent, the client can be forcibly medicated by order of the judge.

Nurses should always be aware of the state laws, policies, and procedures for their jurisdiction relative to the administration of medications to refusing clients. It is extremely important for nurses to check frequently for side-effects relating to medications and to listen carefully to client complaints. The reason for the refusal of medications should be carefully analyzed and documented in all cases. Education of the client and a reassuring therapeutic relationship can assist in diminishing a client's refusal.

Another important right has to do with educating the client. **All clients have a right to be educated regarding the medication they are taking.**

TEACHING THE CLIENT

One of the most important nursing functions is teaching the client. Teaching clients about their medications is imperative in preventing errors and improving the quality of health care. Educating clients regarding medications plays a role in preventing adverse reactions and achieving adherence to prescribed therapy; taking the correct dose of the right medication at the right time helps prevent problems with medication administration. Remember, clients cannot be expected to follow a medication regimen—taking the correct dose of the right medication at the right time—if they haven't been taught. Not knowing what to do results in noncompliance, inaccurate dosages, and other problems. Nurses are in a unique position to teach the client, and this has been a traditional activity of nursing practice. Teaching should begin in the hospital and be a major part of discharge planning because, once discharged, clients need to have been educated about their medications to continue taking them safely and correctly at home. With today's emphasis on outpatient treatment and early discharge, thorough client education regarding medications is necessary.

When the nurse is teaching clients, it is important to thoroughly assess the clients' needs. Determine what the client knows about the medication prescribed, how to take the medication, and the frequency, time, and dose. Identify the client's learning needs, including literacy level and language most easily and clearly understood. Identify relevant ethnic, cultural, and socioeconomic factors that may influence medication use; consider factors such as age and physical capabilities. A variety of teaching techniques may have to be used to facilitate and enhance learning. Return demonstrations on proper use of medication equipment and reading doses, in addition to repeated instructions and directions, may be necessary, especially regarding management at home.

What a client needs to know about a medication varies with that drug. There may be numerous pieces of information clients should learn regarding their medications. The items discussed here relate particularly to dose administration. To ensure that the client takes the right medication in the right dose, by the right route at the right time, client education should include the following:

• Both the brand and generic names of the drug or drugs they are taking.
• Clear explanation of the amount of the drug to be taken (for example, one tablet or 1/2 tablet).

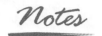

- Clear explanation of when to take the drug. (Prepare a chart created with the client's lifestyle in mind. For example, if the medications is to be taken with meals, perhaps the chart can indicate the client's mealtime and the medication scheduled accordingly.)
- Clear demonstration of measuring oral doses such as liquids. (Encourage the use of measuring devices.)
- Clear explanation of the route of administration (for example, place under tongue).

Although nurses cannot ensure clients will act on or retain everything they are taught, we are responsible for providing information to the client that will prevent error-prone situations and enable safe drug administration. Nurses need to evaluate retention, provide follow-up, and, if necessary, find alternative ways of dealing with a client who has a "no way" attitude.

HOME CARE CONSIDERATIONS

Home health nursing has become a large part of the health care delivery system and continues to grow. This is due to factors such as the promotion of cost-effective health care and early discharge. Home care nursing may involve many activities, such as providing treatments, dressing changes, hospice care, client/family teaching, and medication administration. Medication administration involves administration of medications in various ways (for example, I.V., p.o., and injection). With the increased movement of nursing into the home of the client, which is not a controlled setting, this has some important nursing implications. Home health nursing increases the autonomy of practice. The nurse must conduct a thorough assessment, communicate effectively, problem solve, and use expert critical thinking skills. Thinking must be rational, reasonable, and based on knowledge.

The principles regarding medication administration are the same as in a structured setting (for example, hospital, acute care facility, or nursing home). It is imperative that the client be well educated about safe administration. Depending on the client's condition, home nursing services may be provided on a scheduled or intermittent basis to monitor the status of a client. Not all clients have a health aide, family member, or continuous nursing services in the home (around the clock). It is essential that the nurse calculate medication administration in a systematic, organized manner and adhere to the six rights of medication administration. The sixth right—documentation—is even more essential in home health care. Documentation of medications is not just for legal purposes, but plays a significant role in cost reimbursement and payments. Correct interpretation of medication orders and validation are imperative. Proper education of the client concerning the medication, dose, and route of administration is crucial in order for the client to manage in the home environment. Some may look at it as "the client being totally at your mercy." Clients depend on the nurse to provide direction for them to ensure safe home administration. The nurse has to be able to teach the client to use appropriate utensils for measuring doses and determining the accuracy of the dose. When possible, encourage clients to use devices that are readily available in many drug stores, such as calibrated oral syringes or plastic cups with measurements. Use of these devices can help avoid errors that often occur when clients measure their medication in home utensils. (As discussed in the chapters on systems of measure, the nurse has to be able to convert doses between the various systems.) The nurse providing services to the client in the home has to be innovative and knowledgeable and demonstrate excellent critical thinking skills.

ROUTES OF MEDICATION ADMINISTRATION

Route refers to how a drug is administered. Medications come in a number of forms for administration.

Oral (p.o.)

Oral medication is administered by mouth (for example, tablets, capsules, and liquid solutions). Some medications are sublingual (placed under the tongue) or buccal (placed against the cheek).

Parenteral

This is medication administered by a route other than by mouth or gastrointestinal tract. Parenteral routes include intravenous (I.V.), intramuscular (I.M.), subcutaneous (s.c.), and intradermal (I.D.)

Insertion

Medication is placed into a body cavity, where the medication dissolves at body temperature (for example, suppositories). Vaginal medications, creams, and tablets may also be inserted using special applicators provided by the manufacturer.

Instillation

Medication is introduced in liquid form into a body cavity. It can also include placing an ointment into a body cavity, such as erythromycin eye ointment, which is placed in the conjunctiva of the eye. Nose drops and ear drops are also instillation medications.

Inhalation

Medication is administered into the respiratory tract, via for example, nebulizers used by clients for asthma. Bronchodilators and corticosteroids may be administered by inhalation through the mouth using an aerosolized, pressurized metered dose inhaler (MDI). In some institutions these medications are administered to the client by special equipment, such as positive pressure breathing equipment or the aerosol mask. Other drugs in inhalation form include pentamidine, which is used to treat *Pneumocystis carinii,* a type of pneumonia found in acquired immunodeficiency syndrome (AIDS) clients. Devices such as "spacers" or "extenders" have been designed for use with inhalers to allow all of the metered dose to be inhaled, particularly in clients who have difficulty using inhalers.

Topical

The medication is applied to the external surface of the skin. They can be in the form of lotions, ointments, or pastes.

Percutaneous.   The application of medications to the skin or mucous membranes for absorption. This includes ointments, powders, or lotions for the skin, instillation of solutions onto the mucous membranes of the mouth, ear, nose, or vagina, and inhalation of aerosolized liquids for absorption through the lungs. The primary advantage is the action of the drug, in general, is localized to the site of application.

Transdermal.   Transdermal medication, which is becoming more popular, is contained in a patch or disk and applied topically. The medication is slowly released and absorbed through the skin and enters the systemic circulation. These topical applications may be applied for 24 hours or as long as 7 days and have systemic effects. Examples include nitroglycerin for chest pain, Nicoderm for stopping smoking, and clonidine for hypertension.

Forms of oral medications (tablets, capsules), oral solutions, and routes for parenteral medications will be discussed in more detail in later chapters.

EQUIPMENT USED FOR DOSE CALCULATION

Medicine cup

Equipment used for oral administration includes a 30-mL or 1-oz medication cup made of plastic, used to measure most liquid medications. The cup has measurements in all three systems of measure (Figure 10-2). By looking at the medicine cup you can see that 30 mL = 1 oz, 5 mL = 1 tsp, and so forth. Remember any volume less than 1 tsp (5 mL) should be measured with a more accurate device, such as a syringe.

Soufflé cup

This is a small paper or plastic cup used for solid forms of medication such as tablets and capsules (Figure 10-3).

Calibrated dropper

This may be used to administer small amounts of medication to an adult or child (Figure 10-4). It is usually marked in milliliters. The size of the drops varies and depends on the dropper. Because the size of drops varies it is important to remember that drops should not be used as a medication measure unless the dropper is calibrated. Droppers used for the administration of eye, nose, and ear medication are designed for that purpose. Certain medications come with a dropper calibrated according to the medication. Examples include children's vitamins and nystatin oral solutions. The calibration allows for accurate dosing, which can be difficult with small doses unless there is an exact measuring device. Use the calibrated dropper with the medicine it is designed for only.

Oral syringe

This may be used to administer liquid medications orally to adults and children. No needle is attached (Figure 10-5).

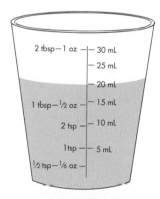

Figure 10-2 Medicine cup. (Modified from Brown M, Mulholland JL: *Drug calculations: process and problems for clinical practice*, ed 6, St Louis, 2000, Mosby.)

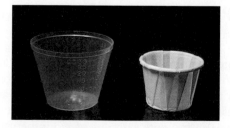

Figure 10-3 Soufflé cup. (Courtesy of Chuck Dresner. From Clayton BD, Stock YN: *Basic pharmacology for nurses*, ed 12, St Louis, 2001, Mosby.)

Notes

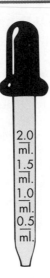

Figure 10-4   Medicine dropper. (From Clayton BD, Stock YN: *Basic pharmacology for nurses,* ed 12, St Louis, 2001, Mosby.)

 Think Critically to Avoid Drug Calculation Errors

Be safe. THINK! Droppers are accurate when used to measure the specific medication they are designed for but not for measuring other medications. Using a dropper for the wrong medication could result in a serious medication error.

Parenteral syringe

This type of syringe is used for I.M., s.c., I.D., and I.V. drugs. These syringes come in various sizes and are marked in mL and units. Some syringes, however, show cubic centimeters as well as minims. It is important to note that many institutions are now ordering syringes that are marked in mL and have no minim markings. Minims are considered inaccurate and their use is discouraged. The specific types of syringes are discussed in more detail in Chapter 17. The barrel of the syringe holds the medication and has calibrations on it. The needle is attached to the tip. The plunger pushes the medication out (Figure 10-6). The size of the needle depends on how the medication is given (for example, s.c. or I.M.), the viscosity of the drug, and the size of the client. See Figure 10-7 for samples of the types of syringes.

EQUIPMENT FOR ADMINISTERING ORAL MEDICATIONS TO A CHILD

Various types of calibrated equipment are on the market for administering medications to children. Most of the available equipment is for oral use. Caregivers should be instructed to always use a calibrated device when administering medications to a child. Household spoons vary in size and are not reliable devices for accurate dosing. Figure 10-8 presents samples of equipment used to administer oral medications to a child.

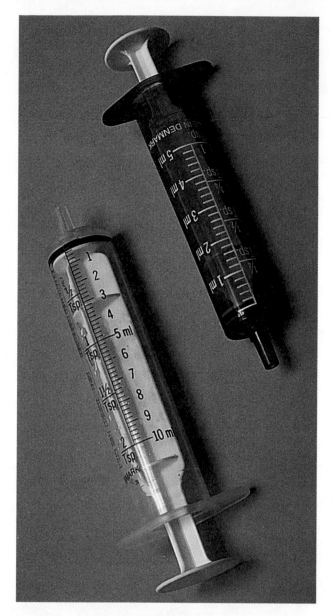

Figure 10-5 Oral syringes. (Courtesy of Chuck Dresner. From Clayton BD, Stock YN: *Basic pharmacology for nurses,* ed 12, St Louis, 2001, Mosby.)

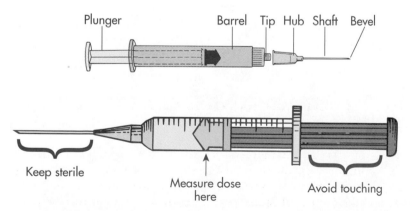

Figure 10-6 Parts of a syringe. (From Potter PA, Perry AG: *Fundamentals of nursing,* ed 5, St Louis, 2001, Mosby.)

Figure 10-7 Types of syringes. **A,** 3-mL syringe. **B,** 1-mL tuberculin syringe (From Potter PA, Perry AG: *Fundamentals of nursing,* ed 5, St Louis, 2001, Mosby.)

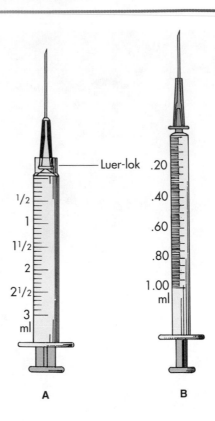

Figure 10-8 **A,** Acceptable devices for measuring and administering oral medication to children (*clockwise*): measuring spoon, plastic syringes, calibrated nipple, plastic medicine cup, calibrated dropper; hollow-handled medicine spoon. **B,** Devices acceptable only for administering premeasured oral medication (clockwise): household teaspoons, paper cups, nipple, uncalibrated dropper. (From Wong DL et al: *Whaley and Wong's nursing care of infants and children,* ed 6, St Louis, 1999, Mosby.)

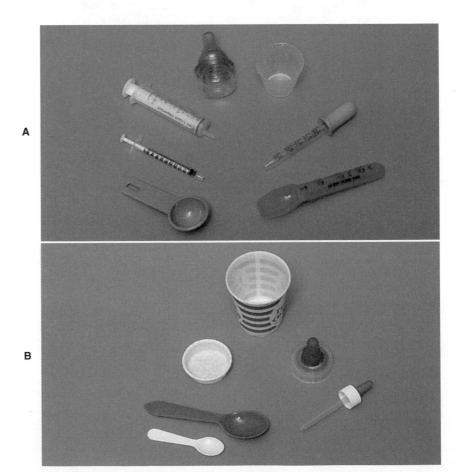

PRACTICE PROBLEMS

Answer the following questions by filling in the correct word or words to complete the sentence.

1. A medicine cup has _____, _____,

   and _____ measures on it.

2. The_____ and _____
   need special considerations regarding medication doses.

3. _____ refers to the way in which a drug is
   administered.

4. Children and the elderly usually require _____
   doses.

5. A _____ cup is used for dispensing solid forms of medication.

6. Application of medication to the external surface of the skin is referred to as

   _____ route.

7. Medication administration is a process that requires critical thinking and the
   nursing process, which includes

   (1) _____ ,

   (2) _____ ,

   (3) _____ ,

   (4) _____ ,

   (5) _____ , and

   (6) _____ .

8. Being an autonomous thinker is an example of _____

   _____ .

9. _____ droppers should be used for medication
   administration.

10. When medications are placed next to the cheek, they are administered by

    the _____ route.

    Answers on p. 499

Notes

POINTS TO REMEMBER

- The six rights of medication administration serve as guidelines for nurses when administering medications. (The right drug, dose, client, route, time, and documentation). Other rights include the right to refuse and the right to be educated.
- Medication administration includes using critical thinking and the nursing process.
- The elderly and children require special considerations with medication administration.
- Home health nursing provides an increase in the autonomy of nursing practice.
- A calibrated dropper should be used when administering medications with a dropper.
- Doses less than a teaspoon should be measured with a device such as a syringe.
- A medication cup has the capacity of 30 mL. A soufflé cup is used to dispense solid forms of medications.
- Medications are administered by various routes.

CHAPTER REVIEW

1. Name the six rights of medication administration

   Right _____

   Right _____

   Right _____

   Right _____

   Right _____

   Right _____

2. Two ways of administering medications to the right client are the following:

   a) _____

   b) _____

3. A medication label should be read _____ times.

4. Medications should be charted _____ you have administered them.

5. The routes of medication administration are _____

   _____ .

   (Name three.)

6. The medicine cup has a _____ capacity.

7. Droppers are calibrated to administer standardized drops regardless of what type of dropper is used. True or false?

8. The syringe used to administer a dose by mouth is referred to as an

   _____ .

9. Volume on a syringe is indicated by _____ .

10. The medicine cup indicates that 2 tablespoons are approximately

    _____ mL.

Answers on p. 499

Chapter 11

Understanding Medication Orders

Objectives

After reviewing this chapter, you should be able to:

1. Identify the components of a medication order
2. Identify the meanings of standard abbreviations used in medication administration
3. Interpret a given medication order

Before a nurse can administer any medication, there must be a written legal order for the medication. Medication orders can be written by physicians, dentists, physician's assistants, midwives, or nurse practitioners, depending on state law. Health care providers use medication orders to communicate to the nurse or designated health care worker which medication or medications to administer to a client. The terms *medication orders* and *doctor's orders* are used interchangeably. Medication orders can be verbal or written. Verbal orders should be taken only in emergencies. In most institutions the verbal order must contain the same things as the written order. For example, the date of the order, name and dosage of the medication, route, frequency, and any special instructions are recorded. The order has to be placed on the doctor's order sheet and repeated back to the doctor for verification. It must be noted that it was a verbal or telephone order and the signature of the nurse taking the order is required. Many institutions have instituted a policy that the order must be signed within 24 hours. Some institutions may require that medication orders written by persons other than a doctor be countersigned by designated personnel. It is important to be familiar with specific policies regarding medication orders because they vary according to the institution or health care facility.

The medication order indicates the drug treatment plan or medication the health care provider has ordered for a client. After a medication order has been written, the nurse is responsible for transcribing the order. This means the order is written on the **MAR** (Medication Administration Record) or entered into a computer system and communicated to the hospital pharmacy. Once the medication is received on the unit, the medication order is implemented and the client receives the drug. Before transcribing an order or preparing a dose, the nurse must be familiar with reading and interpreting an order. To interpret a medication order the nurse must be knowledgeable in the components of a medication order and the standard abbreviations and symbols used in writing a medication order. The nurse therefore must memorize the abbreviations and symbols commonly used in medication orders. The abbreviations include units of measure, route, and frequency for the medication ordered. The common abbreviations and symbols used in medication administration are listed in Tables 11-1 and 11-2.

In writing medication orders, some health care providers may use capital letters, others may use lower case letters; some may place a period after an abbreviation or symbol, others do not. These variations often reflect writing styles.

 Think Critically to Avoid Drug Calculation Errors

It is important for you to concentrate on understanding what abbreviations or symbols mean in the context of the order.

Some abbreviations may be capitalized to indicate different meanings. For example: o.d. lower case letters means once a day, every day; OD in capital letters indicates right eye.

WRITING A MEDICATION ORDER

The health care provider writes a medication order in a special book for doctor's orders or on a form called the *doctor's order sheet* in the client's chart or hospital record. Doctor's order sheets vary from institution to institution. The order sheet should have the client's name on it. A prescription blank is used to write medication orders for clients who are being discharged from the hospital or are seeing the doctor in an outpatient facility. Nurses often have to explain these orders to clients so they understand the dosages they will be taking.

COMPONENTS OF A MEDICATION ORDER

When a medication order is written, it must contain the following seven important parts or it is considered invalid or incomplete.

TABLE 11-1   Symbols and Abbreviations for Units of Measure Used in Medication Administration

Abbreviation/Symbol	Meaning	Abbreviation/Symbol	Meaning
c	cup	oz, ʒ̄	ounce
cc	cubic centimter	pt	pint
dr, ʒ	dram	qt	quart
g	gram	T, tbs	tablespoon
gr	grain	t, tsp	teaspoon
gtt	drop	U†	unit
IU	international unit	/	per
kg	kilogram	<	less than
L	liter	>	more than
m	minim	≅	approximately
mcg	microgram	↑	increase
mEq*	milliequivalent	↓	decrease
mg	milligram	Δ	change
mL	milliliter	+/−, ±	plus or minus
MU	milliunits		

*mEq (milliequivalent) is a drug measure in which electrolytes are measured; it expresses the ionic activity of a drug.
†U (Unit) is a basic quantity used to indicate strength of medication; it is unique for each drug. It is recommended that the abbreviation *U* not be used when writing an order; write out the word *units*.

TABLE 11-2 Commonly Used Medication Abbreviations

Abbreviation	Meaning	Abbreviation	Meaning
ā	before	OS	left eye
aa, āā	of each	OU	both eyes
a.c.	before meals	p̄	after
A.D., AD	right ear	p.c.	after meals
ad.lib.	as desired, freely	per	through or by
amp	ampule	per os, p.o.	by or through mouth
aq	aqueous, water	p.r.	by rectum
A.S., AS	left ear	p.r.n.	when necessary/ required
A.U., AU	both ears		
b.i.d., bid	twice a day	q.	every, each
b.i.w.	twice a week	q.a.m.	every morning
c̄	with	q.d., qd	every day, once a day
c	cup	q.h., qh	every hour
cap, caps	capsule	q2h, q4h, q6h, q8h, q12h	every two hours, every four hours, every six hours, every eight hours, every twelve hours
CD	controlled dose		
CR	controlled release		
d.c., D/C	discontinue		
dil.	dilute		
DS	double strength	qhs, q.h.s.	every night at bedtime
EC	enteric coated	q.i.d., qid	four times a day
elix.	elixir	q.n.	every night
fl, fld.	fluid	q.o.d., qod	every other day
gt, GT	gastrostomy tube	q.s.	a sufficient amount/as much as needed
gtt	drop		
h, hr	hour	r	right
h.s.	hour of sleep, at bedtime	rect	rectum
		s̄	without
I.D.	intradermal	s̄s̄, ss	one half
I.M.	intramuscular	s.c., S.C., s.q.	subcutaneous
I.V.	intravenous	sl, SL	sublingual
IVPB	intravenous piggyback	sol, soln	solution
IVSS	intravenous soluset	s.o.s.	once if necessary
kvo	keep vein open (a very slow infusion rate)	SR	sustained release
		S&S	swish and swallow
L	left	stat, STAT	immediately, at once
LA	long-acting	supp	suppository
LOS	length of stay	susp	suspension
min	minute	syp, syr	syrup
mix	mixture	tab	tablet
NGT, ng	nasogastric tube	t.i.d., tid	three times a day
noc, noct	at night	t.i.w.	three times a week
n.p.o., NPO	nothing by mouth	tr., tinct	tincture
NS, N/S	normal saline	ung., oint	ointment
o.d., od*	once a day	vag, v	vaginally
OD	right eye	XL	long acting
o.n.	every night	XR	extended release
os	mouth		

Note:

Abbreviations may be written with or without the use of periods; this does not alter the meaning.

*Abbreviation od is still used at some institutions to indicate frequency of medication. (Use of abbreviation is regional.)

Client's Full Name

This avoids confusion of the client with another, thereby preventing error in administering the wrong medication to the wrong client. Many institutions use a nameplate to imprint the client's name and record number on the order sheet. In institutions that use computers, the computer screen may also show identifying information for the client, such as age and known drug allergies.

Date and Time the Order Was Written

This includes the month, day, year, and the time the order was written. This will help in determining the start and stop of the medication order. In many institutions the health care provider (or person legally authorized to write a medication order) is required to include the length of time the medication is to be given (for example, 7 days) or he may use the abbreviation LOS (length of stay), which means the client is to receive the medication during the entire stay in the hospital. Even when not written as part of the order, LOS is implied unless stated otherwise. In some institutions there are automatic cutoff times for certain medications even if not specified (for example, 5 to 7 days for a specific antibiotic).

Note: A record of the time the order was written is preferred in many institutions, but omission does not invalidate the order.

Name of the Medication

The medication may be ordered by the generic or brand name (Figures 11-1 and 11-2). To avoid confusion with another medication, the medication should be written clearly and spelled correctly.

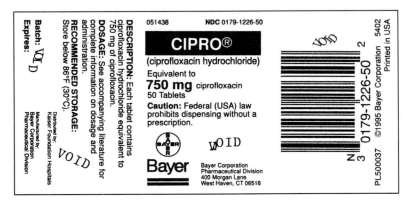

Figure 11-1   Cipro label. Notice two names. The first, *Cipro*, is the trade name, identified by the registration symbol ®. The name in smaller and different print is *ciproflaxacin hydrochloride*, the generic or official name.

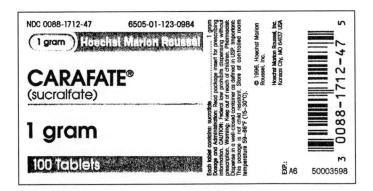

Figure 11-2   Carafate label. Notice the two names. The first, *Carafate*, is the trade name, identified by the registration symbol ®. The name in smaller and different print is *sucralfate*, the generic or official name.

generic name—the proper name, or chemical compound. It is usually designated in lower case letters or a different typeface. Occasionally only the generic name will appear on the label. Each medication has only one generic name.

trade name—the brand name, or the name under which a manufacturer markets the drug. This is usually designated by capital letters and indicated first on a drug label. The trade name is followed by the registration symbol, ®. A drug may have several trade names, based on the manufacturer.

Checking the name of medications even when generic is essential in preventing error. Some very different drugs have similar generic names, such as Mestonin (pyridostigmine bromide), which is used in clients with myasthenia gravis, and Daraprim (pyrimethamine), used to treat parasitic disorders such as toxoplasmosis.

To ensure correct drug identification nurses should cross-check trade and generic names as needed. When reading the name of a medication, never assume. Sometimes orders may be written abbreviating drug names. This has been discouraged unless the abbreviation is common and approved.

I A case of mistaken identity can have tragic results.

For example, achronym AZT may be used. AZT 100 mg p.o. (intended drug order zidovudine [Retrovir] 100 mg, which is used for HIV), can be misunderstood as azathioprine (Imuran), an immunosuppressant.

Dose of the Medication

The amount and strength of the medication should be written clearly to avoid confusion. Dose indicates the amount you are giving at a single time.

To avoid misinterpretation many institutions require that the abbreviation "U," which stands for units, not be used when writing insulin orders, but rather to write out the word. Errors have occurred due to the confusion of "U" with an "O" in a hand written order.

Example: 60 s.c. stat of Humulin Regular. The U is almost completely closed and could be misread as 60 units. The Institute for Safe Medication Practices has recommended that the word *units* be written in full. The hand written letters "q.d.," when used in prescription writing, can be misinterpreted as "q.i.d" if the period is raised and the tail of "q" interferes. Example: Lasix 40 mg *q'd*.

Route of Administration

This is a very important part of a medication order, because medications can be administered by several routes. Never assume that you know which route is appropriate. Standard abbreviations should be used to indicate the route.

Examples: p.o. (oral, by mouth)

I.D. (intradermal)

I.M. (intramuscular)

I.V. (intravenous)

Administering a drug by a route other than what the form indicates, regardless of the source of an error, if you administer the wrong dose, or give a medication by a route other than it is intended for, you are legally responsible for it.

Time and/Frequency of Administration

Standard abbreviations should be used to indicate the times a medication is to be given.

Notes

Example: q.i.d (four times a day), stat (immediately)

The time intervals at which a medication is administered are determined by the institution, and most health care facilities have routine times for administering medications.

Example: t.i.d (three times a day) may be 9 AM, 1 PM, and 5 PM, or 10 AM, 2 PM, and 6 PM.

Factors such as the purpose of the drug, drug interactions, absorption of the drug, and side effects should be considered when scheduling medication times. It is important to realize that when abbreviations such as b.i.d. and t.i.d. are used, the amount you calculate is for one dose, and not for the day's total. The frequency is indicating the dose (amount) of medication given at a single time.

Signature of the Person Writing the Order

For a medication order to be legal it must be signed by the health care provider. The health care provider writing the order must include his or her signature on the order, and it should be legible. In some institutions, depending on the rank of the doctor or the person writing the order, an order may have to be cosigned by a senior doctor.

Example: Residents or interns and persons other than a doctor writing an order must secure the signature of an attending physician.

In addition to the seven required components of a medication order already discussed, any special instructions for certain medications need to be clearly written.

Examples: 1. Hold if blood pressure (B/P) is below 100 systolic.
   2. Administer a half hour before meals (1/2 hour a.c.).

Medications ordered as needed or whenever necessary (p.r.n.) should indicate the purpose of administration as well.

Example: 1. For chest pain
   2. Temperature above 101° F (T↑ 101° F)
   3. For blood pressure greater than 140 systolic and 90 diastolic. (For B/P > 140 systolic and 90 diastolic).

In instances where specific instructions are not stated, nursing judgment must be used to determine whether it is appropriate to administer a medication.

For dose calculations the nurse is usually concerned with the drug name, dose of the drug, route, and time or frequency of administration. This information is necessary in determining a safe and reasonable dosage for a client.

INTERPRETING A MEDICATION ORDER

Medication orders are written in the following order:
   1. Name of the drug
   2. The dose, expressed in standard abbreviations or symbols
   3. Route
   4. Frequency

Example:

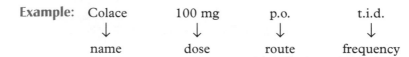

Colace	100 mg	p.o.	t.i.d.
↓	↓	↓	↓
name	dose	route	frequency

Notes

This order means the health care provider wants the client to receive Colace (name of drug), which is a stool softener, 100 milligrams (dose) by mouth (route), three times a day (frequency). The use of abbreviations in a medication order is a form of shorthand. When interpreting orders it is important to commit to memory the abbreviations as well as abbreviations related to the systems of measure. Refer to Tables 11-1 and 11-2 for medical abbreviations and symbols used commonly in medication administration. Be systematic when interpreting the order to avoid an error. In other words, because the drug order follows a specific sequence when written correctly (the name of the drug first, followed by the dose, route, and frequency), interpret the order in this manner as well; avoid "scrambling the order."

Depending on the policy of the institution, the nurse or trained personnel such as the unit secretary (ward clerk) transcribes the medication order to the appropriate MAR or ticket. In facilities where personnel other than the nurse transcribe orders, the nurse is still responsible for double-checking and cosigning the order, indicating it has been correctly transcribed.

Orders are transcribed in institutions where the unit dose is used. In some institutions more transcribing may be necessary because the MAR may have the capacity to be used for only a 5-day period. It is therefore necessary to transcribe orders again at the end of the designated time period.

In facilities that use computers, the medication order is placed into the computer and a printout lists the currently ordered medication.

The use of the computer in some institutions allows the prescriber to enter the order, thus eliminating the need for nurses to transcribe orders. Through the use of computers, the medication order can be transmitted quickly to the pharmacy for rapid filling of the order. In most institutions the computer is able to scan for information such as drug incompatibilities, safe dose ranges, recommended administration times, and allergies, and it can indicate when a new order for a medication is required.

The charting of medications administered is also done directly into the computer at some institutions, whereas at others, charting is done on a computerized printout. Computerized charting does not eliminate the responsibility of the nurse to double-check medication orders.

POINTS TO REMEMBER

- A primary responsibility of the nurse is the safe administration of medications to a client.

- Interpret the order systematically, the way in which it is written.

- The seven components of a medication order are as follows:
  1. The full name of the client
  2. Date and time the order was written
  3. Name of the medication to be administered
  4. Dose of the medication
  5. Route of administration
  6. Time or frequency of administration
  7. Signature of the person writing the order.

- All medication orders must be legible and use standard abbreviations and symbols.

- If any of the seven components of a medication order are missing or seem incorrect, don't assume—clarify the order!

PRACTICE PROBLEMS

Interpret the following abbreviations.

1. q.d. _____

2. pc _____

3. AD _____

4. h _____

5. q12h _____

Interpret the following orders. Use *administer* or *give* at the beginning of the sentence.

6. Zidovudine 200 mg p.o. q4h. _____

   _____

7. Procaine Penicillin G 400,000 U I.V. q8h._____

   _____

8. Gentamycin Sulfate 45 mg IVPB, q12h. _____

   _____

9. Regular Humulin insulin 5 U s.c., a.c. and h.s._____

   _____

10. Vitamn B$_{12}$ 1,000 mcg I.M., q.o.d. _____

    _____

11. Prilosec 20 mg p.o. bid._____

    _____

12. Tofranil 75 mg p.o. h.s. _____

    _____

13. Restoril 30 mg p.o. h.s. _____

    _____

14. Mylanta 1 oz p.o. q4h p.r.n. _____

    _____

15. Synthroid 200 mcg p.o. q.d._____

    _____

Answers on p. 499

✓ CHAPTER REVIEW

Notes

List the seven components of a medication order.

1. _____   5. _____

2. _____   6. _____

3. _____   7. _____

4. _____

Write the meaning of the following abbreviations.

8. b.i.d. _____   16. h.s. _____

9. OU _____   17. o.d. _____

10. ad.lib. _____   18. elix. _____

11. s.c. _____   19. OS _____

12. c̄ _____   20. syr _____

13. a.c. _____   21. n.p.o. _____

14. q.i.d. _____   22. sl _____

15. b.i.w. _____

Give the abbreviations for the following.

23. after meals _____   31. immediately _____

24. three times a day _____   32. right eye _____

25. intramuscular _____   33. ointment _____

26. every eight hours _____   34. one half _____

27. suppository _____   35. milliequivalents _____

28. intravenous _____   36. every night at bedtime _____

29. once if necessary _____   37. by rectum _____

30. without _____

Interpret the following orders. Use *administer* or *give* at the beginning of the sentence.

38. Methergine 0.2 mg p.o. q4h × 6 doses. _____

_____

39. Digoxin 0.125 mg p.o. o.d. _____

_____

40. Regular Humulin insulin 14 U. s.c. q.d. 7:30 A.M. _____

_____

41. Demerol 50 mg I.M. and atropine gr 1/150 I.M. on call to the operating

room. _____

42. Ampicillin 500 mg p.o. stat, and then 250 mg p.o. q.i.d. thereafter. _____

_____

43. Lasix 40 mg I.M. stat. _____

_____

44. Librium 50 mg p.o. q4h p.r.n. for agitation. _____

_____

45. Potassium chloride 20 mEq I.V. $\times$ 2 L. _____

_____

46. Tylenol gr x p.o. q4h p.r.n. for pain. _____

_____

47. Mylicon 80 mg p.o. pc and hs. _____

_____

48. Folic acid 1 mg p.o. o.d. _____

_____

49. Nembutal 100 mg p.o. h.s. p.r.n. _____

_____

50. Aspirin gr x p.o. q4h p.r.n. for temperature $>101°$ F. _____

_____

51. Dilantin 100 mg p.o. t.i.d. _____

_____

52. Minipress 2 mg p.o. b.i.d.; hold for systolic b/p (blood pressure) <120. ___

_____

53. Compazine 10 mg I.M. q4h p.r.n. for nausea and vomiting. _____

_____

54. Ampicillin 1 g I.V.P.B. q6h × 4 doses. _____

_____

55. Heparin 5,000 U. s.c. q12h. _____

_____

56. Dilantin susp 200 mg per NGT q a.m. and 300 mg per NGT h.s. _____

_____

57. Benadryl 50 mg p.o. stat. _____

_____

58. Vitamin B$_{12}$ 1,000 mcg IM t.i.w. _____

_____

59. Milk of magnesia 1 oz p.o. h.s. p.r.n. for constipation. _____

_____

60. Septra DS tab 1 p.o. qd. _____

_____

61. Neomycin ophthalmic ointment 1% OD tid. _____

_____

62. Carafate 1 g via NGT qid. _____

_____

63. Morphine sulfate 15 mg s.c. stat and 10 mg s.c. q4h p.r.n. for pain. _____

_____

64. Ampicillin 120 mg IVSS q6h × 7 days. _____

_____

65. Prednisone 10 mg po qod. _____

_____

Notes

Identify the missing part from the following medication orders. Assume the date, time, and signature are included on the orders.

66. Dicloxacillin 250 mg q.i.d. _____

67. Synthroid 0.05 mg p.o. _____

68. Nitrofurantoin p.o. q6h × 10 days. _____

69. 25 mg p.o. q12h, hold if B/P <100 systolic. _____

70. Solu-Cortef 100 q6h. _____

Answers on pp. 500-501

Chapter 12

Medication Administration Records

Objectives

After reviewing this chapter, you should be able to:

1. Identify the necessary information that must be transcribed to a MAR
2. Read a MAR and identify medications that are given on a routine basis, including the name of the medication, the dose, the route of administration, and the time of administration
3. Transcribe medication orders to a MAR (Medication Administration Record)

The medication record system is the most widely used system for drug administration. The medication record is a way of keeping track of medications a client has received and is currently receiving. The name of each medication, as well as the dose, route, and frequency, is written on the client's medication record. A complete schedule is written out for all the administration times for medications given on a continuous or routine basis. Each time a dose is given the nurse initials the record next to the time. In some institutions separate records are maintained for routine, I.V., and p.r.n. medications, and for medications administered on a one-time basis, whereas in others these are kept on the same record in a designated area. The medication record system is the same as the Medication Administration Record (MAR).

For medication records and charting, some institutions use a Kardex, a MAR, or a combination of both. Other institutions use a computerized system in which medication-charting information is entered into the computer, which automatically generates a list of all the medications to be given and the times.

After a doctor's order has been verified, the order is transcribed to the official record used at the institution. Some institutions attach the actual medication order to the MAR, thereby eliminating the need for written transcription.

The various medication forms used at different institutions represent differences in form only; essential information is common to all.

Notes

ESSENTIAL INFORMATION ON A MEDICATION RECORD

All of the information on the mediation record must be legible and transcribed carefully to avoid a medication error. In addition to client information, the following information is necessary on all medication forms:

1. **Dates.** This information usually includes the date the order was written and the date the medication is to be started (if different from the order date).
2. **Medication Information.** This includes the drug's full name, the dose, the route, and the frequency. Abbreviations used on the medication record should be standard abbreviations.
3. **Time of Administration.** This will be based on the desired administration schedule stated on the order, such as "t.i.d." The desired administration time is placed on the medication record and converted to time periods based on the institution's time intervals for scheduled or routine medications. (Thus t.i.d. may mean 9 AM, 1 PM, and 5 PM at one institution and 10 AM, 2 PM, and 6 PM at another.) A nurse should always become familiar with the hours for medication administration designated by a specific institution. Medication times for p.r.n. and one-time doses are recorded at the time they are administered.
4. **Initials.** Most medication records have a place for the initials of the person transcribing the medication to the MAR and the person administering the medication. The initials are then written under the signature section to identify who gave the medication. Some forms may request the title as well as the signature of the nurse (Figures 12-1 and 12-2).
5. **Special Instructions.** Any special instructions relating to a medication should be indicated on the medication record. For example, "Hold if blood pressure <100 systolic" or "p.r.n. for pain."

In addition to this information, some medication records may include legends, as well as an area for charting to indicate when a medication is omitted or a dose is not given. See Figure 12-2 for a legend of omitted doses. Other medication records may have an area where the nurse can document the reason for omission of a medication directly on the medication record (see Figure 12-1). Other information may include injection codes so the nurse may indicate the injection site for parenteral medications (see Figure 12-2). In cases where there are no injection codes indicated it is still expected that the nurse indicate the injection site. Space may also be allotted for charting information such as pulse and blood pressure if this information is relevant to the medication.

DOCUMENTATION OF MEDICATIONS ADMINISTERED

Medication records include an area for documenting medications administered. After administering the medication, the nurse or other qualified personnel must sign his or her initials next to the time the drug was given. For scheduled medications, a complete schedule is written out, and the initials are recorded next to each given time. With one-time doses and p.r.n. medication, *the time of administration* is written and again initialed by the person administering it. The medication form has a place for the full name of each person administering medications, along with the identifying initials. This allows for immediate identification of the person's initials if necessary. When medications are not administered, some records have notations, such as an asterisk (*), a circle, or a number corresponding to a legend on the medication administration record, to indicate this, or there may be an area on the back or at the bottom of the MAR for charting medications not given (see Figure 12-1). The type of notation used will depend on the institution. In addition to notations made on the medication record, most institutions require documentation in the nurse's notes.

THE JACK D. WEILER
HOSPITAL OF THE ALBERT EINSTEIN
COLLEGE OF MEDICINE
BRONX, NEW YORK 10461

A DIVISION OF MONTEFIORE MEDICAL CENTER

*Addressograph with
Client Identification*

ADDRESSOGRAPH

MEDICATION ADMINISTRATION RECORD

START DATE 4/2/01

STOP DATE _____

MEDICATION ORDER RENEWAL POLICY

All medication orders and orders for I.V. solutions shall have a maximum effective duration of fourteen (14) days except as noted below. These orders shall be automatically cancelled unless renewed in writing. To allow for continuity of administration, the last dose of a drug will be the morning dose following the day of automatic expiration.

The following are exceptions to the above:

	Duration
• Schedule II drugs administered at specific times	72 hours
• Schedule II drugs when a treatment duration is specified	7 days
• Schedule III, IV and V drugs administered at specific times	7 days
• PRN orders for all controlled drugs	72 hours
• Anticoagulants	24 hours
• Anticoagulants when a treatment duration is specified	14 days
• Antineoplastic drugs	24 hours
• Antineoplastic drugs when a treatment duration is specified	7 days
• Antibiotics	10 days
• Parenteral nutrition	4 days

Figure 12-1 MAR for practice exercise 1. (Used with permission from Montefiore Medical Center, Jack D. Weiler Hospital of the Albert Einstein College of Medicine Division, Bronx, New York.)

Continued

WEILER HOSPITAL BRONX, NEW YORK 10461		MEDICATION ADMINISTRATION RECORD	

			T I M E	DATE 4|2|01	DATE 4|3|01
ALLERGY:	☒ NONE			INIT.	INIT.
MEDICATION Keflex	Addressograph with Client Identification		10A	DG	JN
DOSE / ROUTE 250 mg po			2p	DG	JN
FREQUENCY / DURATION q.id x 7 days.			6p	NN	NN
SPECIAL INSTRUCTIONS			10p	NN	NN
PRACTITIONER'S SIGNATURE Sarah Jenkins MD DATE/TIME 4|2|01 8⁵⁰ (A.M.) P.M.					
M.D. COUNTER SIGNATURE DATE/TIME A.M. P.M.					
NOTED BY Deborah C gray RN DATE/TIME 4|2|01 9⁰⁰ (A.M.) P.M. ①					
MEDICATION M V I	Addressograph with Client Identification		10A	DG	JN
DOSE / ROUTE 1 tab po					
FREQUENCY / DURATION QD					
SPECIAL INSTRUCTIONS					
PRACTITIONER'S SIGNATURE Sarah Jenkins MD DATE/TIME 4|2|01 8⁵⁰ (A.M.) P.M.					
M.D. COUNTER SIGNATURE DATE/TIME A.M. P.M.					
NOTED BY Deborah C. gray RN DATE/TIME 4|2|01 9⁰⁰ (A.M.) P.M. ②					
MEDICATION Colace	Addressograph with Client Identification		10A	DG	JN
DOSE / ROUTE 100mg po			6p	NN	NN
FREQUENCY / DURATION bid					
SPECIAL INSTRUCTIONS					
PRACTITIONER'S SIGNATURE Sarah Jenkins MD DATE/TIME 4|2|01 8⁵⁰ (A.M.) P.M.					
M.D. COUNTER SIGNATURE DATE/TIME A.M. P.M.					
NOTED BY Deborah C. gray RN DATE/TIME 4|2|01 9⁰⁰ (A.M.) P.M. ③					
④ ATTACH ORIGINAL HERE					
⑤ ATTACH ORIGINAL HERE					

Note:

MVI =
multi-
vitamin

Figure 12-1, cont'd   MAR for practice exercise 1. (Used with permission from Montefiore Medical Center, Jack D. Weiler Hospital of the Albert Einstein College of Medicine Division, Bronx, New York.)

MEDICATION ADMINISTRATION RECORD

SIGNATURE	INIT.	TITLE	SIGNATURE	INIT.	TITLE
Deborah C. gray	DG	RN			
Nancy Nurse	NN	RN			
Jane Nightingale	JN	RN			

DATE	TIME	MEDICATION	REASON HELD	INIT.	TITLE	DATE	TIME	MEDICATION	REASON HELD	INIT.	TITLE

Figure 12-1, cont'd MAR for practice exercise 1. (Used with permission from Montefiore Medical Center, Jack D. Weiler Hospital of the Albert Einstein College of Medicine Division, Bronx, New York.)

EXPLANATION OF MEDICATION ADMINISTRATION RECORDS

A wide variety of medication records are used, and they vary from institution to institution. However, despite the variety, medication records contain essential information that is common to all and to their purpose. The MAR is used to determine what medications are ordered, the dose, route, and when each is to be given. The MAR is also verified with the doctor's orders. Any MAR requiring transcription of orders should always be checked against the doctor's orders. In institutions where personnel other than the nurse transcribe orders, the nurse should double-

ST. BARNABAS HOSPITAL
BRONX, NY 10457
DEPARTMENT OF NURSING
MEDICATION ADMINISTRATION RECORD

DIAGNOSIS: CHF

ALLERGIC TO: Aspirin   DATE: 5/1/01

Addressograph or printed label with client identification.

LEGEND
Omitted doses (use red pen):
Document in Medication Omission Record
1. NPO   3. I.V. Out   5. Other
2. Off-Unit   4. Pt. Refused

PAGE _____ OF _____

ORDER DATE / EXP. DATE	STANDING MEDICATIONS — MED-DOSE-FREQ-ROUTE	DATE 2001 HOUR	5/1 INIT.	5/2 INIT.	5/3 INIT.	5/4 INIT.	5/5 INIT.	5/6 INIT.	5/7 INIT.	5/8 INIT.	5/9 INIT.
NN 5/1/01 R.N. INIT. — 6/1/01	Vasotec 5mg po daily. hold fu SBP <100	9A / Blp	NN / 130/80								
NN 5/1/01 R.N. INIT. — 6/1/01	Colace 100mg p.o. tid	9A / 1P / 5P	NN								
NN 5/1/01 R.N. INIT. — 6/1/01	Digoxin 0.125mg p.o. daily	9A / AP	NN / 78								
NN 5/1/01 R.N. INIT. — 6/1/01	Lasix 20mg po. daily hold fu SBP <100	9A / Blp.	NN / 130/80								
NN 5/1/01 R.N. INIT. — 5/3/01	Benadryl 25mg po. hs x 3 nights	(9p)	JD								
			①	②	③						

INJECTION CODES:
RT = RIGHT THIGH   RA = RIGHT ARM   LU = LEFT UPPER GLUTEAL   ↑ RAB = UPPER RIGHT ABDOMEN   ↑ LAB = UPPER LEFT ABDOMEN
LT = LEFT THIGH   LA = LEFT ARM   RU = RIGHT UPPER GLUTEAL   ↓ RAB = LOWER RIGHT ABDOMEN   ↓ LAB = LOWER LEFT ABDOMEN

Figure 12-2   MAR showing transcription of medication orders to a medication administration record. (Used with permission of St. Barnabas Hospital, Bronx, New York.)

ST. BARNABAS HOSPITAL
BRONX, NY 10457
DEPARTMENT OF NURSING
MEDICATION ADMINISTRATION RECORD

DIAGNOSIS:

ALLERGIC TO:	DATE:

Addkerograph or printed label with client identification.

ORDER DATE / EXP. DATE	REORDER DATE / EXP. DATE	P.R.N. MEDICATION MED-DOSE-FREQ-ROUTE		DOSES GIVEN
R.N. INIT.			DATE	
			TIME	
			SITE	
REORD INIT.			INIT.	
R.N. INIT.			DATE	
			TIME	
			SITE	
REORD INIT.			INIT.	
R.N. INIT.			DATE	
			TIME	
			SITE	
REORD INIT.			INIT.	
R.N. INIT.			DATE	
			TIME	
			SITE	
REORD INIT.			INIT.	
R.N. INIT.			DATE	
			TIME	
			SITE	
REORD INIT.			INIT.	

INITIAL IDENTIFICATION

INITIAL	PRINT NAME, TITLE	INITIAL	PRINT NAME, TITLE	INITIAL	PRINT NAME, TITLE
1 NN	Nancy News RN	5		9	
2		6		10	
3		7		11	
4		8		12	

Figure 12-2, cont'd (Used with permission of St. Barnabas Hospital, Bronx, New York.)

Notes

check the transcription to make sure there are no discrepancies. Regardless of the variation in format for MARs, the information common to all is:

a) The name of the client
b) Medication (the dose, route)
c) Time/frequency desired for administration
d) A place to indicate allergies
e) A place for date, the initials of the person who administers the medication, and a section to identify the initials of the person administering the medication

Samples of the various MARs are included in this chapter. As you look at the sample records, it is important to locate and identify the information common to all with focus on medications that are given on a continuous basis.

Regardless of the type of MAR, when the drug orders are transcribed to a MAR, the nurse uses the record to check the drug order, prepare the correct dose, and record the drug administered.

COMPUTERIZED MEDICATION RECORDS

Similar to other businesses, the use of computers in health care facilities is increasing. There are various ways that computers may be used in nursing. Many health care facilities are using computers to process drug orders. In some institutions that use a computerized system, orders of the "prescriber" are either electronically transmitted or manually entered into the system along with all other essential information relating to the client, such as allergies. The computerized medication record can be viewed at the computer or from a computer printout. The institution generates its own medication record, following a specific format. The use of computers has become an essential tool for medication administration at some institutions. Through the use of computers, orders can be quickly transmitted and filled by the pharmacy. At some institutions the computer can retrieve information relating to medications, such as the range of dosage and recommended administration times, which increases the importance of computers to the safe administration of medication. It is important to note that the use of computers in reference to medication administration times varies from one institution to the next.

Computer Controlled Dispensing System

This system (Figure 12-3) is gaining increased popularity in many institutions and health care facilities. The computer controlled dispensing system is supplied by the pharmacy daily with stock medications. Controlled drugs are also kept in the cart and the system provides a detailed record relating to the controlled substances used, and by whom. The drug order is received by the pharmacy for the client and then entered into the system. To access medications in this system, the nurse uses a security code and password.

UNIT DOSE SYSTEM

Many institutions have adopted a system of medication administration referred to as *unit dose*. This system has decreased medication preparation time because the medications are prepared daily in the pharmacy and sent to the unit. The type of medication forms used for this system varies from one institution to another. In some instances this system has decreased the amount of transcription of orders. In other institutions, however, transcription of medication orders to the MAR is still required. The doctor's orders are therefore written

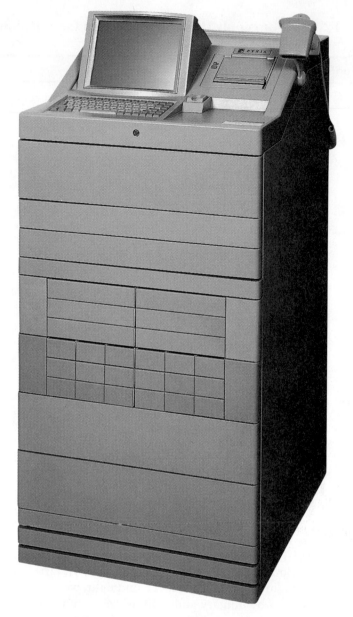

Figure 12-3 Electronic dispensing system—the Pyxis system. (From Clayton BD, Stock YN: *Basic pharmacology for nurses,* ed 12, St Louis, 2001, Mosby.)

on a separate order sheet. Figure 12-2 illustrates the transcription of orders to the MAR.

At some institutions the original prescriber's order is attached to the left side of the medication record, eliminating the need for transcription. Copies of the order remain in the client's chart, and one is sent to the pharmacy.

SCHEDULING MEDICATION TIMES

Many health care facilities have routine schedules for administering medications, which vary from one institution to another. Common abbreviations are used when scheduling and prescribing medications. As previously mentioned in this chapter,

Note:

Times vary according to the institution.

TABLE 12-1 **Commonly Used Abbreviations for Scheduling Medications**

Abbreviation	Meaning
a.c.*	before meals
b.i.d	twice a day
h.s.	at bedtime (hour of sleep)
o.d.	once a day
p.c.*	after meals
p.r.n.	as needed (when necessary/required)
q.d.	once a day/everyday
q.h.	every hour
q2h, q3h, q4h	every two hours, three hours, four hours
q6h, q8h, q12h, q24h	six hours, eight hours, twelve hours, and twenty-four hours
q.i.d.	four times a day
q.o.d.	every other day
stat	immediately (at once)
t.i.d.	three times a day

*Based on meal times.

the nurse must become familiar with the administration schedule used at a specific institution. Table 12-1 shows some examples of commonly used abbreviations in relation to scheduling of medications.

MILITARY TIME

Military time (international time) is a 24-hour clock. The main advantage of using military time is it helps prevent errors because numbers are not repeated. The times 7 AM and 7 PM may look very similar if the A and P are not clear. In military time the colon and AM and PM are omitted. Military hours starts at 1 AM, or 0100 in the morning, and ends at 12 midnight, which is 0000 or 2400. 0000 is commonly used by military and read as "zero hundred" Although still referred to as military time, a more accurate term is "computer time." The reason for using the 24-hour clock in computers was that computers could not understand AM and PM.

Many health care facilities are using military time in documentation such as nursing notes and on medication administration records. Military times are being increasingly used as opposed to traditional time (ante meridiem [AM] and post meridiem [PM]).

Rules for Conversion to Military Time (Computer Time)

▎ To convert AM time: omit the colon and AM.

Example: 8:45 AM = 0845

To convert PM time omit the colon and PM; add 1200 to time.

Example: 7:50 PM = 750 + 1200 = 1950

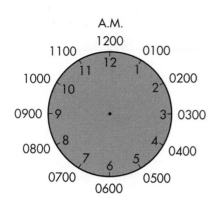

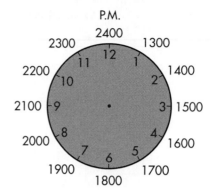

Rules for Converting to Traditional Time

❙ To convert AM time: insert the colon and AM.

Example: 0845 = 8:45 AM

❙ To convert PM time: subtract 1200, insert colon and pm.

Example: 1950 = 1950 − 1200 = 7:50 PM

PRACTICE PROBLEMS

Convert the following to military time.

1. 7:30 AM _____   4. 5:45 PM _____

2. 10:30 AM _____   5. 12:16 AM _____

3. 8:10 PM _____

Convert the following military times to traditional time.

6. 0207 _____   8. 0004 _____

7. 1743 _____   Answers on p. 501

PRACTICE EXERCISE 1

Using the MAR in Figure 12-1, list the medication, dosage, route, and time for the medications given by DG (Deborah C. Gray) on 4/2/01 and by NN (Nancy Nurse) on 4/3/01.

Date

4/2/01	Medication	Dosage	Route	Time
1.	_____	_____	_____	_____
2.	_____	_____	_____	_____

Notes

3. _____   _____   _____   _____

4. _____   _____   _____   _____

**Date
4/3/01   Medication   Dosage   Route   Time**

1. _____   _____   _____   _____

2. _____   _____   _____   _____

3. _____   _____   _____   _____

Answers on p. 501

POINTS TO REMEMBER

- The system used for medication administration plays a role in determining the type of medication record used and whether transcription of orders is necessary.

- Regardless of the type of medication record used at an institution, the nurse should know the data that is essential for the medication record and understand the importance of the accuracy and clarity of medication orders.

- Persons transcribing orders should transcribe them in ink and write legibly to avoid medication errors. All essential notations or instructions should be clearly written on the medication record.

- Documentation of medications administered should be done accurately and only by the person administering them.

- To avoid errors in administration, always check transcribed orders against the prescriber's orders.

- Military time is also referred to as international time. A more accurate term is "computer time."

- To change traditional AM time to military time, omit colon and AM.

- To change traditional PM time to military time omit colon, PM, and add 1200 to time.

- To convert military time to traditional AM time, insert colon and add AM.

- To convert military time to traditional PM time, subtract 1200, insert the colon and PM.

 CHAPTER REVIEW

Convert the following military times to traditional times.

1. 0032 = _____   4. 1345 = _____

2. 0220 = _____   5. 2122 = _____

3. 1650 = _____

Convert the following traditional times to military times.

6. 5:20 AM = _____   9. 4:30 PM = _____

7. 12:00 midnight = _____   10. 1:35 PM = _____

8. 12:05 AM = _____

State whether AM or PM is represented by the following times.

11. 0154 _____

12. 1450 _____

13. If a client had an IV therapy for 8 hours, ending at 1100, when on the 24 hour clock was the IV started? _____

14. Who determines the medication administration times? _____

15. Do b.i.d. and q2h have the same meaning? _____

Explain. _____

Answers on p. 501

 CHAPTER REVIEW EXERCISE 1

Transcribe the following orders to the practice medication sheet (Figure 12-4). When you have completed this, place your initials and signature in the appropriate space on the medication form. Use the times indicated and the date 4/9/01. Indicate client has no known drug allergies (NKDA). Diagnosis: pancreatitis.

1. Norvasc 5 mg p.o. daily, hold for SBP < 100 (9A), expiration date 5/9/01. Leave space for recording B/P.

2. Thiamine 100 mg p.o. daily (9A), expiration 5/9/01.

3. Heparin 5,000 units s.c. q12h 9A, site, 9P, site, expiration 4/16/01.

4. $FeSO_4$ 325 mg p.o. t.i.d. (9A, 1P, 5P), expiration 5/9/01.

Answers on p. 502

 CHAPTER REVIEW EXERCISE 2

Use Figure 12-5 PRN Medication Record for orders 5 and 6. Date ordered 4/10/01. Be sure to include order, date, and expiration date. Use the same client information provided in Exercise 1.

5. Percocet 2 tabs p.o. q4h p.r.n. for pain × 3 days. Chart that you administered it on 4/10/01 at 2 PM (start date 4/10/01, expiration date 4/13/01).

6. Tylenol 650 mg p.o. q4h p.r.n. temp > 101° F. Start date 4/10/01, expiration date 4/17/01.

Answers on p. 503

Note:

Be sure to include order date, expiration date, and complete the initial identification portion on the MAR, and place title as RN.

ST. BARNABAS HOSPITAL

BRONX, NY 10457

DEPARTMENT OF NURSING
MEDICATION ADMINISTRATION RECORD

DIAGNOSIS:

ALLERGIC TO: DATE:

LEGEND
Omitted doses (use red pen):
Document in Medication Omission Record

1. NPO	3. I.V. Out	5. Other
2. Off-Unit	4. Pt. Refused

PAGE _____ OF _____

A Addressograph or printed label
B with client identification.

ORDER DATE / EXP. DATE	STANDING MEDICATIONS MED-DOSE-FREQ-ROUTE	DATE / HOUR	INIT.	INIT.	INIT.	INIT.	INIT.	INIT.	INIT.	INIT.	INIT.
R.N. INIT.											
R.N. INIT.											
R.N. INIT.											
R.N. INIT.											
R.N. INIT.											

INJECTION CODES:

RT = RIGHT THIGH	RA = RIGHT ARM	LU = LEFT UPPER GLUTEAL	↑ RAB = UPPER RIGHT ABDOMEN	↑ LAB = UPPER LEFT ABDOMEN
LT = LEFT THIGH	LA = LEFT ARM	RU = RIGHT UPPER GLUTEAL	↓ RAB = LOWER RIGHT ABDOMEN	↓ LAB = LOWER LEFT ABDOMEN

Figure 12-4 MAR for Chapter Review exercise 1. (Used with permission of St. Barnabas Hospital, Bronx, New York.)

ST. BARNABAS HOSPITAL

BRONX, NY 10457

DEPARTMENT OF NURSING

MEDICATION ADMINISTRATION RECORD

DIAGNOSIS:

ALLERGIC TO: DATE:

Addressograph or printed label with client identification.

ORDER DATE	REORDER DATE	P.R.N. MEDICATION		
EXP. DATE	EXP. DATE	MED-DOSE-FREQ-ROUTE	DOSES GIVEN	

R.N. INIT.			DATE	
			TIME	
			SITE	
REORD INIT.			INIT.	
R.N. INIT.			DATE	
			TIME	
			SITE	
REORD INIT.			INIT.	
R.N. INIT.			DATE	
			TIME	
			SITE	
REORD INIT.			INIT.	
R.N. INIT.			DATE	
			TIME	
			SITE	
REORD INIT.			INIT.	
R.N. INIT.			DATE	
			TIME	
			SITE	
REORD INIT.			INIT.	

INITIAL IDENTIFICATION

INITIAL	PRINT NAME, TITLE		INITIAL	PRINT NAME, TITLE		INITIAL	PRINT NAME, TITLE
1		5			9		
2		6			10		
3		7			11		
4		8			12		

Figure 12-5   MAR for Chapter Review exercises 1 and 2. (Used with permission of St. Barnabas Hospital, Bronx, New York.)

Chapter 13

Reading Medication Labels

Objectives

After reviewing this chapter, you should be able to:

1. Identify the trade and generic names of medications
2. Identify the dose strength of medications
3. Identify the form in which a medication is supplied
4. Identify the total volume of a medication container where indicated
5. Identify directions for mixing or preparing a drug where necessary

To administer medications safely to a client, nurses must be able to read and interpret the information on a medication label. Medication labels indicate the dose contained in the package. It is important to read the label carefully and recognize essential information.

READING MEDICATION LABELS

The nurse should be able to recognize the following information on a medication label.

Generic Name

This is a name given by the manufacturer that first develops the medication. Medications have only one generic name. Doctors are ordering medications more often by the generic name, so nurses need to know the generic name as well as the trade name. Pharmacists in many institutions are dispensing medications by generic name to decrease costs. Sometimes only the generic name may appear on a medication label or package. This is common for drugs that have been used for many years and are well known and do not require marketing under a different trade name.

Examples include morphine, phenobarbital, and atropine (Figure 13-1). Another example of a drug commonly used in the clinical setting and often seen with only the generic name on the label is Demerol. Demerol is the trade or brand name, however, it is often seen with the generic name only (meperidine). Figure

13-2 shows Demerol labels with various strengths. Note that only meperidine is indicated on the label.

> It is important for the nurse to cross check all medications, whether just the generic name or both the trade and generic names are indicated on the label, to accurately identify a drug. Failure to cross check medications could lead to choosing the wrong medication, a violation of the rights of medication administration (the "right" medication).

Remember, even drugs with similar names may have markedly different chemical structures and actions. For example, hydroxyzine (Vistaril), which is an anti-anxiety medication, and hydralazine (Apresoline), which is used to treat hypertension.

Notice that on both labels shown in Figures 13-1 and 13-2 the acronym *USP* appears after the name of the drug. USP is the acronym for United States Pharmacopoeia, which is one of the two official national listing of drugs. The other is the National Formulary, N.F. You will see these initials on drug labels.

Trade Name

The trade name is also referred to as the *brand name* or *proprietary name;* it is the manufacturer's name for the drug. Notice the brand name is very prominent on the label, and the first letter is capitalized. It is important to remember that dif-

Note:

It is important to avoid confusing these official listings with other initials or abbreviations on a drug label, which may serve to identify additional drugs or specific actions of or reactions to a drug.

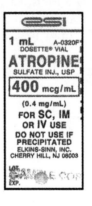

Figure 13-1 Atropine label.

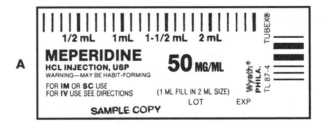

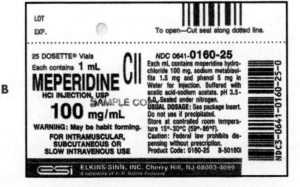

Figure 13-2 **A,** Meperidine 50 mg/mL. **B,** Meperidine 100 mg/mL.

ferent manufacturers may market a drug under different trade names. The trade name is followed by an ®, which is the registration symbol. Some medications may have the abbreviation ™ after the trade name, which stands for trademark. See Figures 13-3 and 13-4 for the labels for Epivir Oral Solution, manufactured by Glaxo Wellcome Inc., and Corvert, manufactured by the Upjohn Company.

Notice the ™ after the names *Epivir* and *Corvert*. The trade name is the name given to the drug by the manufacturer and therefore cannot be used by any other company. The drug name is a trademark for that company. Once the Patent and Trademark Office formally registers the trademark, the symbol ® then appears on the medication label.

Figure 13-5 shows the label for Zocor. Zocor is a trade name identified by the ® registration symbol. The name underneath in smaller print, Simvastatin is the generic or official name of the drug.

Dose Strength

This refers to the weight or amount of the medication per unit of measure (the weight per tablet, capsule, milliliter, etc.).

Examples: In solution the medication may be stated as 80 mg/2 mL (80 mg in 2 mL), whereas in solid form (tablets, capsules) it may be stated as 50 mg/tablet (50 mg in 1 tablet) or 250 mg/capsule (250 mg in 1 capsule).

Dose strength can be expressed in different systems of measure. Some labels may state the dose strength in apothecary and metric measures (e.g., nitroglycerin). Some oral liquids may state household measures (e.g., each 15 mL [tablespoon] contains 80 mg).

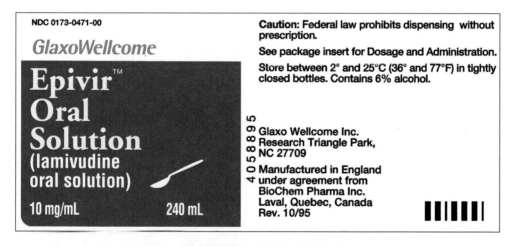

Figure 13-3 Epivir label.

⚠ Think Critically to Avoid Errors in Administration

Always read a drug label carefully to avoid errors. Drug names can be deceptively similar. Similarity in name doesn't mean the same action. For example, *Inderal* and *Inderide* are similar names, but the action and the contents of the medications are different. Inderal delivers a certain dose of propranolol hydrochloride; Inderide combines two antihypertensive agents (propranolol hydrochloride and hydrochlorothiazide, a diuretic-antihypertensive).

Notes

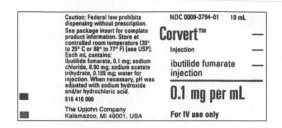

Figure 13-4 Corvert label.

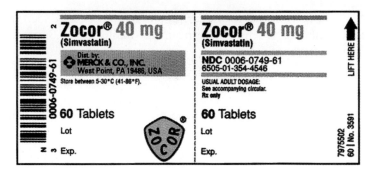

Figure 13-5 Zocor label.

Form

The form specifies the type of preparation available.

- Examples of forms include tablets, capsules, liquids, suppositories, or ointments. Solutions may be indicated by milliliters (mL) and described as oral suspension or aqueous solution. Some medications are available in powder, granular form, and patches.
- Labels may also indicate abbreviations or words that describe the form of the drug. Examples include CR (controlled release), LA (long acting), DS (double strength), SR (sustained release), and XL (long acting).
- Abbreviations that describe the form of drugs indicate whether the drug has been prepared in a form that allows extended action, or slow release, of a drug. Often these drugs are given less frequently. Examples are Procardia XL, Inderal LA, and Verapamil SR.

Route of Administration

The route of administration describes how the medication is to be administered.

Example: Oral, I.M., I.V., topical

It is important to realize that on some labels the route may not be stated directly (Figure 13-6). However, unless specified otherwise tablets, capsules, and caplets are always intended for oral use. Any form intended for oral use should be administered orally. Certain forms shouldn't be crushed or dissolved for use through a nasogastric, gastrostomy, or jejunostomy tube without first consulting a pharmacist.

Total Volume

On solutions for injections or oral liquids, total volume as well as dose strength is stated. Total volume refers to the quantity contained in a package, bottle, or vial. For solid forms of medication such as tablets or capsules, it is the total number of tablets or capsules in the container. On injectable solutions or oral liquids, total volume and dose strength are stated. The total volume is also included on solid forms of medication such as tablets or capsules.

Examples: A bottle may contain 100 tablets; however, the dose strength is the number of mg per tablet. In Figure 13-5 (Zocor tablets), the total volume is 60 tablets, whereas the dose strength is 40 mg per tablet.

On the Epivir label shown in Figure 13-3, 240 mL is the total volume, and the dose strength is 10 mg/mL.

1 mL is the total volume of the Atropine injectable shown in Figure 13-1, but the solution or liquid contains 0.4 mg per mL (400 mcg/mL).

Note:

It is important to recognize the difference between the amount per mL and the total volume to avoid confusion and errors.

Directions for Mixing or Reconstituting a Medication

When medication comes in a powdered form, the directions for how to mix or reconstitute it and with what solution are found on the label. It is important that the directions for reconstitution are followed exactly as stated on the label for accuracy in administration.

Precautions

Specific instructions related to safety, effectiveness, or administration that need to be adhered to are included on the label. Medication labels also contain information such as the expiration date (which may be indicated with the abbreviation "EXP"). Expiration dates indicate the last date in which a medication should be used. This information can be found on the back or side of a label. Other information includes storage information, lot numbers, the name of the drug manufacturer, and a National Drug code (NDC) number. Some medication labels are more detailed than others; however, recognition of pertinent information on a medication label is an absolute requirement before calculation and administration.

Note:

It is imperative that nurses check the expiration dates on medications as a routine habit.

Remember to always read the expiration date. After the expiration date, the drug may lose its potency or cause adverse or different effects on a client's body. Discard expired drugs according to agency policy. For some medications, such as narcotics, disposal must be witnessed. Never give expired drugs to a client! Clients must be educated in *all* aspects of medication administration, so teach them to check medications for expiration dates.

Let's examine some medication labels.
1. In Figure 13-6, note the following:
   a) *Indocin SR* is the brand name.

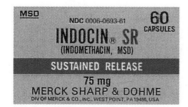

Figure 13-6 Indocin label.

b) *Indomethacin MSD* is the generic name.
c) The drug form is sustained-release capsule.
d) The dose strength is 75 mg per capsule.
e) The drug manufacturer is Merck Sharp & Dohme.

> ## Think Critically to Avoid Drug Calculation Errors
>
> Read labels carefully. Read the total volume on a medication container carefully. Confusing volume with dose strength can cause a serious medication error.

2. In figure 13-7, note the following:

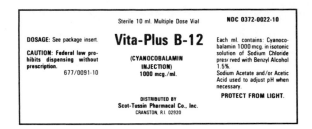

Figure 13-7   Vita-Plus B-12 label.

a) *Vita-Plus B-12* is the trade name.
b) *Cyanocobalamin* is the generic name.
c) Injection is the drug form or route.
d) 10 mL is the total volume of the vial.
e) 1000 mcg/mL is the dose strength.
f) The directions for storage are to "protect from light."
g) Scot-Tussin Pharmacal Co, Inc. is the drug manufacturer.
h) The NDC is 0372-0022-10.

3. The label in Figure 13-8 includes the following information:

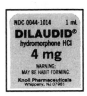

Figure 13-8   Dilaudid label.

a) *Dilaudid* is the trade name.
b) *Hydromorphone HCl* is the generic name.
c) The total volume of the ampule is 1 mL.
d) The dose strength is 4 mg/mL.
e) The NDC is 0044-1014.
f) Knoll Pharmaceuticals is the drug manufacturer.
g) "May be habit forming" is the warning.

4. The following information is indicated on the label in Figure 13-9:
a) *Vancocin HCl* is the trade name.
b) *Vancomycin hydrochloride* is the generic name.
c) "Dilute with 10 mL of sterile water for injection" are the directions for mixing.
d) The dose strength (50 mg/mL) is 500 mg/10 mL.
e) Injection is the form. The label specifies I.V. use.
f) "After dilution, refrigerate" are the directions after reconstitution.
g) Eli Lilly & Co is the drug manufacturer.

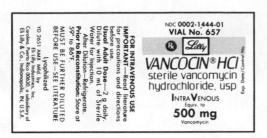

Figure 13-9   Vancocin HCl label.

In this chapter, sample medication labels are presented to help you learn to recognize essential information on a drug label. It is important to note that some drugs may not indicate their strength but are ordered by the number of tablets (for example, multivitamin tablet 1 p.o. every day, Bactrim DS 1 tablet p.o. b.i.d., Percocet 1 tablet p.o. q4h p.r.n). This is because these medications are available in one strength only. This is also common with some medications that contain a combination of drugs.

Most of the medications administered in the hospital setting are available in unit dose. The pharmacy provides a 24-hour supply of each drug for the client. In unit dose, the medications will come to the unit in individually wrapped packets that are labeled for an individualized dose for a specific client. The label includes the generic name or trade name or sometimes both. The strength is indicated on the medication label. The nurse must read the label on unit-dose packages and note that sometimes, even with this method, calculation may be necessary. The pharmacy in some institutions provides the unit with a supply of medications available in multidose containers. These medications may be in unit-dose packaging but are used a great deal by the clients on the unit. Examples include Tylenol and aspirin. Some medications may also be dispensed in bottles—for example, 100 tablets of aspirin 325 mg.

Most hospital units have a combination of unit dose and multidose. Figure 13-10 shows examples of unit-dose packaging.

A new administration system called the Pyxis system, is also available and used at some institutions. All medications are kept in the system and the nurse has a user ID and password to access the system to get a client's medications.

MEDICATION LABELS FOR COMBINED DRUGS

Some medication labels may indicate that a medication contains two drugs. These are usually indicated in the generic name of the drug, and the label specifies the dose strength for each next to the name.

Example 1:   The label for Sinemet, which is the trade name for an antiparkinsonian drug, indicates the medication contains carbidopa and levodopa. The first number specifies the amount of carbidopa, and the second number represents the amount of levodopa. This is further indicated on the bottom of the label. See sample labels in Figures 13-11 and 13-12. Combined drugs such as Sinement, which comes in several strengths, cannot be ordered without a specific dosage; the number of tablets alone is insufficient to fill the order. **It must include the dosage!**

Example 2:   Septra, an antibacterial that is also manufactured under the trade name Bactrim, is a combination of trimethoprim and sulfamethoxazole. For example, a Septra tablet contains 80 mg trimethoprim and 400 mg sulfamethoxazole. Septra DS is 160 mg trimethoprim and 800 mg sulfamethoxazole. See the labels for Septra in Figures 13-13 and 13-14.

Notes

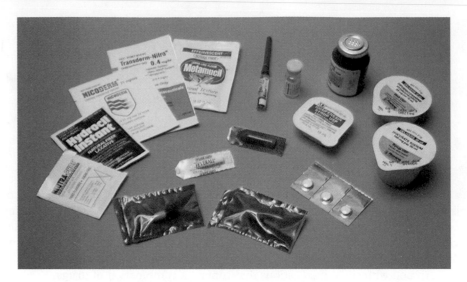

Figure 13-10 Unit dose packages. (Courtesy of Chuck Dresner. From Clayton BD, Stock YN: *Basic pharmacology for nurses,* ed 12, St Louis, 2001, Mosby.)

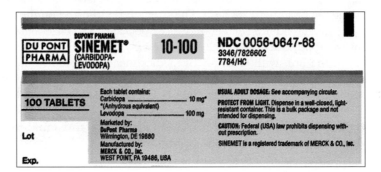

Figure 13-11 This label indicates the strength of carbidopa as 10 mg and levodopa as 100 mg.

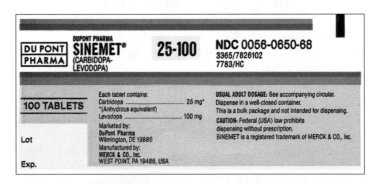

Figure 13-12 The dose strength of carbidopa is 25 mg and levodopa is 100 mg.

Remember extra initials or abbreviations after a drug name identify additional drugs in the preparation or a special action. For example, in Figure 13-14 Septra DS is a double strength tablet.

Although tablets and capsules that contain more than one drug are often ordered by the brand name and number of tablets to be given (for example, Septra

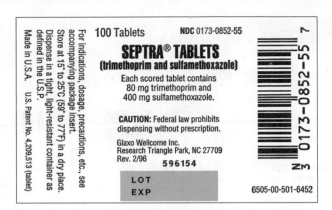

Figure 13-13 Septra label.

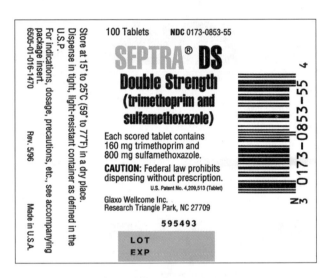

Figure 13-14 Septra DS.

DS 1 tab p.o. b.i.d), the health care provider may order this medication by another route, for example, I.V. With the I.V. order, the nurse calculates the dose to be given based on the strength of the trimethoprim. The nurse would learn such information described by using appropriate resources such as a reference drug book (PDR), pharmacist, or hospital formulary.

Example: Medication available: 10 mL multidose vial containing 160 mg trimethoprim (16 mg/mL) and 800 mg sulfamethoxazole (80 mg/mL)
Order: Septra 320 mg IVPB q8h. (In calculating the dose, the nurse would calculate the amount to be given based on the trimethoprim [16 mg/mL].)

Think Critically to Avoid Drug Calculation Errors

Read the label carefully to validate you have the correct medication and dose for combined drugs.

Notes

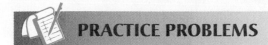

PRACTICE PROBLEMS

Use the labels to identify the information requested.

AUGMENTIN®
125mg/5mL

125mg/5mL
NDC 0029-6085-23

NSN 6505-01-408-8181
Directions for mixing:
Tap bottle until all powder
flows freely. Add approximately 2/3 of total water
for reconstitution
(total = 90 mL); shake
vigorously to wet powder.
Add remaining water; again
shake vigorously.
Dosage: See accompanying
prescribing information.

AUGMENTIN®
AMOXICILLIN/
CLAVULANATE
POTASSIUM
FOR ORAL SUSPENSION
When reconstituted,
each 5 mL contains:
AMOXICILLIN, 125 MG,
as the trihydrate
CLAVULANIC ACID, 31.25 MG,
as clavulanate potassium

100mL
(when reconstituted)

Keep tightly closed.
Shake well before using.
Must be refrigerated.
Discard after 10 days.

SB SmithKline Beecham

Use only if inner seal is intact.
Net contents: Equivalent to 2.5 g amoxicillin
and 0.625 g clavulanic acid.
Store dry powder at room temperature.
SmithKline Beecham Pharmaceuticals
Philadelphia, PA 19101

Rx only

3 0029-6085-23 2

LOT

EXP.

9405705-D

1. Trade name ————————   Dose strength (when reconstituted)

   Generic name ————————   ————————————————————

   Form ————————————   Total volume (when reconstituted)

   ————————————————————

NDC 0049-5460-74
Vistaril®
hydroxyzine hydrochloride
50 mg / ml
10ml
INTRAMUSCULAR SOLUTION
CAUTION: Federal law prohibits
dispensing without prescription.
ROERIG *Pfizer*

9249

PATIENT:
ROOM NO.:

2. Trade name ————————   Dose strength ————————

   Generic name ————————   Total volume ————————

   Form ————————————

NOTE TO PHARMACIST–
Do not dispense capsules which are discolored.

Dosage–Adults, 1 capsule three or four times daily or as directed.

See package insert under cap for complete prescribing information.

Keep this and all drugs out of the reach of children.

Dispense in a tight, light-resistant container as defined in the USP.

Store below 30°C (86°F). Protect from light and moisture.

Exp date and lot

0362G420

N 0071-0362-32
KAPSEALS®
Dilantin®
(Extended Phenytoin
Sodium Capsules, USP)
100 mg
℞ Only
1000 CAPSULES

6505-00-584-2338

N 0071-0362-32
3

© 1997-'98, Warner-Lambert Co.

PARKE-DAVIS
Div of Warner-Lambert Co
Morris Plains, NJ 07950 USA

Ⓟ **PARKE-DAVIS**

3. Dose strength _____   Total volume _____

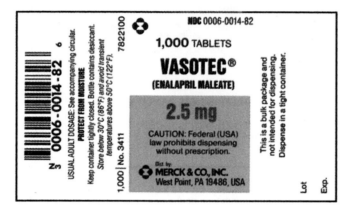

NDC 0006-0014-82

1,000 TABLETS

VASOTEC®

(ENALAPRIL MALEATE)

2.5 mg

CAUTION: Federal (USA) law prohibits dispensing without prescription.

Dist. by
❂ **MERCK & CO., INC.**
West Point, PA 19486, USA

USUAL ADULT DOSAGE: See accompanying circular.
PROTECT FROM MOISTURE. Bottle contains desiccant.
Keep container tightly closed. Store below 30°C (86°F) and avoid transient temperatures above 50°C (122°F).

1,000 | No. 3411

7822100

N 3 0006-0014-82 6

This is a bulk package and not intended for dispensing. Dispense in a tight container.

Lot   Exp.

4. Generic name _____   Total volume _____

   Dose strength _____

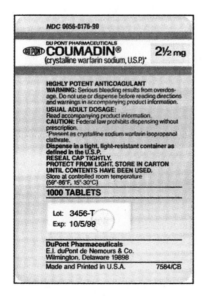

NDC 0056-0176-98

DU PONT PHARMACEUTICALS
⏍DUPONT **COUMADIN®**   **2½ mg**
(crystalline warfarin sodium, U.S.P.)*

HIGHLY POTENT ANTICOAGULANT
WARNING: Serious bleeding results from overdosage. Do not use or dispense before reading directions and warnings in accompanying product information.
USUAL ADULT DOSAGE:
Read accompanying product information.
CAUTION: Federal law prohibits dispensing without prescription.
*Present as crystalline sodium warfarin isopropanol clathrate.
Dispense in a tight, light-resistant container as defined in the U.S.P.
RESEAL CAP TIGHTLY.
PROTECT FROM LIGHT. STORE IN CARTON UNTIL CONTENTS HAVE BEEN USED.
Store at controlled room temperature
(59°-86°F, 15°-30°C)

1000 TABLETS

Lot: 3456-T
Exp: 10/5/99

DuPont Pharmaceuticals
E.I. duPont de Nemours & Co.
Wilmington, Delaware 19898
Made and Printed in U.S.A.   7584/CB

5. Trade name _____   Form _____

   Dose strength _____   NDC number _____

Answers on p. 504

Notes

POINTS TO REMEMBER

- Read medication labels three times.
- Check expiration dates; never administer expired drugs to a client.
- Read directions for mixing when indicated.
- Read labels carefully and don't confuse medication names; they are often deceptively similar. When in doubt, check appropriate resources such as a reference book or the hospital pharmacist. Always cross reference drug names.
- Differentiate among dose strength, total volume, form, and route.
- Read the label on combined drugs carefully to ascertain whether you're administering the correct medication dose.
- Extra abbreviations or initials after a drug name may identify additional drugs in the preparation or a special action.

✓ CHAPTER REVIEW

Read the label and identify the information requested.

NDC 0663-4310-71

250 Capsules

Minipress®

prazosin hydrochloride

1 mg†

CAUTION: Federal law prohibits dispensing without prescription.

Distributed by
LABORATORIES DIVISION
New York, N.Y. 10017

RECOMMENDED STORAGE
STORE BELOW 86°F (30°C)
Dispense in tight, light resistant
containers (USP).

†Each capsule contains prazosin
hydrochloride equivalent to
1 mg of prazosin.

Manufactured by
Pfizer Pharmaceuticals, Inc., Barceloneta, P.R. 00617

6505-01-039-6320

READ ACCOMPANYING
PROFESSIONAL INFORMATION

DOSAGE: See accompanying
prescribing information.

IMPORTANT: This closure is
not child-resistant.

1. Generic name _____   Form _____

   Trade name _____   Dose strength _____

LANOXIN® 2mL
(digoxin) Injection
500 µg (0.5 mg) in 2 mL
(250 µg [0.25 mg] per mL)
Store at 15° to 25°C (59° to 77°F).
PROTECT FROM LIGHT.
Glaxo Wellcome Inc.
Research Triangle Park, NC 27709
Rev. 1/96

542308

LOT
EXP

2. Generic name _____   Form _____

   Trade name _____   Dose strength _____

   Total volume _____

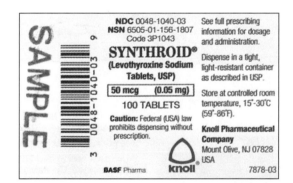

3. Generic name _____   Form _____

   Trade name _____   Dose strength _____

NDC 0048-1040-03
NSN 6505-01-156-1807
Code 3P1043

SYNTHROID®
(Levothyroxine Sodium
Tablets, USP)

50 mcg   (0.05 mg)

100 TABLETS

Caution: Federal (USA) law
prohibits dispensing without
prescription.

SAMPLE

See full prescribing
information for dosage
and administration.

Dispense in a tight,
light-resistant container
as described in USP.

Store at controlled room
temperature, 15°-30°C
(59°-86°F).

**Knoll Pharmaceutical
Company**
Mount Olive, NJ 07828
USA

BASF Pharma   knoll®   7878-03

4. Generic name _____   Form _____

   Trade name _____   Dose strength _____

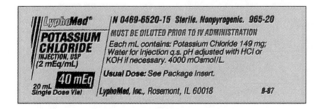

LyphoMed® N 0469-6520-15 Sterile. Nonpyrogenic. 965-20
**POTASSIUM
CHLORIDE**
INJECTION, USP
(2 mEq/mL)

MUST BE DILUTED PRIOR TO IV ADMINISTRATION

Each mL contains: Potassium Chloride 149 mg;
Water for Injection q.s. pH adjusted with HCl or
KOH if necessary. 4000 mOsmol/L.

40 mEq

20 mL
Single Dose Vial

Usual Dose: See Package Insert.

LyphoMed, Inc., Rosemont, IL 60018   8-87

5. Generic name _____   Form _____

   Trade name _____   Dose strength _____

Notes

An aid in the treatment of temporary constipation.
Keep this and all medication out of the reach of children.
Warning: As with any drug, if you are pregnant or nursing a baby, seek the advice of a health professional before using this product.
Caution: If cramping pain occurs, discontinue the medication.
Manufactured by R.P. Scherer
Clearwater, Florida 33518
Expressly for:
HOECHST-ROUSSEL Pharmaceuticals Inc.
Somerville, New Jersey 08876
℞ REG TM HOECHST AG
60210-2/85

NDC 0039-0002-10
Surfak®
docusate calcium USP
STOOL SOFTENER
Seal Under Cap
Printed Hoechst-Roussel
100 CAPSULES
50 MG EACH

Each capsule contains 50 mg docusate calcium USP and the following inactive ingredients: alcohol USP up to 1.3% (w/w), corn oil NF, FD&C Red #3, FD&C Red #40, gelatin NF, glycerin USP, parabens NF, sorbitol NF, soybean oil USP and other ingredients.
Usual Dosage: Adults—two or three capsules daily; children 6 to 12 and adults with minimal needs — one to three capsules daily. Continue for several days or until bowel movements are normal. For children under 6 consult a physician. Preserve in a tight container. Store at controlled room temperature (59°-86°F) in a dry place.

6. Generic name _____ Form _____

   Trade name _____ Dose strength _____

MADE IN U.S.A. 2
RECOMMENDED STORAGE IN DRY FORM
STORE BELOW 86° F (30° C)
Sterile reconstituted solutions should be protected from light and may be stored at room temperature for four weeks without significant loss of potency.

Sterile
Streptomycin Sulfate, USP
Equivalent to 5.0 g of Streptomycin Base
5.0 g
FOR INTRAMUSCULAR USE ONLY
CAUTION: Federal law prohibits dispensing without prescription.
ROERIG *Pfizer*
A Division of Pfizer Inc., N.Y., N.Y. 10017

Usual Daily Dosage
Adults: Varies with infection— consult package insert.
Adult average single injection:
0.5 to 1.0 g
ml Diluent added
9.0 ml
mg/ml of Solution
400 mg/ml
The dry powder is dissolved by adding Water for Injection, USP or Sodium Chloride for Injection, USP in an amount to yield the desired concentration.

PATIENT:
ROOM NO.:
DATE DILUTED:

7. Generic name _____ Directions for mixing _____

   Trade name _____ Dose strength after reconstitution

   _____

   Form _____ Storage instructions _____

NDC 0173-0471-00

GlaxoWellcome

Epivir™
Oral
Solution
(lamivudine
oral solution)
10 mg/mL   240 mL

Caution: Federal law prohibits dispensing without prescription.
See package insert for Dosage and Administration.
Store between 2° and 25°C (36° and 77°F) in tightly closed bottles. Contains 6% alcohol.

4058895

Glaxo Wellcome Inc.
Research Triangle Park,
NC 27709
Manufactured in England under agreement from BioChem Pharma Inc.
Laval, Quebec, Canada
Rev. 10/95

8. Generic name _____ Form _____

   Trade name _____ Dose strength _____

   Total volume _____

ZOVIRAX® STERILE POWDER   **1000 mg**   NDC 0173-0952-01
(ACYCLOVIR SODIUM) **equivalent to 1000 mg acyclovir**
FOR INTRAVENOUS INFUSION ONLY
CAUTION: Federal law prohibits dispensing without prescription.
Preparation of Solution: inject 20 mL Sterile Water for Injection into vial. Shake vial until a clear solution is
achieved and use within 12 hours. DO NOT USE BACTERIOSTATIC WATER FOR INJECTION CONTAINING
BENZYL ALCOHOL OR PARABENS.
Dilute to 7 mg/mL. or lower prior to infusion. See package insert for additional reconstitution and dilution instructions.
For indications, dosage, precautions, etc., see accompanying package insert.
Store at 15° to 25°C (59° to 77°F).
                   U.S. Patent No. 4199574
Glaxo Wellcome Inc.   Rev. 2/96
Research Triangle Park, NC 27709   Made in U.S.A.

647627

9. Generic name _____   Form _____

    Trade name _____   Dose strength _____

    Directions for mixing _____

    _____

    Storage _____

NDC 0173-0363-00

Glaxo Pharmaceuticals

Zantac®
(ranitidine
hydrochloride)
Injection

25 mg/mL*

40-mL Pharmacy Bulk Package—
Not for Direct Infusion

Sterile
Caution: Federal law prohibits
dispensing without prescription.

Contents should be used as soon as possible following initial closure
puncture. Discard any unused portion within 24 hours of first entry.

* Each 1 mL of aqueous solution contains ranitidine 25 mg
(as the hydrochloride); phenol 5 mg as preservative;
monobasic potassium phosphate and dibasic sodium
phosphate as buffers.

See package insert for Dosage and Administration and
directions for use of Pharmacy Bulk Package.

Store between 4° and 30°C (39° and 86°F). Protect
from light. Store vial in carton until time of use.

Zantac® Injection tends to exhibit a yellow color that
may intensify over time without adversely affecting
potency.

Glaxo Pharmaceuticals, Division of Glaxo Inc.
Research Triangle Park, NC 27709
Manufactured
in England
4/93

4043014

10. Generic name _____   Form _____

    Trade name _____   Dose strength _____

    NDC number _____

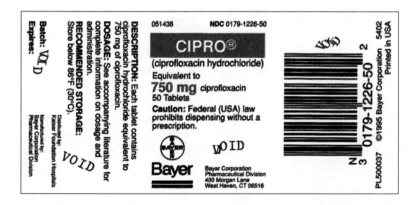

051436   NDC 0179-1226-50

CIPRO®
(ciprofloxacin hydrochloride)
Equivalent to
750 mg ciprofloxacin
50 Tablets
Caution: Federal (USA) law
prohibits dispensing without a
prescription.

Bayer
Bayer Corporation
Pharmaceutical Division
400 Morgan Lane
West Haven, CT 06516

DESCRIPTION: Each tablet contains
ciprofloxacin hydrochloride equivalent to
750 mg of ciprofloxacin.
DOSAGE: See accompanying literature for
complete information on dosage and
administration.
RECOMMENDED STORAGE:
Store below 86°F (30°C).

Batch: VOID
Expires: VOID

Distributed by:
Kaiser Foundation Hospitals

Manufactured by:
Bayer Corporation
Pharmaceutical Division

VOID

VOID

0179-1226-50 2

PL500037   ©1995 Bayer Corporation   5402
Printed in USA

N 3

11. Generic name _____   Form _____

    Trade name _____   Dose strength _____

    Total volume _____

Notes

> NDC 0003-0437-30
> NSN 6505-01-084-9453
> 50 mg
> **FUNGIZONE®** Rx only
> **INTRAVENOUS**
> Amphotericin B for Injection USP
> STOP: Verify product name & dosage
> if dose exceeds 1.5 mg/kg
>
> For intravenous infusion
> in hospitals only
> Sterile • See insert
> for reconstitution and
> dosage information
> REFRIGERATE
>
> Manufactured for: APOTHECON®
> A Bristol-Myers Squibb Co.
> Princeton, NJ 08540 USA
> by E. R. Squibb & Sons, Inc.
> A Bristol-Myers Squibb Co.
> Princeton, NJ 08543 USA
>
> C02170 / 43730

12. Generic name _____   Form _____

    Trade name _____   Drug manufacturer _____

> NDC 0009-7376-01
> 1 mL Single Dose Syringe
> **Depo-Provera®**
> **Contraceptive Injection**
> sterile medroxyprogesterone
> acetate suspension, USP
> **150 mg per mL**
> **Intramuscular Use Only**
> **Shake vigorously before use**
> 816 289 000   504711/1
> **The Upjohn Company**
> Lot:
> EXP:
> S L

13. Generic name _____   Form _____

    Trade name _____   Dose strength _____

    Directions for use _____

> See package insert for complete
> product information.
> Shake vigorously immediately
> before each use.
> Store at controlled room temperature
> 15° to 30° C (59° to 86° F).
> Each mL contains: Medroxyproges-
> terone acetate, 400 mg.
> Also, polyethylene glycol 3350, 20.5 mg;
> sodium sulfate anhydrous, 11 mg;
> myristyl-gamma-picolinium chloride,
> 1.69 mg added as preservative. When
> necessary, pH was adjusted with
> sodium hydroxide and/or hydrochloric
> acid.
> 813 279 203
> The Upjohn Company
> Kalamazoo, Michigan 49001, USA
>
> NDC 0009-0626-02
> 10 mL Vial
> **Depo-Provera®**
> Sterile Aqueous Suspension
> sterile medroxyprogesterone
> acetate suspension, USP
> For intramuscular use only
> **400mg per mL**
> Caution: Federal law prohibits
> dispensing without prescription.

14. Generic name _____   Dose strength _____

    Trade name _____   Directions for use _____

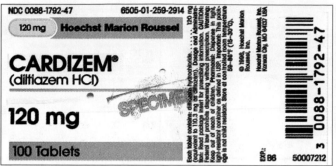

15. Generic name _____   Form _____

    Trade name _____   Dose strength _____

    Total volume _____

16. Generic name _____   Form _____

    Trade name _____   Dose strength _____

    Directions for use _____

17. Generic name _____   Dose strength _____

    Trade name _____   Total volume _____

    Directions for use _____

Notes

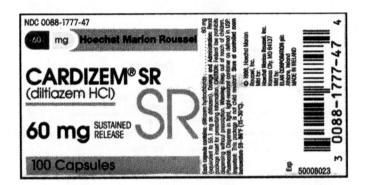

Zocor® 10 mg
(Simvastatin)
Dist. by:
MERCK & CO., INC.
West Point, PA 19486, USA
Store between 5 - 30°C (41 - 86°F).
0006-0735-61
60 Tablets
Lot
Exp.

Zocor® 10 mg
(Simvastatin)
NDC 0006-0735-61
6505-01-354-4545
USUAL ADULT DOSAGE:
See accompanying circular.
Rx only
60 Tablets
Lot
Exp.

LIFT HERE

18. Trade name _____   Dose strength _____

Generic name _____   NDC number _____

NDC 0088-1777-47

60 mg Hoechst Marion Roussel

CARDIZEM® SR
(diltiazem HCl)

SR

60 mg SUSTAINED RELEASE

100 Capsules

0088-1777-47

Exp 50008023

19. Generic name _____   Dose strength _____

Form _____

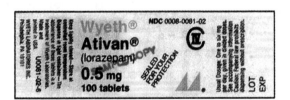

Wyeth®   NDC 0008-0081-02

Ativan®
(lorazepam)
0.5 mg
100 tablets

SEALED FOR YOUR PROTECTION

LOT
EXP

20. Trade name _____   Total volume _____

Dose strength _____

Answers on pp. 504-505

Calculating Doses Using Ratio-Proportion

Several methods are used for calculating doses. The most common methods are *ratio-proportion* and *use of a formula.* After presentation of the various methods, students can choose the method they find easiest to use. First, let's discuss calculating using ratio-proportion. If necessary, review Chapter 4 on ratio-proportion.

USE OF RATIO-PROPORTION IN DOSE CALCULATION

Ratio-proportion is useful and easy to use in dose calculation, because it is often necessary to find only one unknown quantity.

For example, suppose you had a medication with a dose strength of 50 mg in 1 mL, and the doctor orders a dose of 25 mg. A ratio-proportion may be used to solve this. The known ratio is 50 mg : 1 mL, and *x* represents the unknown number of mL that would contain 25 mg. Therefore, to set this problem up in a ratio-proportion, the known ratio (50 mg : 1 mL) is stated first, then the unknown ratio (25 mg : *x* mL). The known ratio is what you have **available,** or the information on the drug label.

It is important to remember when stating ratios that the units of measure should be stated in the same sequence (in the example, mg : mL = mg : mL).

Example 1:   50 mg : 1 mL = 25 mg : *x* mL
                  (known)   (unknown)

Solution: To solve for *x* use the principles presented in Chapter 4 on ratio-proportion.

$$50 \text{ mg} : 1 \text{ mL} = 25 \text{ mg} : x \text{ mL}$$

$$50x = \text{product of extremes}$$

$$25 = \text{product of means}$$

$$50x = 25 \text{ is the equation}$$

$$\frac{50x}{50} = \frac{25}{50} \quad \begin{array}{l}\text{(Divide both} \\ \text{sides by 50,} \\ \text{the number in} \\ \text{front of } x.)\end{array}$$

$$x = 0.5 \text{ mL}$$

Note:

As shown in Chapter 4 on ratio-proportion, this proportion could also be stated in fraction format.

IMPORTANT POINTS WHEN CALCULATING DOSES USING RATIO-PROPORTION

1. Make sure all terms are in the same unit and system of measure before calculating. If they are not, a conversion will be necessary before calculating the dose. Conversions can be made by changing what is ordered to the units in which the medication is available or by changing what is available to the units in which the medication is ordered. Try to be consistent as to how you make conversions. It is usual to convert what is ordered to the same unit and system of measure you have available.
2. Before calculating the dose, make a mental estimate of the approximate and reasonable answer.
3. Set up the proportion, labeling all terms in proportion. This includes x. State the known ratio first (what is available or on the drug label).
4. Make sure the terms of the ratios are stated in the same sequence.
5. Label the value you obtain for x (for example, mL, tabs).

Let's use ratio-proportion to solve some more problems.

Example 2:   Order: 40 mg p.o. of a drug.
                    Available: 20 mg tablets

Solution: $20 \text{ mg} : 1 \text{ tab} = 40 \text{ mg} : x \text{ tab}$

                    (known)   (unknown)

$$\frac{20x}{20} = \frac{40}{20}$$

$$x = 2 \text{ tabs}$$

Note: When setting up the ratios, follow the sequence in stating the terms for both.

For example, mg : tab = mg : tab

This proportion could also be stated as a fraction and solved by cross multiplication.

$$\begin{array}{cc}\text{Known} & \text{Unknown} \\ \dfrac{20 \text{ mg}}{1 \text{ tab}} & = \dfrac{40 \text{ mg}}{x \text{ tab}}\end{array}$$

Here the known is stated as the first fraction and the unknown as the second.

Example 3:   Order: 1 g p.o. of an antibiotic

Available: 500 mg capsules. How many capsules will you give?

Solution: Notice the dose ordered is a different unit from what is available. Proceed first by changing the units of measure so they are the same. As shown in Chapter 8, ratio-proportion can be used for conversion.

After making the conversion, set up the problem and calculate the dose to be given. In this example the conversion required is within the same system (metric).

In this example g is converted to mg by using the equivalent 1,000 mg = 1 g. After making the conversion of 1 g to 1,000 mg, the ratio is stated as follows:

$$500 \text{ mg} : 1 \text{ cap} = 1,000 \text{ mg} : x \text{ cap}$$

(known)   (unknown)

$$x = 2 \text{ caps}$$

An alternate method of solving might be to convert mg to g. In doing this, 500 mg would be converted to g using the same equivalent: 1,000 mg = 1 g. However, decimals are common when measures are changed from smaller to larger in the metric system: 500 mg = 0.5 g. Even though converting the mg to g would net the same final answer, *conversions that net decimals are often the source of calculation errors.* Therefore, if possible, avoid conversions that require their use. As a rule, it is best to convert to the measure stated on the drug label. Doing this consistently can prevent confusion. As with the other examples, this proportion could be stated as a fraction as well.

For the purpose of learning to calculate doses using ratio-proportion, this chapter emphasizes the mathematics used to calculate the answer. Determining whether an answer is logical is essential and necessary in the calculation of medication. An answer *must make sense.* Determining whether an answer is logical will be discussed further in later chapters covering the calculation of doses by various routes.

POINTS TO REMEMBER

- When stating ratios, the known ratio is stated first. The known ratio is what is available, on hand, or the information obtained from the drug label.

- The unknown ratio is stated second. The unknown ratio is the dose desired, or what the prescriber has ordered.

- The terms of the ratios in a proportion must be written in the same sequence of measurement.

- Label all terms of the ratios in the proportion, including x.

- When conversion of units is required, it is usually easier to convert to the unit of measure on the drug label, or what the medication is available in. A problem cannot be solved if the units of measurement are not the same.

- Estimate the answer.

- Label all answers obtained.

Continued

Notes

Notes

POINTS TO REMEMBER—cont'd

- A proportion may be stated in horizontal fashion or as a fraction.
- Double check all work.
- Be consistent in how ratios are stated and conversions are done.
- An error in the set up of the ratio proportion can cause an error in calculation.

PRACTICE PROBLEMS

Answer the following problems by indicating whether you need less than 1 tab or more than 1 tab. Refer to Chapter 4, Ratio-Proportion, if you have difficulty with problems in this area.

1. A client is to receive gr 1/300 of a drug. The tablets available are gr 1/150.

   How many tablets do you need? _____

2. A client is to receive 1.25 mg of a drug. The tablets available are 0.625 mg.

   How many tablets do you need? _____

3. A client is to receive gr 1/8 of a drug. The tablets available are gr 1/4.

   How many tablets do you need? _____

4. A client is to receive 10 mg of a drug. The tablets available are 20 mg.

   How many tablets do you need? _____

5. A client is to receive 100 mg of a drug. The tablets available are 50 mg.

   How many tablets do you need? _____

Answers on p. 505

Solve the following problems using ratio-proportion calculations. Express your answer to the nearest tenth where indicated, and include the units of measure in the answer.

6. Order: 7.5 mg p.o. of a drug.

   Available: Tablets labeled 5 mg. _____

7. Order: gr 3/4 p.o. of a drug.

   Available: Tablets labeled 30 mg. _____

8. Order: gr 1 1/2 p.o. of a drug.

   Available: Capsules labeled 100 mg. _____

9. Order: 0.25 mg I.M. of a drug.

   Available: 0.5 mg per mL. _____

10. Order: 100 mg p.o. of a liquid medication.

    Available: 125 mg per 5 mL. _____

11. Order: 20 mEq I.V. of a drug.

    Available: 40 mEq per 10 mL. _____

12. Order: 5,000 U s.c. of a drug.

    Available: 10,000 U per mL. _____

13. Order: 50 mg I.M. of a drug.

    Available: 80 mg per 2 mL. _____

14. Order: 0.5 g p.o. of an antibiotic.

    Available: Capsules labeled 250 mg. _____

15. Order: 400 mg p.o. of a liquid medication.

    Available: 125 mg per 5 mL. _____

16. Order: 50 mg I.M. of a drug.

    Available: 80 mg per mL. _____

17. Order: gr 1 I.M. of a drug.

    Available: gr $\frac{1}{2}$ per mL. _____

18. Order: gr xv of a drug.

    Available: Tablets labeled gr v. _____

19. Order: 0.24 g p.o. of a liquid medication.

    Available: 80 mg per 7.5 mL. _____

20. Order: 20 g p.o. of a liquid medication.

    Available: 10 g per 15 mL. _____

21. Order: 0.125 mg I.M. of a drug.

    Available: 0.5 mg per 2 mL. _____

22. Order: 0.75 mg I.M. of a drug.

    Available: 0.25 mg per mL. _____

23. Order: 375 mg p.o. of a liquid medication.

    Available: 125 mg per 5 mL. _____

24. Order: 10,000 U s.c. of a drug.

    Available: 7,500 U per mL. _____

25. Order: 0.45 mg p.o. of a drug.

    Available: Tablets labeled 0.3 mg. _____

26. Order: 20 mg I.M. of a drug.

    Available: 25 mg per 1.5 mL. _____

27. Order: 150 mg I.V. of a drug.

    Available: 80 mg per mL. _____

28. Order: 2 mg I.M. of a drug.

    Available: 1.5 mg per 0.5 mL. _____

29. Order: 500 mcg I.V. of a drug.

    Available: 750 mcg per 3 mL. _____

30. Order: 0.15 mg I.M. of a drug.

    Available: 0.2 mg per 1.5 mL. _____

31. Order: 1,100 U s.c. of a drug.

    Available: 1,000 U per 1.5 mL. _____

32. Order: 0.6 g I.V. of a drug.

    Available: 1 g per 3.6 mL. _____

33. Order: 3 g I.V. of a drug.

    Available: 1.5 g per mL. _____

34. Order: 35 mg I.M. of a drug.

    Available: 40 mg per 2.5 mL. _____

35. Order: 0.3 mg s.c. of a drug.

    Available: 1,000 mcg per 2 mL. _____

36. Order: 200 mg I.M. of a drug.

    Available: 0.5 g per 2 mL. _____

37. Order: 10 mEq I.V. of a drug.

    Available: 20 mEq per 10 mL. _____

38. Order: 165 mg I.V. of a drug.

    Available: 55 mg per 1.1 mL. _____

39. Order: 35 mg s.c. of a drug.

    Available: 45 mg per 1.2 mL. _____

40. Order: 700 mg I.M. of a drug.

    Available: 1,000 mg per 2.3 mL. _____

Answers on pp. 505-509

✓ CHAPTER REVIEW

Part I

Directions: Read the medication labels where available, and calculate the tablets or capsules necessary to provide the dose ordered. Include the unit of measure in your answer.

1. Order: gr 1/4 p.o. of phenobarbital t.i.d.

    Available: Phenobarbital tablets labeled 15 mg. _____

2. Order: Ampicillin 0.25 g p.o. q.i.d

    Available: _____

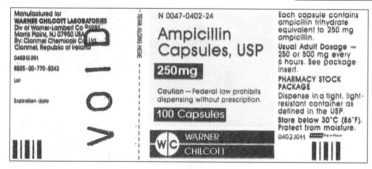

3. Order: Ampicillin 1 g p.o. q6h.

    Available: _____

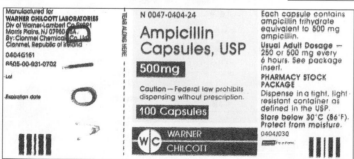

Notes

4. Order: Phenobarbital 60 mg p.o. h.s.

   Available: Phenobarbital tablets labeled 30 mg. _____

5. Order: Baclofen 20 mg p.o. t.i.d.

   Available: _____

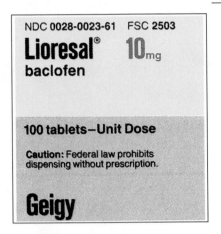

6. Order: Isosorbide dinitrate 20 mg p.o. t.i.d.

   Available: Isosorbide dinitrate tablets labeled 40 mg. _____

7. Order: Dexamethasone 4 mg p.o. q6h.

   Available: _____

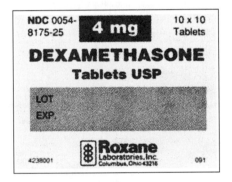

8. Order: Diabinese 250 mg p.o. q.d.

   Available: _____

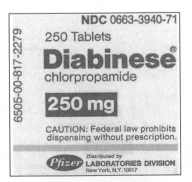

9. Order: Digoxin 125 mcg p.o. q.d.

   Available: _____

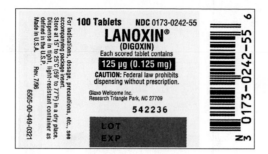

10. Order: Synthroid 0.05 mg p.o. q.d.

    Available: _____

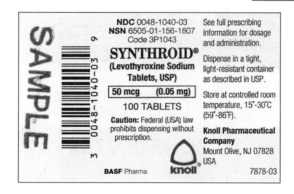

11. Order: Restoril 30 mg p.o. h.s. p.r.n.

    Available: _____

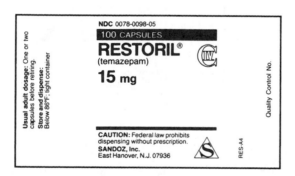

12. Order: Phenobarbital gr i p.o. h.s.

    Available: Phenobarbital tablets labeled 60 mg. _____

13. Order: Macrodantin 100 mg p.o. t.i.d.

    Available: Capsules labeled 50 mg. _____

Notes

14. Order: Keflex 0.5 g p.o. q.i.d.

Available: _____

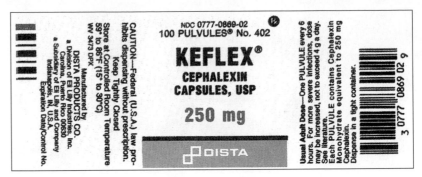

15. Order: Cogentin 2 mg p.o. b.i.d.

Available: Cogentin tablets labeled 1 mg.   _____

16. Order: Augmentin 0.5 g p.o. q8h.

Available: _____

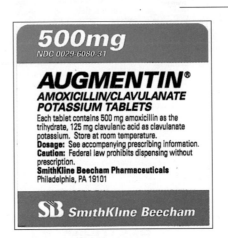

17. Order: Zovirax 400 mg p.o. b.i.d. × 7 days.

Available: _____

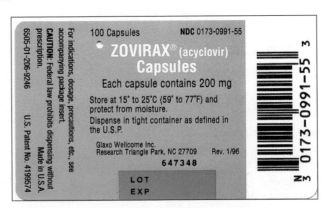

18. Order: Rifampin 0.6 g p.o. o.d.

    Available: _____

NDC 0068-0508-30

300 mg   MARION MERRELL DOW INC.

RIFADIN®
(rifampin capsules)

300 mg

30 Capsules

Each capsule contains: rifampin.....................300 mg
Usual Dose: See accompanying product information.
CAUTION: Federal law prohibits dispensing without prescription.
Keep tightly closed. Store in a dry place. Avoid excessive heat.
Dispense in tight, light-resistant container with child-resistant
closure.

© 1993 Marion Merrell Dow Inc.

Merrell Dow Pharmaceuticals Inc.
Subsidiary of Marion Merrell Dow Inc.
Kansas City, MO 64114   H 3 6 4 C

19. Order: Carafate 1,000 mg p.o. b.i.d.

    Available: _____

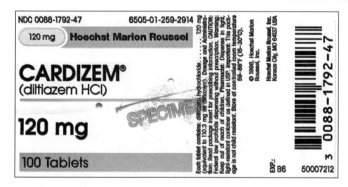

20. Order: Cardizem 240 mg p.o. daily.

    Available: _____

21. Order: Xanax 0.25 mg p.o. b.i.d.

    Available: _____

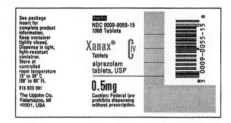

Notes

22. Order: Septra DS 1 tab p.o. 3 × a week.

Available: _____

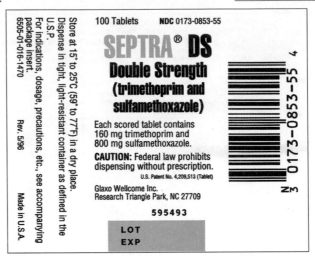

23. Order: Sinemet 25-100 2 tabs p.o. t.i.d.

Available: _____

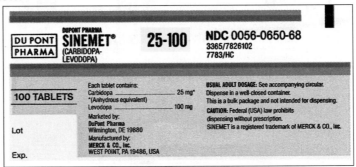

24. Order: Retrovir 0.2 g p.o. t.i.d.

Available: _____

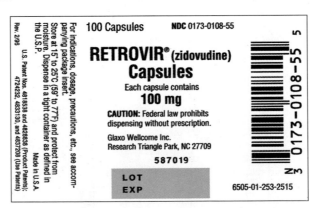

25. Order: Lanoxicaps 0.05 mg p.o. q.o.d.

    Available: _____

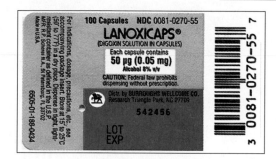

26. Order: Risperdal 3 mg p.o. b.i.d.

    Available: Risperdal scored tablets labeled 1 mg. _____

27. Order: Flagyl 0.5g p.o. q8h.

    Available: Flagyl tablets labeled 500 mg. _____

28. Order: Lopressor 100 mg p.o. b.i.d.

    Available: _____

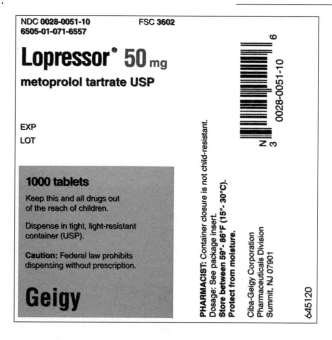

Notes

29. Order: Lasix 60 mg p.o. q.d.

    Available: Scored tablets.   _____

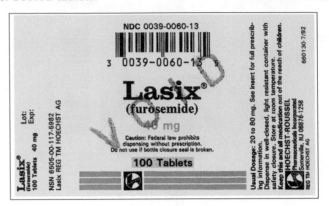

30. Order: Motrin 600 mg p.o. q6h p.r.n. for pain.

    Available: Motrin tablets labeled 300 mg.   _____

31. Order: Potassium chloride extended release 16 mEq p.o. q.d.

    Available: Potassium chloride extended-release
    tablets labeled 8 mEq.   _____

32. Order: Mevacor 20 mg p.o. q.d. at 6 PM.

    Available: Mevacor tablets labeled 10 mg.   _____

33. Order: Effexor 75 mg p.o. b.i.d.

    Available: Scored Effexor tablets
    labeled 37.5 mg.   _____

Answers on p. 509

Part II

Directions: Calculate the volume necessary (in mL) to provide the dose ordered, using medication labels where available. Express your answer as a decimal fraction to the nearest tenth where indicated.

34. Order: Dilantin 100 mg via gastrostomy tube t.i.d.

    Available: Dilantin 125 mg per 5 mL.   _____

35. Order: Benadryl 50 mg p.o. h.s.

    Available: Benadryl elixir 12.5 mg/5 mL.   _____

36. Order: Gentamicin 50 mg I.M. q8h.

    Available: Gentamicin labeled 80 mg/2 mL.   _____

37. Order: Vibramycin 100 mg p.o. q12h.

Available: _____

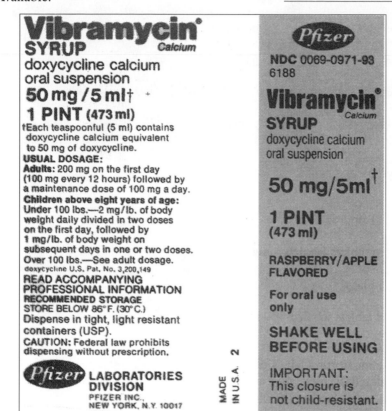

38. Order: Meperidine hydrochloride 50 mg I.M. q4h p.r.n. for pain.

Available: Meperidine 75 mg/mL. _____

39. Order: Gentamicin 90 mg I.V. q8h.

Available: Gentamicin 40 mg/mL. _____

40. Order: Morphine gr 1/4 s.c. q4h p.r.n.

Available: Morphine 15 mg/mL. _____

41. Order: Vitamin B_{12} 1,000 mcg I.M. once monthly.

Available: _____

42. Order: Morphine 10 mg s.c. stat. Express answer in hundredths.

    Available: Morphine 15 mg/mL. _____

43. Order: Kaon-Cl 20 mEq p.o. q.d.

    Available: Kaon-Cl 40 mEq/15 mL. _____

44. Order: Nystatin oral suspension 100,000 U swish and swallow q6h.

    Available: Nystatin oral suspension
    labeled 100,000 U per/mL. _____

45. Order: Heparin 5,000 U s.c. o.d.

    Available: _____

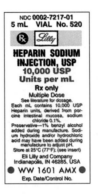

46. Order: Atropine 0.2 mg s.c. stat.

    Available: _____

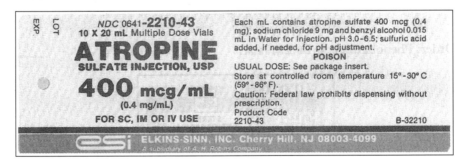

47. Order: Amoxicillin 500 mg p.o. q6h × 7 days.

    Available: _____

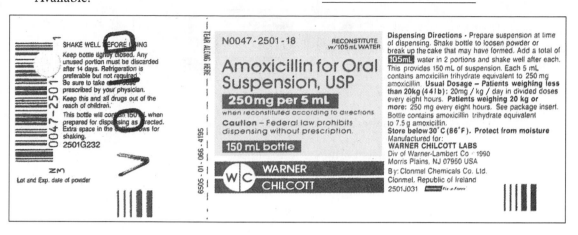

48. Order: Heparin 7,500 U s.c. o.d. Express answer in hundredths.

    Available: Heparin 10,000 U/mL. _____

49. Order: Solu-Medrol 70 mg I.V. o.d.

    Available: _____

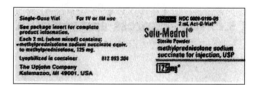

50. Order: Ativan 2 mg I.M. q4h p.r.n. agitation.

    Available: _____

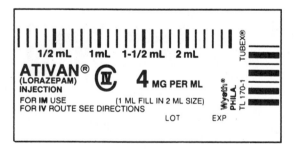

51. Order: Vistaril 25 mg I.M. on call to operating room (OR).

    Available: _____

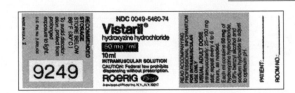

52. Order: Phenobarbital gr iss I.M. stat.

    Available: Phenobarbital 130 mg/mL.   _____

53. Order: Aminophylline 100 mg I.V. q6h.

    Available: Aminophylline 25 mg/mL   _____

54. Order: Zantac 150 mg I.V. q.d.

    Available: _____

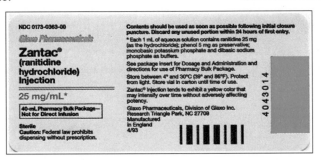

55. Order: Augmentin 0.5 g p.o. q8h.

    Available: _____

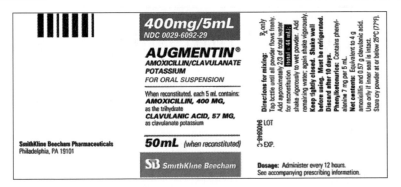

56. Order: Thorazine concentrate 75 mg p.o. q.d.

Available: _____

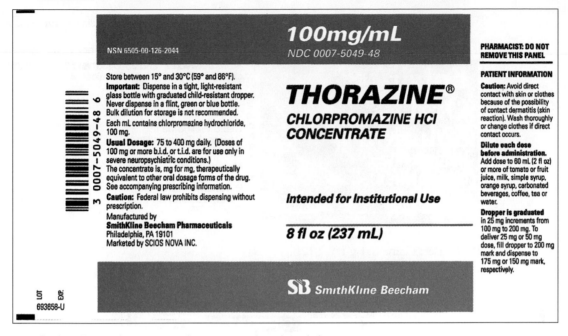

57. Order: Retrovir 200 mg via nasogastric tube t.i.d.

Available: _____

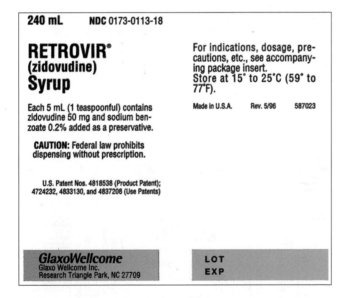

Notes

58. Order: Epivir 0.3 g p.o. b.i.d.

     Available: _____

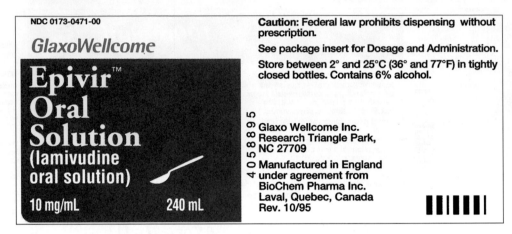

59. Order: Cipro 0.4 g I.V. q12h.

     Available: _____

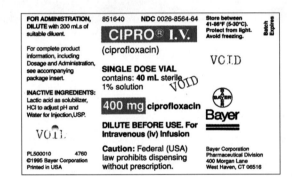

60. Order: Prozac 40 mg p.o. q.d.

     Available: _____

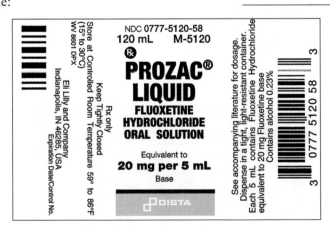

Notes

61. Order: Depo-Provera 0.4 g I.M. once a week.

    Available: _____

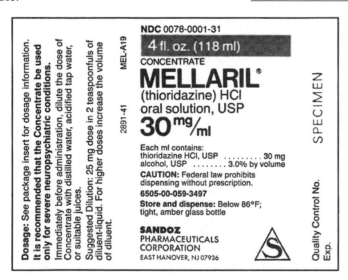

62. Order: Thorazine concentrate 500 mg p.o. b.i.d.

    Available: Thorazine Concentrate
    labeled 30 mg/mL.   _____

63. Order: Lactulose 30 g p.o. t.i.d.

    Available: Lactulose Syrup
    labeled 10g/15 mL.   _____

64. Order: Mellaril 40 mg p.o. b.i.d.

    Available: _____

65. Order: Compazine 7 mg I.M. q4h p.r.n. for vomiting.

    Available: _____

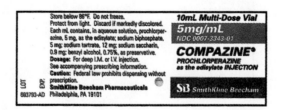

Notes

66. Order: Ceclor 0.5 g p.o. q8h.

Available:

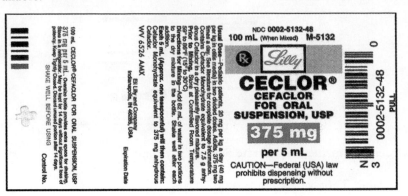

Answers on pp. 509-510

Chapter 15

Dose Calculation Using the Formula Method

Objectives

After reviewing this chapter, you should be able to:

1. **Identify the information from a calculation problem to place into the formulas given**
2. **Solve problems using one of the stated formulas**

This chapter shows how to use a formula for dose calculation, which requires substituting information from the problem into the formula. There are two formulas that may be used to calculate doses. **The nurse should choose a formula and consistently use it in its entirety to avoid calculation errors.**

 Think Critically to Avoid Drug Calculation Errors

Do not rely solely on formulas when calculating doses to be administered. Use critical thinking skills such as considering what the answer should be, reasoning, problem solving, and finding rational justification for your answer. Formulas should be used as a tool for validating the dose you THINK should be given.

FORMULAS FOR CALCULATING DOSES

The formulas presented in this chapter can be used when calculating doses in the same system of measurement. When the dose desired and the dose on hand are in different systems, convert them to the same system before using the formulas. We can write the first formula as

$$\frac{D}{H} \times Q = x$$

where

D = The dose desired, or what the doctor has ordered, including the weights. Example: mg, g, etc.

H = The dose strength available, what is on hand, or the weight of the drug on the label, including the weights. Example: mg, g, etc.

Q = The quantity or the unit of measure that contains the dose that is available. In other words the number of tablets, capsules, milliliters, etc., that contains the available dosage. "Q" is labeled accordingly as tablet, capsule, milliliter, etc.

Note:

It is important to note that the unknown "*x*" and "*Q*" will always be stated in the same unit of measure. It is critical that the formula is always set up with all of the terms in the formula labeled with the correct units of measure.

Note:

As with the previous formula, it is critical that the formula be set up with all units of measure labeled. In this formula, the DV, which is the unknown "*x*," is stated in the same unit of measures as SV.

When solving problems that involve solid forms of medication (tabs, caps), Q is always 1 and can be eliminated from the equation. **For consistency and to avoid chances of error when Q is not 1, always include Q even with tablet and capsule problems.** When solving problems for medications in solution, the amount for Q varies and must always be included.

x = The unknown, the dose you are looking for, the dosage you are going to administer, how many mL, tab, etc. you will give.

The second formula (Copyright Research Foundation, New York) is a ratio-proportion; the terms in the proportion are labeled differently and set up as a fraction. We can write it as

$$\frac{DW}{SW} = \frac{DV}{SV}$$

where:

DW = Dose weight—The dose desired, or what the doctor has ordered, including the weights. Example; mg, g, etc.

SW = Stock weight—The dose strength available, what is on hand, or the weight of the drug on the label, including the weights. Example; mg, g, etc.

DV = Dose volume—The unknown, the dose you are looking for, the dose you are going to administer—*x* is used to represent this value. The number of mL, tab, caps, etc. *x* is always labeled.

SV = Stock volume—The quantity of unit of measure that contains the dose available. For solid forms of medication (tabs, caps) the SV is always 1 (for example, 1 tab, 1 caps). For medications in solution the amount for SV varies. To avoid errors in calculation always include the SV even if the value is 1.

STEPS FOR USE OF THE FORMULAS

Either of the formulas presented may be used to calculate a dose to administer. The nurse should choose a formula and use it consistently. Regardless of which formula is used, remember the steps for using the formula (Box 15-1).

Now we will look at sample problems illustrating the use of the formulas.

Example 1:   Order: 0.375 mg p.o. of a drug. The tablets available are labeled 0.25 mg.

Solution: The dose 0.375 mg is desired, the dose strength available is 0.25 mg per tablet. No conversion is necessary. What is desired is in the same system and unit of measure as what you have on hand.

➡️ Formula Setup

$$\frac{D}{H} \times Q = x$$

The desired (D) is 0.375 mg. You have on hand (H) 0.25 mg per (Q) 1 tablet. The label on x is tablet. Notice the label on x is always the same as Q.

$$\frac{\text{(D) } 0.375 \text{ mg}}{\text{(H) } 0.25 \text{ mg}} \times \text{(Q) 1 tab} = x \text{ tab}$$

$$\frac{0.375}{0.25} \times 1 = x$$

$$\frac{0.375}{0.25} = x$$

OR

$$\frac{DW}{SW} = \frac{DV}{SV}$$

The desired (DW) is 0.375 mg. You have on hand (SW) 0.25 mg per (SV) 1 tablet. The label on x is tablet (DV). Notice the label on x is always the same as SV.

$$\frac{\text{(DW) } 0.375 \text{ mg}}{\text{(SW) } 0.25 \text{ mg}} = \frac{\text{(DV) } x \text{ tab}}{\text{(SV) } 1 \text{ tab}}$$

$$0.25 \times (x) = 0.375 \times 1$$

$$\frac{0.25 \text{ x}}{0.25} = \frac{0.375}{0.25} \qquad \frac{0.375}{0.25} = x$$

Therefore, $x = 1.5$ tabs, or 1 1/2 tabs. (Because 0.375 mg is larger than 0.25 mg, you will need more than 1 tab to administer 0.375 mg.) Note: Although 1.5 tabs is the same as 1 1/2 tabs, for administration purposes it would be best to state it as 1 1/2 tabs.

Example 2: Order: 7,000 U I.M. of a drug. The drug is available 10,000 U in 2 mL.

Solution:

$$\frac{\text{(D) } 7,000 \text{ U}}{\text{(H) } 10,000 \text{ U}} \times \text{(Q) 2 mL} = x \text{ mL}$$

$$\frac{7,000}{10,000} \times 2 = x$$

$$\frac{14,000}{10,000} = x$$

OR

$$\frac{\text{(DW) } 7,000 \text{ U}}{\text{(SW) } 10,000 \text{ U}} = \frac{\text{(DV) } x \text{ mL}}{\text{(SV) } 2 \text{ mL}}$$

$$10,000 \times (x) = 7,000 \times 2$$

$$\frac{10,000x}{10,000} = \frac{14,000}{10,000} \qquad \frac{14,000}{10,000} = x$$

Therefore, $x = 1.4$ mL. (Because 7,000 U $\times$ 2 is more than 10,000 U, it will take more than 1 mL to administer the dose.)

Note:

Omitting Q here could result in an error. A liquid medication is involved; Q must be included.

Note:

SV here is 2 mL and is important to include, because with liquid medications this can vary.

> ### BOX 15-1   Steps for Using a Formula
>
> 1. Memorize the formula, or verify the formula from a resource.
> 2. Place the information from the problem into the formula in the correct position, with all terms in the formula labeled correctly.
> 3. Make sure all measures are in the same units and system of measure or a conversion must be done *before* calculating the dose.
> 4. Think logically and consider what a reasonable amount would be to administer.
> 5. Calculate your answer.
> 6. Label all answers—tabs, caps, mL, etc.

Note:

What is desired and what is available must be in the *same units and system of measure.* Remember it is usual to convert what is desired to what is available. Therefore change gr to mg; this will also eliminate the fraction and decrease the chance of error in calculation.

Example 3:   Order: gr 1/2 p.o. Available are tablets labeled 15 mg.

Rule for Different Units or Systems of Measure

Whenever the desired amount and the dose on hand are in different units or systems of measure, follow these steps:

1. Choose the identified equivalent.
2. Convert what is ordered to the same units or system of measure as what is available on hand by using one of the methods presented in the chapter on converting.
3. Use the formula $\dfrac{D}{H} \times Q = x$ or $\dfrac{DW}{SW} = \dfrac{DV}{SV}$ to calculate the dose to administer.

Solution: Convert gr 1/2 to mg. The equivalent to use is 60 mg = gr 1. Therefore gr 1/2 = 30 mg.

Now that you have everything in the same system and units of measure, use either formula presented to calculate the dose to be administered.

Solution: $\dfrac{\text{(D) 30 mg}}{\text{(H) 15 mg}} \times \text{(Q) 1 tab} = x \text{ tab}$

$$\frac{30}{15} \times 1 = x \qquad\qquad \frac{30}{15} = x$$

OR

$$\frac{\text{(DW) 30 mg}}{\text{(SW) 15 mg}} = \frac{\text{(DV) } x \text{ tab}}{\text{(SV) 1 tab}}$$

$$15 \times (x) = 30 \times 1$$

$$\frac{15x}{15} = \frac{30}{15} \qquad\qquad \frac{30}{15} = x$$

Therefore, x = 2 tabs. (Because 30 mg is a larger dose than 15 mg, it will take more than 1 tab to administer the desired dose.)

Example 4:   Order: gr 1/6 s.c. of a drug. The drug is available gr 1/2 per mL. (Express the answer to the nearest tenth.)

Solution: $\dfrac{\text{(D) gr } \dfrac{1}{6}}{\text{(H) gr } \dfrac{1}{2}} \times \text{(Q) 1 mL} = x \text{ mL}$

$$\frac{1}{6} \div \frac{1}{2} = x \qquad \frac{1}{6} \times \frac{2}{1} = \frac{2}{6} = \frac{1}{3} \qquad \frac{1}{3} = x$$

OR

$$\frac{\text{(DW) gr } \dfrac{1}{6}}{\text{(SW) gr } \dfrac{1}{2}} = \frac{\text{(DV) } x \text{ mL}}{\text{(SV) 1 mL}}$$

$$\frac{1}{2} \times (x) = \frac{1}{6} \times 1 \qquad \frac{\dfrac{1}{2}}{\dfrac{1}{2}}x = \frac{\dfrac{1}{6}}{\dfrac{1}{2}} \qquad \frac{1}{6} \div \frac{1}{2} = x$$

$$\frac{1}{6} \times \frac{2}{1} = \frac{2}{6} = \frac{1}{3} \qquad\qquad \frac{1}{3} = x$$

Therefore, $x = 0.33$ mL $= 0.3$ mL. (Because 1/2 is a larger dose than 1/6, it will take less than 1 mL to administer the required dose.)

Critical Thinking

Always think critically, even when using a formula. It is an essential step to estimate what is reasonable and logical in terms of a dosage. This will avoid error in calculation from setting up the problem incorrectly or careless math, and will trigger your thinking to double check your calculation and identify any error.

Note:

As you will learn in a later chapter, stating the answer as 1/3 mL (fraction) would be incorrect, because if this was being administered using a small syringe, the only fraction on the syringe is 1/2, and all other values are expressed as decimal numbers or whole numbers.

POINTS TO REMEMBER

- The formula $\dfrac{D}{H} \times Q = x$ or $\dfrac{DW}{SW} = \dfrac{DV}{SV}$ can be used to calculate the dose to be administered.

- The Q and SV are always 1 for solid forms of medications (tabs, caps, etc.) but vary when medications are in liquid form.

- Always set up the formula with the units of measure included.

- Before the dose to be given is calculated, the dose desired must be in the same units and system of measure as the dose available or a conversion is necessary.

- Double check all of your math and think logically about the answer obtained.

- Label all answers obtained.

- The use of a formula does not eliminate the need to think critically.

 ## PRACTICE PROBLEMS

Calculate the following problems using one of the formulas presented in this chapter.

1. Order: 0.4 mg p.o.

   Available: Tablets labeled 0.2 mg. _____

Notes

2. Order: 0.75 g p.o.

   Available: Capsules labeled 250 mg. _____

3. Order: 90 mg p.o.

   Available: Tablets labeled 60 mg. _____

4. Order: 7.5 mg p.o.

   Available: Tablets labeled 2.5 mg. _____

5. Order: 0.05 mg p.o.

   Available: Tablets labeled 25 mcg. _____

6. Order: 0.4 mg p.o.

   Available: Tablets labeled 200 mcg. _____

7. Order: 1,000 mg p.o.

   Available: Tablets labeled 500 mg. _____

8. Order: 0.6 g p.o.

   Available: Capsules labeled 600 mg. _____

9. Order: 1.25 mg p.o.

   Available: Tablets labeled 625 mcg. _____

Answers on pp. 510-511

Calculate the following in mL; round to the nearest tenth where indicated.

10. Order: 10 mg s.c.

    Available: 15 mg per mL. _____

11. Order: 400 mg p.o.

    Available: Oral solution labeled 200 mg/5 mL. _____

12. Order: 15 mEq p.o.

    Available: Oral solution labeled 20 mEq/10 mL. _____

13. Order: 125 mg p.o.

    Available: Oral solution labeled 250 mg/5 mL. _____

14. Order: 0.025 mg p.o.

    Available: Oral solution labeled 0.05 mg/5 mL. _____

15. Order: 375 mg p.o.

    Available: Oral solution labeled 125 mg/5 mL. _____

Answers on pp. 511-512

CHAPTER REVIEW

Calculate the following doses using the medication label or information provided. Label answers correctly; tabs, caps, mL. Answers expressed in mL; round to the nearest tenth where indicated.

1. Order: Phenobarbital gr 1/2 p.o. t.i.d.

   Available: Phenobarbital tablets labeled 30 mg. _____

2. Order: Gantrisin 500 mg p.o. q.i.d.

   Available: _____

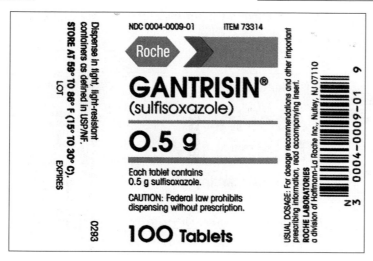

3. Order: Indocin 50 mg p.o. t.i.d.

   Available: _____

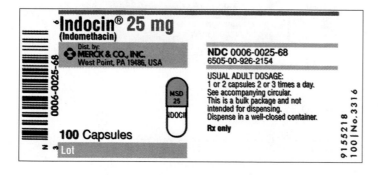

Notes

4. Order: Hydrochlorothiazide 50 mg p.o. b.i.d.

   Available: _____

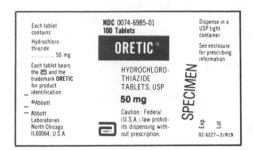

5. Order: Aspirin gr x p.o. q4h p.r.n. for pain.

   Available: _____

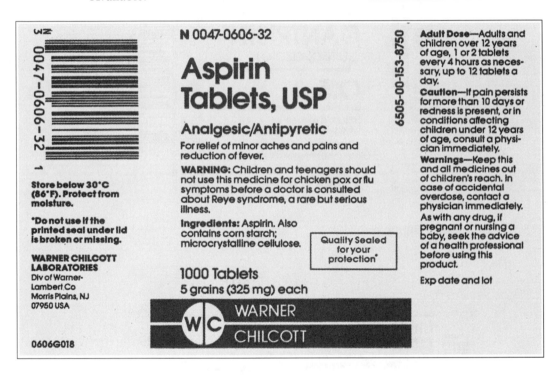

6. Order: Digoxin 0.375 mg p.o. o.d.

   Available: Digoxin 250 mcg (0.25 mg) per tab. _____

7. Order: Keflex 0.25 g p.o. q6h.

   Available: _____

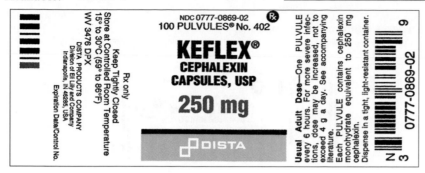

8. Order: Seconal 100 mg p.o. h.s.

   Available: Seconal capsules labeled 100 mg. _____

9. Order: Minipress 2 mg p.o. b.i.d. × 2 days.

   Available: _____

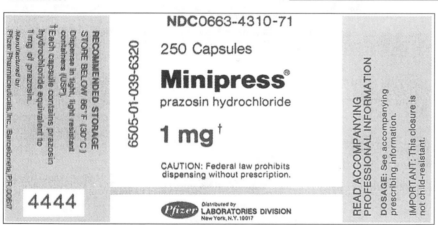

10. Order: Motrin 0.8 g p.o. q8hr p.r.n. for pain.

    Available: Tablets labeled 400 mg. _____

11. Order: Codeine gr ³/₄ p.o. q4h p.r.n. for pain.

    Available: _____

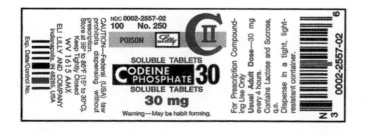

Notes

12. Order: Cephradine 0.5 g p.o. q6h.

    Available: Cephradine 250 mg caps.   _____

13. Order: Cogentin 0.5 mg p.o. h.s.

    Available: _____

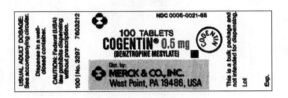

14. Order: Thorazine 75 mg p.o. b.i.d.

    Available: _____

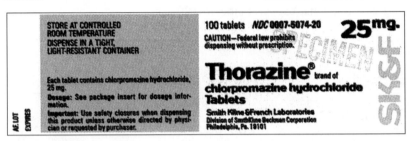

15. Order: Dilantin 60 mg p.o. b.i.d.

    Available: _____

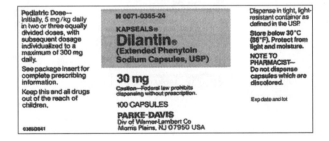

16. Order: Meperidine hydrochloride 50 mg I.M. q4h p.r.n. for pain.

    Available: Meperidine 75 mg/mL.   _____

17. Order: Solu-Medrol 60 mg I.V. o.d.

    Available: _____

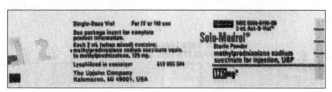

18. Order: Amikacin 90 mg I.M. q12h.

    Available: _____

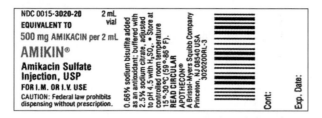

19. Order: Amoxicillin 300 mg p.o. q8h.

    Available: Amoxicillin 125 mg/5 mL.   _____

20. Order: Amoxicillin 0.5 g via nasogastric tube q6h.

    Available: _____

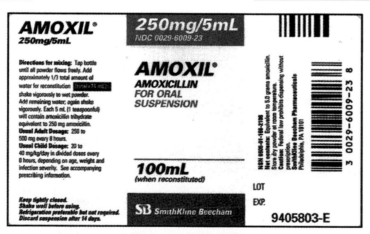

21. Order: Phenobarbital elixir 45 mg p.o. b.i.d.

    Available: Phenobarbital elixir 20 mg/5 mL.   _____

Notes

22. Order: Heparin 3,000 U s.c. b.i.d.

Available: _____

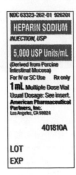

23. Order: Procaine penicillin 600,000 U I.M. q12h.

Available: _____

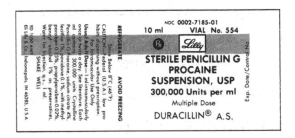

24. Order: Gentamicin 70 mg I.V. q8h.

Available: Gentamicin 80 mg/2 mL. _____

25. Order: Add potassium chloride 20 mEq to each I.V. bag.

Available: Potassium chloride 2 mEq/mL. _____

26. Order: Depo-Medrol 60 mg I.M. q. Monday × 2 weeks.

Available: _____

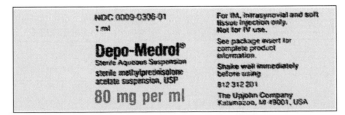

27. Order: Vistaril 100 mg I.M. stat.

Available: Vistaril 50 mg/mL. _____

28. Order: Morphine sulfate 6 mg s.c. q4h p.r.n. for pain.

Available: Morphine 10 mg/mL. _____

29. Order: Atropine 0.3 mg I.M. stat.

    Available: Atropine 0.4 mg/mL. _____

30. Order: Stadol 1 mg I.M. q4h p.r.n. for pain.

    Available: _____

31. Order: Ativan 1 mg I.M. stat.

    Available: Ativan 4 mg/mL. _____

32. Order: Kanamycin 250 mg I.M. q6h.

    Available: _____

33. Order: Robinul 0.4 mg I.M. stat on call to OR.

    Available: _____

34. Order: Aminophylline 80 mg I.V. q6h.

    Available: Aminophylline 25 mg/mL. _____

35. Order: Lithium citrate oral solution 300 mg t.i.d.

    Available: Lithium citrate 300 mg/5 mL. _____

Notes

36. Order: Sinemet 25/100 p.o. q.i.d.

Available: _____

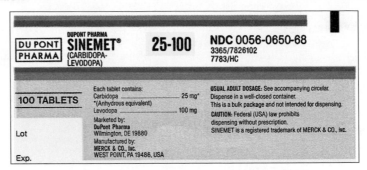

37. Order: Lopid 0.6 g p.o. b.i.d. 30 minutes before meals.

Available: _____

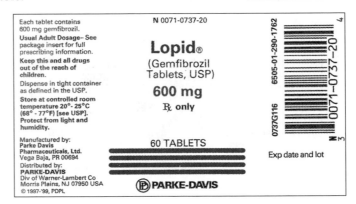

38. Order: Prozac 20 mg p.o. q.d.

Available: _____

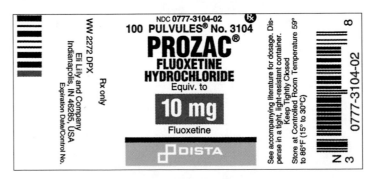

39. Order: Potassium chloride 10 mEq I.V. $\times$ 2 L.

    Available: _____

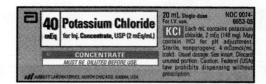

40. Order: Augmentin 0.875 g p.o. q12h.

    Available: _____

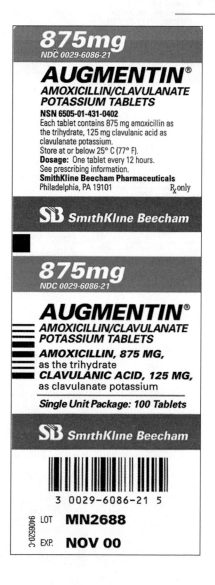

Notes

41. Order: Tagamet 800 mg p.o. h.s.

    Available: _____

    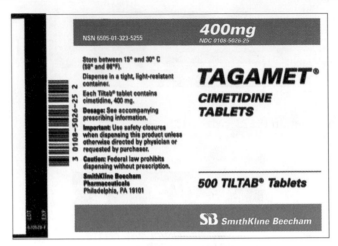

42. Order: Depo-Provera 500 mg I.M. once a week.

    Available: _____

    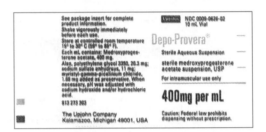

43. Order: Tagamet 300 mg I.V. q8h.

    Available: Tagamet 300 mg/2 mL.   _____

44. Order: Nembutal 150 mg I.M. h.s. p.r.n.

    Available: _____

    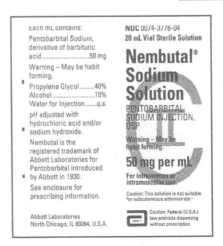

45. Order: Cipro 1.5 g p.o. q12h.

    Available: _____

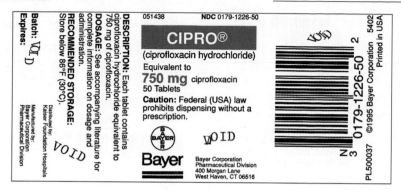

46. Order: Vasotec 5 mg p.o. q.d.

    Available: _____

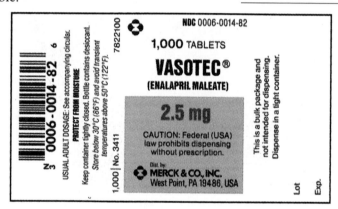

47. Order: Clozaril 50 mg p.o. b.i.d.

    Available: Tablets labeled 25 mg.   _____

48. Order: Clindamycin 450 mg p.o. q.i.d. × 5 days.

    Available: Oral solution labeled 75 mg/mL.   _____

49. Order: Benadryl 30 mg p.o. t.i.d.

    Available: Oral solution labeled 12.5 mg/5 mL. _____

50. Order: Primidone 125 mg p.o. q.d.

    Available: Oral solution labeled 250 mg/5 mL. _____

51. Order: Glucophage 0.5 g p.o. b.i.d.

Available:

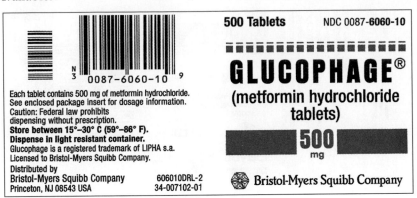

Answers on p. 513

UNIT FOUR

Oral and Parenteral Doseforms, Insulin, and Pediatric Dose Calculations

Oral medications are the easiest, most economical, and most frequently used medications, but sometimes parenteral (non-gastrointestinal tract) dosage routes are necessary. Both oral and parenteral drugs can be administered in liquid or powder form. In addition to oral and parenteral doseforms, this unit examines the varying types of insulin, as well as pediatric dose calculations.

Chapter 16
Calculation of Oral Medications

Chapter 17
Parenteral Medications

Chapter 18
Powdered Drugs

Chapter 19
Insulin

Chapter 20
Pediatric Dose Calculation

Calculation of Oral Medications

Objectives

After reviewing this chapter, you should be able to:

1. Identify the forms of oral medication
2. Identify the terms on the medication label to be used in calculation of doses
3. Calculate doses for oral and liquid medications using ratio-proportion or the formula method
4. Apply principles learned concerning tablet and liquid preparations to obtain a rational answer

The easiest, most economical, and most commonly used method of medication administration is p.o. Drugs for oral administration are available in solid forms such as tablets and capsules or as liquid preparations. To calculate doses appropriately the nurse needs to understand the principles that apply to administration of medications by this route.

FORMS OF SOLID MEDICATIONS

Tablets

Tablets are preparations of powdered drugs that have been molded into various sizes and shapes. Tablets come in a variety of doses that can be expressed in apothecaries' or metric measure—for example, milligrams and grains. There are different types of tablets (Figure 16-1, *A*).

Caplets

A caplet is a tablet that has an elongated shape like a capsule and is coated for ease of swallowing. Tylenol is available in caplet form.

Scored Tablets

These are tablets designed to administer a dose that is less than what is available in a single tablet. In other words, scored tablets have indentations or markings that allow you to break the tablet into halves or quarters. Only scored tablets should be broken because there is no way to determine the dose being administered when a nonscored tablet is broken. Breaking a tablet that is not scored could lead to the administration of an inaccurate dose if the table isn't divided equally. The purpose for the groove or indentation is to provide a guide for breaking a whole tablet into a fractional part (Figure 16-1, *B*). **Breaking an unscored tablet is risky, dangerous, and can lead to the administration of an unintended dose.** Examples of scored tablets are Lanoxin and Capoten (Figure 16-2).

Enteric-Coated Tablets

These are tablets with a special coating that protects them from the effects of gastric secretions and prevents them from dissolving in the stomach. They are dissolved and absorbed in the intestines.

The enteric coating also prevents the drug from becoming a source of irritation to the gastric mucosa, thereby preventing gastrointestinal upset. Examples include enteric-coated aspirin and iron tablets such as ferrous gluconate. **Enteric-coated tablets should never be crushed, because crushing them destroys the special coating and defeats its purpose.** Always consult a drug reference or the pharmacist when in doubt about the safety of crushing a tablet or opening capsules.

Sublingual Tablets

These tablets are designed to be placed under the tongue, where they dissolve in saliva and the medication is absorbed. Sublingual tablets should never be swallowed because this will prevent them from achieving their desired effect. Nitroglycerine, which is used for the relief of acute chest pain, is usually administered sublingually.

In addition to the types of tablets mentioned, "timed release" and extended release tablets are available. Medication from these tablets is released over a period of time, at specific time intervals. These types of preparations should be swallowed whole.

Capsules

A capsule is a form of medication that contains a powder, liquid, or oil enclosed in a hard or soft gelatin. Capsules come in a variety of colors, sizes, and doses. Some capsules have special shapes and colorings to identify which company produced them. Capsules are also available as timed release, sustained release, and spansules and work over a period of time.

Figure 16-1 **A,** Various shapes of tablets. **B,** Tablets scored in halves and fourths. (From Kee J and Hayes ER: *Pharmacology: a nursing process approach,* ed 3, Philadelphia, 2000, W.B. Saunders.)

Figure 16-2 Lanoxin tablet scored in half. (From Brown M and Mulholland J: *Drug calculations: process and problems for clinical practice,* ed 6, St Louis, 2000, Mosby.)

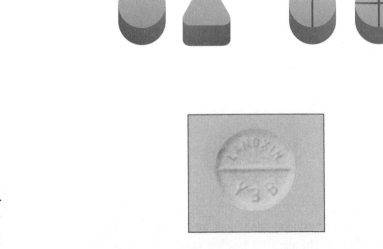

Capsules should always be administered whole to achieve the desired result (e.g., sustained release). Sustained-release and timed-release capsules cannot be divided or crushed (Figure 16-3). Always consult an appropriate reference or pharmacist when in doubt as to whether to open a capsule.

Examples of medications that come in capsule form are ampicillin, tetracycline, Colace, and lanoxicaps. Lanoxicap is an example of a capsule that has liquid medication contained in a gelatin capsule (Figure 16-4, *A*).

Although there are other forms of solid preparations for oral administration—such as lozenges and troches—tablets, capsules, and pulvules are the most common forms of solids requiring calculation encountered by the nurse. Figure 16-4 shows forms of solid oral medications, including capsules. Figures 16-4 through 16-6 show various types of capsules.

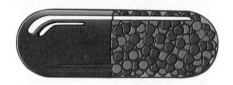

Figure 16-3 Timed-release capsule. (From Clayton B and Stock Y: *Basic pharmacology for nurses,* ed 12, St Louis, 2001, Mosby.)

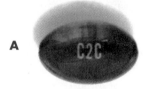

A

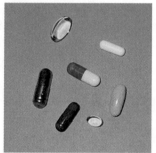

B

Figure 16-4 Various types of capsules. **A,** Lanoxicap. **B,** Different types of capsules. (From Brown M and Mulholland J: *Drug calculations: process and problems for clinical practice,* ed 6, St Louis, 2000, Mosby. **A,** Reproduced with permission of Glaxo Wellcome Inc. **B,** Courtesy Amanda Sunderman, St Louis, Mo.)

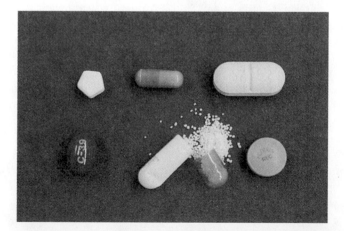

Figure 16-5 Forms of solid oral medications. Top row, unique by shaped tablet, capsule, scored tablet; bottom row, gelatin-coated liquid capsule, extended-release capsule, enteric-coated tablet. (From Potter PA and Perry AG: *Fundamental of nursing,* ed 5, St Louis, 2001, Mosby.)

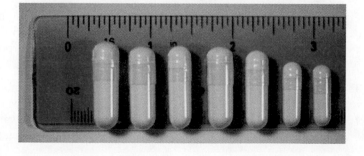

Figure 16-6 Various sizes and numbers of gelatin capsules. Courtesy of Oscar H. Allison (From Clayton B and Stock Y: *Basic pharmacology for nurses,* ed 12, St Louis, 2001, Mosby.)

CALCULATING DOSES INVOLVING TABLETS AND CAPSULES

When administering medications, you will have to calculate the number of tablets or capsules needed to administer the dose ordered. To help determine if your calculated dose is sensible, accurate, and safe, remember the following points:

POINTS TO REMEMBER

- Converting drug measures from one system to another and one unit to another to determine the dose to be administered can result in discrepancies, depending on the conversion factor used.

- Example: Aspirin may indicate on the label 5 grains (325 mg). This is based on the equivalent 65 mg = gr 1. On the other hand, another label on aspirin may indicate 5 grains (300 mg). Here the equivalent 60 mg = gr 1 was used. Both of the equivalents are correct. **Remember, equivalents are not exact.** Use the common equivalents when making conversions—for example, 60 mg = gr 1.

- When the precise number of tablets or capsules is determined and you find that administering the amount calculated is unrealistic or impossible, always use the following rule to avoid an error in administration: *No more than 10% variation should exist between the dose ordered and the dose administered.* For example, you may determine a client should receive 0.9 tablet or 0.9 capsule. Administration of such an amount accurately would be impossible. Following the stated rule, if you determined that 0.9 tablet or 0.9 capsule should be given, you could safely administer 1 tab or 1 cap.

- Capsules are not scored and cannot be divided. They are administered in whole amounts only. If a client has difficulty swallowing a capsule, check to see if a liquid preparation of the same drug is available. Never crush or open a timed-release capsule or empty its contents into a liquid or food; this may cause release of all the medication at once. There are, however, some instances in which a soft gelatin capsule filled with liquid may be pierced with a small sterile needle and the medication squeezed out for sublingual use. For example, Procardia (nifedipine) has been used in this way for severe hypertension. This drug is not approved by the FDA for use in this manner. When used in this manner, the action of the drug is erratic and shortterm. When administered in this manner, it can cause a hypotensive effect that is not easy to control. Precipitous drops in blood pressure can spell disaster for some clients. Over the years there have been reports of stroke and other complications resulting from lowering the blood pressure too much. It is important to note that administration of this medicine in this manner is not a practice.

- Pulvules are proprietary capsules containing a dose of a drug in powder form. For example, the popular and new antidepressant, Prozac, comes in pulvule form (proprietary capsules owned by a corporation under a trademark or patent).

- Tablets and capsules may be available in different strengths for administration, and you may have a choice when giving a dose. For example, 75 mg of a drug may be ordered. When you check what is available, it may be in tablet or capsule form as 10, 25, or 50 mg. In deciding the

Note:

This rule is often applied with adults, but not necessarily in the pediatric setting.

POINTS TO REMEMBER—cont'd

best combination of tablets or capsules to give, the nurse should always choose the strength that would allow the least number of tablets or capsules to be administered without breaking a tablet, if possible, because breaking is found to result in variations in dosage. In the example given, the best combination for administering 75 mg is one 50-mg tablet or capsule and one 25-mg tablet or capsule.

• The maximum number of tablets or capsules given to a client to achieve a certain dose is usually three. It is important to note that although the maximum number of tablets or capsules given to a client to administer a full dose is usually three, for some medications the client may have to take more than three to achieve the desired dose. This is true with some of the solid forms of HIV medications (e.g., tablets, capsules). Examples: Viracept 1,250 mg p.o. bid (available 250 mg/tab) and Ritonavir 400 mg p.o. q12h (available 100 mg/tab). Although many HIV medications come in liquid, many clients prefer to take tablets or capsules. **Remember:** Except for special medications, any more than 3 capsules or tablets to achieve a certain dose is unusual and may indicate an error in interpreting the order, transcribing, or in calculation. Think! Always question any order that exceeds this amount.

• When using the formula or ratio-proportion method to calculate tablet and capsule problems, remember that each tablet and capsule contains a certain weight of the drug. The weight indicated on a label is per tablet or per capsule. This is particularly important when reading a medication label on bottles or single unit-dose packages.

• In calculating oral doses you may encounter measures other than apothecaries' or metric measure. For example, electrolytes such as potassium will indicate the number of milliequivalents (mEq) per tablet. Units is another measure you may see for oral antibiotics or vitamins. For example, a vitamin E capsule will indicate 400 U per capsule. Units and milliequivalents measurements are specific to the drug they are being used for. There is no conversion between these and apothecaries' or metric measure. (These will be discussed in Chapter 17.)

• Always consult a drug reference or pharmacist when in doubt as to whether a capsule may be opened or pierced or whether a tablet can be crushed.

Remembering the points mentioned will be helpful before starting to calculate doses. Any of the methods presented in Chapters 14 and 15 can be used to determine the dose to be administered.

To compute doses accurately it is necessary to review a few reminders that were presented in previous chapters.

Critical Thinking

Question a dose that seems unreasonable or requires administering a drug by a route other than what the form indicates. Regardless of the source of error, if you administer the wrong dose or give a medication by a route other than it is intended you are legally responsible for the error.

Reminders

1. Read the problem carefully and
   a) Identify known factors
   b) Identify unknown factors
   c) Eliminate unnecessary information that is not relevant
2. Make sure that what is ordered and what is available are in the same system of measurement and units, or a conversion will be necessary. When a conversion is necessary, it is usual to convert what is ordered into what you have available or what is indicated on the drug label. You can, however, convert the measure in which the drug is available into the same units and system of measure as the dose ordered. The choice is usually based upon whichever is easier to calculate. Use any of the methods presented in Chapter 8 to make conversions consistent to avoid confusion. If necessary, go back and review these methods.
3. Consider what would be a reasonable answer based on what is ordered.
4. Set up the problem using ratio-proportion or the formula method.
5. Label the final answer (tablet, capsule).
6. For administration purposes, state answers to problems in fractions. Example: 1/2 tab, 1 1/2 tabs, instead of 0.5 tabs, 1.5 tabs.

Let's look at some sample problems calculating the number of tablets or capsules to administer.

Example 1: Order: Digoxin 0.375 mg p.o. o.d.

Available: Digoxin (scored tablets) labeled 0.25 mg

▶ Problem Setup

1. No conversion is necessary; the units are in the same system of measure.
   Order: 0.375 mg
   Available: 0.25 mg
2. Think critically: Tablets are scored; 0.375 mg is larger than 0.25 mg; therefore you will need more than 1 tab to administer the correct dose.
3. Solve using ratio-proportion or the formula method.

▶ Solution Using Ratio-Proportion Method

$$0.25 \text{ mg} : 1 \text{ tab} = 0.375 \text{ mg} : x \text{ tab}$$

(Known)   (Unknown)

(What's available)   (What's ordered)

$$\frac{0.25x}{0.25} = \frac{0.375}{0.25}$$

$$x = \frac{0.375}{0.25}$$

Therefore, $x = 1.5$ tabs or $1\frac{1}{2}$ tabs. (It is best to state it as $1\frac{1}{2}$ tabs for administration purposes.)

▶ Solution Using the Formula Method

$$\frac{(D)0.375 \text{ mg}}{(H)0.25 \text{ mg}} \times (Q) \ 1 \text{ tab} = x \text{ tab}$$

$$\frac{0.375}{0.25} \times 1 = x$$

$$x = 1\frac{1}{2} \text{ tabs}$$

Note:

You can administer $1\frac{1}{2}$ tabs because the tablets are scored. The above ratio-proportion could have been written as a fraction as well. (If necessary, review Chapter 4 on ratio-proportion.)

OR

$$\frac{(DW)\ 0.375\ mg}{(SW)\ 0.25\ mg} = \frac{(DV)x\ tab}{(SV)\ 1\ tab}$$

$$\frac{0.25x}{0.25} = \frac{0.375}{0.25}$$

$$x = \frac{0.375}{0.25}$$

$$x = 1\frac{1}{2}\ tabs$$

Example 2:   Order: Ampicillin 0.5 g p.o. q6h.

Available: Ampicillin capsules labeled 250 mg per capsule.

1. Order: 0.5 g
   Available: 250-mg capsules
2. After making the necessary conversion, think, what is a reasonable amount to administer?
3. Calculate the dose to be administered using ratio-proportion or the formula method.
4. Label your final answer (tablets, capsules).

➤ Problem Setup

1. Convert g to mg. Equivalent: 1,000 mg = 1 g

$$1,000\ mg : 1\ g = x\ mg : 0.5\ g$$

$$x = 1,000 \times 0.5$$

$$x = 500\ mg$$

Therefore 0.5 g is equal to 500 mg. Converting the g to mg eliminated a decimal, which is often the source of calculation errors. Converting mg to g would necessitate a decimal. Whenever possible, conversions that result in a decimal should be avoided to decrease the chance of error in calculating. Remember, a ratio-proportion could also be stated as a fraction. If necessary, review Chapter 4 on ratio-proportion. Because the measures are metric in this problem (g, mg), the other method that can be used is to move the decimal the desired number of places (0.5 g = 500 mg).

2. After making the conversion, you are now ready to calculate the dose to be given, using ratio-proportion or the formula method. In this problem we will use the answer obtained from converting what was ordered to what's available (0.5 g = 500 mg).

➤ Solution Using Ratio-Proportion Method

$$250\ mg : 1\ cap = 500\ mg : x\ cap$$

$$\frac{250x}{250} = \frac{500}{250}$$

$$x = \frac{500}{250}$$

$$x = 2\ caps$$

Note:

A conversion is necessary. The ordered dose and the available dose are in the same system of measurement (metric), but the units are different (g and mg). Before calculating the dose to be administered, you must have the ordered dose and the available dose in the same units.

Note:

2 caps is a logical answer. Capsules are administered in whole amounts; they are not dividable. Using the conversion obtained from converting mg to g in this problem would also net a final answer of 2 caps.

▶ Solution Using the Formula Method

$$\frac{(D)500 \text{ mg}}{(H)250 \text{ mg}} \times (Q) \; 1 \text{ cap} = x \text{ cap}$$

$$\frac{500}{250} \times 1 = x$$

$$x = 2 \text{ cap}$$

OR

$$\frac{(DW)500 \text{ mg}}{(SW)250 \text{ mg}} = \frac{(DV)x \text{ cap}}{(SV)1 \text{ cap}}$$

$$x = \frac{500}{250}$$

$$x = 2 \text{ caps}$$

Example 3:   Order: Nitroglycerin gr 1/150 sublingual p.r.n. for chest pain.

Available: Sublingual nitroglycerin tablets labeled 0.4 mg.

▶ Problem Setup

1. Conversion is required.
   Order: gr 1/150
   Available: 0.4 mg
   Equivalent 60 mg = gr 1. Convert what is ordered to the same system and units as what is available (gr is apothecaries', mg is metric).

$$60 \text{ mg} : \text{gr } 1 = x \text{ mg} : \text{gr } \frac{1}{150}$$

$$x = 60 \times \frac{1}{150}$$

$$x = \frac{60}{150}$$

$$x = 0.4 \text{ mg}$$

Note:

In this problem it was easier to change gr to mg; gr 1/150 is equal to 0.4 mg.

2. Think critically—it's obvious after making the conversion that you will give 1 tab.
3. Solve to obtain the desired dose.

▶ Solution Using Ratio-Proportion Method

$$0.4 \text{ mg} : 1 \text{ tab} = 0.4 \text{ mg} = x \text{ tab}$$

$$\frac{0.4x}{0.4} = \frac{0.4}{0.4}$$

$$x = \frac{0.4}{0.4}$$

$$x = 1 \text{ tab}$$

▶ Solution Using the Formula Method

$$\frac{(D) \; 0.4 \text{ mg}}{(H) \; 0.4 \text{ mg}} \times Q \; (1 \text{ tab}) = x \text{ tab}$$

$$\frac{0.4}{0.4} \times 1 = x$$

$$x = 1 \text{ tab}$$

OR

$$\frac{(DW)0.4\ mg}{(SW)0.4\ mg} = \frac{(DV)x\ tab}{(SV)1\ tab}$$

$$x = \frac{0.4}{0.4}$$

$$x = 1\ tab$$

Note:

This involved the division of decimals. Remember the rule for dividing decimals. If necessary, review Chapter 3 on decimals.

➡ Alternative Method of Doing Example 3

An alternative way of solving the problem in Example 3 is to eliminate the decimal and therefore convert 0.4 mg to gr. In doing this, more mathematical steps are involved. The same equivalent would be used.

$$60\ mg : gr\ 1 = 0.4\ mg : x\ gr$$

$$60x = 0.4$$

$$x = \frac{0.4}{60}$$

Remember: Apothecaries' measures are expressed using fractions. Therefore 0.4 must be divided by 60. To divide 0.4 by 60, the decimal point in the numerator is eliminated by moving the decimal point one place to the right to make it 4. For every place the decimal point is moved to make the numerator a whole number, a zero is added to the denominator; therefore the calculation is as follows:

$$\frac{0.4}{60} = \frac{4}{600}$$

$$\frac{4}{600} = \frac{1}{150}$$

Converting this way will net the same answer when calculating the dose to be given.

➡ Alternative Solution Using Ratio-Proportion Method

$$gr\ \frac{1}{150} : 1\ tab = gr\ \frac{1}{150} : x\ tab$$

$$\frac{\frac{1}{150}x}{\frac{1}{150}} = \frac{\frac{1}{150}}{\frac{1}{150}}$$

$$x = \frac{1}{150} \div \frac{1}{150}$$

$$x = \frac{1}{150} \times \frac{150}{1}$$

$$x = \frac{150}{150}$$

$$x = 1\ tab$$

➡ Alternative Solution Using the Formula Method

$$\frac{(D)\ gr\ \dfrac{1}{150}}{(H)\ gr\ \dfrac{1}{150}} \times Q\ (1\ tab) = x\ tab$$

Notes

$$\frac{\dfrac{1}{150}}{\dfrac{1}{150}} \times 1 = x$$

$$x = 1 \text{ tab}$$

OR

$$\frac{(DW) \text{ gr } \dfrac{1}{150}}{(SW) \text{ gr } \dfrac{1}{150}} = \frac{(DV)x \text{ tab}}{(SV)1 \text{ tab}}$$

$$x = \frac{\dfrac{1}{150}}{\dfrac{1}{150}}$$

$$x = 1 \text{ tab}$$

Example 4:   Order: Nembutal gr 1 1/2 p.o. h.s. p.r.n.

Available: Nembutal capsules labeled 100 mg

▶ **Problem Setup**

1. Convert gr 1 1/2 to mg. Equivalent: 60 mg = gr 1

$$60 \text{ mg} : \text{gr } 1 = x \text{ mg} : \text{gr } 1\frac{1}{2}$$

$$60 \text{ mg} : \text{gr } 1 = x \text{ mg} : \text{gr } \frac{3}{2}$$

$$x = 60 \times \frac{3}{2} = \frac{180}{2}$$

$$x = 90 \text{ mg}$$

2. Solve for the dose to be administered.

▶ **Solution Using Ratio-Proportion Method**

$$100 \text{ mg} : 1 \text{ cap} = 90 \text{ mg} : x \text{ cap}$$

$$\frac{100x}{100} = \frac{90}{100}$$

$$x = \frac{90}{100}$$

$$x = 0.9 \text{ cap}$$

Administer 1 cap.

Think Critically to Avoid Drug Calculation Errors

Capsules are not dividable; 0.9 is closest to 1 cap. It is safe to administer 1 cap; 1 cap falls within the 10% variation allowed between the dose ordered and the dose given.

▶ Solution Using the Formula Method

$$\frac{\text{(D) 90 mg}}{\text{(H) 100 mg}} \times Q \ (1 \ \text{cap}) = x \ \text{cap}$$

$$\frac{90}{100} \times 1 = x$$

$$x = 0.9 \ \text{cap}$$

Administer 1 capsule.

OR

$$\frac{\text{(DW) 90 mg}}{\text{(SW) 100 mg}} = \frac{\text{(DV)}x \ \text{cap}}{\text{(SV)}1 \ \text{cap}}$$

$$x = \frac{90}{100}$$

$$x = 0.9 \ \text{cap}$$

Administer 1 capsule.

As already discussed, alternative equivalents may be used to achieve the same answer. For example, if the equivalent 65 mg = gr 1 is used to convert gr 1 1/2 to mg, the answer for the conversion is 97.5 mg.

Therefore, in calculating the dose to administer, the precise answer would have been 0.975 cap. This would still require that 1 cap be administered. Remember, there is a 10% margin because of approximate equivalents.

Another alternative to the conversion for this problem might be to think 1,000 mg = 1 g. Therefore, because gr 15 = 1 g, 100 mg could be converted to gr as follows:

$$1,000 \ \text{mg} : \text{gr} \ 15 = 100 \ \text{mg} : x \ \text{gr}$$

$$1,000x = 1,500$$

$$x = \frac{1,500}{1,000}$$

$$x = \text{gr} \ 1\frac{1}{2}$$

Converting in this manner will give the same answer of 1 cap as illustrated using the ratio-proportion method to calculate the dose to be given.

$$\text{gr} \ 1\frac{1}{2} : 1 \ \text{cap} = \text{gr} \ 1\frac{1}{2} : x \ \text{cap}$$

$$\text{gr} \ \frac{3}{2} : 1 \ \text{cap} = \text{gr} \ \frac{3}{2} : x \ \text{cap}$$

$$\frac{3}{2}x = \frac{3}{2}$$

$$x = \frac{3}{2} \div \frac{3}{2}$$

$$x = \frac{3}{2} \times \frac{2}{3}$$

$$x = \frac{6}{6}$$

$$x = 1 \ \text{cap}$$

Note:

gr 1 1/2 can be changed to an improper fraction for the purpose of calculating.

Example 5:   Order: Thorazine 100 mg p.o. t.i.d.

Available: Thorazine tablets labeled 25 mg and 50 mg

➤ Problem Setup

1. No conversion is necessary.
2. Thinking critically: 100 mg is larger than 25 or 50 mg. Therefore more than 1 tab is needed to administer the dose. The client should always be given the strength of tablets or capsules that would require the least number to be taken.
3. In this problem, selection of the 50-mg tablets would require the client to receive 2 tabs, whereas using 25-mg tablets would require 4 tabs to be administered.

➤ Solution Using Ratio-Proportion Method

$$50 \text{ mg} : 1 \text{ tab} = 100 \text{ mg} : x \text{ tab}$$

$$\frac{50x}{50} = \frac{100}{50}$$

$$x = 2 \text{ tabs (50 mg each)}$$

➤ Solution Using the Formula Method

$$\frac{\text{(D) } 100 \text{ mg}}{\text{(H) } 50 \text{ mg}} \times Q \, (1 \text{ tab}) = x \text{ tab}$$

$$\frac{100}{50} \times 1 = x$$

$$x = 2 \text{ tabs (50 mg each)}$$

OR

$$\frac{\text{(DW)} 100 \text{ mg}}{\text{(SW)} 50 \text{ mg}} = \frac{\text{(DV)} x \text{ tab}}{\text{(SV)} 1 \text{ tab}}$$

$$x = \frac{100}{50}$$

$$x = 2 \text{ tabs (50 mg each)}$$

Note:

In Example 5, not only is the number of tablets specified, but the strength of tablets chosen is specified as well. This could have been done without placing it into a formula or using ratio-proportion.

Variation of Tablet and Capsule Problems

You will at times find it necessary to decide how many tablets or capsules are needed. This requires knowing the dosage and frequency. Numerous scenarios could arise, but for the purpose of illustration we will use one: A client is going out of town on vacation and needs to know whether it's necessary to refill the prescription before leaving.

Example 1:   A client has an order for Valium 10 mg p.o. q.i.d. and has 5 mg tablets. The client is going out of town for 7 days, and wants to know how many tablets to take along.

Solution: To obtain 10 mg the client requires two 5-mg tablets each time. Therefore eight 5-mg tablets are necessary to administer the dose q.i.d. (four times a day).
(Number of days ordered for) ×
(Number of tablets needed per day)
= Total number of tablets needed

$$8 \times 7 = 56$$

Answer: Total number of tablets needed for 7 days would be 56 tabs

Determining the Dose to Be Given Each Time

Example 2: A client is to receive 1 g of a drug p.o. daily. The drug should be given in four equally divided doses.

How many mg should the client receive each time the medication is administered?

Solution: $\dfrac{\text{Total daily allowance}}{\text{Number of doses per day}} = \text{Dose to be administered}$

Answer: $\dfrac{1 \text{ g } (1{,}000 \text{ mg})}{4} = 250 \text{ mg}$

POINTS TO REMEMBER

- The maximum number of tablets and capsules to administer to achieve a desired dose is usually three. Question any order for more than this before administering.

- Before calculating a dose, make sure that the dose ordered and what's available are in the same system of measurement and units. When a conversion is required, it is usually best to convert the dose ordered to what's available.

- No more than a 10% variation should exist between the dose ordered and the dose administered.

- Regardless of the method used to calculate a dose, it is important to develop the ability to think critically about what is a reasonable amount.

- State doses as you are actually going to administer them. Example: 0.5 tab = 1/2 tab.

PRACTICE PROBLEMS

Directions: Calculate the correct number of tablets or capsules to be administered in the following problems using the labels or information provided. Use any of the methods presented to calculate the dose.

Remember to label your answers.

Notes

1. Order: Synthroid 0.025 mg p.o. q.d.

   Available: Scored tablets.   _____

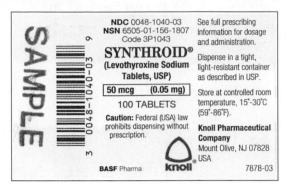

2. Order: Capoten 6.25 mg p.o. b.i.d.

   Available: Tablets scored in fourths.   _____

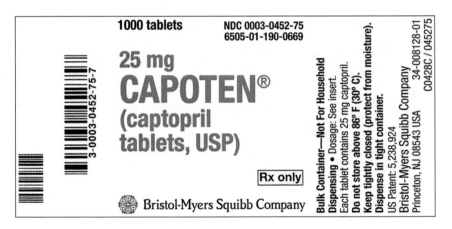

3. Order: Ethambutol 1.2 g p.o. o.d.

   Available: _____

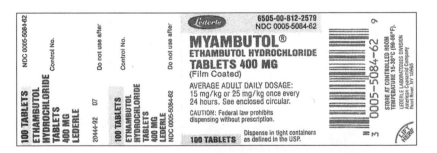

Notes

4. Order: Coumadin 7.5 mg p.o. h.s.

   Available: Scored tablets.

   a) What would be the appropriate
      strength tablet to use?   _____

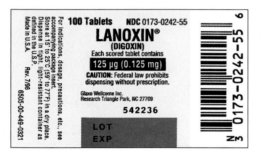

   COUMADIN®   2½ mg
   (Warfarin Sodium Tablets, USP)
   Crystalline
   DuPont Pharma
   Wilmington, Delaware 19880
   LOT JJ275A
   EXP

   COUMADIN®   5 mg
   (Warfarin Sodium Tablets, USP)
   Crystalline
   DuPont Pharma
   Wilmington, Delaware 19880
   LOT KA009A
   EXP

5. Order: Lanoxin 0.125 mg p.o. q.d.

   Available: Scored tablets.

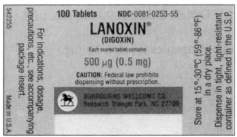

   a) What is the appropriate strength tablet to use? _____

   b) What will you prepare to administer?   _____

6. Order: Ampicillin 1 g p.o. q6h.

   Available: Ampicillin capsules labeled 500 mg and 250 mg.

   a) Which strength capsule is appropriate
      to use?   _____

   b) How many capsules are needed for one dose? _____

   c) What is the total number of capsules needed
      if the medication is ordered for 7 days?   _____

7. Order: Reglan 10 mg p.o. t.i.d. 1/2 hr a.c.

   Available: Reglan tablets labeled 5 mg.   _____

8. Order: Baclofen 15 mg p.o. t.i.d. × 3 days.

   Available: Scored tablets.

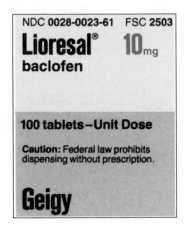

   a) How many tablets are needed for one dose?　_____

   b) What is the total number of mg the client
      will receive in 3 days?　_____

9. Order: Synthroid 0.075 mg p.o. q.d.

   Available: Synthroid scored tablets
   labeled 50 mcg.　_____

10. Order: Calcium carbonate 1.3 g p.o. o.d.

    Available: Calcium carbonate tablets
    labeled 650 mg.　_____

11. Order: Dilantin 90 mg p.o. t.i.d.

    Available: Dilantin capsules labeled 30 mg.　_____

12. Order: Tegretol 200 mg p.o. t.i.d.

    Available:

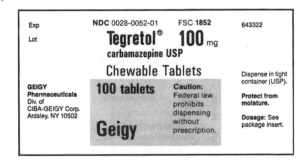

    a) How many tablets will you administer for
       each dose?　_____

13. Order: Dicloxacillin 1 g p.o. as an initial dose and 0.5 g p.o. q6h thereafter.

Available:

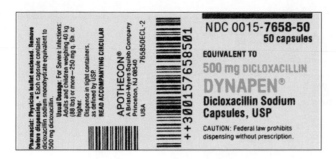

   a) How many capsules will you need for the
      initial dose?   _____

   b) How many capsules are needed for each
      subsequent dose?   _____

14. Order: Aldomet 250 mg p.o. b.i.d.

Available:

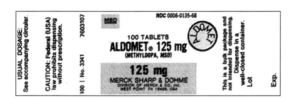

   a) How many tablets will you administer for
      each dose?   _____

15. Order: Phenobarbital gr $1\frac{1}{2}$ p.o. h.s.

Available: Phenobarbital 15-mg tabs and
30-mg tabs.   _____

   a) Which strength tablet is best to administer?   _____

   b) How many tablets of which strength will
      you prepare to administer?   _____

Notes

16. Order: Decadron 3 mg p.o. b.i.d. × 2 days.

    Available:

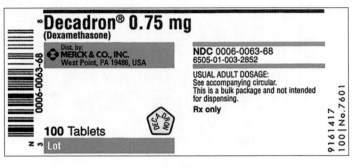

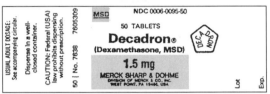

    a) Which is the best strength to administer? _____

    b) How many tablets of which strength will
       you prepare to administer? _____

17. Order: Thorazine 100 mg p.o. t.i.d.

    Available:

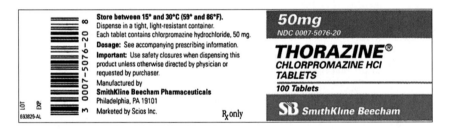

    a) How many tablets are needed for 3 days? _____

18. Order: Verapamil 120 mg p.o. t.i.d. Hold for systolic blood pressure <100,
    heart rate <55.

    Available: Verapamil scored tablets labeled
    80 mg and 40 mg.

    a) Which is the best strength tablet to use? _____

    b) How many of which strength tablet will
       you administer? _____

19. Order: Acetaminophen grx p.o. q4h p.r.n. for a temp >101° F.

    Available: _____

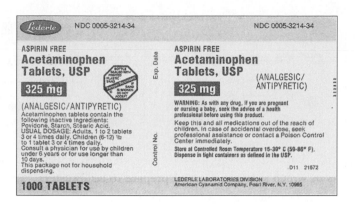

20. Order: Cogentin 1 mg p.o. t.i.d.

    Available: _____

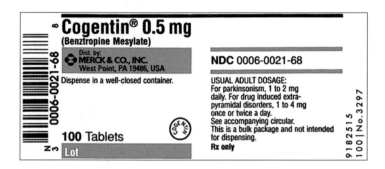

21. Order: Prazosin hydrochloride 3 mg p.o. b.i.d.

    Available: Prazosin hydrochloride capsules
    labeled 1 mg.   _____

22. Order: Nitroglycerin gr 1/150 SL p.r.n.

    Available: _____

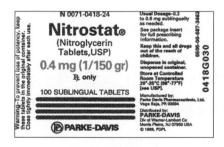

23. Order: Dexamethasone 6 mg p.o. o.d.

Available: Scored tablets.

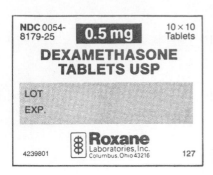
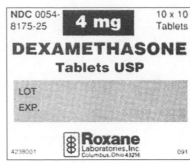
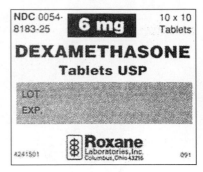

a) How many of which strength tablets will
you give?   _____

24. Order: Pyridium 0.2 g p.o. q8h.

Available: Pyridium tablets labeled 100 mg.   _____

25. Order: Lasix 60 mg p.o. stat.

Available: Scored tablets.   _____

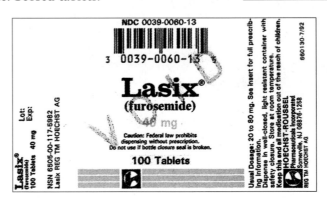

26. Order: Glyburide 2.5 mg p.o. o.d.

Available: Scored Glyburide tablets labeled 5 mg.

a) How many tablets will you administer
for each dose?   _____

27. Order: Tagamet 400 mg p.o. b.i.d.

Available: Tagamet tablets labeled 200 mg.

a) How many tablets will you administer
for each dose?   _____

28. Order: Indocin SR 150 mg p.o. b.i.d.

    Available:

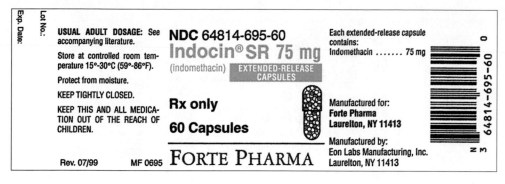

a) How many capsules will you administer for each dose? _____

29. Order: Sulfasalazine 1 g p.o. q6h.

    Available:

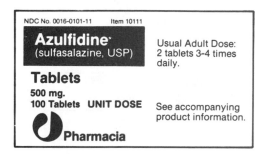

a) How many tablets will you administer for each dose? _____

30. Order: Capoten 12.5 mg p.o. b.i.d.

    Available: Scored capoten tablets (quarters) labeled 25 mg.

a) How many tablets will you administer for each dose? _____

31. Order: Synthroid 100 mcg p.o. o.d.

    Available: Synthroid tablets labeled 75 mcg and 25 mcg.

a) How many tablets of which strength will you use to administer the dose? _____

Notes

32. Order: Capoten 25 mg p.o. q8h.

    Available: _____

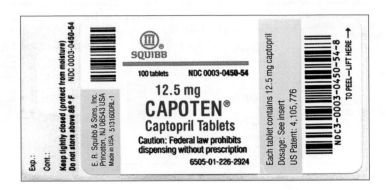

33. Order: Clonazepam 0.25 mg p.o. b.i.d. and h.s.

    Available: Clonazepam scored tablets
    labeled 0.5 mg. _____

34. Order: Augmentin 0.25 g p.o. q8h.

    Available: _____

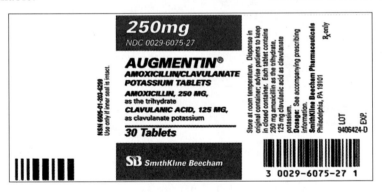

35. Order: Synthroid 25 mcg p.o. o.d.

    Available: Synthroid tablet labeled
    0.025 mg (25 mcg). _____

36. Order: Aspirin 650 mg p.o. q4h p.r.n.

    Available: Aspirin tablets 325 mg. _____

37. Order: Dilantin extended capsules 0.2 g p.o. t.i.d.

    Available: _____

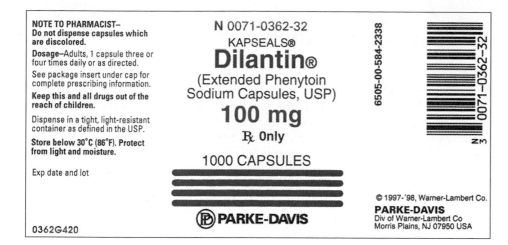

38. Order: Motrin 800 mg p.o. q6h p.r.n.

    Available: _____

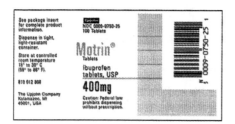

39. Order: Procardia XL 60 mg p.o. q.d.

    Available: Procardia XL labeled
    30 mg per tablet.   _____

40. Order: Isoniazid 0.3 g p.o. q.d.

    Available: _____

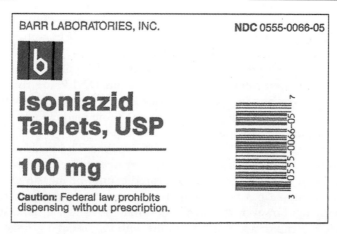

Notes

41. Doctor's Order: Inderal LA 160 mg p.o. q.d.

Available: Inderal LA capsules labeled 80 mg. _____

Answers on pp. 513-517

CALCULATING ORAL LIQUIDS

Medications are also available in liquid form for oral administration. Liquid medications are desirable to use for clients who have dysphagia (difficulty swallowing) or who are receiving medications by tubes such as nasogastric (tube in nose to stomach), gastrostomy (tube placed directly into stomach), or jejunostomy (tube directly into intestines). Liquid medications are also desired for use in young children, infants, and elderly clients. When medications are ordered that cannot be crushed for administration, the availability of the medication in liquid form should be investigated. Medications in liquid form contain a specific amount or weight of a drug in a given amount of solution that is indicated on the label. Liquid medications are prepared in different forms, as follows:

1. Elixir—Alcohol solution that is sweet and aromatic.
   Example: Phenobarbital elixir.
2. Suspension—One or more drugs finely divided into a liquid such as water.
   Example: Penicillin suspension.
3. Syrup—Medication dissolved in concentrated solution of sugar and water.
   Example: Colace.

Liquid medications also come as tincture and extract preparations for oral use. Although oral liquids may be administered by means other than p.o., as already discussed, they should **never** be given by any other route, such as I.V. or by injection.

In solving problems that involve oral liquids, the methods presented in Chapters 14 and 15 can be used; however, you must calculate the volume or amount of liquid that contains the dose of the medication. This information is usually indicated on the medication label and can be expressed per milliliter, ounce, etc.—for example, 25 mg per mL. The amount may also be expressed in terms of multiple milliliters. Example: 80 mg per 2 mL, 125 mg per 5 mL.

When calculating liquid medications, the stock or what you have available is in liquid form; therefore the label on your answer will always be expressed in liquid measures such as mL.

MEASURING ORAL LIQUIDS

Liquid medications can be measured in several ways:

1. The standard measuring cup (plastic), which is calibrated in metric, apothecaries', and household measures, can be used. When pouring liquid medications, pour them at eye level and read at the meniscus (a curvature made by the solution) while the cup is on a flat surface (Figure 16-7).
2. Calibrated droppers are also used for measuring liquid medications (Figure 16-8). **A calibrated dropper should be used ONLY for medication intended; they are not interchangeable.** If a dropper comes with a medication, it can only be used for that medication. Some medicine droppers are calibrated in mL or by actual dose.
3. Syringes may also be used to measure medications. The medication is poured in a medication cup and drawn up in the syringe without the use of a needle. This is often done when the amount desired cannot be measured accurately in a cup. For example 6.3 mL cannot be measured accurately in the standard medication cup; however, the medication may be drawn up in a syringe, then squirted into a cup or administered orally with the use of a syringe without the

needle. Solutions can also be measured using a specially calibrated *oral syringe* (Figure 16-9). Oral syringes are not sterile, are often available in colors, and have an off-center tip. These features make it easy to distinguish from the hypodermic syringe. Oral syringes may also have markings such as teaspoon and tablespoon. Figure 16-10 demonstrates how to fill a syringe from a medicine cup. Some oral liquid medications come in containers that allow the client to drink right out of the container, therefore eliminating the need to transfer it to a medication cup.

Before we proceed to calculate liquid medications, let's review some helpful pointers.

1. The label on the medication container must be read carefully to determine the dose strength in the volume of solution, because it varies. **Do not confuse dose strength with the total volume.** For example: the label on a medication may indicate a total volume of 100 mL, but the dose strength may be 125 mg per 5 mL. Important to note, dose strength can be written on solutions in several ways to indicate the same thing. For example, 125 mg per 5 mL may be written as 125 mg/5 mL or 125 mg = 5 mL. Other examples of dose strength: 20 mg per mL, 20 mg/mL, 200 mg/5 mL, 200 mg per 5 mL.

2. Answers are labeled using liquid measures. Example: mL.

3. Calculations can be done using the same methods (formula, ratio-proportion) and the same steps as for solid forms of oral medications.

Now let's look at some sample problems that involve the calculation of oral liquids.

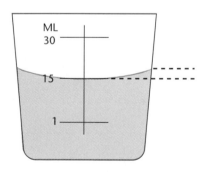

Figure 16-7 Reading meniscus. The meniscus is caused by the surface tension of the solution against the walls of the container. The surface tension causes the formation of a concave or hollowed curvature on the surface of the solution. Read the level at the lowest point of the concave curve. (From Clayton B and Stock Y: *Basic pharmacology for nurses,* ed 12, St Louis, 2001, Mosby.)

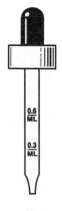

Figure 16-8 Medicine dropper. (From Brown M and Mulholland J: *Drug calculations: process and problems for clinical practice,* ed 6, St Louis, 2000, Mosby.)

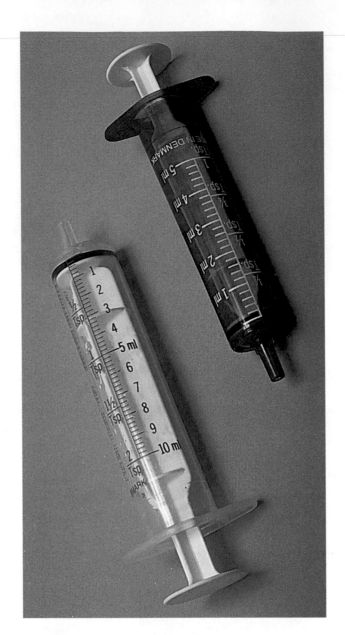

Figure 16-9 Oral syringes. (Courtesy Chuck Dresner. From Clayton B and Stock Y: *Basic pharmacology for nurses,* ed 12, St Louis, 2001, Mosby.)

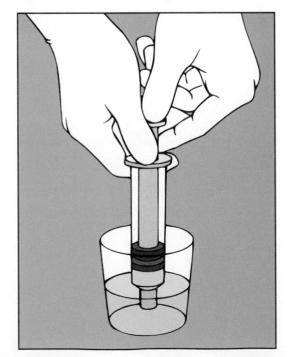

Figure 16-10 Filling a syringe directly from medicine cup. (From Clayton B and Stock Y: *Basic pharmacology for nurses,* ed 12, St Louis, 2001, Mosby.)

Example 1: Order: Dilantin 200 mg p.o. t.i.d.

Available: Dilantin suspension labeled 125 mg per 5 mL.

▶ Problem Setup

1. No conversion is required. Everything is in the same units of measure and the same system.
   Order: 200 mg.
   Available: 125 mg per 5 mL.
2. Think critically: What would be a logical answer? Looking at Example 1, you can assume the answer will be greater than 5 mL.
3. Set up the problem using the ratio-proportion or formula method.
4. Label the final answer with the correct unit of measure. In this case the label will be mL. Remember: The answer has no meaning without the appropriate label.

▶ Solution Using Ratio-Proportion Method

$$125 \text{ mg} : 5 \text{ mL} = 200 \text{ mg} : x \text{ mL}$$

$$\text{(Known)} \qquad \text{(Unknown)}$$

$$125x = 200 \times 5$$

$$\frac{125x}{125} = \frac{1{,}000}{125}$$

$$x = \frac{1{,}000}{125}$$

$$x = 8 \text{ mL}$$

▶ Solution Using the Formula Method

$$\frac{\text{(D)}200 \text{ mg}}{\text{(H)}125 \text{ mg}} \times \text{(Q) } 5 \text{ mL} = x \text{ mL}$$

$$\frac{200}{125} \times 5 = x$$

$$\frac{1{,}000}{125} = x$$

$$x = 8 \text{ mL}$$

OR

$$\frac{\text{(DW)}200 \text{ mg}}{\text{(SW)}125 \text{ mg}} = \frac{\text{(DV)}x \text{ mL}}{\text{(SV)}5 \text{ mL}}$$

$$\frac{125x}{125} = \frac{1{,}000}{125}$$

$$x = \frac{1{,}000}{125}$$

$$x = 8 \text{ mL}$$

Example 2: Order: Lactulose 30 g p.o. b.i.d.

Available: Lactulose labeled 10 g = 15 mL.

Note:

When possible, the numbers may be reduced to make them smaller and easier to deal with.

> **Solution Using Ratio-Proportion Method**

$$10 \text{ g} : 15 \text{ mL} = 30 \text{ g} : x \text{ mL}$$

$$\frac{10x}{10} = \frac{450}{10}$$

$$x = \frac{450}{10}$$

$$x = 45 \text{ mL}$$

> **Solution Using the Formula Method**

$$\frac{(D)30 \text{ g}}{(H)10 \text{ g}} \times (Q) \ 15 \text{ mL} = x \text{ mL}$$

$$\frac{30 \times 15}{10} = x$$

$$x = \frac{450}{10}$$

$$x = 45 \text{ mL}$$

OR

$$\frac{(DW)30 \text{ g}}{(SW)10 \text{ g}} = \frac{(DV)x \text{ mL}}{(SV)15 \text{ mL}}$$

$$\frac{10x}{10} = \frac{450}{10}$$

$$x = \frac{450}{10}$$

$$x = 45 \text{ mL}$$

Note:

A conversion is necessary before calculating the dose. What the doctor has ordered is different from what's available.

Example 3: Order: Elixir of phenobarbital gr iss p.o. o.d.

Available: Elixir of phenobarbital labeled 20 mg per 5 mL.

Order: gr 1 1/2.

Available: 20 mg per 5 mL.

Equivalent: 60 mg = gr 1

$$60 \text{ mg} : \text{gr } 1 = x \text{ mg} : \text{gr } 1\frac{1}{2} \left(\frac{3}{2} \right)$$

$$60 \text{ mg} : \text{gr } 1 = x \text{ mg} : \text{gr } \frac{3}{2}$$

$$x = \frac{180}{2}$$

$$x = 90 \text{ mg}$$

> **Solution Using Ratio-Proportion Method**

$$20 \text{ mg} : 5 \text{ mL} = 90 \text{ mg} : x \text{ mL}$$

$$\frac{20x}{20} = \frac{450}{20}$$

$$x = \frac{450}{20}$$

$$x = 22.5 \text{ mL} \quad \text{or} \quad 22\frac{1}{2} \text{ mL}$$

➡ Solution Using the Formula Method

$$\frac{\text{(D)90 mg}}{\text{(H)20 mg}} \times \text{(Q) 5 mL} = x \text{ mL}$$

$$\frac{90 \times 5}{20} = x$$

$$x = \frac{450}{20}$$

$$x = 22.5 \text{ mL or } 22\frac{1}{2} \text{ mL}$$

OR

$$\frac{\text{(DW)90 mg}}{\text{(SW)20 mg}} = \frac{\text{(DV)}x \text{ mL}}{\text{(SV)5 mL}}$$

$$\frac{20x}{20} = \frac{450}{20}$$

$$x = \frac{450}{20}$$

$$x = 22.5 \text{ mL or } 22\frac{1}{2} \text{ mL}$$

Note:

Some medication orders state the specific amount to be given and therefore require no calculation. Examples: milk of magnesia (1 ounce) p.o. h.s.; Robitussin 15 mL p.o. q4h p.r.n.; multivitamin 1 tab p.o. o.d.; Fer-In-Sol 0.2 cc p.o. o.d.

POINTS TO REMEMBER ✛ ─ > ≡

- Liquid medications can be calculated using the same methods as those used for solid forms (tabs, caps).

- Read labels carefully on medication containers; identify the dose strength contained in a certain amount of solution.

- Administration of accurate doses of liquid medications may require the use of calibrated droppers or syringes. Oral syringes are designed for oral use; they are not sterile.

- The use of ratio-proportion or a formula is a means of validating an answer; however, it still requires thinking in terms of the dose you will administer and applying principles learned to calculate doses that are sensible and safe.

- Dose strength on solutions can be written several ways. Do not confuse it with total volume (total amount in container).

- For accurate measurement oral solutions are poured at eye level, and read at eye level while resting on a flat surface.

- Calibrated droppers should be used only for the medication they are intended for.

 ## PRACTICE PROBLEMS

Calculate the following doses for oral liquids in mL. Don't forget to label your answer. Labels have been included when possible. Round answers to the nearest tenth where indicated.

Notes

42. Order: Colace syrup 100 mg by jejunostomy tube t.i.d.

    Available: Colace syrup 50 mg/15 mL.   _____

43. Order: Ascorbic acid 1 g by nasogastric tube b.i.d.

    Available: Ascorbic acid solution
    500 mg = 10 mL.   _____

44. Order: Kaon-Cl 40 mEq p.o. qd.

    Available: Potassium oral solution
    40 mEq = 15 mL.   _____

45. Order: Theophylline elixir 80 mg/15 mL p.o. b.i.d.

    Available: Theophylline elixir 80 mg/5 mL.   _____

46. Order: Erythromycin oral suspension 250 mg po q6h.

    Available: _____

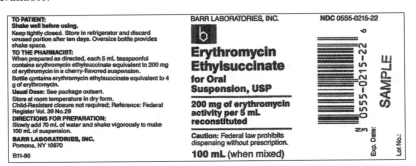

47. Order: Dilantin 100 mg p.o. t.i.d.

    Available: Dilantin suspension 125 mg/5 mL.   _____

48. Order: Digoxin 125 mcg p.o. o.d.

    Available: _____

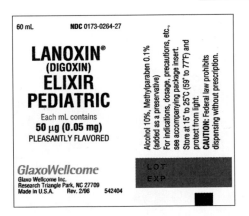

49. Order: Keflex 250 mg p.o. q6h.

    Available: Keflex suspension 125 mg/5 mL.   _____

50. Order: Amoxicillin 0.5 g p.o. q6h.

    Available: _____

AMOXIL®
125mg/5mL

125mg/5mL
NDC 0029-6008-23

AMOXIL®
AMOXICILLIN
FOR ORAL
SUSPENSION

Directions for mixing: Tap bottle until all powder flows freely. Add approximately 1/3 total amount of water for reconstitution (total=78 mL); shake vigorously to wet powder. Add remaining water; again shake vigorously. Each 5 mL (1 teaspoonful) will contain amoxicillin trihydrate equivalent to 125 mg amoxicillin.
Usual Adult Dosage: 250 to 500 mg every 8 hours.
Usual Child Dosage: 20 to 40 mg/kg/day in divided doses every 8 hours, depending on age, weight and infection severity. See accompanying prescribing information.

100mL
(when reconstituted)

Rx only

NSN 6505-01-153-3862
Net contents: Equivalent to 2.5 grams amoxicillin.
Store dry powder at room temperature.
SmithKline Beecham Pharmaceuticals
Philadelphia, PA 19101

3 0029-6008-23 1

Keep tightly closed.
Shake well before using.
Refrigeration preferable but not required.
Discard suspension after 14 days.

SB SmithKline Beecham

LOT

EXP.

9405793-F

51. Order: Phenobarbital 60 mg p.o. h.s.

    Available: Phenobarbital elixir 20 mg/5 mL. _____

52. Order: Mellaril 150 mg p.o. b.i.d.

    Available: Mellaril 30 mg/mL. _____

53. Order: Diphenhydramine HCl 25 mg p.o. b.i.d. p.r.n. for agitation.

    Available: Diphenhydramine hydrochloride
    elixir 12.5 mg/5 mL. _____

54. Order: Lithium carbonate 600 mg p.o. h.s.

    Available: Lithium citrate syrup. Each 5 mL contains lithium carbonate 300 mg. (Each unit dose container contains 5 mL.)

    a) How many mL are needed to administer
       the required dose? _____

    b) How many containers of the drug will you need
       to prepare the dose? _____

55. Order: Haldol 10 mg p.o. b.i.d.

    Available: Haldol concentrate labeled 2 mg/mL. _____

Notes

56. Order: Dicloxacillin sodium 0.5 g by gastrostomy tube q6h.

    Available: Dicloxacillin suspension 100 mL, labeled 62.5 mg per 5 mL.   _____

57. Order: V-Cillin K suspension 500,000 U p.o. q.i.d.

    Available: V-Cillin K oral solution 200,000 Units per 5 mL.   _____

58. Order: Keflex 1 g by nasogastric tube q6h.

    Available: Keflex oral suspension 125 mg/5 mL.   _____

59. Order: Trilafon 24 mg p.o. b.i.d.

    Available: Trilafon concentrate labeled 16 mg/5 mL.   _____

60. Order: Acetaminophen elixir 650 mg by nasogastric tube q4h p.r.n. for temperature greater than 101° F.

    Available: Acetaminophen elixir labeled 500 mg/15 mL.   _____

61. Order: Tagamet 400 mg p.o. q6h.

    Available: Tagamet labeled 300 mg/5 mL.   _____

62. Order: Epivir 150 mg p.o. b.i.d.

    Available: _____

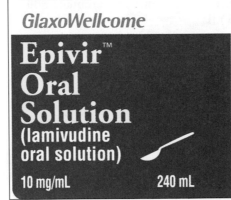

63. Order: Retrovir 0.3 g p.o. b.i.d.

    Available: _____

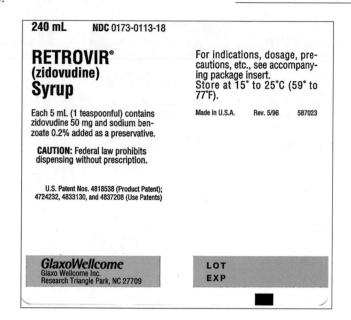

64. Order: Mycostatin suspension 200,000 U p.o. b.i.d.

    Available: _____

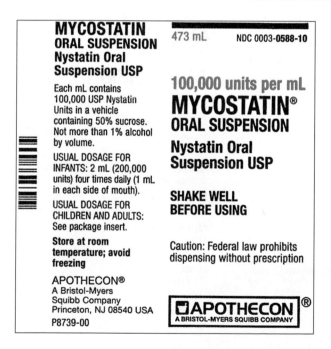

65. Order: Thorazine concentrate 150 mg p.o. b.i.d.

    Available: Thorazine concentrate 100 mg/mL. _____

Notes

66. Order: Augmentin 0.25 g p.o. q8h.

Available: _____

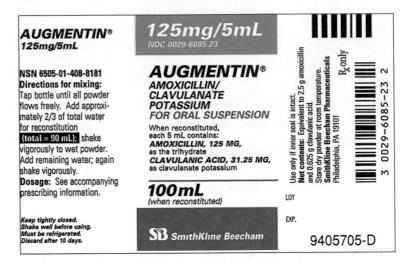

67. Order: Zovirax 200 mg p.o. q4h × 5 days.

Available: _____

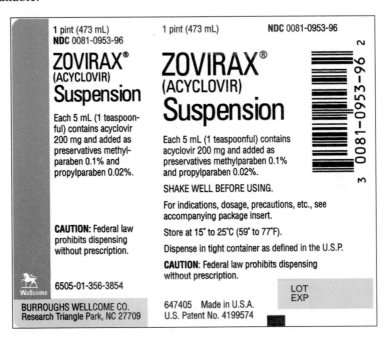

68. Order: Prozac 30 mg p.o. q.d. in AM.

    Available: _____

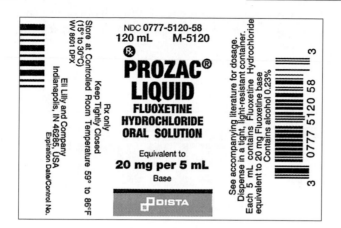

69. Order: Zantac 150 mg b.i.d. via nasogastric tube.

    Available: _____

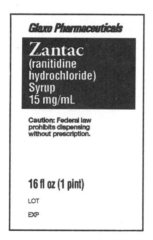

70. Order: Mellaril 50 mg p.o. t.i.d.

    Available: _____

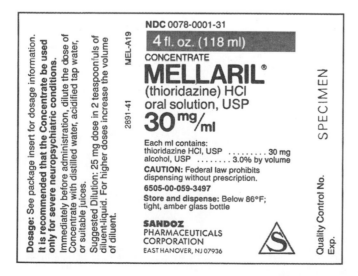

Answers on pp. 517-520

Notes

✓ **CHAPTER REVIEW**

Calculate the following doses using the medication label or information provided. Express volume answers in mL; round answers to the nearest tenth as indicated.

1. Order: Tylenol 975 mg p.o. q6h p.r.n. for earache.

   Available: _____

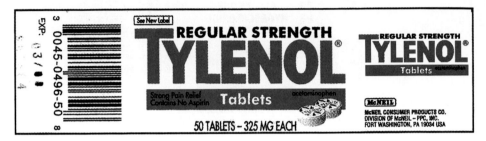

2. Order: Dilantin 300 mg p.o. q.d.

   Available: _____

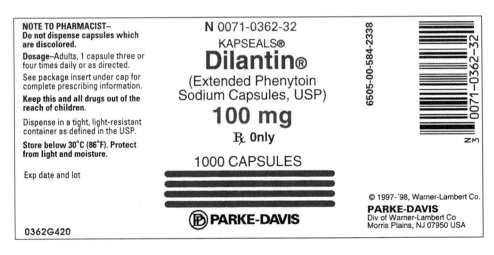

3. Order: Lopressor 100 mg p.o. b.i.d., hold for B/P <100/60.

   Available: Lopressor tablets 50 mg.   _____

4. Order: Pravachol 30 mg p.o. qhs.

   Available: _____

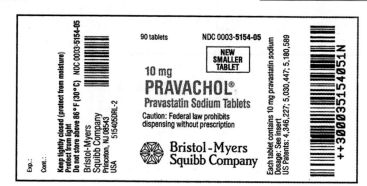

5. Order: Atacand 16 mg p.o. o.d. Hold if SBP <100.

   Available: Atacand tablets 8 mg. _____

6. Order: Depakote 500 mg p.o. h.s.

   Available: Depakote syrup labeled
   200 mg/5 mL. _____

7. Order: Glucophage 0.85 g p.o. b.i.d. after meals.

   Available: Glucophage 850 mg/tab. _____

8. Order: Ativan 1 mg p.o. q4h p.r.n. for agitation.

   Available: _____

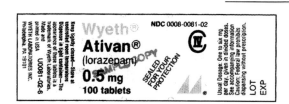

9. Order: Lopressor 25 mg per ngt b.i.d.

   Available: Scored Lopressor tablets
   labeled 50 mg. _____

10. Order: Norvasc 10 mg per ngt q.d. Hold for SBP <100.

    Available: Norvasc tablets labeled 5 mg. _____

Notes

11. Order: Digoxin 0.1 mg p.o. o.d.

    Available: _____

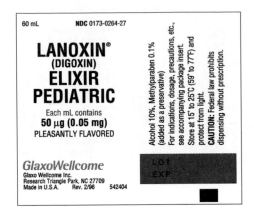

12. Order: Amoxicillin 0.75 g p.o. q6h.

    Available: _____

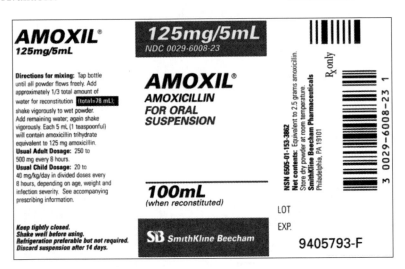

13. Order: Hydrochlorothiazide 12.5 mg p.o. o.d. Hold for B/P <90/60.

    Available: (scored tablets) _____

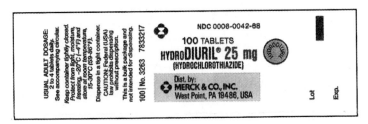

14. Order: Tylenol 650 mg via ngt. q4h p.r.n. for temp >101.4.

Available: Tylenol Elixir 160 mg/5 mL.   _____

15. Order: Dilantin 200 mg via gt b.i.d.

Available: Dilantin 125 mg/5 mL.   _____

16. Order: Elixophyllin Elixir 300 mg via ngt b.i.d.

Available: Elixophyllin 80 mg/15 mL.   _____

17. Order: Xanax 0.75 mg p.o. t.i.d.

Available: Xanax tabs labeled 0.25 mg.   _____

18. Order: Mevacor 20 mg p.o. o.d.

Available: Mevacor tablets labeled 10 mg.   _____

19. Order: Antivert 25 mg p.o. q.d.

Available: Antivert tablets labeled 12.5 mg.   _____

20. Order: Erythromycin suspension 0.25 g p.o. q.i.d.

Available: _____

TO PATIENT:
Shake well before using.
Keep tightly closed. Store in refrigerator and discard unused portion after ten days. Oversize bottle provides shake space.
TO THE PHARMACIST:
When prepared as directed, each 5 mL teaspoonful contains erythromycin ethylsuccinate equivalent to 200 mg of erythromycin in a cherry-flavored suspension.
Bottle contains erythromycin ethylsuccinate equivalent to 4 g of erythromycin.
Usual Dose: See package outsert.
Store at room temperature in dry form.
Child-Resistant closure not required; Reference: Federal Register Vol. 39 No. 29
DIRECTIONS FOR PREPARATION:
Slowly add 70 mL of water and shake vigorously to make 100 mL of suspension.
BARR LABORATORIES, INC.
Pomona, NY 10970
R11-90

BARR LABORATORIES, INC.   NDC 0555-0215-22

Erythromycin Ethylsuccinate
for Oral Suspension, USP

200 mg of erythromycin activity per 5 mL reconstituted

Caution: Federal law prohibits dispensing without prescription.

100 mL (when mixed)

21. Order: Clonidine 0.5 mg p.o. t.i.d. hold for B/P <100/60.

Available: Clonidine tablets labeled 0.1 mg, 0.2 mg, 0.3 mg.

Which would be the best combination to
administer to the client?   _____

22. Order: Nitrostat 0.3 mg sl stat.

Available: Nitrostat tablets labeled gr 1/200.   _____

23. Order: Procan SR 1 g p.o. q6h.

Available: Procan SR 1,000 mg.   _____

24. Order: Lactulose 20 g via gt b.i.d.

Available: Lactulose syrup 10 g/15 mL.   _____

25. Order: Kanamycin (Kantrex) 1 g p.o. q6h × 5 days.

Available: Kanamycin capsules labeled 500 mg.   _____

Answers on p. 520

Parenteral Medications

Objectives

After reviewing this chapter, you should be able to:

1. Identify the various types of syringes used for parenteral administration
2. Read and measure doses on a syringe
3. Read medication labels on parenteral medications
4. Calculate doses of parenteral medications already in solution
5. Identify appropriate syringes to administer doses calculated

The term *parenteral* is used to indicate medications that are administered by any route other than through the digestive system. However, the term parenteral is commonly used to refer to the administration of medications by injection with the use of a needle and syringe. Examples of common parenteral routes are I.M., s.c., I.D., and I.V. Medications administered by the parenteral route act more quickly than oral medications because they are absorbed more rapidly into the bloodstream. The parenteral route may be desired when rapid action of a drug is necessary, for a client who is unable to take a medication orally due to emesis (vomiting), or if a client is in an unconscious state.

Under special circumstances, such as with the psychiatric client, the parenteral injection can be advantageous if the client is refusing to take medications. A judicial hearing must be held and the client mandated to take medications if it is deemed the client can be harmful to self or others. The court, acting in the best interest of the client, can give an order for medication to be given by mouth (p.o.) with the stipulation that if the client refuses the p.o. medication it can be administered by injection.

Medications for parenteral use are available in liquid (solution) or powder. When medications are available in powder form, they must be diluted with a liquid or solvent (reconstituted) before they can be used. Reconstitution of drugs in powder form will be covered in Chapter 18.

PACKAGING OF PARENTERAL MEDICATIONS

Parenteral medications are packaged in various forms:
1. Ampule—This is a sealed glass container designed to hold a single dose of medication. Ampules have a particular shape with a constricted neck. They are

designed to snap open. The neck of the ampule may be scored or have a darkened line or ring around it to indicate where it should be broken to withdraw medication (Figure 17-1).

To withdraw the medication from an ampule the neck is snapped off by grasping the neck with an alcohol wipe or sterile gauze and breaking it off. Aspiration of the medication into a syringe occurs easily and may be completed with a filter needle, if required by institutional policy (Potter, Perry, *Fundamentals of Nursing,* St Louis, 2001, Mosby).

When inserting the needle into an ampule care must be taken to prevent the shaft and tip of the needle from touching the rim of the ampule. Medication is aspirated into the syringe by gently pulling back on the plunger, which creates a negative pressure and allows the fluid to be pulled into the syringe.

2. Vial—This is a plastic or glass container that has a rubber stopper (diaphragm) on the top. The rubber stopper is covered with a metal lid to maintain sterility until the vial is used for the first time (Figure 17-2). Vials are available in different sizes. Multidose vials contain more than one dose of the medication. The label on the vial will specify the amount of medication in a certain amount of solution, for example, 60 mg per mL, 0.2 mg per 0.5 mL. Single-dose vials contain a single dose of medication for injection. Many vials are single dose, because it is safer. The medication in a vial may be in liquid (solution) form, or it may contain a powder that has to be reconstituted before administration.

To withdraw medication from a vial, the top is wiped with alcohol, air equal to the amount of solution being withdrawn is injected into the air space between the solution and the rubber stopper, the vial is inverted, and the desired volume of medication is withdrawn.

In contrast with the ampule, the vial is a closed system, and air must be injected into it to allow for withdrawal of the medication. If air is not injected into the vial before withdrawing medication a vacuum remains in the vial that makes the withdrawal of medication difficult. When withdrawing large volumes of solution from a vial, less air is required to initiate the flow of medication. Injecting large volumes of air into the vial can create too much pressure in the vial and cause the top of the vial to be popped off, or the plunger of the syringe could be rapidly forced backward by the air pressure within the vial.

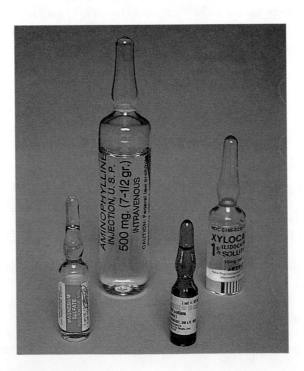

Figure 17-1 Medication in ampules. (From Elkin M, Perry A, and Potter P: *Nursing interventions and clinical skills,* ed 2, St Louis, 2000, Mosby.)

It is important to note that for both single-dose vials and ampules, there is a little extra medication present; it is most important to measure the amount of medication carefully.

3. Mix-o-vial—Some medications come in mix-o-vials (Figure 17-3); for example, Solu-Medrol, Solu-Cortef. The vial usually contains a single dose of medication. The mix-o-vial has two compartments separated by a rubber stopper. The top compartment contains the sterile liquid (diluent), and the bottom compartment contains the powdered medication. When pressure is applied to the top of the vial, the rubber stopper that separates the medication and liquid is released. This allows the liquid and medication to be mixed, thereby dissolving the drug (Figure 17-4).

   A needle is inserted to withdraw the medication.

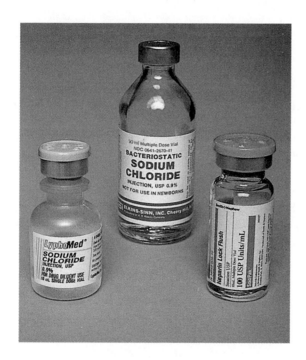

Figure 17-2 Medication in vials. (From Elkin M, Perry A, and Potter P: *Nursing interventions and clinical skills,* ed 2, St Louis, 2000, Mosby.)

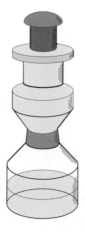

Figure 17-3 Mix-o-vial. (From Clayton B and Stock Y: *Basic pharmacology of nurses,* ed 12, St Louis, 2001, Mosby.)

Notes

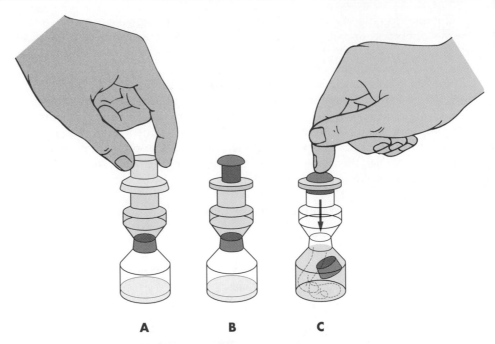

Figure 17-4 Mix-o-vial directions. **A,** Remove plastic lid protector. **B,** Powdered drug is in lower half; diluent is in upper half. **C,** Push firmly on the diaphragm-plunger. Downward pressure dislodges the divider between the two chambers. (From Clayton B and Stock Y: *Basic pharmacology of nurses,* ed 12, St Louis, 2001, Mosby.)

4. Cartridge—Some medications are packaged in a prefilled glass or plastic container. The cartridge is clearly marked, indicating the amount of medication in it. Certain cartridges require a special holder called a *Tubex* or *Carpuject* to release the medication from the cartridge. The cartridge contains a single dose of medication.

    If the dose to be administered is less than the amount contained in the unit, discard the unneeded portion if any, then administer the medication (Figure 17-5).
5. Prepackaged syringe—The medication comes prepared for administration in a syringe with the needle attached. A specific amount of medication is contained in the syringe. The amount desired is calculated, the excess disposed of, and the calculated dose is administered. These syringes are for single use only. Valium comes in prepackaged syringes.

SYRINGES

Various sized syringes are available for use. They have different capacities and specific calibrations. Syringes are made of plastic and glass, but plastic syringes are most commonly used. They are disposable and designed for one-time use only. Syringes have three parts (Figure 17-6):
1. The barrel—The outer calibrated portion that holds the medication.
2. The plunger—The inner device that is moved backward to withdraw and measure the medication and is pushed to eject the medication from the syringe.
3. The tip—The end of the syringe that holds the needle. The tip can be plain or Luer-Lok (Figure 17-7).

    Syringes are classified as being Luer-Lok or non–Luer-Lok. They are disposable and designed for one-time use. Luer-Lok syringes require special needles, which are twisted onto the tip and lock themselves in place, which prevents inadvertent

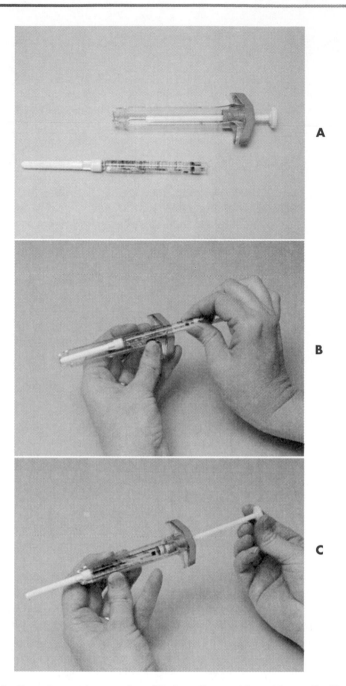

Figure 17-5 **A,** Carpuject syringe and prefilled sterile cartridge with needle. **B,** Assembling the Carpuject. **C,** Cartridge locks at needle end; plunger screws into opposite end. (From Elkin M, Perry A, and Potter P: *Nursing interventions and clinical skills,* ed 2, St Louis, 2000, Mosby.)

removal of the needle. Non-Luer-Lok syringes require needles that slip onto the tip (Elkin, Potter, Perry: *Fundamentals of nursing concepts, process and practice,* ed 2, 2000). The needle fits onto the tip of the syringe. Needles come in various lengths and diameters. The nurse chooses the needle according to the client's size, the type of tissue being injected into, and the viscosity of the medication to be injected.

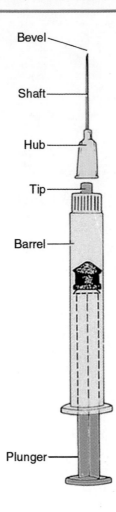

Bevel

Shaft

Hub

Tip

Barrel

Plunger

Figure 17-6   Parts of syringe. (From Elkin M, Perry A, and Potter P: *Nursing interventions and clinical skills,* ed 2, St Louis, 2000, Mosby.)

It is important to note that needle-stick prevention has become increasingly important in preventing transmission of blood-borne infections from contaminated needles. Consequently, this has resulted in special prevention techniques (e.g., no recapping of a needle after use) and development of special equipment, such as syringes with a sheath or guard that covers the needle after it is withdrawn from the skin, thereby decreasing the chance of needle-stick injury (Figure 17-8).

Types of Syringes

The three types of syringes are hypodermic, tuberculin, and insulin.

Hypodermic Syringes

Hypodermic syringes come in a variety of sizes. Syringes are calibrated or marked in cc but hold varying capacities. The smaller-capacity syringes (1, 2, $2\frac{1}{2}$, 3 cc/mL) are used most often for the administration of medication; however, hypodermic syringes are also available in larger sizes (10, 20, 50 cc/mL). Although some syringes are labeled in mL, there are many syringes still labeled with cc rather than mL. **It is important to note that milliliter (mL) is more correct. The mL is a measure of volume, cc is a three-dimensional measure of space and represents the space that a mL occupies. The terms, although**

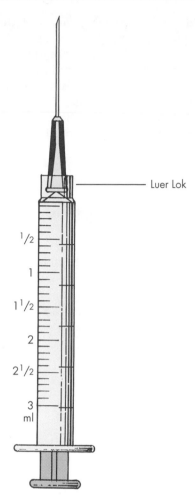

Luer Lok

1/2

1

1 1/2

2

2 1/2

3
ml

Figure 17-7 Small hypodermic. (From Elkin M, Perry A, and Potter P: *Nursing interventions and clinical skills,* ed 2, St Louis, 2000, Mosby.)

A   **B**

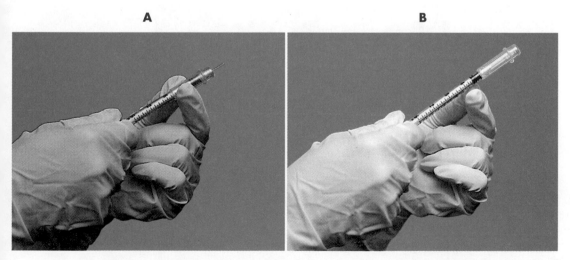

Figure 17-8 Needle with plastic guard to prevent needle sticks. **A,** Position of guard before injection. **B,** After injection the guard locks in place, covering the needle. (From Elkin M, Perry A, and Potter P: *Nursing interventions and clinical skills,* ed 2, St Louis, 2000, Mosby.)

Notes

sometimes used interchangeably, are not the same. Many institutions are now purchasing syringes that indicate mL as opposed to cc. This text shows mL on syringes, not cc. The smaller-capacity syringes (1, 2, 2½, 3 cc/mL) are also calibrated in minims (m). 16 minims = 1 mL. The use of minim scale is rare and discouraged because of its inaccuracy. Although many syringes still have minim markings, more institutions are purchasing syringes that do not have minim markings on them to discourage their use (Figure 17-9).

It has been found that most errors in dose measurement occur from misreading the minim scale.

It is critical that the scale on small hypodermics be read carefully, and that the minim (m) scale not be misread as the metric scale cubic centimeter (cc) or milliliter (mL). This mistake could lead to a medication error.

For small hypodermics decimal numbers are used to express doses (e.g., 1.2 mL, 0.3 mL). Notice that small hypodermics up to 3-mL size also have fractions on them, allowing doses involving a decimal to be stated as fractions (e.g., 0.5 mL as ½ mL) (Figure 17-9, diagram A). There are, however, some syringes that indicate 0.5 mL, 1.5 mL, etc., instead of fractions.

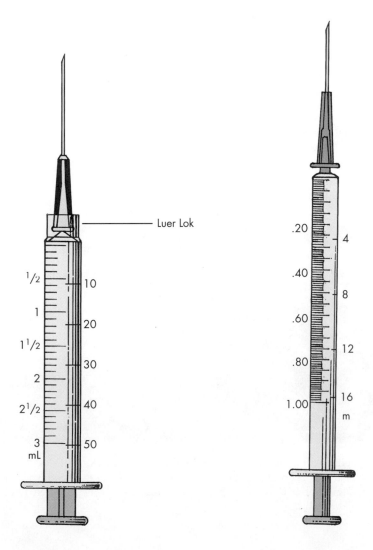

Figure 17-9 3-mL & 1-mL syringes. Note: mL is the correct term; technically cc, although still on some syringes, is incorrect. (From Elkin M, Perry A, and Potter P: *Nursing interventions and clinical skills,* ed 2, St Louis, 2000, Mosby.)

Notes

Notice the side that indicates mL. There are 10 spaces between the largest markings. This indicates the syringe is marked in tenths of a mL. Each of the lines is 0.1 mL. The longer lines indicate $\frac{1}{2}$ (0.5) and full mL measures. On the other side of the syringe are minim markings. Each small line counts as 1 minim, and the longer lines represent 5-minim increments—5, 10, etc.

When looking at the syringe shown in Figure 17-10, notice the rubber ring. When measuring medication and reading the medication withdrawn, the forward edge of the plunger head indicates the amount of medication withdrawn. Do not become confused by the second, bottom ring or by the raised section (middle) of the suction tip. The point where the rubber plunger tip makes contact with the barrel is the spot that should be lined up with the amount desired.

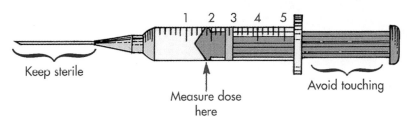

Figure 17-10 Reading measured amount of medication in a syringe. (From Elkin M, Perry A, and Potter P: *Nursing interventions and clinical skills,* ed 2, St Louis, 2000, Mosby.)

Let's examine the syringes below to illustrate specific amounts in a syringe.

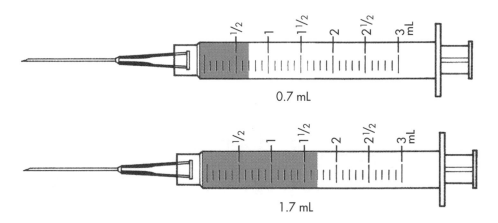

Because the smaller-capacity syringes are used most often to administer medications, it is very important to know how to read them to draw amounts accurately.

POINTS TO REMEMBER

- Small-capacity hypodermics (2, $2\frac{1}{2}$, 3 mL) are calibrated in 0.1 mL and minims. Doses administered with them must correlate to the calibration. Minims should not be used.

- Do not confuse the minim scale with the metric scale (mL); doing so can cause a serious medication error.

Continued

Notes

POINTS TO REMEMBER—cont'd

- Syringes are labeled using the abbreviations cc and mL. More and more syringes are being manufactured with mL and no minim markings.

- mL is the correct measure for volume. Although some syringes still indicate cc, technically it is incorrect.

PRACTICE PROBLEMS

Shade in the indicated amounts on the syringes in mL.

1. 0.8 mL

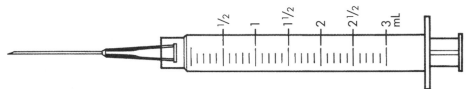

2. 1.2 mL

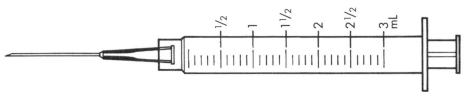

3. 1.5 mL

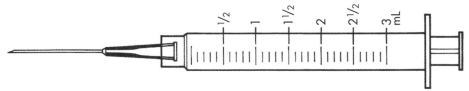

4. 2.4 mL

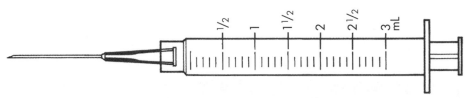

Indicate the number of mL shaded in on the following syringes.

5.

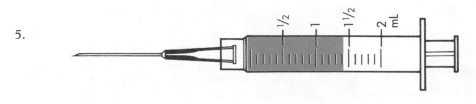

6.

7.

8.

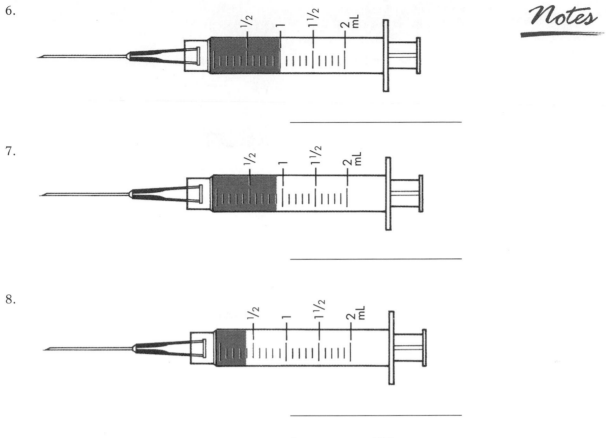

Answers on p. 521

The larger hypodermics (5, 6, 10, and 12 mL) are used when volumes larger than 3 mL are desired. These syringes are used to measure whole numbers of mL as opposed to smaller units such as a tenth of a mL. There are no minim markings on the larger syringes. Syringes 5, 6, 10, and 12 mL in size are calibrated in increments of fifths of an mL (0.2 mL), with the whole numbers indicated by the long lines. Figure 17-11, *A* shows 0.8 mL of medication drawn, and Figure 17-11, *B* shows 7.8 mL drawn. Syringes that are 20 mL and larger are calibrated in whole mL increments and can have other measures, such as ounces, on them. **Remember: The larger the syringe, the larger the calibration. Example: 5 mL and 10 mL each shorter calibration measures two tenths of a mL (0.2 mL).**

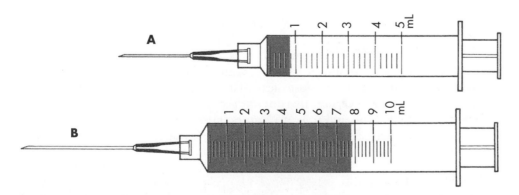

Figure 17-11   Large hypodermics. **A,** 5-mL syringe filled with 0.8 mL. **B,** 10-mL syringe filled with 7.8 mL.

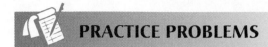

PRACTICE PROBLEMS

Indicate the number of mL shaded in on the following syringes.

9.

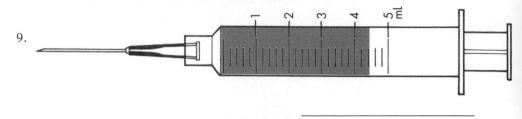

_____

10.

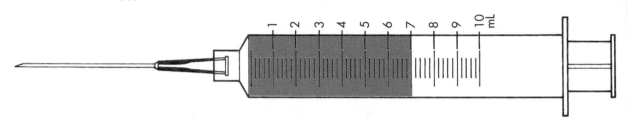

_____

11.

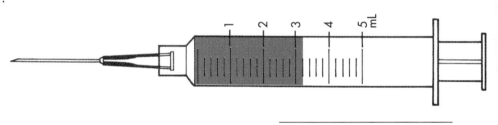

_____

Answers on p. 521

Tuberculin Syringe

This is a narrow syringe that has a capacity of 0.5 mL and 1 mL. The 1-mL size is used most often. The volume of a tuberculin syringe can be measured on the mL or the minim scale. On the minim side of the syringe, the lines represent 1 minim. On the mL side of the syringe the syringe is calibrated in tenths and hundredths of a mL (0.01 mL) and tenths (0.1 mL). The markings on the syringe (lines) are closer together to indicate how small the calibrations are (Figure 17-12). Although minim markings are on the syringe, remember their use is discouraged.

Tuberculin syringes are used to accurately measure medications given in very small volumes (for example, heparin). This syringe is also often used in pediatrics and for diagnostic purposes (for example skin testing, test for tuberculosis). It is recommended that doses less than 1 mL be measured using a tuberculin syringe to make certain that the correct dose is administered to a client. Doses such as 0.42 mL and 0.37 mL can be measured accurately using a tuberculin syringe. When using a tuberculin syringe, it is important to read it carefully to avoid error.

Insulin Syringes

These syringes are designed for the administration of insulin only. Insulin doses are measured in units (U). Insulin syringes are calibrated to match the dose strength of the insulin being used. They are marked U-100 and are designed to be used with insulin that is marked U-100. **U-100 Insulin should be measured**

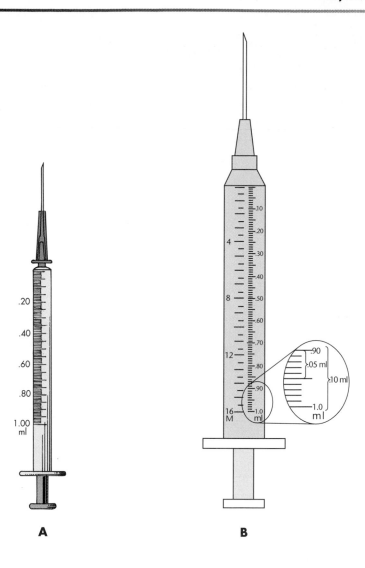

Figure 17-12 **A,** Tuberculin syringe. **B,** Diagram showing tuberculin syringe calibration. (**A,** From Potter PA, and Perry AG: *Fundamentals of nursing,* ed 5, St Louis, 2001, Mosby. **B,** From Clayton B and Stock Y: *Basic pharmacology of nurses,* ed 12, St Louis, 2001, Mosby.)

only in a U-100 insulin syringe. It is important to note that for U-100 Insulin, 100 units = 1 mL. There are two types of insulin syringes: Lo-Dose and 1-mL size.

The *Lo-Dose syringe* is used to measure small doses and is 0.5 mL in size. It may be used for clients receiving 50 U or less of U-100 insulin. It has a capacity of 50 U. The scale on the Lo-Dose syringe is easy to read. Each calibration (shorter lines) measures 1 U, and each 5-U increment is numbered (long lines) (Figure 17-13, *A*).

A 30 U syringe, which is also a Lo-Dose syringe, is available for use with U-100 insulin only and is designed for small doses of 30 U or less. Each increment on the syringe represents 1 U (Figure 17-14). A 30-unit insulin syringe is commonly used in pediatrics to administer insulin.

The *1-mL size syringe* is designed to hold 100 U. There are currently two types on the market. One type of 1 mL (100 U) capacity has each 10-U increment numbered. This syringe is calibrated in 2-U increments (Figure 17-13, *B*). Odd-numbered units are therefore measured between the even calibrations. Use of this syringe should be avoided if possible because accuracy of the dose is questionable. The second type of 1 mL-capacity syringe has two scales on it. The odd number are on the left of the syringe and the even are on the right. The calibrations are in 1 U increments. The best method for using this type of syringe is the following: Measure uneven doses on the left, and measure even doses using the scale on the right (Figure 17-13). The calculation of insulin doses and reading of the calibrations are discussed in more detail in Chapter 19.

Note:

It is important to note that insulin syringes do not have detachable needles. The needle, hub, and barrel are inseparable.

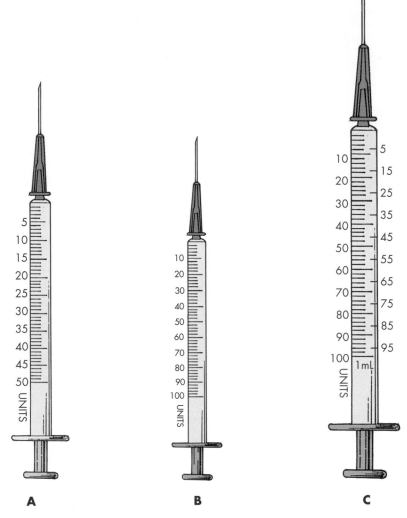

Figure 17-13 Insulin syringes. **A,** Lo-Dose (50 units). **B,** 1-mL size 100 U. **C,** 1-mL capacity with odd and even calibration. (**A** and **C** from Elkin M, Perry A, and Potter P: *Nursing interventions and clinical skills,* ed 2, St Louis, 2000, Mosby. **B,** From Potter PA and Perry AG: *Fundamentals of nursing,* ed 5, St Louis, 2001, Mosby.)

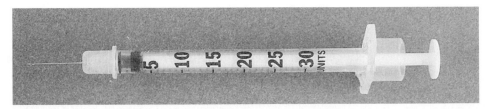

Figure 17-14 Lo-Dose syringe—30 units/mL. (Courtesy Becton Dickinson Consumer Products. From Brown M and Mulholland JL: *Drug calculations: process and problems for clinical practice,* ed 6, 2000, St Louis, Mosby.)

Think Critically to Avoid Drug Calculation Errors

- Doses must be measurable and appropriate for the syringe used.
- When reading syringes with both minim (m) and milliliter calibration (mL), remember they are not the same measurement. It is critical to avoid making errors with m and mL.
- The insulin syringe and the tuberculin syringe are different. Confusion of the two can cause a medication error.
- If the dose cannot be accurately measured, don't give it.

POINTS TO REMEMBER

- When preparing parenteral medications for administration it is important to use the correct syringe for accurate administration of the dose.
- Most syringes are marked in cubic centimeters (cc) whereas most drugs are prepared and labeled with the dosage strength given per milliliter (mL). Remember, although you may see these terms used interchangeably and as equivalent measures (1 cc = 1 mL), technically they are not equivalents; mL should be used instead of cc.
- Syringes are available with mL and without minims.
- Hypodermic syringes—2, 2 1/2, and 3 mL—are marked in minims and 0.1 mL. These small-capacity syringes are most often used for medication administration. It is *important* not to confuse minim scale with metric scale. The use of m is discouraged.
- Hypodermic syringes—5, 6, 10, and 12 mL—are marked in increments of 0.2 mL and 1 mL.
- Hypodermic syringes—20 mL and larger—are marked in 1 mL increments and may have other markings, such as ounces.
- Tuberculin syringes—small syringes marked in minims, tenths, and hundredths of a mL. They are used to administer small doses and are recommended for use with a dose less than 0.5 mL.
- Insulin syringes—marked U-100 for administration with U-100 insulin only. Insulin is measured in units, and should be administered only with an insulin syringe.
- For small hypodermics, doses involving the decimal 0.5 should be expressed as a fraction 1/2 mL up to 3 mL in size. Other values are expressed as decimal numbers.

Before proceeding to discuss calculation of parenteral doses, it is necessary to review some specifics in terms of reading labels. Reading the label and understanding what information is essential is important in determining the correct dose to administer.

READING PARENTERAL LABELS

The information contained on the parenteral label is similar to the information on an oral liquid label. It contains the total volume of the container and the dose

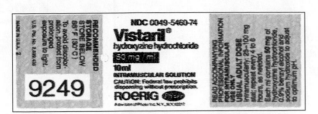

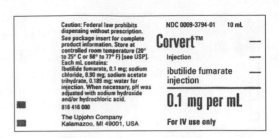

Figure 17-15   Vistaril label.   **Figure 17-16   Corvert label.**

strength (amount of medication in solution) expressed in cc or mL. It is important to read the label carefully to determine the dose strength and volume. Example: 25 mg per mL. Let's examine some labels.

The Vistaril label in Figure 17-15 tells us the total size of the vial is 10 mL. The dose strength is 50 mg/mL. The Corvert label shown in Figure 17-16 shows that the total vial size is 10 mL and there are 0.1 mg per mL.

Some labels may contain two systems of measurement (e.g., apothecary and metric). The dose strength on parenteral labels can be expressed in either metric or apothecary or a combination of both. When apothecary measures are indicated on a label, the equivalent in metric is indicated as well.

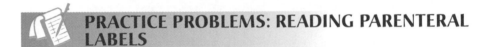

PRACTICE PROBLEMS: READING PARENTERAL LABELS

Use the labels provided to answer the questions.

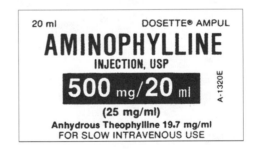

Using the aminophylline label above, answer the following questions:

12. What is the total volume of the ampule?   _____

13. What is the dose strength?   _____

14. If 250 mg were ordered, how many mL
    would this be?   _____

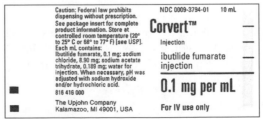

Using the Corvert label above, answer the following questions:

15. What is the total volume of the vial?   _____

16. What is the dose strength? _____

17. What is the route of administration? _____

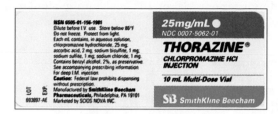

Using the Thorazine label above, answer the following questions:

18. What is the total volume of the vial? _____

19. What is the dose strength? _____

20. If 50 mg were ordered, how many mL would this be? _____

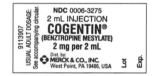

Using the Cogentin label above, answer the following questions:

21. What is the total volume of the ampule? _____

22. What is the dose strength? _____

23. If 1 mg were ordered, how many mL would this be? _____

Answers on p. 521

Parenteral labels can express medications in percentage strengths, as well as units and milliequivalents.

DRUGS LABELED IN PERCENTAGE STRENGTHS

Drugs that are labeled as percentage solutions give information such as the percentage of the solution and the total volume of the vial or ampule. Although percentage is used, metric measures are used as well. Example: In the figure below, which shows a label of Lidocaine 1%, notice there are 10 mg/mL.

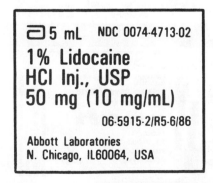

Often no calculation is necessary when giving medications expressed in percentage strength. The doctor usually states the number of mL to prepare or may state it in the number of ampules or vials. Example: Calcium gluconate 10% may be ordered as "Administer one vial of 10% calcium gluconate or 10 mL of 10% calcium gluconate" (see Figure below).

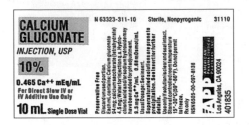

SOLUTIONS EXPRESSED IN RATIO STRENGTH

A medication commonly expressed in terms of ratio strength is epinephrine. Drugs expressed this way include metric measures as well, and are often ordered by the number of mL. Example: Epinephrine may state 1:1,000 and indicate 1 mg/mL.

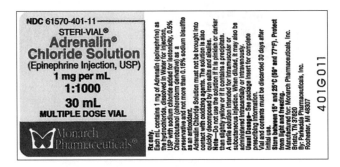

PARENTERAL MEDICATIONS MEASURED IN UNITS

Some medications measured in units for parenteral administration are heparin, pitocin, insulin, and penicillin. Notice the labels indicate how many units per mL. Example, Pitocin 10 U/mL, Heparin 1,000 U/mL. Units express the amount of drug present in 1 mL of solution, and they are specific to the drug for which they are used. Units measure a drug in terms of its action (see heparin and insulin label below).

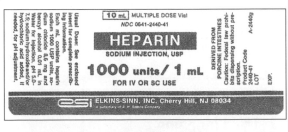

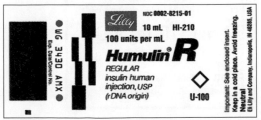

PARENTERAL MEDICATIONS IN MILLIEQUIVALENTS

Notes

Potassium and sodium bicarbonate are drugs that are expressed in milliequivalents. Like units, milliequivalents are specific measurements that have no conversion to another system and are specific to the medication used. Milliequivalents (mEq) are used to measure electrolytes, (for example, potassium) and the ionic activity of a drug. Milliequivalents (mEq) are also defined as an expression of the number of grams of a drug contained in 1 mL of a normal solution. This definition is often used by a chemist or pharmacist.

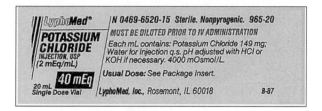

PRACTICE PROBLEMS

Use the labels provided to answer the questions.

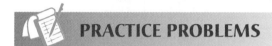

Use the potassium chloride label above to answer the following questions:

24. What is the total volume of the vial?   _____

25. What is the dose in mEq/mL?   _____

Use the sodium bicarbonate label to answer the following questions:

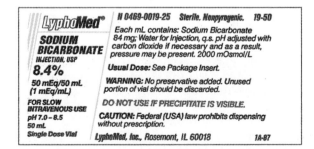

26. What is the total volume of the vial?   _____

27. What is the dose strength expressed in mEq/mL?   _____

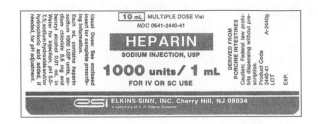

Use the heparin label to answer the following questions:

28. What is the total volume of the vial? _____

29. What is the dose strength? _____

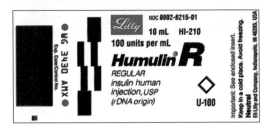

Use the insulin label to answer the following questions:

30. What is the total volume of the vial? _____

31. What is the dose strength? _____

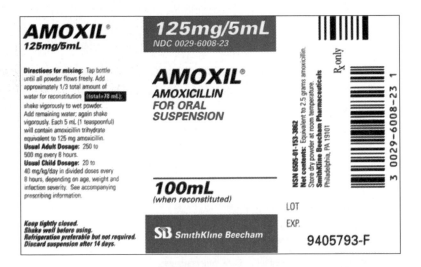

Use the Amoxil label to answer the following questions:

32. What is the total volume of the oral solution when reconstituted? _____

33. What is the dose strength? _____

Answers on p. 521

Note:

It is important to read the label on parenteral medications carefully. Labels on parenteral medications include a variety of units to express dose strengths. To calculate doses to administer it is important to know the strength of the medication in solution per mL. Confusing dose strength with total volume can lead to a medication error.

CALCULATING PARENTERAL DOSAGES

Parenteral doses can be calculated using the same rules and methods used to compute oral doses. The ratio-proportion and formula methods have been presented in earlier chapters. The following guidelines will help you calculate a dose that is logical, reasonable, and accurate.

Guidelines for Calculating Parenteral Dosages

1. Use the ratio-proportion or formula method to calculate the dose to be administered.
2. The rules and the steps for calculating parenteral doses are the same as those used for computing oral doses.
3. Remember, the stock volume varies and is not always per 1 mL. Read the label carefully to determine the dose strength contained in a certain volume of solution.
4. Although cc and mL are used interchangeably, labels to answers should be expressed in mL. Dose strength on labels are often expressed per milliliter.
5. Accuracy in calculating parenteral doses depends on the syringe used. Therefore it is important to be able to understand syringes.
6. Small-capacity syringes—2, 2 1/2, and 3 mL—are marked in minims and tenths (0.1) of a mL. These syringes are used most often for the administration of I.M. medications. Doses are stated using decimal numbers. Doses involving decimal 0.5 are stated as fractions. The syringe has fraction markings.
7. Tuberculin syringes are used for small doses and are calibrated in tenths (0.1) and hundredths (0.01) of a mL. Tuberculin syringes have a maximum capacity of 1 mL; they are designed to administer small doses and potent medications. They are often used in pediatrics.
8. **Insulin syringes are designed for insulin only.** Measuring insulin in an insulin syringe requires no calculation or conversion. It is safest to measure insulin with an insulin syringe! Insulin will be discussed in more detail in Chapter 19.

CALCULATING INJECTABLE MEDICATIONS ACCORDING TO THE SYRINGE

Now that you have an understanding of syringes, let's discuss obtaining an answer that is measurable according to the syringe being used.

Note:

It is critical to choose the correct size syringe to ensure accurate measurement.

POINTS TO REMEMBER

- When using a 2, 2 $\frac{1}{2}$, or 3 mL syringe, round answers in mL to the nearest tenth, never to a whole unit.

- mL and cc are used interchangeably; however, mL is a more correct term, and should be used rather than cc.

Continued

Notes

POINTS TO REMEMBER—cont'd

- When calculating a dose for a syringe marked in hundredths (0.01) of a mL, if the math calculation does not work out evenly to the hundredths place, then the division goes to the thousandths place and is rounded to the hundredths place. For example, 0.876 mL = 0.88 mL.

  a) For an answer in mL, math is carried two decimal places and rounded to the nearest tenth. Example: 1.75 mL = 1.8 mL.

  b) Minims **are rarely** used and are discouraged because of their inaccuracy. When mL is changed to m, the equivalent m 16 = 1 mL is preferred and gives a more accurate answer. Minim is an apothecaries' measure and is not exact. It is better to express answers in metric measures such as mL.

- When administering less than 1 mL, a tuberculin syringe is used. When using a tuberculin syringe to calculate a dose in mL, math is carried to the thousandth place and rounded to the nearest hundredth because the syringe is marked in hundredths (0.01) of a mL (if math doesn't work out evenly to hundredths place). Example: 0.876 mL = 0.88 mL.

- For injectable medications there are guidelines as to the amount of medication that can be administered. When the dose exceeds these guidelines, the dose should be questioned and the calculation double checked.

  a) According to Potter and Perry (*Fundamentals of nursing*, 2001, Mosby), the normal well-developed client can tolerate 3 mL of medication into a large muscle without severe muscle discomfort. Children, older adults, and thin clients can tolerate only 2 mL of an intramuscular injection. Whaley and Wong *(Essentials of pediatric nursing*, 2000, Mosby), recommends giving no more than 1 mL to small children and older infants.

  b) Subcutaneous—The volume that can be administered safely is 0.5 mL to 1 mL.

- In administering medications by injection, the absorption and consistency of the medication is also considered. For example, a dose of 3 mL of a thick oily substance may be divided into two injections of 1.5 mL (1 1/2 mL) each.

- Doses administered should be measured in mL, therefore the answer is labeled accordingly.

- Proceed with calculations in a logical and reasonable manner.

- Injectables that are added to an I.V. solution may have a volume greater than 5 mL.

Notes

Now, with the guidelines in mind, let's look at some sample problems. Regardless of what method you use to calculate, the following steps are used.
1. Check to make sure everything is in the same system and unit of measure.
2. Think critically about what the answer should logically be.
3. Consider the type of syringe being used. **The cardinal rule should always be any dose given must be able to be measured accurately in the syringe you are using.**
4. Use the ratio-proportion or formula method to calculate the dose. Let's look at some sample problems calculating parenteral doses.

Example 1: Order: Gentamicin 75 mg I.M. q8h.

Available: Gentamicin labeled 40 mg = 1 mL.

Note: No conversion is necessary here. Think—The dose ordered is going to be more than 1 mL but less than 2 mL. Set up and solve.

➤ Solution Using Ratio-Proportion Method

$$40 \text{ mg} : 1 \text{ mL} = 75 \text{ mg} : x \text{ mL}$$

$$\frac{40x}{40} = \frac{75}{40}$$

$$x = 1.87 \text{ mL} = 1.9 \text{ mL}$$

Answer: 1.9 mL

The answer here is rounded to the nearest tenth of a mL. Remember, you are using a small hypodermic syringe marked in tenths of a mL.

➤ Solution Using the Formula Method

$$\frac{(D)75 \text{ mg}}{(H)40 \text{ mg}} \times (Q) \ 1 \text{ mL} = x \text{ mL} \quad \textbf{OR} \quad \frac{(DW)75 \text{ mg}}{(SW)40 \text{ mg}} = \frac{(DV)x \text{ mL}}{(SV)1 \text{ mL}}$$

$$x = \frac{75}{40} \qquad\qquad \frac{40 \ x}{40} = \frac{75}{40}$$

$$x = 1.87 \text{ mL} = 1.9 \text{ mL} \qquad x = \frac{75}{40}$$

$$x = 1.87 \text{ mL} = 1.9 \text{ mL}$$

Answer: 1.9 mL

The answer to Example 1 could have also been expressed as minims because small hypodermics have minims on them. Remember, however, it is always preferable to express the answer in metric measures, because apothecaries' measures are not exact. **Minims are rarely used.**

Refer to the syringe below, illustrating 1.9 mL shaded in on the syringe.

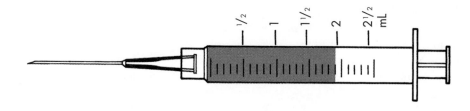

Notes

Example 2: Order: Kantrex 500 mg I.M. q12h.

Available: Kanamycin (Kantrex) labeled 0.5 g per 2 mL.

In this problem a conversion is necessary. Equivalent: 1,000 mg = 1 g. Convert what is ordered to what is available: 500 mg = 0.5 g. To get rid of the decimal point, convert what's available to what's ordered: 0.5 g = 500 mg. Remember, either way will net the same final answer.

Think—The dose you will need to give is greater than 1 mL, and it's being given I.M. The dose therefore should fall within the range that is safe for I.M. The solution, after making conversion, is as follows:

▶ **Solution Using Ratio-Proportion Method**

$$0.5 \text{ g} : 2 \text{ mL} = 0.5 \text{ g} : x \text{ mL}$$

$$\frac{\cancel{0.5}x}{\cancel{0.5}} = \frac{1.0}{0.5}$$

$$x = \frac{1.0}{0.5}$$

$$x = 2 \text{ mL}$$

▶ **Solution Using the Formula Method**

$$\frac{(D)0.5 \text{ g}}{(H)0.5 \text{ g}} \times (Q)2 \text{ mL} = x \text{ (mL)} \quad \textbf{OR} \quad \frac{(DW)500 \text{ mg}}{(SW)500 \text{ mg}} = \frac{(DV)x \text{ mL}}{(SV)2 \text{ mL}}$$

$$x = \frac{0.5 \times 2}{0.5} \qquad\qquad \frac{\cancel{500}x}{\cancel{500}} = \frac{1,000}{500}$$

$$x = \frac{1.0}{0.5} \qquad\qquad x = \frac{1,000}{500}$$

$$x = 2 \text{ mL} \qquad\qquad x = 2 \text{ mL}$$

Refer to the syringe below illustrating 2 mL drawn up.

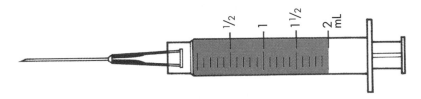

Example 3: Order: Morphine sulfate gr 1/2 I.M. stat.

Available: Morphine sulfate in a 20-mL vial, labeled 15 mg per mL.

▶ **Problem Setup**

1. A conversion is necessary. Convert gr 1/2 to mg using the equivalent 60 mg = gr 1; gr 1/2 therefore is 30 mg.
2. Think—You will need more than 1 mL to administer the dose.
3. Set up the problem, and calculate the dose to be administered.

Notes

Solution Using Ratio-Proportion Method

$$15 \text{ mg} : 1 \text{ mL} = 30 \text{ mg} : x \text{ mL}$$

$$\frac{\cancel{15}x}{\cancel{15}} = \frac{30}{15}$$

$$x = 2 \text{ mL}$$

Solution Using the Formula Method

$$\frac{(D)30 \text{ mg}}{(H)15 \text{ mg}} \times (Q)1 \text{ mL} = x \text{ (mL)} \quad \textbf{OR} \quad \frac{(DW)30 \text{ mg}}{(SW)15 \text{ mg}} = \frac{(DV)x \text{ mL}}{(SV)1 \text{ mL}}$$

$$x = \frac{30}{15} \qquad\qquad \frac{\cancel{15}x}{\cancel{15}} = \frac{30}{15}$$

$$x = 2 \text{ mL} \qquad\qquad x = \frac{30}{15}$$

$$x = 2 \text{ mL}$$

Note: Refer to the Example 2 to visualize 2 mL in a syringe.

Example 4: Order: Atropine sulfate gr 1/100 I.M. stat.

Available: Atropine sulfate in 20-mL vial labeled 0.4 mg per mL.

Problem Setup

1. A conversion is necessary. Convert gr 1/100 to mg using the equivalent 60 mg = gr 1; gr 1/100 is therefore 0.6 mg
2. Think—The dose will be greater than 1 mL to administer the required dose.
3. Set up the problem and calculate the dose to be administered.

Solution Using Ratio-Proportion Method

$$0.4 \text{ mg} : 1 \text{ mL} = 0.6 \text{ mg} : x \text{ mL}$$

$$\frac{0.4x}{0.4} = \frac{0.6}{0.4}$$

$$x = \frac{0.6}{0.4}$$

$x = 1.5$ mL or $1\frac{1}{2}$ mL (For purposes of administering medication it is best to state this answer as $1\frac{1}{2}$ mL. Note that the small hypodermics have fraction markings.)

Solution Using the Formula Method

$$\frac{(D)0.6 \text{ mg}}{(H)0.4 \text{ mg}} \times (Q) 1 \text{ mL} = x \text{ (mL)} \quad \textbf{OR} \quad \frac{(DW)0.6 \text{ mg}}{(SW)0.4 \text{ mg}} = \frac{(DV) \, x \text{ mL}}{(SV)1 \text{ mL}}$$

$$x = \frac{0.6}{0.4} \qquad\qquad \frac{0.\cancel{4}x}{0.\cancel{4}} = \frac{0.6}{0.4}$$

$$x = 1.5 \text{ mL, } 1 \ 1/2 \text{ mL} \qquad\qquad x = \frac{0.6}{0.4}$$

$$x = 1.5 \text{ mL, } 1 \ 1/2 \text{ mL}$$

Notes

Refer to the syringe below illustrating 1 1/2 mL shaded in on the syringe.

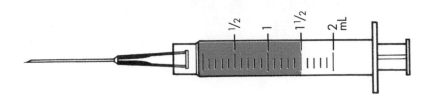

CALCULATING DOSES FOR MEDICATIONS IN UNITS

As previously mentioned, certain drugs are measured in units. Some medications measured in units include vitamins, antibiotics, insulin, and heparin. The calculation of insulin will be discussed in Chapter 19. Insulin syringes are used for insulin only. In determining the dose to administer when medications are measured in units, use the same steps as with other parenteral medications. Doses of certain medications such as heparin are administered with a tuberculin syringe, as opposed to a hypodermic (2, 2 1/2, 3 mL). Because of its effects, heparin is never rounded off, but rather exact doses are given. Heparin will also be discussed in more detail in Chapter 22. Let's look at sample problems with units.

Example 1:   Order: Heparin 750 U. s.c. o.d.

Available: Heparin 1,000 U per mL

Using a 1-mL (tuberculin) syringe, calculate the dose to be administered.

▶ Problem Setup

1. No conversion is required. No conversion exists for units.
2. Think—The dosage to be given is less than 1 mL. This dose can be accurately measured in a 1-mL tuberculin syringe. To administer in a hypodermic (2, 2 1/2, 3 mL) the dose would have to be expressed to the nearest tenth of a mL. Heparin is administered in exact doses.
3. Set up the problem, and calculate the dose to be given.

 Think Critically to Avoid Drug Calculation Errors

Due to the action of heparin, an exact dose is crucial; the dose should not be rounded off.

▶ Solution Using Ratio-Proportion Method

$$1{,}000 \text{ U} : 1 \text{ mL} = 750 \text{ U} : x \text{ mL}$$

$$\frac{1{,}000x}{1{,}000} = \frac{750}{1{,}000}$$

$$x = \frac{75}{1{,}000}$$

$$x = 0.75 \text{ mL}$$

➤ Solution Using the Formula Method

$$\frac{(D)750 \text{ U}}{(H)1,000 \text{ U}} \times (Q)1 \text{ mL} = x \text{ mL} \quad \textbf{OR} \quad \frac{(DW)750 \text{ U}}{(SW)1,000 \text{ U}} = \frac{(DV)x \text{ mL}}{(SV)1 \text{ mL}}$$

$$x = \frac{750}{1,000} \qquad\qquad \frac{1,000x}{1,000} = \frac{750}{1,000}$$

$$x = 0.75 \text{ mL} \qquad\qquad x = \frac{750}{1,000}$$

$$x = 0.75 \text{ mL}$$

Refer to the syringe illustrating 0.75 mL shaded in.

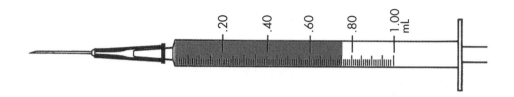

Example 2:   Order: Penicillin G procaine, 500,000 U I.M. b.i.d.

   Available: Penicillin G procaine labeled 300,000 U per mL.

➤ Problem Setup

1. No conversion is required.
2. Think—The dose ordered is more than what is available. Therefore more than 1 mL would be required to administer the dose.
3. Set up the problem in ratio-proportion or formula to calculate the dose.

➤ Solution Using the Ratio-Proportion Method

$$300,000 \text{ U} : 1 \text{ mL} = 500,000 \text{ U} : x \text{ mL}$$

$$300,000x = 500,000$$

$$x = \frac{500,000}{300,000}$$

$$x = 1.66 \text{ mL} = 1.7 \text{ mL}$$

Answer: 1.7 mL

Note:

The division here is carried two decimal places. This answer is then rounded off to 1.7 mL. Remember the hypodermic syringe (2, 2 1/2, 3 mL) is marked in tenths of a mL.

➤ Solution Using the Formula Method

$$\frac{(D)500,000 \text{ U}}{(H)300,000 \text{ U}} \times (Q)1 \text{ mL} = x \text{ (mL)} \quad \textbf{OR} \quad \frac{(DW)500,000 \text{ U}}{(SW)300,000 \text{ U}} = \frac{(DV)x \text{ mL}}{(SV)1 \text{ mL}}$$

$$x = \frac{500,000}{300,000} \qquad\qquad x = \frac{300,000x}{300,000} = \frac{500,000}{300,000}$$

$$x = 1.66 \text{ mL} = 1.7 \text{ mL} \qquad\qquad x = 1.66 \text{ mL} = 1.7 \text{ mL}$$

Answer: 1.7 mL

Notes

Refer to the syringe illustrating 1.7 mL shaded in.

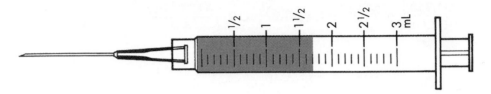

Caution

Read orders carefully when the order is expressed in units. Do not confuse the "U" when written in an order with an "0." To avoid confusion some institutions require doctors to write out the word *units* to avoid misinterpretation of an order—for example, "50 () " as "500 units." (Notice that the U is almost closed and could be read as 500 units.)

 PRACTICE PROBLEMS

Calculate the doses for the problems below and indicate the number of mL you will administer. Shade in the dose on the syringe provided. Use labels where provided to calculate the volume necessary to administer the dose ordered. Express your answers to the nearest tenth except where indicated.

34. Order: Compazine 10 mg I.M. q4h p.r.n.

    Available: _____

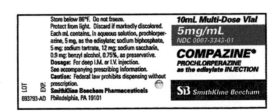

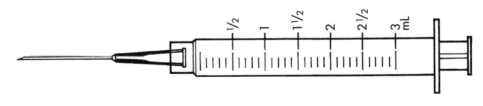

35. Order: Aquamephyton 5 mg sc q.d. × 3 days.

    Available: _____

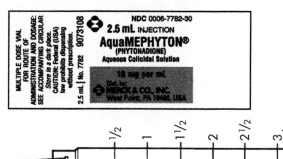

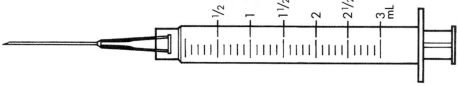

36. Order: Cogentin 1 mg I.M. stat.

    Available: Cogentin labeled 2 mg/mL. _____

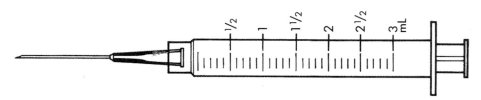

37. Order: Valium 8 mg I.M. q4h p.r.n. for agitation.

    Available: 10 mL vial labeled 5 mg/mL. _____

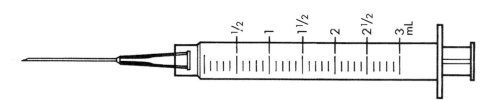

38. Order: Sandostatin 0.05 mg s.c. o.d.

    Available: Sandostatin labeled 1 mL =
    100 mcg. _____

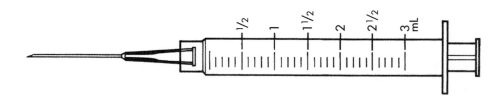

Notes

39. Order: Demerol 50 mg I.M. and Vistaril 25 mg I.M. q4h p.r.n. for pain.

Available: Demerol labeled 75 mg/mL.
Vistaril labeled 50 mg/mL.   _____

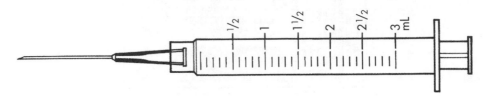

40. Order: Reglan 5 mg I.M. b.i.d. 1/2 hour a.c.

Available: Reglan labeled 10 mg per 2 mL.   _____

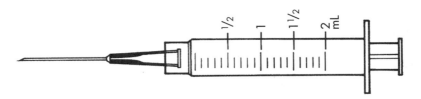

41. Order: Heparin 5,000 U s.c. b.i.d.

Available:

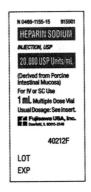

Express your answer in hundredths.   _____

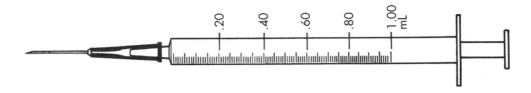

42. Order: Morphine sulfate gr 1/4 I.M. q4h p.r.n.

Available: _____

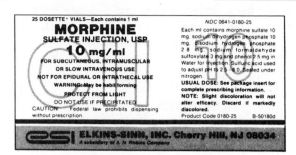

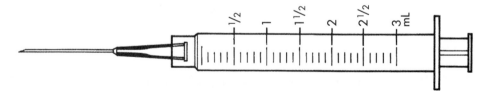

43. Order: Lasix (furosemide) 20 mg I.M. stat.

Available: _____

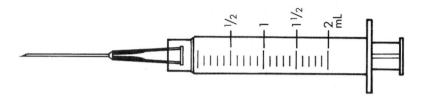

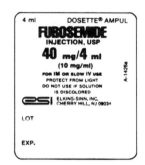

Answers on pp. 522-524

Notes

✓ CHAPTER REVIEW

Calculate the doses for the problems below and indicate the number of mL you will administer. Shade in the dose on the syringe provided. Use labels where provided to calculate the volume necessary to administer the dose ordered. Express your answers to the nearest tenth except where indicated. Problems requiring conversions reflect converting what was ordered to what is available.

1. Order: Clindamycin 0.3 g I.M. q6h.

   Available: _____

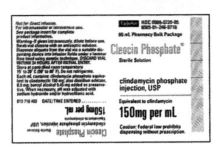

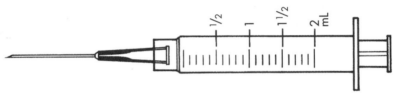

2. Order: Atropine gr 1/150 I.M. stat.

   Available: Atropine 0.4 mg per mL.   _____

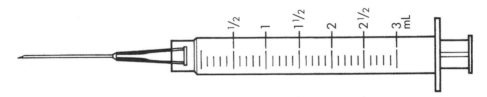

3. Order: Ketzol 0.5 g I.M. q6h.

   Available: Ketzol after reconstitution
   labeled 225 mg/mL.   _____

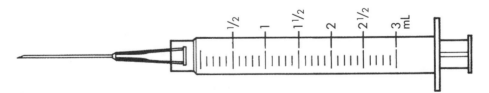

4. Order: Digoxin 100 mcg I.M. q.d.

   Available: Digoxin injection 0.5 mg/2 mL.   _____

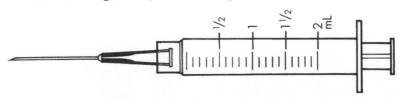

5. Order: Dilaudid 2 mg s.c. q4h p.r.n. for pain.

Available: _____

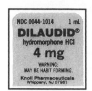

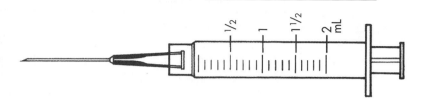

6. Order: Penicillin G 250,000 U I.M. q6h.

Available: _____

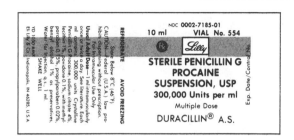

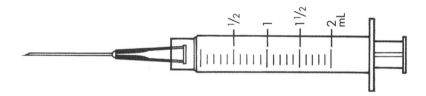

7. Order: Solu-Medrol 100 mg I.M. q8h × 2 doses.

Available: _____

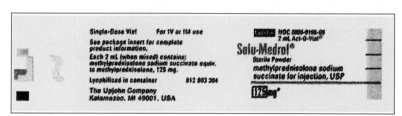

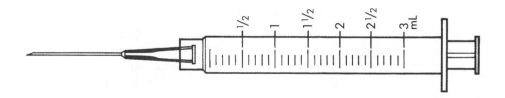

Notes

8. Order: Methergine 0.4 mg I.M. q4h × 3 doses.

    Available: Methergine labeled 0.2 mg/mL.   _____

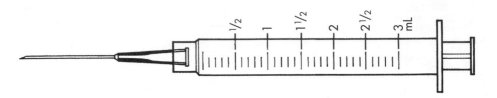

9. Order: Heparin 8,000 U s.c. q12h.

    Available: _____

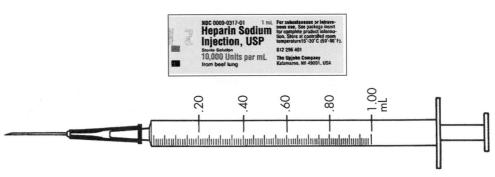

10. Order: Morphine sulfate 4 mg I.M. q4h p.r.n.

    Available: Morphine 10 mg per mL.   _____

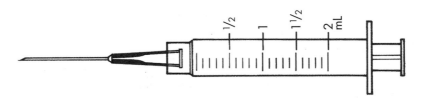

11. Order: Vitamin K 10 mg I.M. q.d. × 3 days.

    Available: Vitamin K labeled 5 mg per mL.   _____

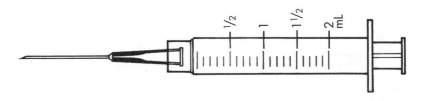

12. Order: Codeine gr 1/4 I.M. q4h p.r.n. for pain.

Available: Codeine phosphate 30 mg (gr 1/2) per mL. _____

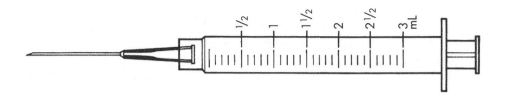

13. Order: Phenergan 25 mg I.M. q4h p.r.n. for nausea.

Available: Phenergan labeled 50 mg per mL. _____

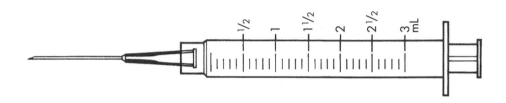

14. Order: Stadol 1.5 mg I.M. q3-4h for pain.

Available: Stadol labeled 2 mg per mL. _____

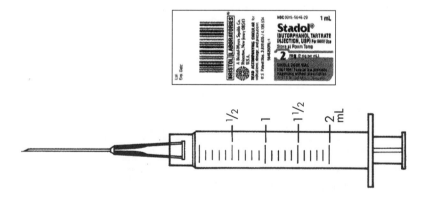

15. Order: Dilaudid 3 mg I.M. q4h prn.

Available: Dilaudid 4 mg per mL. _____

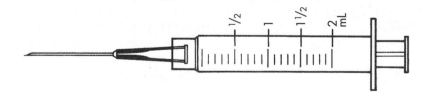

Notes

16. Order: Scopolamine gr 1/300 s.c. stat.

    Available: Scopolamine hydrobromide injection labeled 0.4 mg/mL.

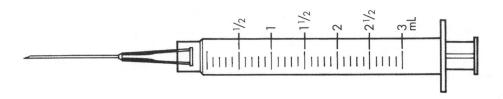

17. Order: Haldol 3 mg I.M. q6h p.r.n.

    Available:

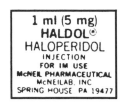

1 ml (5 mg)
HALDOL®
HALOPERIDOL
INJECTION
FOR IM USE
McNEIL PHARMACEUTICAL
McNEILAB, INC
SPRING HOUSE PA 19477

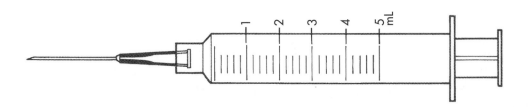

18. Order: Solu-Cortef 400 mg I.V. o.d. for a severe inflammation.

    Available:

Single-Dose Vial   For IV or IM use
Contains Benzyl Alcohol as a Preservative
See package insert for complete
product information.
Per 2 mL (when mixed):
* hydrocortisone sodium succinate equiv.
to hydrocortisone, 250 mg. Protect
solution from light. Discard after 3 days.

814 070 205   Reconstituted . . . .

The Upjohn Company
Kalamazoo, MI 49001, USA

2 mL Act-O-Vial®   NDC 0009-0909-08
Solu-Cortef® Sterile Powder
hydrocortisone sodium succinate
for injection, USP
250 mg*

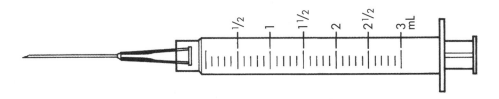

19. Order: Solu-Medrol 40 mg I.V. q6h × 3 days.

    Available: Solu-Medrol 125 mg per 2 mL. _____

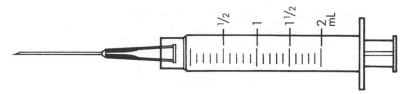

20. Order: Robinul 200 mcg I.M. on call to the O.R.

    Available: _____

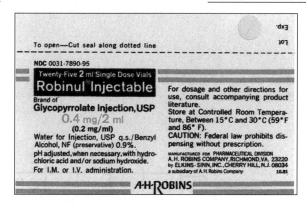

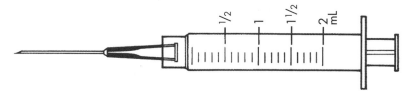

21. Order: Heparin 2,500 U s.c. o.d.

    Available: _____

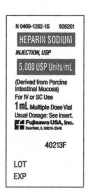

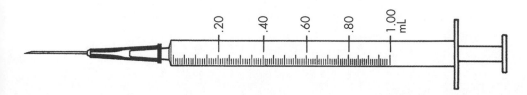

Notes

22. Order: Vistaril 35 mg I.M. stat.

Available: Vistaril labeled 50 mg/mL. _____

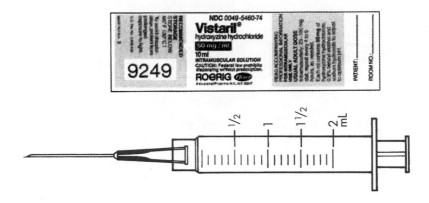

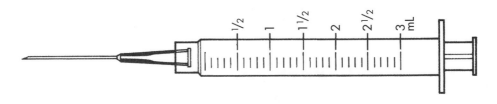

23. Order: Meperidine 60 mg I.M. q3-4h p.r.n. for pain.

Available: Meperidine 75 mg per mL. _____

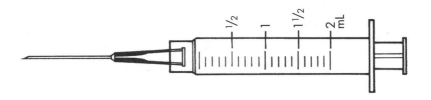

24. Order: Bicillin 400,000 U I.M. q4h.

Available: _____

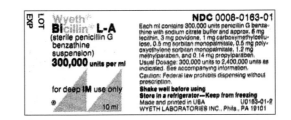

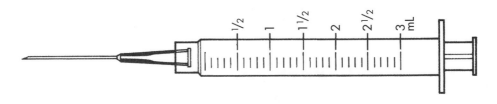

25. Order: Lanoxin 0.4 mg I.M. stat.

    Available: _____

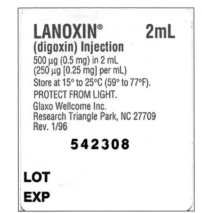

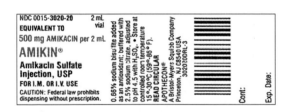

26. Order: Amikin 100 mg I.M. q8h.

    Available: _____

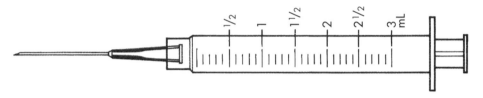

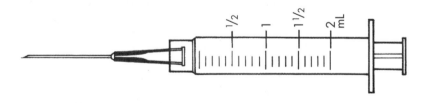

Notes

27. Order: Depo-Medrol 60 mg I.M. b.i.d. × 3 days.

    Available: _____

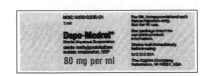

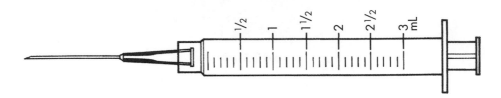

28. Order: Ativan 2 mg I.M. b.i.d. p.r.n. for agitation.

    Available: _____

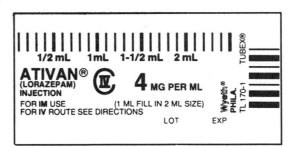

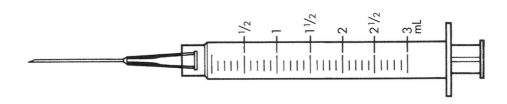

Chapter 17 *Parenteral Medications* **287**

29. Order: Thorazine 75 mg I.M. q4h p.r.n.

Available: _____

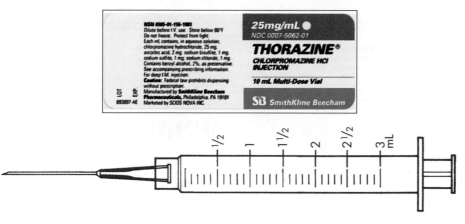

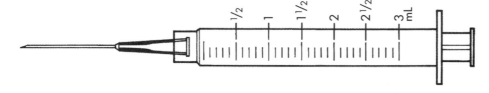

30. Order: Nembutal sodium 120 mg I.M. h.s. p.r.n.

Available: _____

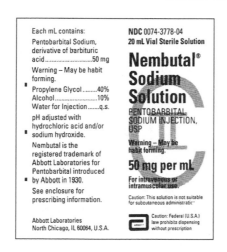

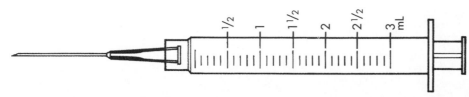

31. Order: Epogen 3,000 U s.c. o.d. every Monday, Wednesday, and Friday.

Available: Epogen labeled 2,000 U per mL. _____

Notes

32. Order: Zantac 50 mg I.M. q8h.

Available: _____

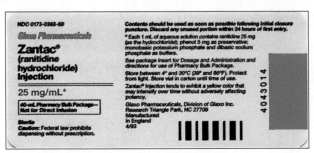

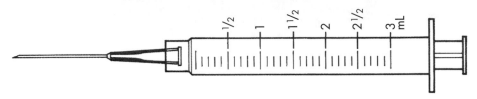

33. Order: Lovenox 30 mg s.c. q12h.

Available: _____

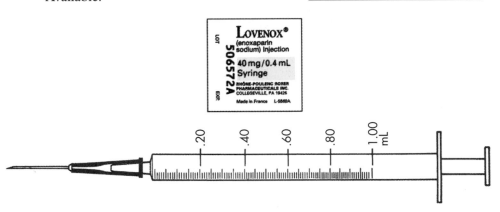

34. Order: Cimetidine 0.3 g I.V. t.i.d.

    Available: _____

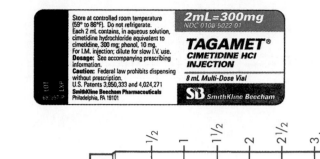

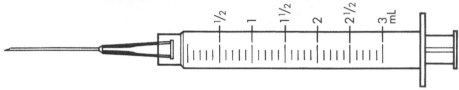

35. Order: Valium 7.5 mg I.M. stat.

    Available: Valium 5 mg per mL.   _____

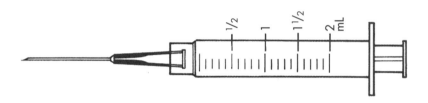

36. Order: Numorphan 1 mg s.c. q4h p.r.n.

    Available: _____

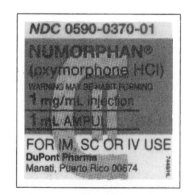

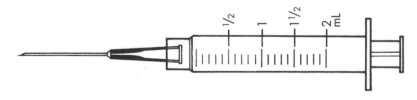

Notes

37. Order: Lasix 30 mg I.V. stat.

    Available: Lasix 20 mg per 2 mL.   _____

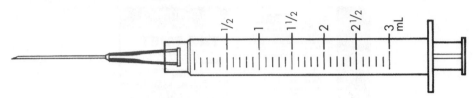

38. Order: Betamethasone 12 mg I.M. q24h × 2 doses.

    Available: Betamethasone 4 mg per mL.   _____

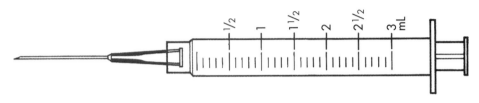

39. Order: Aminophylline 0.25 g I.V. q6h.

    Available: Aminophylline 500 mg per 20 mL._____

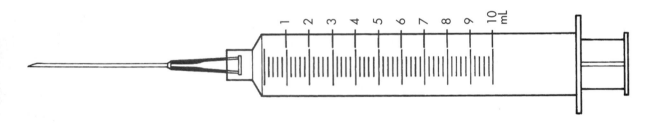

40. Order: Pronestyl 0.5 g I.V. stat.

    Available: Pronestyl 500 mg per mL.   _____

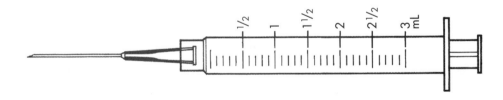

Answers on pp. 525-533

Chapter 18

Powdered Drugs

Objectives

After reviewing this chapter, you should be able to:

1. Prepare a solution from a powdered medication according to directions on the vial or other resources
2. Identify essential information to be placed on the vial of a medication after it is reconstituted
3. Determine the best concentration strength for medications ordered when there are several directions for mixing
4. Calculate doses from reconstituted medications

Some drugs are unstable when stored in liquid form for long periods of time and therefore are packaged in powdered form. When medications come in powdered form, they must be diluted with a liquid referred to as a *diluent* or *solvent* before they can be administered to a client. Once a liquid is added to a powdered drug, the solution may be used for only 1 to 14 days, depending on the type of medication. The process of adding a solvent or diluent to a medication in powdered form to dissolve it and form a solution is referred to as *reconstitution*. Reconstitution is necessary for medications that come in powdered form before they can be measured and administered. If you think about it, this process is something you do in everyday situations. For example, when you make Kool-Aid or iced tea (powdered form), what you're doing in essence is reconstituting. The Kool-Aid, for example, is the powder, and the water you add to it is considered the diluent, or solvent. Medications requiring reconstitution can be for oral or parenteral use.

BASIC PRINCIPLES FOR RECONSTITUTION

The initial step in preparing a powdered medication is to carefully read the information on the vial or the package insert; directions for reconstituting are indicated there.

1. The drug manufacturer provides directions for reconstitution, including information regarding the number of mL of diluent or solvent that should be added, as well as the type of solution that should be used to reconstitute the medication. The concentration (or strength) of the medication after it has been reconstituted according to the directions is also indicated on some medications. The directions for reconstituting must be read carefully and followed.
2. The diluent (solvent, liquid) commonly used for reconstitution is sterile water or sterile normal saline, prepared for injection. Other solutions that may be

used are 5% dextrose and water and bacteriostatic water. Some powdered medications for oral use may be reconstituted with tap water. The manufacturer's directions will tell you which solution to use. If the medication requires a special solution for reconstitution, it is usually supplied by the drug manufacturer and packaged with the medication.

3. Once you have located the reconstitution directions on the label, you need to identify the following information:

   a) The type of diluent to use for reconstitution.

   b) The amount of diluent to add. This is essential because directions relating to the amount can vary based on the route of administration. There may be different dilution instructions for I.V. versus I.M.

   c) The length of time the medication is good once it is reconstituted. The length of time a medication can be stored once reconstituted can vary depending on how stored.

   d) Directions for storing the medication after mixing.

   e) The strength or concentration of the medication after it's reconstituted.

   Refer to Figure 18-1 showing the oxacillin sodium reconstitution procedure. Note that directions on the label say to add 2.7 mL sterile water for injection and that each 1.5 mL contains 250 mg. The available dosage after reconstitution is 250 mg of oxacillin per 1.5 mL solution (500 mg/3 mL).

4. If there are no directions for reconstitution on the label or on a package insert, or if any of the information (listed in number 3) is missing, consult appropriate resources such as the *Physician's Desk Reference* (PDR), a pharmacology text, the hospital drug formulary, or the pharmacy.

5. After mixing the powdered drug, you must place the following information on the medication vial.

   a) **Your initials.**

   b) **The date and time prepared and the expiration date and time.** Note: If all of the solution that is mixed is used, this information is not necessary. Information regarding the date and time of preparation and date and time for expiration is crucial when all of the medication is not used. Powdered medications once reconstituted must be used within a certain time period. For example, ampicillin once reconstituted must be used within an hour.

6. When reconstituting medications that are in multiple-dose vials or have several directions as to how they can be prepared, **information regarding the dose strength or final concentration (what the medication's strength or concentration is after you mixed it) must be on the label; for example, 500 mg/mL. This is important because others using the medication after you need this information to determine the dose.**

7. After adding the diluent to a powder, some drugs completely dissolve and there is no additional volume added. Often, however, the powdered medication adds volume to the solution. The powdered drug takes up space as it dissolves and results in an increase in the amount of total (fluid) volume once it has dissolved. This is sometimes referred to as the *displacement factor*, or just *displacement*. The reconstituted material represents the diluent and powder. For ex-

Critical Thinking

Always determine both the type and amount of diluent to be used for reconstituting medications. Read and follow the label or package insert directions carefully to ensure that your client receives the intended dose. Consult a pharmacist or other appropriate resources if there are any questions. Never assume!

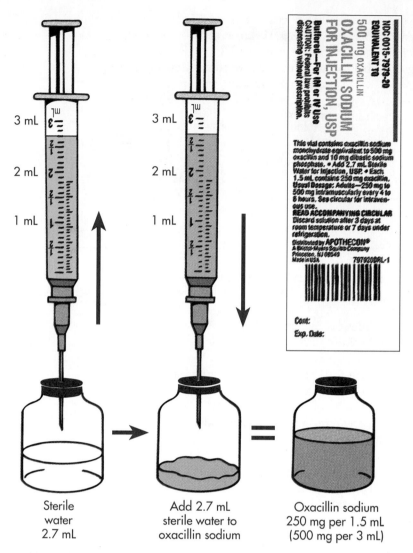

NDC 0015-7979-20
EQUIVALENT TO
500 mg OXACILLIN
OXACILLIN SODIUM
FOR INJECTION, USP
Buffered—For IM or IV Use
CAUTION: Federal law prohibits
dispensing without prescription.

This vial contains oxacillin sodium
monohydrate equivalent to 500 mg
oxacillin and 10 mg dibasic sodium
phosphate. • Add 2.7 mL Sterile
Water for Injection, USP. • Each
1.5 mL contains 250 mg oxacillin.
Usual Dosage: Adults—250 mg to
500 mg intramuscularly every 4 to
6 hours. See circular for intravenous use.
READ ACCOMPANYING CIRCULAR
Discard solution after 3 days at
room temperature or 7 days under
refrigeration.
Distributed by **APOTHECON®**
A Bristol-Myers Squibb Company
Princeton, NJ 08540
Made in USA   7979200RL-1

Cont:
Exp. Date:

Sterile	Add 2.7 mL	Oxacillin sodium
water	sterile water to	250 mg per 1.5 mL
2.7 mL	oxacillin sodium	(500 mg per 3 mL)

Figure 18-1 Oxacillin reconstitution procedure. (Modified from: Brown M, Mulholland J: *Drug calculations: process and problems for clinical practice,* ed 6, St Louis, 2000, Mosby.)

ample, directions for a 1 g powdered medication may state to add 2.5 mL sterile water to provide an approximate volume of 3 mL (330 mg/mL). When the
2.5 mL of diluent is added, the 1 g of powdered drug displaces an additional
0.5 mL for a total volume of 3 mL. The available dose after reconstitution is
330 mg per mL of solution.

Important: If displacement occurs as illustrated in the example, it must be considered when calculating the correct dose of medication. Whether a drug causes displacement will be indicated on the medication label or in the package insert.

Let's do some practice problems answering questions relating to single-strength
solutions.

Notes

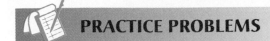

PRACTICE PROBLEMS

Using the label for ampicillin, answer the following questions.

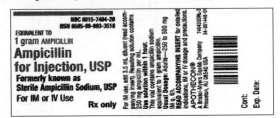

1. What is the total strength of ampicillin in this vial? _____

2. How much diluent is added to the vial to prepare the drug for I.M. use? _____

3. What diluent is recommended for reconstitution? _____

4. What is the final concentration of the prepared solution for I.M. administration? _____

5. How long will reconstituted material retain its potency? _____

6. 500 mg I.M. q6h is ordered. How many mL will you give? Shade the dose in on the syringe provided. _____

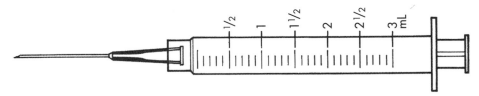

Using the label for oxacillin, answer the following questions.

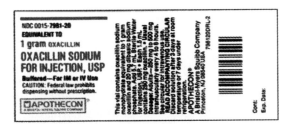

7. What is the total strength of oxacillin in the vial? _____

8. How many mL of diluent are needed to prepare the solution? _____

9. What diluent is recommended for reconstitution? _____

10. What is the final concentration of the prepared
    solution? _____

11. How long does the medication retain its potency
    at room temperature? _____

12. How long does the medication retain its potency
    if it is refrigerated? _____

13. 400 mg I.M. q6h is ordered. How many mL
    will you give? Shade the dose in on the syringe
    provided. _____

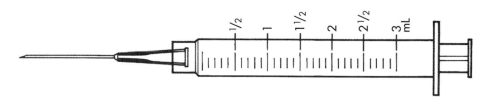

Use the label for Ticar to answer the following questions.

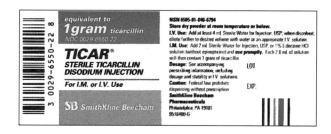

14. What is the total strength of Ticar in the vial? _____

15. What diluent is recommended to prepare
    for I.V. dose? _____

16. How many mL of diluent are needed to prepare
    for I.M. dose? _____

17. What is the final concentration of the prepared
    solution I.M.? _____

18. Ticar 500 mg I.M. q8h is ordered. How many
    mL will you give? Shade the amount in on the
    syringe provided. _____

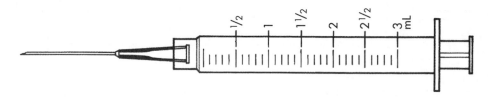

Using the label for Cefobid, answer the following questions.

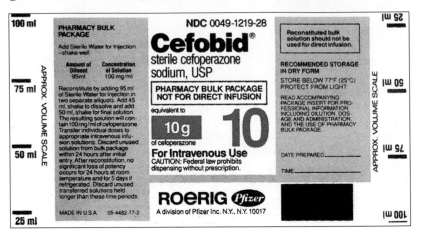

19. What is the total strength of Cefobid in this vial? _____

20. For what route of administration is the medication indicated? _____

21. How much diluent must be added to prepare the solution? _____

22. What kind of diluent is recommended for reconstitution? _____

23. What is the final concentration of the prepared solution? _____

24. How long does the medication maintain its potency at room temperature? _____

25. How long does the medication maintain its potency if refrigerated? _____

26. 1 g I.V. q6h is ordered. How many mL will you give? Shade the amount in on the syringe provided.

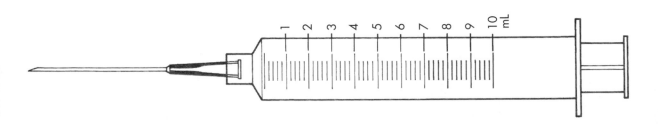

Using the label for Augmentin, answer the following questions.

Notes

Product No. 609064 **NOT FOR SALE**
Store dry powder at or below 25°C (77°F).
After mixing, refrigerate, keep tightly
closed and use within 24 hours. Shake
well before using.
Directions for mixing: Tap bottle until
all powder flows freely. Add approximately
1 teaspoonful (5 mL) of water; shake
vigorously. When reconstituted, each 5 mL
will contain 250 mg amoxicillin as the
trihydrate and 62.5 mg clavulanic acid as
clavulanate potassium. **9406441-E**

250mg/5mL *Patient Starter Package*

AUGMENTIN®
AMOXICILLIN/CLAVULANATE POTASSIUM
FOR ORAL SUSPENSION

1 x 5mL *(when reconstituted)*

SB *SmithKline Beecham*

SmithKline Beecham Pharmaceuticals, Philadelphia, PA 19101

27. How much diluent must be added to prepare the solution? _____

28. What type of solution is used for the diluent? _____

29. What is the final concentration of the prepared solution? _____

30. How should the medication be stored after it is reconstituted? _____

Using the label for Zovirax and a portion of the package insert, answer the following questions.

ZOVIRAX® STERILE POWDER   1000 mg   NDC 0173-0952-01
(ACYCLOVIR SODIUM) **equivalent to 1000 mg acyclovir**
FOR INTRAVENOUS INFUSION ONLY
CAUTION: Federal law prohibits dispensing without prescription.
Preparation of Solution: Inject 20 mL Sterile Water for Injection into vial. Shake vial until a clear solution is
achieved and use within 12 hours. DO NOT USE BACTERIOSTATIC WATER FOR INJECTION CONTAINING
BENZYL ALCOHOL OR PARABENS.
Dilute to 7 mg/mL or lower prior to infusion. See package insert for additional reconstitution and dilution instructions.
For indications, dosage, precautions, etc., see accompanying package insert.
Store at 15° to 25°C (59° to 77°F).

Glaxo Wellcome Inc.
Research Triangle Park, NC 27709

U.S. Patent No. 4199574
Rev. 2/96
Made in U.S.A.

647627

Method of Preparation: Each 10 mL vial contains acyclovir sodium equivalent to 500 mg of acyclovir. Each
20 mL vial contains acyclovir sodium equivalent to 1000 mg of acyclovir. The contents of the vial should be
dissolved in Sterile Water for Injection as follows:

Contents of Vial	Amount of Diluent
500 mg	10 mL
1000 mg	20 mL

The resulting solution in each case contains 50 mg acyclovir per mL (pH approximately 11). Shake the vial well
to assure complete dissolution before measuring and transferring each individual dose. DO NOT USE BACTE-
RIOSTATIC WATER FOR INJECTION CONTAINING BENZYL ALCOHOL OR PARABENS.

31. What is the total strength of Zovirax in this vial? _____

32. How much diluent must be added to prepare the solution? _____

33. What diluent is recommended for reconstitution? _____

34. What is the final concentration of the prepared solution? _____

35. What is the route of administration? _____

Using the label for erythromycin, answer the following questions.

TO PATIENT:
Shake well before using.
Keep tightly closed. Store in refrigerator and discard unused portion after ten days. Oversize bottle provides shake space.
TO THE PHARMACIST:
When prepared as directed, each 5 mL teaspoonful contains erythromycin ethylsuccinate equivalent to 200 mg of erythromycin in a cherry-flavored suspension.
Bottle contains erythromycin ethylsuccinate equivalent to 8 g of erythromycin.
Usual Dose: See package outsert.
Store at room temperature in dry form.
Child-Resistant closure not required; Reference: Federal Register Vol.39 No.29.
DIRECTIONS FOR PREPARATION: Slowly add 140 mL of water and shake vigorously to make 200 mL of suspension.
BARR LABORATORIES, INC.
Pomona, NY 10970
R11-90

BARR LABORATORIES, INC.

Erythromycin Ethylsuccinate
for Oral Suspension, USP

200 mg of erythromycin activity per 5 mL reconstituted

Caution: Federal law prohibits dispensing without prescription.

200 mL (when mixed)

NDC 0555-0215-23
NSN 6505-00-080-0653

0555-0215-23

SAMPLE

Exp. Date:
Lot No.:

36. How much diluent must be added to prepare the solution? _____

37. What is the volume of the solution after it is mixed? _____

38. What is the final concentration of the prepared solution? _____

39. How long is the reconstituted solution good? _____

Answers on pp. 534-535

Calculation of Medications When the Final Concentration (Dose Strength) Is Not Stated

Sometimes medications come with directions for only one way to reconstitute them, and the label does not indicate the final dose strength after it is mixed, such as "becomes 250 mg per mL." Example: A particular medication is available in 1 g in powder. Directions tell you that adding 2.5 mL of sterile water yields 3 mL of solution. When you add 2.5 mL of sterile water, the solution expands to 3 mL. The concentration is not changing; you will get 3 mL of solution; however, it will be equal to 1 g.
The problem is therefore calculated using 1 g = 3 mL.

RECONSTITUTING MEDICATIONS WITH MORE THAN ONE DIRECTION FOR MIXING

Some medications come with a choice of how to reconstitute them, thereby providing a choice of dose strengths. In this case the nurse must choose the concentration or dose strength appropriate for the dose ordered. A common medication that has a choice of dose strengths is penicillin. When a medication comes with several directions for preparation or offers a choice of dose strengths, you must choose the strength most appropriate for the dosage ordered. The following guidelines may be used.

Guidelines for Choosing Appropriate Concentrations

1. Consider the route of administration.
   a) I.M.—You are concerned that the amount does not exceed the maximum allowed I.M. However you don't want to choose a concentration that will result in irritation when injected into a muscle. When a choice of strengths can be made, do not choose an amount that would exceed the amount allowed I.M. or that is very concentrated.
   b) I.V.—Keep in mind that this medication is usually further diluted because once reconstituted, the reconstituted material is then placed in additional fluid of 50 to 100 mL, depending on the medication being administered. Example: Erythromycin requires that the reconstituted solution be placed in 250 mL of fluid before administration to a client. In pediatrics a medication may be given in a smaller volume of fluid depending on the age, the child's size, and the medication.
2. Choose the concentration or dose strength that comes closest to what the doctor has ordered. The dose strengths are given for the amount of diluent used. Example: If the doctor orders 300,000 U of a particular medication I.M., and the choices of strength are 200,000 U/mL, 250,000 U/mL, and 500,000 U/mL, the strength closest to 300,000 U/mL is 250,000 U/mL. It allows you to administer a dose within the range for I.M., and it is not the most concentrated.
3. The word *respectively* may be used sometimes on a medication label for directions on reconstitution. For example, reconstitute with 23 mL, 18 mL, 8 mL of diluent to provide concentrations of 200,000 U, 250,000 U, 500,000 U per mL, respectively. The word *respectively* means in the order given. In terms of the directions for reconstitution, this means if you add 23 mL diluent, it will provide 200,000 U per mL, 18 mL diluent will provide 250,000 U per mL, etc. In other words, the amounts of diluent correspond to the order in which the concentrations are written. Remember: **When you are mixing a medication that is a multiple-strength solution, the dose strength that you prepare must be written on the vial.** Let's look at a sample label that shows a multiple-strength solution.

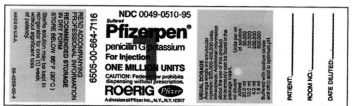

When looking at the penicillin label, notice that it states one million U. This means there is a total of 1,000,000 U of penicillin in the vial. The directions for reconstitution and the dose strengths that can be obtained are listed on the right side of the label. If the dosage ordered for the client was, for example, 200,000 U q6h, the most appropriate strength to mix would be 200,000 U per mL. When reading the directions, if you look across next to the dose strength, you will notice that 4.6 mL of diluent must be added to obtain a concentration of solution 200,000 U per mL. Because this is a multiple-strength solution, the dose strength you choose must be indicated on the vial after you reconstitute it. Since the type of diluent is not indicated on the label, other resources such as those recommended previously must be consulted.

> **Thinking Critically**
>
> If a multiple-strength solution is prepared and not used in its entirety, the dose strength (final concentration) you mixed must be indicated on the label to verify the dose strength of the reconstituted solution. Proper labeling is a crucial detail.

Notes

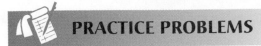

PRACTICE PROBLEMS

Using the label for penicillin G potassium, answer the following questions.

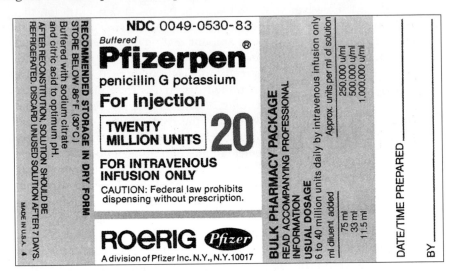

40. What is the total number of units of penicillin contained in the vial? (Write out in numbers.) _____

41. If you add 33 mL of diluent to the vial, what dose strength will you print on the label? _____

42. If 2,000,000 U I.V. is ordered, which dose strength would be appropriate to use? _____

43. How many mL will you administer? _____

44. How long will the medication maintain its potency if refrigerated? _____

Using the label for penicillin G potassium, answer the following questions.

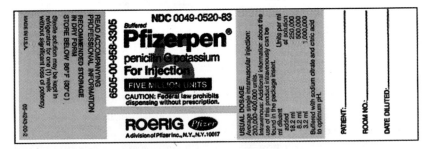

45. What is the total number of units of penicillin contained in the vial? (Write out in numbers.) _____

46. If 700,000 U I.M. is ordered, which dose strength would be appropriate to use? _____

47. How many mL will you administer? _____

48. Where will you store any unused medication? _____

49. How long will the medication maintain its potency? _____

50. What concentration strength would be obtained if you added 18.2 mL of diluent? (Write out in numbers.) _____

51. How long can the potency of the medication be maintained if it is refrigerated? _____

RECONSTITUTION FROM PACKAGE INSERT DIRECTIONS

If the label does not contain reconstitution directions you must obtain directions from the information insert that accompanies the vial. Refer to the Tazicef label and insert provided.

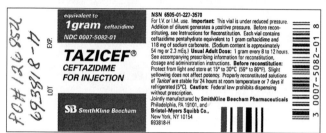

RECONSTITUTION

Single Dose Vials:
For I.M. injection, I.V. direct (bolus) injection, or I.V. infusion, reconstitute with Sterile Water for injection according to the following table. The vacuum may assist entry of the diluent. SHAKE WELL.

Table 5

Vial Size	Diluent to Be Added	Approx. Avail. Volume	Approx. Avg. Concentration
Intramuscular or Intravenous Direct (bolus) Injection			
1 gram	3.0 ml.	3.6 ml.	280 mg./ml.
Intravenous Infusion			
1 gram	10 ml.	10.6 ml.	95 mg./ml.
2 gram	10 ml.	11.2 ml.	180 mg./ml.

Withdraw the total volume of solution into the syringe (the pressure in the vial may aid withdrawal). The withdrawn solution may contain some bubbles of carbon dioxide.

NOTE: As with the administration of all parenteral products, accumulated gases should be expressed from the syringe immediately before injection of 'Tazicef'.

These solutions of 'Tazicef' are stable for 18 hours at room temperature or seven days if refrigerated (5°C.). Slight yellowing does not affect potency.

For I.V. infusion, dilute reconstituted solution in 50 to 100 ml. of one of the parenteral fluids listed under COMPATIBILITY AND STABILITY

52. How much diluent must be added to this vial for I.M. reconstitution? _____

53. What kind of diluent must be used? _____

54. What is the concentration per mL of this solution? _____

55. What is the dosage of the total vial? _____

Answers on p. 535

Before we proceed to calculate doses, let's review the steps to use with medications that have been reconstituted.

1. The formula or the ratio-proportion method may be used to calculate the dose. What's available becomes the dose strength you obtain after mixing the medication according to the directions.
2. Powdered medications may increase in volume after a liquid is added (diluent + powder). The volume to which the medication expands must be considered when calculating.
3. When the final concentration is not stated, the total weight of the medication in powdered form is used, and the number of mL produced is indicated after the solvent or liquid has been added.

4. As with all calculation problems, check to make sure that the ordered and the available medications are in the same system of measurement and the same units.
5. Don't forget to label your answer.

CALCULATION OF DOSES

To calculate the dose to administer after reconstituting a medication, the ratio-proportion or formula method may be used, as with other forms of medication. However, the H (have or what's available) is the dose strength you obtain when you mix the medication according to the directions. If using ratio-proportion, therefore, the known ratio is also the dose strength obtained when you mix the medication.

In $\dfrac{D}{H} \times Q = x$, Q is the volume of solution that contains the dose strength.

In $\dfrac{DW}{SW} = \dfrac{DV}{SV}$, SV is the volume of solution that contains the dose strength.

To illustrate, let's calculate the dose you would administer if you mixed penicillin and made a solution containing 1,000,000 U/mL. Order: 2,000,000 U I.M. q6h.

➡ Solution Using the Ratio-Proportion Method

$$1,000,000 \text{ U} : 1 \text{ mL} = 2,000,000 \text{ U} : x \text{ mL}$$

$$(\text{Known}) \qquad\qquad (\text{Unknown})$$

$$\frac{1,000,000 \, x}{1,000,000} = \frac{2,000,000}{1,000,000}$$

$$x = \frac{2,000,0000}{1,000,000}$$

$$x = 2 \text{ mL}$$

➡ Solution Using the Formula Method

$$\frac{D}{H} \times Q = x$$

$$\frac{2,000,000 \text{ U}}{1,000,000 \text{ U}} \times 1 \text{ mL} = x \text{ mL}$$

$$x = \frac{2,000,000}{1,000,000}$$

$$x = 2 \text{ mL}$$

OR

$$\frac{DW}{SW} = \frac{DV}{SV}$$

$$\frac{2,000,000 \text{ U}}{1,000,000 \text{ U}} = \frac{x \text{ mL}}{1 \text{ mL}}$$

$$\frac{1,000,000x}{1,000,000} = \frac{2,000,000}{1,000,000}$$

$$x = \frac{2,000,000}{1,000,000}$$

$$x = 2 \text{ mL}$$

Sample Problem: Order: 0.5 g of an antibiotic I.M. q4h.

Available: 1 g of the drug in powdered form; the label reads: Add 1.7 mL of sterile water; each mL will then contain 500 mg.

▶ Problem Setup

1. A conversion is necessary. Equivalent 1,000 mg = 1 g. Convert what's ordered into the available units. This will eliminate a decimal point. Therefore 0.5 g = 500 mg.
2. Think: What would a logical answer be?

▶ Solution Using the Ratio-Proportion Method

$$500 \text{ mg} : 1 \text{ mL} = 500 \text{ mg} : x \text{ mL}$$

$$\text{(Known)} \qquad \text{(Unknown)}$$

$$\frac{500x}{500} = \frac{500}{500}$$

$$x = \frac{500}{500}$$

$$x = 1 \text{ mL}$$

▶ Solution Using the Formula Method

$$\frac{D}{H} \times Q = x$$

$$\frac{500 \text{ mg}}{500 \text{ mg}} \times 1 \text{ mL} = x \text{ mL}$$

$$x = \frac{500}{500}$$

$$x = 1 \text{ mL}$$

OR

$$\frac{DW}{SW} = \frac{DV}{SV}$$

$$\frac{500 \text{ mg}}{500 \text{ mg}} = \frac{x \text{ mL}}{1 \text{ mL}}$$

$$\frac{\cancel{500}x}{\cancel{500}} = \frac{500}{500}$$

$$x = 1 \text{ mL}$$

Note:

If there is no area on the label for this information to be indicated, the information can be written directly on the vial in an area that can be read clearly.

POINTS TO REMEMBER

- If the medication is not used entirely after it is mixed, any medication remaining for use must have the following information clearly written on the label.

a) Initials of the preparer

b) Dose strength (if multichoice strengths/multiple strength)

c) Date and time of preparation and the date and time of expiration

- Read all directions carefully; if there are no instructions on the vial, then the package insert, pharmacy, or other reliable resources may be used to find the necessary information for reconstitution.

- When directions on the label are for I.M. and I.V. reconstitution, read the label carefully for the solution you are preparing.

- The type and amount of diluent to be used for reconstitution must be followed exactly.

- Read directions relating to storage (room temperature, refrigeration) and the time period for maintaining potency.

- When diluting powdered medication results in an increase volume, this must be considered in calculating the dose.

CHAPTER REVIEW

Use the labels where provided to obtain the necessary information; shade the dosage on syringes where provided. Round the answers to the nearest tenth where indicated. Note: For problems where conversion is indicated, answers are shown with order changed to what's available.

1. Order: Ampicillin 400 mg I.M. q4h.

   Available:

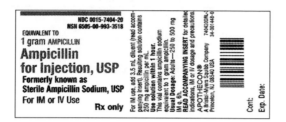

   a) How many mL will you administer? _____

   b) Shade the dose calculated on the syringe provided.

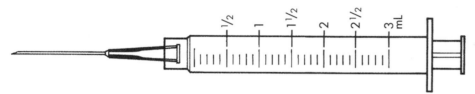

2. Order: Ampicillin 1 g I.V. q6h.

   Available: 1 g vial. Directions for I.V. administration state: Reconstitute with 10 mL of diluent.

   a) How many mL will you administer? _____

   b) Shade the dose calculated on the syringe provided.

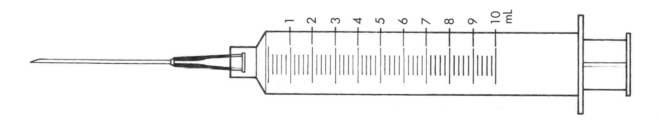

Notes

3. Order: Oxacillin 300 mg I.M. q6h.

   Available:

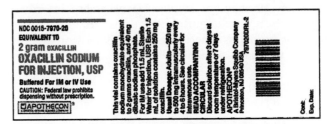

   a) How many mL will you give? _____

   b) Shade the dose calculated on the syringe provided.

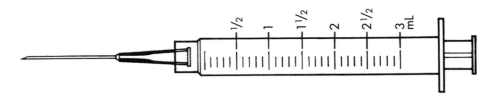

4. Order: Mezlocillin 1.5 g I.V. q6h.
   Label states: For I.V. use reconstitute with 30 mL sterile water for injection.
   Each 30 mL of reconstituted solution will contain 3 g mezlocillin.

   a) How many mL will you administer? _____

5. Order: Ticar 1 g I.M. q6h.

   Available:

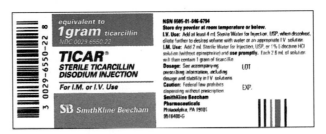

   a) How many mL of diluent must be added? _____

   b) What diluent is recommended for
      reconstitution? _____

   c) What is the dose strength of the
      reconstituted solution? _____

   d) How many mL will you administer? _____

   e) Shade the dose calculated on the syringe provided.

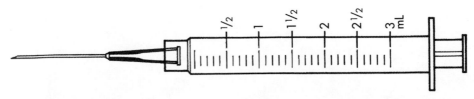

6. Order: Penicillin G 600,000 U I.V. q4h.

   Available:

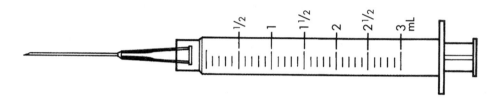

   a) Which dose strength would be best
      to choose?   _____

   b) How many mL of diluent would be needed
      to make the dose strength?   _____

   c) How many mL will you administer?   _____

   d) Shade the dose calculated on the syringe provided.

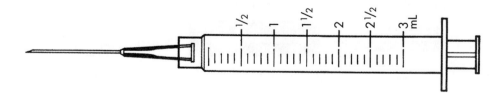

7. Order: Solu-Cortef 200 mg I.V. q6h × 1 week.

   Available:

Single-Dose Vial For IV or IM use	2 mL Act-O-Vial® NDC 0009-0909-08
Contains Benzyl Alcohol as a Preservative	**Solu-Cortef®** Sterile Powder
See package insert for complete product information.	hydrocortisone sodium succinate
Per 2 mL (when mixed):	for injection, USP
• hydrocortisone sodium succinate equiv. to hydrocortisone, 250 mg. Protect solution from light. Discard after 3 days.	**250 mg***
814 070 205 Reconstituted	
The Upjohn Company Kalamazoo, MI 49001, USA	

   a) How many mg per mL is the reconstituted
      material?   _____

   b) How many mL will you administer?   _____

   c) Shade the dose calculated on the syringe provided.

Notes

8. Order: Carbenicillin 1 g I.M. q6h.

   Available:

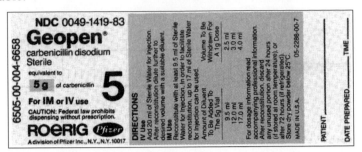

   a) What is the total strength of Geopen in this vial? _____

   b) What diluent is recommended for reconstitution? _____

   c) If you reconstitute with 9.5 mL of diluent, how many mL will you administer? _____

   d) Shade the dose calculated on the syringe provided.

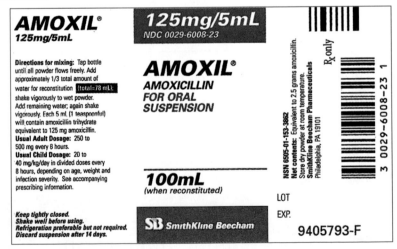

9. Order: Amoxicillin 500 mg p.o. q6h.

   Available:

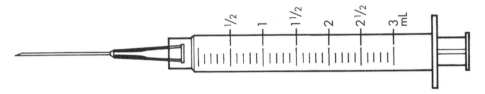

   a) How many mL of diluent must be added? _____

   b) What is the dose strength after reconstitution? _____

   c) How many mL are needed to administer the required dose? _____

10. Order: Ancef 500 mg I.M. q8h.

Available:

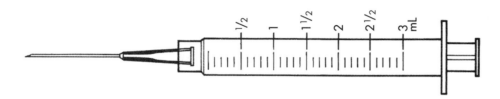

a) How many mL of diluent should be used to reconstitute? _____

b) What will be the dose strength of the reconstituted Ancef? _____

c) How many mL will you administer? _____

d) Shade the dose calculated on the syringe provided.

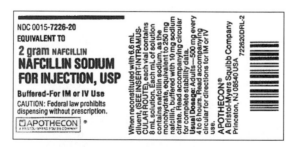

11. Order: Nafcillin 0.5 g I.M. q6h.

Available:

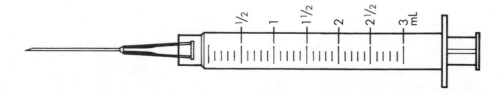

a) What is the dose strength of the reconstituted nafcillin? _____

b) How many mL will you administer? _____

c) Shade the dose calculated on the syringe provided.

12. Order: Cefotaxime 750 mg I.M. q8h.

Available: Cefotaxime with the package insert below.

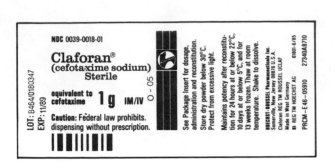

PREPARATION OF CLAFORAN STERILE

Claforan for IM or IV administration should be reconstituted as follows:

Strength	Diluent (mL)	Withdrawable Volume (mL)	Approximate Concentration (mg/mL)
1g vial (IM)*	3	3.4	300
2g vial (IM)*	5	6.0	330
1g vial (IV)*	10	10.4	95
2g vial (IV)*	10	11.0	180
1g infusion	50-100	50-100	20-10
2g infusion	50-100	50-100	40-20
10g bottle	47	52.0	200
10g bottle	97	102.0	100

*in conventional vials

Shake to dissolve; inspect for particulate matter and discoloration prior to use. Solutions of Claforan range from very pale yellow to light amber, depending on concentration, diluent used, and length and condition of storage.

a) How many grams of cefotaxime are in the vial? _____

b) According to the package insert, what volume of diluent is used for I.M. reconstitution? _____

c) What is the dose strength of the reconstituted cefotaxime? _____

d) How many mL will you administer? _____

e) Shade the dose calculated on the syringe provided.

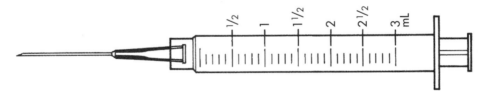

13. Order: Streptomycin 0.5 g I.M. q6h.

    Available:

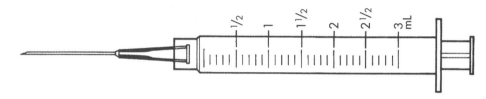

a) How many grams of streptomycin are
   in the vial? _____

b) What is the volume of diluent used for
   reconstitution? _____

c) What is the dose strength of the reconstituted
   streptomycin? _____

d) How many mL will you give? _____

e) Shade the dose calculated on the syringe provided.

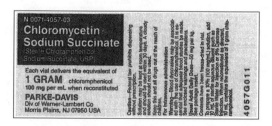

14. Order: Chloromycetin 0.5 g I.V. q6h.

    Available:

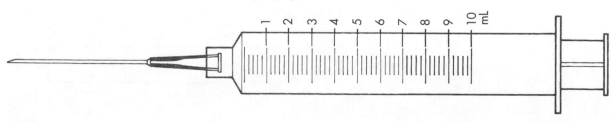

a) What is the volume of diluent used for
   reconstitution? _____

b) What is the dose strength of the reconstituted
   Chloromycetin? _____

c) How many mL will you administer? _____

d) Shade the dose calculated on the syringe provided.

Notes

15. Order: Penicillin G potassium 400,000 U I.M. q4h.

    Available: Penicillin G 5,000,000 U. Directions state: Add 8.2 mL diluent to provide 500,000 U/mL.

    a) How many mL will you administer?   _____

    b) Shade the dose calculated on the syringe provided.

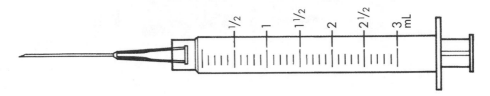

16. Order: Ceftazidime 250 mg I.M. q12h.

    Available: Ceftazidime 600 mg. Directions for I.M. use state: Add 1.5 mL of an approved diluent to provide 300 mg/mL.

    a) How many mL will you administer?   _____

    b) Shade the dose calculated on the syringe provided.

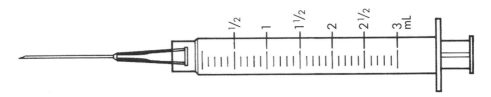

17. Order: Ticar 0.5 g I.M. q6h.

    Available:

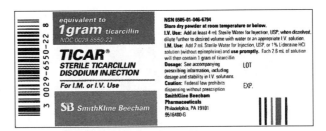

    a) How many mL of diluent would be used
       to reconstitute?   _____

    b) What is the dose strength of the
       reconstituted Ticar?   _____

    c) How many mL will you administer?   _____

    d) Shade the dose calculated on the syringe provided.

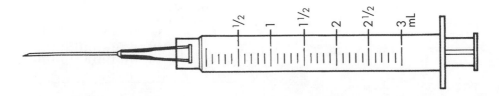

18. Order: Tazicef 0.4 g I.V. q8h.

    Directions for I.V. state: Add 10 mL sterile water. Each mL of solution contains 95 mg/mL

    a) How many mL will you administer? _____

    b) Shade the dose calculated on the syringe provided.

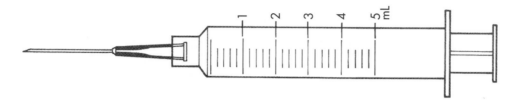

19. Order: Vancomycin 0.5 g I.V. q12h.
    Use the directions below from insert.

    Available:

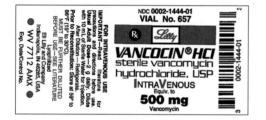

PREPARATION AND STABILITY
At the time of use, reconstitute by adding either 10 mL of Sterile Water for Injection to the 500-mg vial or 20 mL of Sterile Water for Injection to the 1-g vial of dry, sterile vancomycin powder. Vials reconstituted in this manner will give a solution of 50 mg/mL. FURTHER DILUTION IS REQUIRED.
After reconstitution, the vials may be stored in a refrigerator for 14 days without significant loss of potency. Reconstituted solutions containing 500 mg of vancomycin must be diluted with at least 100 mL of diluent. Reconstituted solutions containing 1 g of vancomycin must be diluted with at least 200 mL of diluent. The desired dose, diluted in this manner, should be administered by intermittent intravenous infusion over a period of at least 60 minutes.

    a) How many mL will you administer? _____

    b) Shade the dose calculated on the syringe provided.

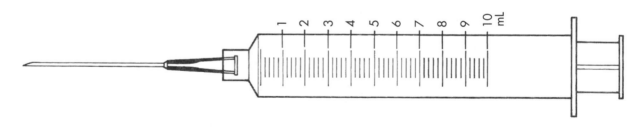

20. Order: Levothyroxine sodium 0.05 mg I.V. o.d.

    Available: Levothyroxine sodium vial with directions that state: Dilute with 5 mL of sodium chloride to produce 200 mcg.

    a) How many mL will you administer? _____

    b) Shade the dose calculated on the syringe provided.

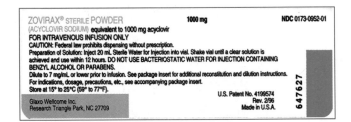

21. Order: Zovirax 0.25 g I.V. q8h × 5 days.
    Directions state: Add 10 mL of sterile water to produce 50 mg/mL.

    Available:

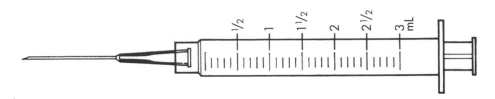

    a) How many mL will you administer? _____

    b) Shade the dose you calculated in on the syringe provided.

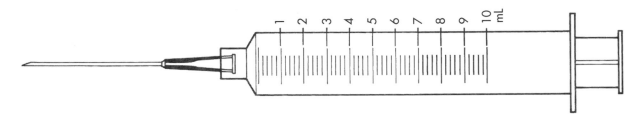

22. Order: Suprax 400 mg p.o. q.d.

    Available:

    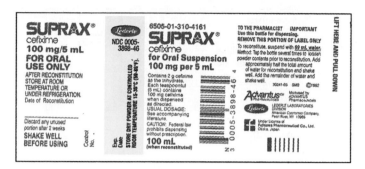

    a) How many mL of water is needed to
    reconstitute the powder? _____

    b) How many mL will you administer using
    an oral syringe? _____

23. Order: Timentin 2 g I.V. q12h.

    Available: Timentin 3.1 g. Directions state: Reconstitute with approximately
    13 mL of sterile water for injection or sodium chloride for injection. The
    concentration will be approximately 200 mg/mL.

    a) How many mL will you administer? _____

    b) Shade the dose on the syringe provided.

    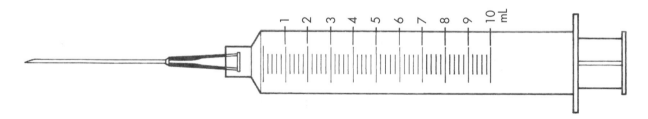

24. Order: Maxipime (cefepime hydrochloride) 2 g I.V. q12h.

    Available:

    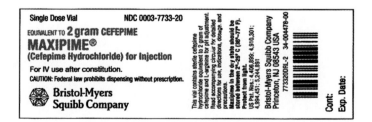

    When reconstituted, yields a concentration of 160 mg/mL.

    How many mL will you administer? _____

Notes

25. Order: Nafcillin 300 mg I.M. q6h.

    Available:

    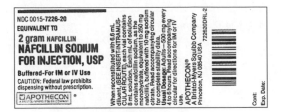

    a) How many mL will you give? _____

    b) Shade the dose on the syringe provided.

    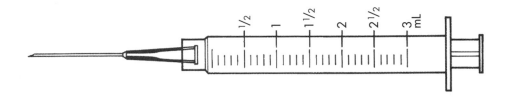

26. Order: Tazicef 1 g I.V. q12h.

    Available: Tazicef 1 g, when reconstituted for I.V. use 95 mg/mL.

    How many mL will you administer? _____

27. Order: Cefadyl 0.75 g I.V. q6h.

    Available:

    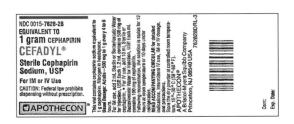

    How many mL will you administer? _____

Answers on pp. 535-542

Insulin

Objectives

After reviewing this chapter, you should be able to:

1. Identify important information on insulin labels
2. Read calibrations on U-100 insulin syringes
3. Measure insulin in single doses
4. Measure combined insulin doses

Insulin, which is used in the treatment of diabetes mellitus, is a hormone secreted by the islets of Langerhans in the pancreas. It is a necessary hormone for glucose use by the body. Individuals who do not produce adequate insulin experience an increase in their blood sugar (glucose) level. These individuals may require the administration of insulin. Accuracy in insulin administration is extremely important because inaccurate doses can lead to serious or life-threatening effects. Insulin doses are measured in units (U) and administered with syringes that correspond to insulin U-100; U-100 insulin means 100 U/mL. The most common type of insulin is supplied in 10-mL vials and labeled U-100. Insulin is also available as U-500 (500 U/mL). U-500 is a more concentrated strength and is used for diabetic clients who have blood sugars that fluctuate to extremely high levels.

TYPES OF INSULIN

Different types of insulin are available today. The choice of dose and insulin preparations are dependent on the needs of the client. Insulin is derived from animal or human sources as indicated on the labels. Human insulin is indicated on the label as of recombinant DNA origin. Humalog insulin (Lispro), a new fast-acting insulin and also a recombinant DNA insulin, acts within 15 minutes. The most common insulin on the market is recombinant DNA, because it has fewer reactions than variety from animal sources. It is essential that the nurse know where to locate this information; when an insulin order is written it may specify the origin. Specification of origin when an order is written is recommended because of variations. Also found on the label is the type of insulin. This is indicated by a letter that follows the trade name. (Figure 19-1 identifies information that can be found on an insulin label.)

The letters that follow the trade name on insulin labels (e.g., Humulin R, Humulin N) identify the type of insulin by action and time (see Figure 19-1). Nurses must be familiar with the onset, peak, and duration of action, which vary depending on the type of insulin. There are three basic action times of insulins: rapid-acting (regular, Semilente, and Lispro); intermediate-acting (Lente, NPH insulins); and long-acting (Ultra Lente). The expiration date and concentration are also indicated on the label and are important to check. For insulins manufactured by Eli Lilly and Com-

Notes

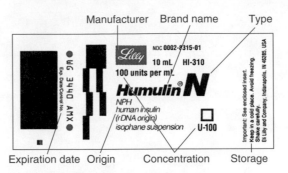

Figure 19-1   Insulin label.

pany under the trade name Humulin, an international symbol is also indicated on the label, so insulins can be identified worldwide.

Example:

($\diamond$) = Regular, ($\square$) = NPH. (See Humulin insulin label in Figure 19-1.) Notice that the label shows Humulin (trade name) followed by the letter N. N = NPH (intermediate acting). Note the international symbol on the label as well.

❚ Be sure to read the label carefully to administer insulin of the correct origin.

PRACTICE PROBLEMS

Using the labels below, identify the type of insulin and its origin. Note that the left side of the label indicates whether the insulin is made from beef or pork.

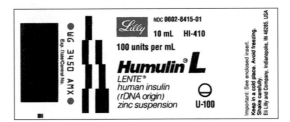

1. _____

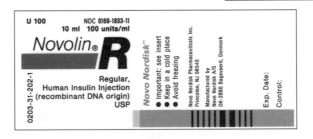

2. _____

⚠ Thinking Critically

Careful reading of insulin labels is essential for correct identification and avoiding of a medication error that could be life threatening. Always read the label and compare it with the medication order. Reading the label carefully ensures selection of the correct action time and species of insulin.

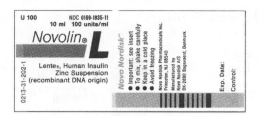

3. _____

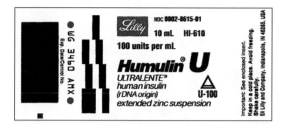

4. _____

Answers on p. 542

Types of U-100 Insulins

Nurses must be familiar with the three types of U-100 insulins. Below are samples of labels according to their action times.

Fast-Acting (Rapid-Acting)

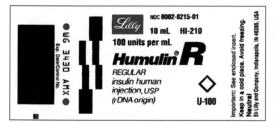

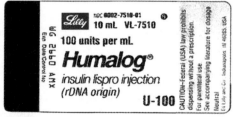

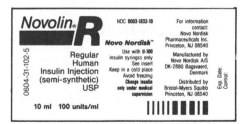

Intermediate-Acting

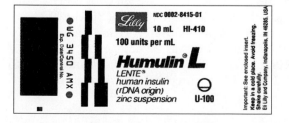

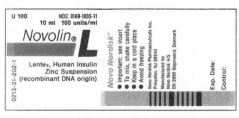

Intermediate-Acting—cont'd

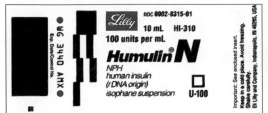
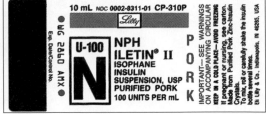

Long-Acting

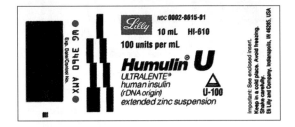

APPEARANCE OF INSULIN

Regular insulin is clear and is the only insulin that may be administered intravenously (I.V.). All other insulin is cloudy. Previously it was recommended that cloudy insulins must be rotated between the hands to mix. A recent article in the *American Journal of Nursing* (February 1999, Vol 99, No. 2, "Challenging Traditional Insulin Injection Practices" by Doris R. Fleming, MSN, NP, CDE) states: "because rolling a vial of insulin doesn't adequately mix a suspension such as NPH or lente, and may result in an inconsistent concentration of insulin it's necessary to vigorously shake the vial. . . . Remember that shaking the vial decreases the risk of an inconsistent concentration of insulin, and consequently minimizes the likelihood of fluctuating blood glucose levels."

FIXED-COMBINATION INSULINS

Fixed-combination insulins are now available: 70/30 U-100 and 50/50 U-100 (Figure 19-2). The purpose of the fixed-combination insulins is to simulate the varying levels of insulin within the bodies of nondiabetic persons. The 70/30 combination insulin is used most often.

To understand fixed-combination insulin orders, it is important for the nurse to understand that, for example, 70/30 concentration means there is 70% NPH insulin (isophane) and 30% regular insulin in each unit. Therefore if the order was 30 units of Humulin 70/30 insulin, the client would receive 21 U of NPH (70% or 0.7 × 30 U = 21 U and 9 U of Regular insulin (30% or 0.3 × 30 U = 9 U).

The 50/50 insulin concentration means there is 50% NPH insulin and 50% Regular insulin in each unit. Therefore if the order was 20 units of 50/50 insulin, the client would receive 10 U of NPH (50% or 0.5 × 20 U = 10 U) and 10 U of Regular insulin (50% or 0.5 × 20 U = 10 U). Figure 19-2 shows labels of fixed-combination insulins.

Figure 19-2 Fixed-combination insulins.

U-100 SYRINGE

The U-100 syringe was discussed in Chapter 17. To review, insulin is supplied in units that denote strength. Insulin is administered with special insulin syringes s.c., usually with a syringe marked U-100. In addition, insulin is given with insulin pens that contain cartridges filled with insulin. CSII pumps (continuous subcutaneous insulin infusion pumps) are used to administer a programmed dose of a rapid-acting 100 U insulin at a set rate of units per hour. We will focus on the administration of insulin with the use of U-100 syringes. There are different types of U-100 syringes.

1. Lo-Dose syringe—It has a capacity of 50 U (1/2 mL). Each calibration on the syringe measures 1 U. There is also a 30-U syringe, which is used to accurately measure very small amounts of insulin. It is marked in units up to 30 units. Each calibration is 1 U (0.3 mL).
2. 1-mL (100 U) capacity syringe—There are two types of 1-mL syringes in current use.
   a) The single-scale syringe is calibrated in 2-U increments. Any dose measured in an odd number of units is measured between the even calibrations. This would not be the desired syringe for clients with vision problems.
   b) The double-scale syringe has odd-numbered units on the left and even units on the right. To avoid confusion, the scale on the left should be used for odd units (e.g., 13 U) and the scale on the right for even numbers of units (e.g., 26 U). When measuring even numbers of units, each calibration then is measured as 2 U. Look carefully at the increments when using a dual syringe.

> *Note:*
>
> Using smaller syringes enables the smaller insulin doses to be more precise.

Remember: Administer insulin in an insulin syringe only. Do not use any other syringe. Use U-100 insulin syringes; 30 and 50 units measure a smaller volume of insulin but are intended for the measurement of U-100 insulin only. Use the smallest capacity insulin syringe available to ensure the accuracy of dose preparation.

To review what the syringes look like, see Figure 19-3 for the four types of insulin syringes discussed.

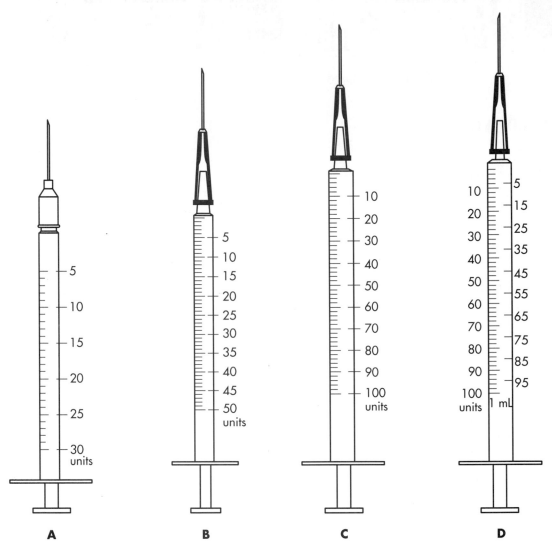

Figure 19-3 Types of insulin syringes. **A,** Lo-Dose insulin syringe (30 U). **B,** Lo-Dose insulin syringe (50 U). **C,** Single-scale syringe (100 U). **D,** Double-scale syringe (100 U).

Lo-Dose Syringe

Let's look at some insulin doses measured in the syringes to help you visualize the amounts in a syringe. Syringe *A* shows 30 U and syringe *B* shows 37 U on a Lo-Dose syringe.

Notes

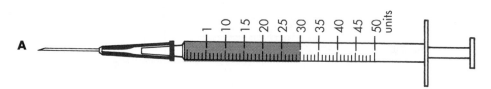

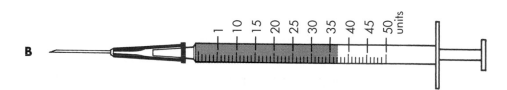

 PRACTICE PROBLEMS

Using the syringes below, indicate the doses shown by the arrows.

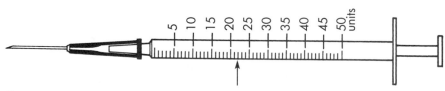

5. _____

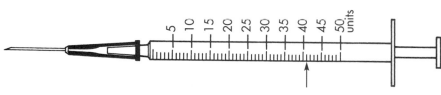

6. _____

Using the syringes below, shade the doses indicated.

7. 17 U

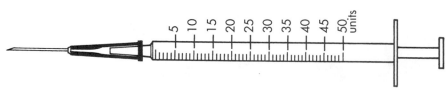

8. 47 U

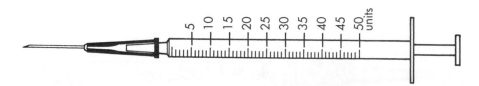

Answers on p. 542

Notes

Single-Scale 1-mL Syringe

Now let's look at what doses would look like on a single-scale 1-mL syringe. The syringes below show 25 U in syringe *A* and 55 U in syringe *B*. Notice that the doses are drawn up in between the even calibrations.

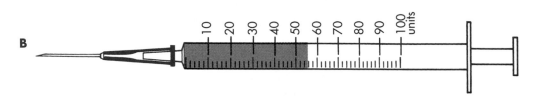

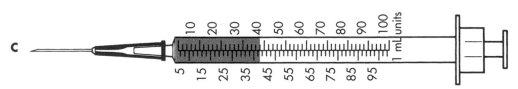

Double-Scale 1-mL Syringe

Now let's look at the dose indicated on a double-scale 1-mL syringe. Syringe *C* shows 37 U; notice that the scale on the left is used. Syringe *D* shows 54 U; notice that the scale on the right is used.

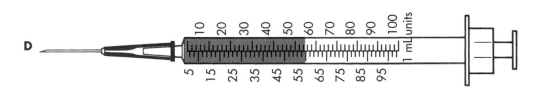

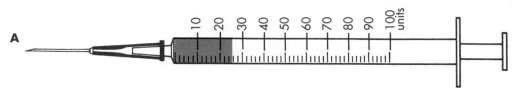

 PRACTICE PROBLEMS

Read the following doses shaded on the U-100 (1-mL) syringes.

9. _____

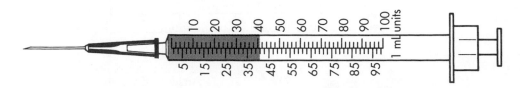

Notes

10. _____

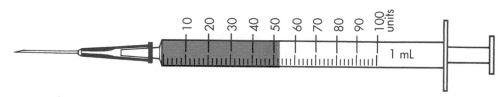

11. _____

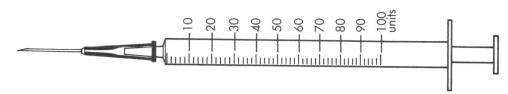

12. _____

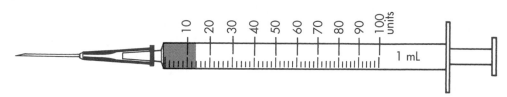

Shade the specified doses on each of the U-100 syringes below.

13. 88 U

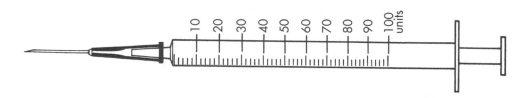

14. 44 U

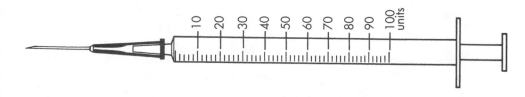

15. 30 U

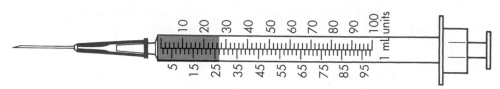

Answers on pp. 542-543

INSULIN ORDERS

Like any written medication order, insulin orders must be written clearly and contain certain information to prevent errors in administration. An error in administration can cause harmful effects to a client. Insulin orders should contain the following information:

a) The brand name of insulin (which implies the origin) and the action time. Example: Humulin R indicates human origin. Regular indicates rapid action. Some orders may be written simply as Humulin Regular.

b) The number of units to be administered. Example: 20 U, Humulin Regular.

c) The route (s.c.). Insulin is usually administered s.c.; however, regular insulin can be administered I.V. as well.

d) The time it should be given. Example: 1/2 hour before meals.

e) The strength of the insulin to be administered. Example: U-100.

Note:

Insulin is given s.c. unless specified I.V.)

Example of Insulin Order: Regular Humulin insulin U-100 20 U s.c. $^1/_2$ hr ā breakfast.

To avoid misinterpretation many institutions require that the abbreviation "U," which stands for units, not be used when writing insulin orders, but instead to write out the word. Errors have occurred due to the confusion of "U" with an "O" in a hand-written order. Example: 6 Ʊ s.c. stat of Humulin Regular. The U is almost completely closed and could be misread as 60 units. The recommendation to write out the word "units" has also been issued by the Institute for Safe Medication Practices.

Coverage Orders

Sometimes, in addition to standing insulin orders, clients may have orders for additional insulin to "cover" their increased blood sugar levels. (This is often referred to as a sliding scale). The sliding scale adds or deletes units of insulin from the client's standard daily dose depending on current blood glucose levels. Regular insulin is used because of its immediate action and short duration. A coverage order specifies the dose of insulin according to the blood sugar level and the frequency. The amount of insulin and the blood sugar level should be specific. The following is a sample coverage order (sliding scale):

Note:

This sliding scale is an example used in one patient. It is not a standard scale. Sliding scales are individualized for clients.

Humulin Regular U-100 according to finger stick q8h.

0-180 mg	no coverage
181-240 mg	2 U s.c.
241-300 mg	4 U s.c.
301-400 mg	6 U s.c.
>400 mg	8 U s.c. stat and notify doctor. Repeat finger stick in 2 hr.

At some institutions there is a special record to document insulins given. A sample of an insulin therapy record is shown in Figure 19-4.

ST. BARNABAS HOSPITAL
BRONX, NY 10457

INSULIN THERAPY RECORD

Addressograph or Label (printed) with Client Identification

DIAGNOSIS:
SIP I&D of Perineal Abscess

| ALLERGIC TO: **NKDA** | DATE 4/1/01 |

USE ASTERISK (*) TO INDICATE DOSES NOT GIVEN-EXPLAIN IN NURSES NOTES.

ORDER DATE / EXP DATE	STANDING INSULIN ORDERS MED-DOSE-FREQ-ROUTE	DATE 2001 HOUR	4/1 INIT.	4/2 INIT.	4/3 INIT.	4/4 INIT.	4/5 INIT.	4/6 INIT.	4/7 INIT.	4/8 INIT.	4/9 INIT.
RN. INIT. DM	NPH 10 units sq	7³⁰A	DM	JN	DG						
4/1/01 / 5/1/01	q AM	site	RA	RT	LA						
RN. INIT. DM	NPH 12 units sq	4³⁰p	NN	NN	JJ						
4/1/01 / 5/1/01	q PM	site	LA	LT	RA						
RN. INIT.											
RN. INIT.											

SINGLE/STAT ORDERS

ORDER DATE	NURSE INIT.	MED-DOSE-ROUTE	TO BE GIVEN DATE	TIME	NURSE INIT.	ORDER DATE	NURSE INIT.	MED-DOSE-ROUTE	TO BE GIVEN DATE	TIME	NURSE INIT.

INJECTION CODES: RT = RIGHT THIGH   LT = LEFT THIGH   RA = RIGHT ARM   LA = LEFT ARM   ▲ RAB = UPPER RIGHT ABDOMEN   ▼ RAB = LOWER RIGHT ABDOMEN   ▲ LAB = UPPER LEFT ABDOMEN   ▼ LAB = LOWER LEFT ABDOMEN

Form 001 3/97

Figure 19-4   MAR for insulin administration. (Used with permission from St. Barnabas Hospital, Bronx, New York.)

Continued

INITIAL IDENTIFICATION

(NORMAL CBG RANGE 80 - 120 MG/DL)

INITIAL	PRINT NAME, TITLE	INITIAL	PRINT NAME, TITLE	INITIAL	PRINT NAME, TITLE
1 DM	Deborah C. Morris RN	5 JJ	Jupiter Jones RN	9	
2 NN	Nancy Nurse RN	6 MS	Mary Smith RN	10	
3 JN	Jane Nightingale RN	7		11	
4 DG	Deborah Gray RN	8		12	

INSULIN COVERAGE

INSULIN COVERAGE ORDERS

ORDER DATE / RN. INIT. 4/1/01 DM	ORDER DATE / RN. INIT.	ORDER DATE / RN. INIT.
CBG bid		
BS 200-250 2 units Reg. Insulin sq		
251-300 4 units Reg. Insulin sq		
301-350 6 units Reg. Insulin sq		
351-400 8 units Reg. Insulin sq		
Call MD if <60 or >400		

DATE	TEST TIME	URINE SUGAR / ACETONE	CBG RESULT	TIME GIVEN	INSULIN TYPE DOSE SITE	SIGNATURE/ TITLE	REMARKS (FBS RESULTS, TPN, ETC.)
4/1/01	6A		314	6A	Regular Insulin 6U sq LA	Mary Smith RN	
4/1/01	4³⁰p		243	4⁴⁰p	Regular Insulin 2U sq LT	Nancy Nurse RN	

Form 001/Back 3/97

Figure 19-4, cont'd   MAR for insulin administration. (Used with permission from St. Barnabas Hospital, Bronx, New York.)

PREPARING A SINGLE DOSE OF INSULIN IN AN INSULIN SYRINGE

Measuring insulin in an insulin syringe requires no calculation or conversion.

Example 1: Order: Humulin Regular U-100 40 U s.c. in AM 1/2 hr before breakfast.

Available: Humulin Regular labeled 100 U.

To measure 40 U, withdraw U-100 insulin to the 40 mark on the U-100 syringe. A Lo-Dose syringe can also be used to draw up this dose, as shown below.

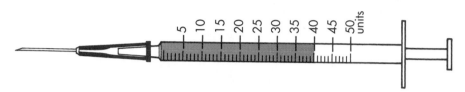

Example 2: Order: Humulin NPH U-100 70 U s.c. o.d. at 7:30 AM.

Available: Humulin NPH labeled 100 U.

There is no calculation or conversion required here. Draw up the required amount using a U-100 (1-mL) syringe.

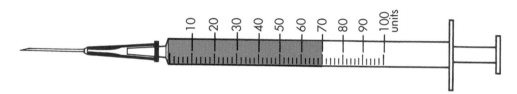

Example 3: Order: Humulin Regular U-100 5 U s.c. stat.

Available: Humulin Regular labeled 100 U.

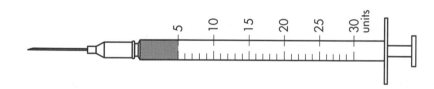

MEASURING TWO TYPES OF INSULIN IN THE SAME SYRINGE

Sometimes individuals may require two different types of insulin for control of their blood sugar levels, for example, NPH and regular. To decrease the number of injections it is common to mix two insulins in a single syringe. To mix insulin in one syringe, remember:

❙ Regular insulin is always drawn up in the insulin syringe first!

The aforementioned article by Doris R. Fleming, MSN, NP, CDE, stated, "the likelihood of frequent or substantial contamination from one vial of insulin to another is minimal compared to the risk of accidentally switching the vials and taking the wrong dose of each insulin. . . This switch in sequence and dosage could cause a hypoglycemic (low blood sugar) episode in the client." According to the article, "the rationale for a standard sequence while mixing insulin is primarily to establish a routine for the patient."

Drawing Regular insulin up first prevents contamination of the Regular insulin with other insulin.

Note:

The cloudy insulin has to be shaken well before drawing up. Recent studies and the article already cited recommend shaking the vial of cloudy insulin vigorously to adequately mix the cloudy insulin to lessen the risk of inconsistent concentration of insulin.

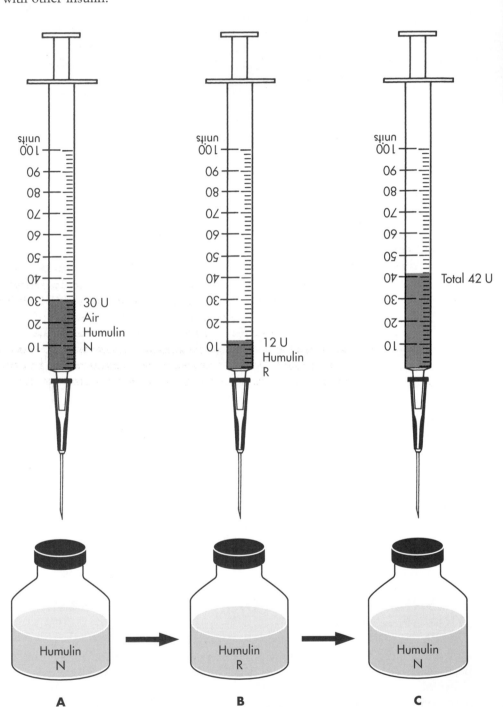

Figure 19-5 Mixing insulins. Order: Humulin N (NPH) U-100 30 U s.c., Humulin R (Regular) U-100, 12 U s.c.. **A,** Insert 30 U air into Humulin N first, do not allow needle to touch insulin. **B,** Inject 12 U of air into Humulin R and withdraw 12 U; withdraw needle. **C,** Insert needle into vial of Humulin N and withdraw 30 U. Total 30 U + 12 U = 42 U. (Modified from Brown M and Mulholland J: *Drug calculations: process and problems for clinical practice,* ed 6, St Louis, 2000, Mosby.)

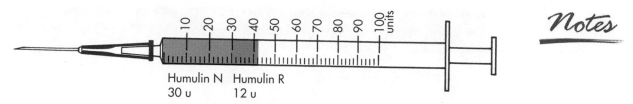

Humulin N   Humulin R
30 u   12 u

Figure 19-6   Sharing total of two insulins. Total = 42 U (30 Humulin NPH + 12 U Humulin R).

To prepare insulin in one syringe (mixing insulin), complete the following steps (Figures 19-5 and 19-6):

1. Cleanse tops of both vials with alcohol wipe.
2. Inject air equal to the amount being withdrawn into the vial of cloudy insulin first. When injecting the air, the tip of the needle should not touch the solution.
3. Remove the needle from the vial of cloudy insulin.
4. Using the same syringe, inject an amount of air into the Regular insulin (clear) equal to the amount to be withdrawn, invert or turn the bottle up in the air, and draw up the desired amount.
5. Remove the syringe from the Regular insulin and check for air bubbles. If air bubbles are present, gently tap the syringe to remove them.
6. Next withdraw the desired dose from the vial of cloudy insulin.
7. The total number of units in the syringe will be the sum of the two insulin orders.

Example: The order is to administer 18 U of Regular U-100 and 22 U of NPH U-100.

The total amount of insulin is 40 U (18 U + 22 U = 40 U).

To administer this dose a Lo-Dose syringe or a U-100 (1-mL) syringe can be used. However, because the dose is 40 U, the Lo-Dose would be more desirable. (See syringes below illustrating this dosage.)

When mixing insulins, it is important to follow the steps outlined. Committing one of the following phrases to memory may help you remember the steps: (1) Last injected is first drawn up; (2) run fast first (Regular), then slow down (NPH); or (3) clear to cloudy. Also remember when mixing insulins, only the same type should be mixed together, for example, Humulin and Humulin.

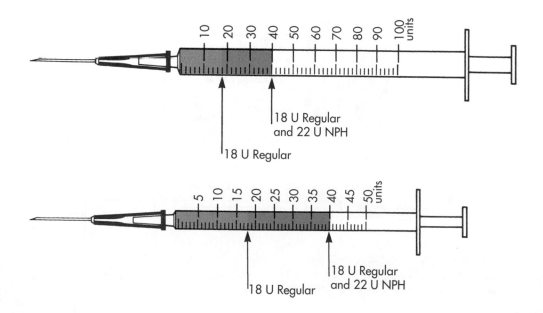

18 U Regular
and 22 U NPH

18 U Regular

18 U Regular
and 22 U NPH

18 U Regular

Notes

POINTS TO REMEMBER

- U-100 means 100 U/mL.

- To ensure accuracy, insulin should be given only with an insulin syringe.

- U-100 insulin is designed to be given with syringes marked U-100.

- Insulin doses must be exact. Read the calibration on the insulin syringes carefully.

- Lo-Dose syringes are desirable for small doses up to 50 U. The Lo-Dose 30 U may be used for doses up to 30 U. Although Lo-Dose insulin syringes 30 U and 50 U can hold a smaller volume, they are intended for U-100 insulin only.

- A U-100 (1-mL capacity) syringe is desirable when the dose exceeds 50 U.

- When mixing insulin, Regular insulin is always drawn up first.

- The total volume when mixing insulins is the sum of the two insulin amounts.

- Read insulin labels to ensure that you have the correct type of insulin and avoid medication errors. Always mix the same types of insulin (e.g., Humulin and Humulin).

- Use the smallest-capacity syringe possible to ensure accuracy.

✓ CHAPTER REVIEW

Using the syringes below and the labels where provided, indicate the dose you would prepare. Indicate the dose on the syringe with an arrow and shade in.

1. Order: Humulin Regular U-100 35 U s.c. o.d.

   Available:

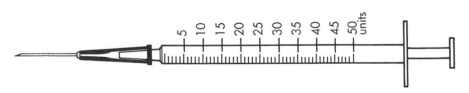

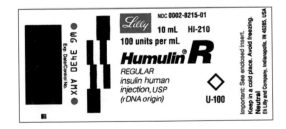

2. Order: Humulin NPH U-100 56 U s.c. o.d.

Available:

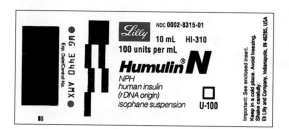

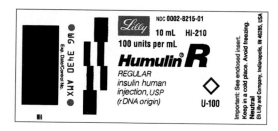

3. Order: Humulin Regular U-100 18 U s.c. and NPH U-100 40 U s.c. o.d.

Available:

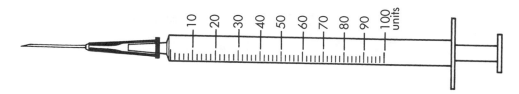

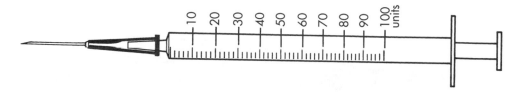

Notes

4. Order: Novolin R U-100 9 U s.c. o.d.

Available:

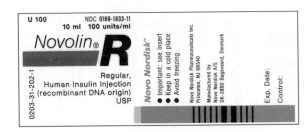

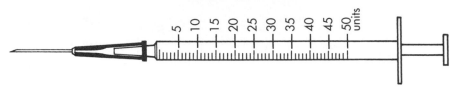

Indicate the number of units measured in the following syringes.

5. Units measured   _____

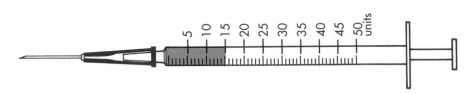

6. Units measured   _____

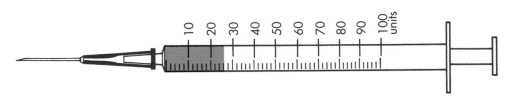

7. Units measured   _____

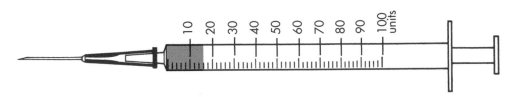

8. Units measured   _____

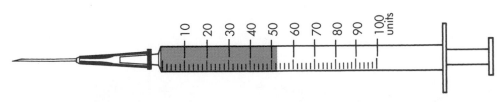

9. Units measured   _____

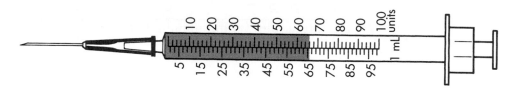

10. Units measured   _____

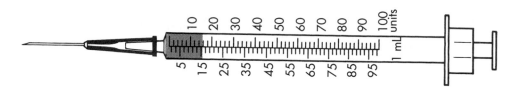

11. Units measured   _____

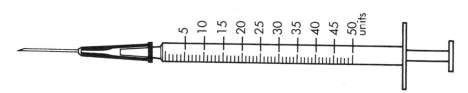

Calculate the dose of insulin where necessary and shade the dose on the syringe provided. Labels have been provided for some problems.

12. Order: Humulin Regular U-100 10 U s.c. a.c. 7:30 AM.

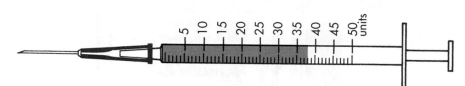

13. Order: Humulin Regular U-100 16 U s.c. and Humulin NPH U-100 24 U s.c. a.c. 7:30 AM.

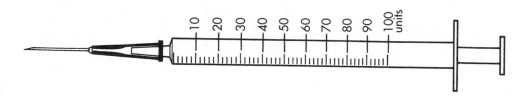

14. Order: Humulin Lente U-100 75 U s.c. a.c. 7:30 AM.

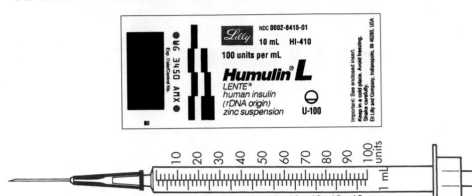

15. Order: Humulin Regular U-100 10 U s.c. and Humulin NPH U-100 15 U s.c. a.c. 7:30 AM.

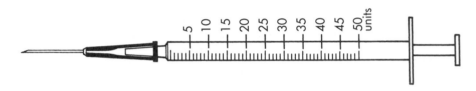

16. Order: Humulin Regular U-100 5 U s.c. and Humulin NPH U-100 25 U s.c. a.c. 7:30 AM.

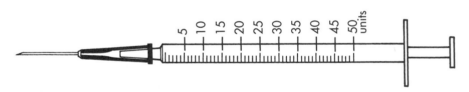

17. Order: Humulin Lente U-100 40 U s.c. and Humulin Regular U-100 10 U s.c. at 7:30 AM.

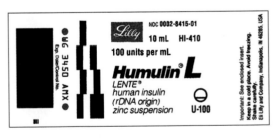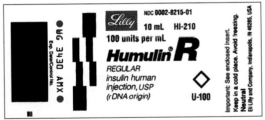

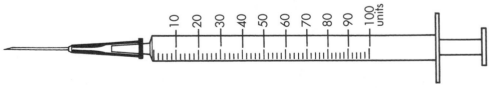

18. Order: Humulin NPH U-100 48 U s.c. and Humulin Regular U-100 30 U s.c. a.c. 7:30 AM.

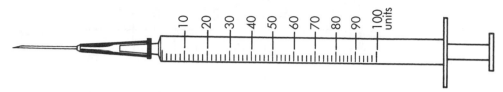

19. Order: Novolin Regular U-100 16 U s.c. and Novolin Lente U-100 12 U s.c. 7:30 AM.

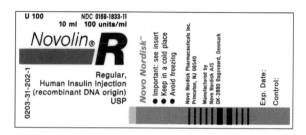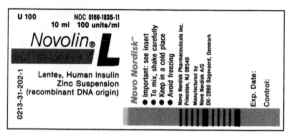

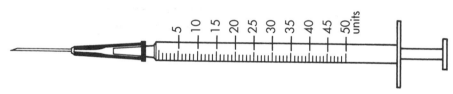

20. Order: Novolin Regular U-100 17 U s.c. 5 PM.

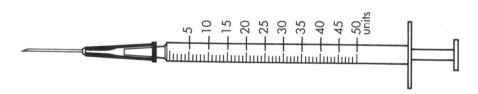

21. Order: Humalog U-100 15 U s.c. q.d. 7:30 AM.

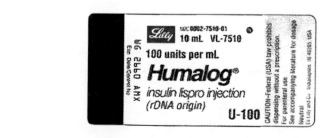

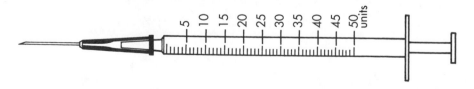

Notes

22. Order: Humulin Regular U-100 26 U s.c. and Humulin NPH U-100 48 U s.c. q.d.

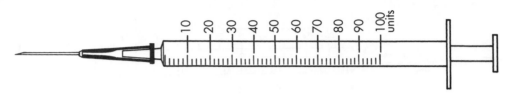

23. Order: Humulin 70/30 U-100 27 U s.c. at 5 PM.

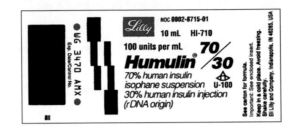

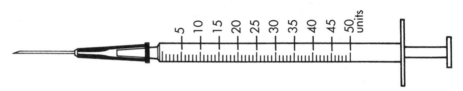

24. Order: Novolin Regular U-100 21 U s.c. and Novolin Lente U-100 35 U s.c. o.d.

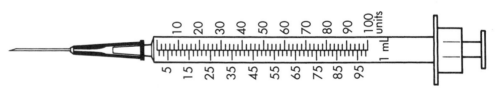

25. Order: Novolin Regular U-100 5 U s.c. and Novolin Lente U-100 35 U s.c. 7:30 AM.

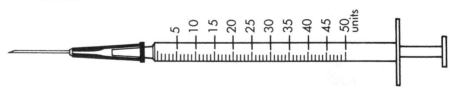

26. Order: Humulin Lente U-100 36 U s.c. 10 PM.

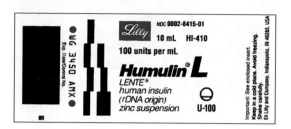

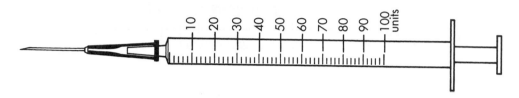

27. A client is on a sliding scale for insulin doses. The order is for Humulin Regular insulin U-100 q6h as follows:

Finger stick		
0-180 mg	no coverage
181 mg-240 mg	2 U s.c.
240 mg-300 mg	4 U s.c.
301 mg-400 mg	6 U s.c.
>400 mg	8 U s.c. and repeat finger stick in 2 hr.

At 11:30 AM the client's finger stick is 364 mg. Shade the syringe to indicate the dose that should be given.

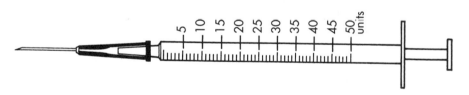

28. Order: Humulin NPH U-100 66 U s.c. 10 PM.

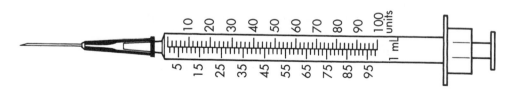

Notes

29. Order: Humulin U U-100 32 U s.c. q AM.

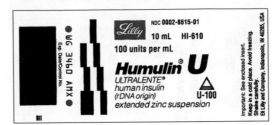

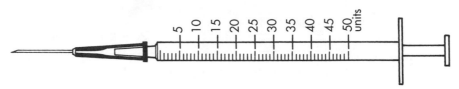

Shade the dose on the insulin syringe.

30. Order: Humulin Lente U-100 35 U s.c. q.d.

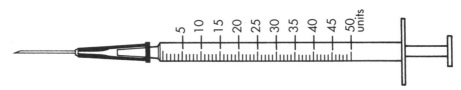

31. Order: Humulin Regular U-100 9 U s.c. 5 PM.

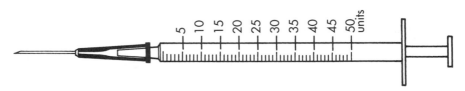

32. Order: Humulin NPH U-100 24 U s.c. 10 PM.

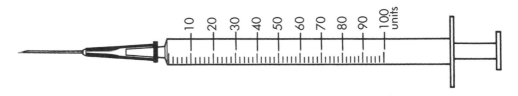

33. Order: Humulin Regular U-100 8 U s.c. in AM, and Humulin NPH U-100 18 U in AM.

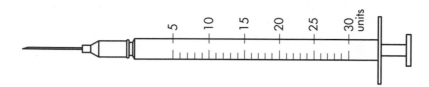

34. Order: Humulin NPH U-100 11 U s.c. h.s.

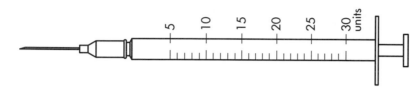

35. Order: Humulin 70/30 U-100 20 U s.c. 1/2 hr ā breakfast.

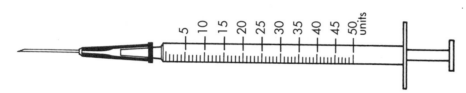

Answers on pp. 543-546

Chapter 20

Pediatric Dose Calculation

Objectives

After reviewing this chapter, you should be able to:

1. Convert body weight from lb to kg
2. Convert body weight from kg to lb
3. Calculate doses based on mg per kg
4. Determine whether a dose is safe
5. Determine body surface area (BSA) using the West nomogram
6. Calculate BSA using formulas according to units of measure
7. Determine doses using the BSA

Body weight is an important factor used to calculate medication doses for both children and adults. The safe administration of medications to infants and children requires knowledge of the methods used in calculating doses. Because children are smaller than adults, calculating doses for children requires exact and careful mathematics. Exact, accurate doses are especially important; even small discrepancies can be dangerous because of the size, weight, BSA (body surface area), and physiological capabilities of pediatric clients (e.g., a lessened ability to metabolize drugs because of immaturity of systems, variations in capabilities of metabolism and excretion).

Although the prescriber is responsible for ordering the medication and dosage, **the nurse remains responsible for verifying the dose to be sure it is correct and safe for administration.** If a dose is higher than normal it may be unsafe, and a dose lower than normal may not have the desired therapeutic effect. It is imperative that nurses check drug labels or package inserts for specific dosage details. Other references that may be checked for more in-depth and additional information on a drug are drug formularies at the institution, *Physician's Desk Reference* (PDR), drug reference books, and the hospital pharmacist.

The two methods currently being used to calculate pediatric doses are as follows:
1. According to the weight of the child (mg per kg)
2. According to the child's BSA

 Critical Thinking:

When in doubt, consult a reliable source. Remember that the nurse administering the medication is responsible for any errors in calculating the dose.

Notes

Determining drug doses according to body weight and BSA is a means of individualizing drug therapy. Although body weight and BSA are common determinants for drug dosing in children, they are also used to calculate adult medication doses, particularly in those who are very old, grossly underweight, and in the administration of cancer medications. Of the two methods, the BSA method has been determined to be the most accurate for calculating doses.

PRINCIPLES RELATING TO BASIC CALCULATIONS

Before calculating medications for the child or infant, there are some guidelines that are helpful to know.
1. Calculation of pediatric doses, as with adult doses, involves the use of ratio-proportion or the formulas $\dfrac{D}{H} \times Q = x$ or $\dfrac{DW}{SW} = \dfrac{DV}{SV}$ to determine the amount of medication to administer.
2. Pediatric doses are much smaller than those for an adult. Micrograms are used a great deal, and minims are rarely used. The tuberculin syringe (1-mL capacity) is used to administer very small doses.
3. I.M. doses are usually not more than 1 mL; however, this can vary with the size of the child.
4. Doses that are less than 1 mL may be measured in minims, in tenths of a mL, or with a tuberculin syringe in hundredths of a mL. However, as with adults, the preference is to express an answer using metric measures such as mL instead of minims because of the inaccuracy of minim measurements.
5. Medications in pediatrics generally are not rounded off to the nearest tenth but may be administered with a tuberculin syringe to ensure accuracy. Again, answers may be changed to minims, but the preference is for metric measures because they are more accurate, and the use of minims is strongly discouraged.
6. All answers must be labeled.

CALCULATION OF DOSES BASED ON BODY WEIGHT

Let's begin our discussion with calculation of doses according to mg/kg of body weight. Before calculating doses according to mg/kg of body weight, it is essential that you be able to convert a child's weight. Most recommendations for drug doses are based on weight in kilograms.

Therefore the most common conversion you will encounter will involve the conversion from lb to kg. To do this, remember the conversion 1 kg = 2.2 lb. Conversions of weights are presented in Chapter 9. It is, however, essential that we review this again.

Remember:

To convert from lb to kg use the conversion 1 kg = 2.2 lb. To convert from lb to kg divide by 2.2, and express your answer to the nearest tenth.

CONVERTING lb TO kg

Let's do some sample problems with the conversion of weights.

Example 1: Convert a child's weight of 30 lb to kg.

$$2.2 \text{ lb} = 1 \text{ kg}$$

$$2.2 \text{ lb} : 1 \text{ kg} = 30 \text{ lb} : x \text{ kg}$$

$$\frac{2.2x}{2.2} = \frac{30}{2.2}$$

$30 \div 2.2 = 13.63$ (rounded to the nearest tenth = 13.6 kg)

Example 2: Convert an infant's weight of 14 lb and 6 oz to kg.

  1. Convert oz to lbs.

$$16 \text{ oz} : 1 \text{ lb} = 6 \text{ oz} : x \text{ lb}$$

$$\frac{16x}{16} = \frac{6}{16}$$

$6 \div 16 = 0.37$ lb (0.4 lb to nearest tenth)

Infant's weight = 14.4 lb

  2. Convert total lb to kg.

$$2.2 \text{ lb} : 1 \text{ kg} = 14.4 \text{ lb} : x \text{ kg}$$

$$\frac{2.2x}{2.2} = \frac{14.4}{2.2}$$

$14.4 \div 2.2 = 6.54$ (6.5 kg to nearest tenth)

Infant's weight = 6.5 kg

Example 3: Convert the weight of a 157 lb adult to kg.

$$2.2 \text{ lb} = 1 \text{ kg}$$

$$2.2 \text{ lb} : 1 \text{ kg} = 157 \text{ lb} : x \text{ kg}$$

$$\frac{2.2x}{2.2} = \frac{157}{2.2}$$

$157 \div 2.2 = 71.36$ (71.4 kg to nearest tenth)

Adult's weight = 71.4 kg

 PRACTICE PROBLEMS

Convert the following weights in lb to kg. Round to the nearest tenth.

1. 15 lb = _____ kg   5. 71 lb   = _____ kg

2. 68 lb = _____ kg   6. 133 lb   = _____ kg

3. 31 lb = _____ kg   7. 8 lb 4 oz = _____ kg

4. 52 lb = _____ kg   8. 5 lb 6 oz = _____ kg

Answers on p. 546

CONVERTING kg TO lb

> Remember:
>
> To convert from kg to lb use the conversion 1 kg = 2.2 lb. To convert from kg to lb multiply by 2.2, and express your weight to the nearest lb.

Note:

Any of the methods presented in Chapter 8 can be used to convert lb to kg and kg to lb, except with decimal movement.

Example 1:   Convert a child's weight of 24 kg to lb.

$$2.2 \text{ lb} = 1 \text{ kg}$$
$$2.2 \text{ lb} : 1 \text{ kg} = x \text{ lb} : 24 \text{ kg}$$
$$x = 24 \times 2.2$$
$$x = 52.8 \ (53 \text{ lb to nearest lb})$$

Child's weight = 53 lb

Example 2:   Convert an adult's weight of 70.2 kg to lb.

$$2.2 \text{ lb} = 1 \text{ kg}$$
$$2.2 \text{ lb} : 1 \text{ kg} = x \text{ lb} : 70.2 \text{ kg}$$
$$x = 70.2 \times 2.2$$
$$x = 154.4 \ (154 \text{ lb to nearest lb})$$

Adult's weight = 154 lb

Example 3:   Convert the weight of a 10.2 kg child to lb.

$$2.2 \text{ lb} = 1 \text{ kg}$$
$$2.2 \text{ lb} : 1 \text{ kg} = x \text{ lb} : 10.2 \text{ kg}$$
$$x = 10.2 \times 2.2$$
$$x = 22.4 \ (22 \text{ lb to nearest lb})$$

Child's weight = 22 lb

 PRACTICE PROBLEMS

Convert the following weights in kg to lb. Round to the nearest lb.

9. 21.3 kg   = _____ lb   13. 34 kg   = _____ lb

10. 17.7 kg   = _____ lb   14. 71.4 kg   = _____ lb

11. 22 kg   = _____ lb   15. 73 kg   = _____ lb

12. 15 kg   = _____ lb   16. 98.3 kg   = _____ lb

Answers on p. 546

Infants 0 to 4 weeks old (neonates) and premature infants may also be placed on medications. The scale will convert the child's weight in grams, or the weight may be reported in grams, rather than kilograms. Therefore it may be necessary for the nurse to convert the weight in grams to kilograms because most dose recommendations are commonly given in kilograms.

As discussed in the chapter on metric conversions, 1 kg = 1,000 g; therefore to convert grams to kilograms, divide by 1,000 or move the decimal point three places to the left.

Note:

Decimal movement may be preferred for converting g to kg; however, the other methods presented in Chapter 8 can also be used.

Remember:

To convert grams to kilograms use the conversion 1 kg = 1,000 g. Divide the number of grams by 1,000 or move the decimal point three places to the left. Round kg to the nearest tenth.

Example 1: Convert an infant's weight of 3,000 g to kg.

$$1 \text{ kg} = 1,000 \text{ g}$$

$$1 \text{ kg} : 1,000 \text{ g} = x \text{ kg} : 3,000 \text{ g}$$

$$\frac{1,000x}{1,000} = \frac{3,000}{1,000}$$

Infant's weight = 3 kg

Decimal movement: 3$\underset{\sim}{000}$ = 3 kg

Example 2: Convert an infant's weight of 1,350 g to kg.

$$1 \text{ kg} = 1,000 \text{ g}$$

$$1 \text{ kg} : 1,000 \text{ g} = x \text{ kg} : 1,350 \text{ g}$$

$$\frac{1,000x}{1,000} = \frac{1,350}{1,000}$$

Infant's weight = 1.35 kg (1.4 kg rounded to the nearest tenth)

Decimal movement: 1$\underset{\sim}{350}$ = 1.35 kg (1.4 kg rounded to the nearest tenth)

Example 3: Convert an infant's weight of 2,700 g to kg.

$$1 \text{ kg} = 1,000 \text{ g}$$

$$1 \text{ kg} : 1,000 \text{ g} = x \text{ kg} : 2,700 \text{ g}$$

$$\frac{1,000x}{1,000} = \frac{2,700}{1,000}$$

Infant's weight = 2.7 kg

Decimal movement: 2$\underset{\sim}{700}$ = 2.7 kg

PRACTICE PROBLEMS

Convert the following weights in grams to kilograms. Round to the nearest tenth.

17. 4,000 g = _____ kg   20. 3,600 g = _____ kg

18. 1,450 g = _____ kg   21. 1,875 g = _____ kg

19. 2,900 g = _____ kg   Answers on p. 546

Remember the Following When Converting Weights

1. 2.2 lb = 1 kg, 1 kg = 1,000 g
2. To convert from lb to kg divide the number of lb by 2.2. Carry the division out to the hundredths place and round off the answer to the nearest tenth. Calculations based on body weight can be rounded off to the nearest tenth.
3. To convert from kg to lb multiply number of kg by 2.2 and express the answer to the nearest pound.
4. If the child's weight is in oz and lb, convert the oz to the nearest tenth of a lb, and then add it to the total lb. Convert the total lb to kg to the nearest tenth.
5. To convert from grams to kilograms, divide by 1,000 or move the decimal point three places to the left. Round kilograms to the nearest tenth as indicated.

Note:

Students should know that although lb is an apothecaries' measure, a decimal may be seen when expressing weight, for example, 65.8 lb.

Medication doses can be calculated based on mg/kg/day, mg/lb/day, or sometimes mcg per kg. References often state the safe amount of the drug in mg/kg/day (24-hour period). Once you have determined the child's weight in kg, you are ready to calculate the medication dose. Calculating the dose involves three steps:

1. Calculation of the daily dose.
2. Division of the daily dose by the number of doses to be administered.
3. Use of either ratio-proportion or the formula method to calculate the number of tablets or capsules or the volume to give to administer the ordered dose.

Example 1: Refer to Dilantin label

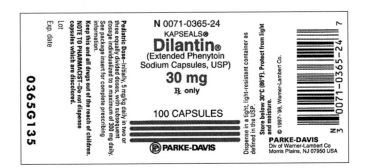

A child weighs 18 kg and requires Dilantin. The recommended dosage is 5 mg/kg/day in two or three equally divided doses. Now that we have the dosage information and the child's weight, we can calculate the dose for this child. Note: The child's weight is in kg (18 kg), and the average dose range is 5 mg/kg. No conversion of weight is required.

Step 1: Start by calculating the safe total daily dosage for this child.

$$5 \text{ mg} \times 18 \text{ kg} = 90 \text{ mg/day}$$

The safe dosage for this child (total) is 90 mg/day.

The calculation of the safe daily dosage could also be done by setting up a ratio-proportion using the format of fractions or colons. Using this example, the setup as a ratio-proportion might be:

$$\frac{5 \text{ mg}}{x \text{ mg}} = \frac{1 \text{ kg}}{18 \text{ kg}} \qquad x = 90 \text{ mg/day}$$

OR

$$5 \text{ mg} : 1 \text{ kg} = x \text{ mg} : 18 \text{ kg}$$

$$x = 90 \text{ mg/day}$$

Step 2: Now determine the amount of each dose.

The dose is to be given in three equally divided doses. Therefore:

$$\frac{90 \text{ mg}}{3} = 30 \text{ mg per dose}$$

After calculating the safe dose for a child, you can assess whether what the doctor ordered is a safe dose.

The order is 30 mg q8h. Is this a safe dose?

$$\text{q8h} = 24 \div 8 = 3 \text{ doses}$$

$30 \times 3 = 90$ mg. Compare the ordered daily dosage with the safe daily dosage you calculated in Step 1. A daily dosage of 90 mg is safe.

Step 3: Use the ratio-proportion or formula method to determine the number of capsules to give.

Dilantin is supplied in 30-mg capsules (refer to label). The ordered dose is 30 mg per dose.

$$30 \text{ mg} : 1 \text{ capsule} = 30 \text{ mg} : x \text{ caps}$$

$$\frac{30x}{30} = \frac{30}{30} \qquad x = 1 \text{ cap}$$

OR

$$\frac{30 \text{ mg}}{30 \text{ mg}} \times 1 \text{ cap} = x \text{ caps};$$

$$x = 1 \text{ cap}$$

OR

$$\frac{30 \text{ mg}}{30 \text{ mg}} = \frac{x \text{ caps}}{1 \text{ cap}}$$

$$x = 1 \text{ cap}$$

You would give 1 caps q8h to administer the ordered dose.

Example 2: Order: gentamicin 50 mg IVPB q8h for a child weighing 40 lb. The recommended dosage for a child is 6-7.5 mg/kg/day divided q8h.

Notes

Step 1: First, a weight conversion is necessary because you have the child's weight in lb and the reference is in kg. Convert the child's weight in lb to kg and round to the nearest tenth.

$$\frac{2.2 \text{ lb}}{40 \text{ lb}} = \frac{1 \text{ kg}}{x \text{ kg}}$$

$$\frac{2.2 \, x}{2.2} = \frac{40}{2.2}$$

$$x = 18.18 \text{ kg}$$

The weight is 18.2 kg.

Step 2: Now that you've converted the weight, you can calculate the safe dose. You must calculate and obtain a range. (The recommended dosage is 6–7.5 mg/kg/day.)

Therefore calculate the lower and upper range:

$$6 \text{ mg} \times 18.2 \text{ kg} = 109.2 \text{ mg}$$

$$7.5 \text{ mg} \times 18.2 \text{ kg} = 136.5 \text{ mg}$$

The safe range for the child weighing 18.2 kg is 109.2-136.5 mg.

Step 3: Now divide the total daily dosage by the number of times the drug will be given in a day.

$$q8h = 24 \div 8 = 3$$

$$109.2 \div 3 = 36.4 \text{ mg per dose}$$

$$136.5 \div 3 = 45.5 \text{ mg per dose}$$

The dose range is 36.4–45.5 mg per dose q8h. The ordered dosage of 50 mg q8h exceeds the dose of 109.2-136.5 mg total dosage for 24 hours.

$$50 \text{ mg q8h} = 50 \text{mg} \times 3 = 150 \text{ mg}$$

Remember that factors such as the child's medical condition might warrant a larger dose. Call the prescriber to verify the dose.

Example 3: The recommended dosage for dicloxacillin sodium for oral suspension is 12.5 mg/kg/day for children weighing less than 40 kg (88 lb) in equally divided doses q6h. What is the dosage for a child weighing 36 lb?

Step 1: First convert the child's weight in lb to the nearest tenth of a kg.

$$2.2 \text{ lb} : 1 \text{ kg} = 36 \text{ lb} : x \text{ kg (or state ratio as a fraction)}.$$

$$\frac{2.2 \, x}{2.2} = \frac{36}{2.2}$$

$$x = 16.36 \text{ kg. To the nearest tenth the weight is 16.4 kg.}$$

Step 2: Now that you've converted the weight to kg, you can calculate the safe dosage for this child.

$$12.5 \text{ mg} \times 16.4 \text{ kg} = 205 \text{ mg}$$

The safe dosage for a child weighing 16.4 kg is 205 mg/day.

Notes

If 50 mg is ordered q6h, is this a safe dosage?

$$24 \text{ h} \div 6 \text{ h} = 4 \text{ doses per day}$$

$$50 \text{ mg} \times 4 \text{ doses} = 200 \text{ mg per day}$$

The ordered dosage is safe.

Although the dosage ordered is safe, it is important to realize that even when small discrepancies exist between the safe dosage and what is ordered (e.g., in this problem, the safe dosage is 205 mg and the child is receiving 200 mg), the difference, though small, can be significant. The prescriber should be notified. The discrepancy may be due to factors such as age of child, medical condition, or other factors.

Step 3: Next, calculate the amount of medication needed to administer the ordered dose.

Dicloxacillin sodium oral suspension is available in a dose strength of 62.5 mg per 5 mL. Use either ratio-proportion or formula method as follows:

$$62.5 \text{ mg} : 5 \text{ mL} = 50 \text{ mg} : x \text{ mL}$$

$$\frac{62.5x}{62.5} = \frac{250 \text{ mg}}{62.5}$$

$$x = 4 \text{ mL}$$

OR

$$\frac{50 \text{ mg}}{62.5 \text{ mg}} \times 5 \text{ mL} = x \text{ mL};$$

$$\frac{250}{62.5} = 4 \text{ mL}$$

OR

$$\frac{50 \text{ mg}}{62.5 \text{ mg}} = \frac{x \text{ mL}}{5 \text{ mL}}$$

$$\frac{250}{62.5} = 4 \text{ mL}$$

You would give 4 mL to administer the ordered dose of 50 mg.

Example 4: The recommended dosage for neonates receiving ceftazidime (Tazidime) is 30 mg/kg q12h. An infant weighs 2,600 g. What is the safe daily dosage for this infant?

Step 1: Change the infant's weight in grams to kg. Reference expressed as mg/kg.

$$1,000 \text{ g} = 1 \text{ kg}$$

$$1,000 \text{ g} : 1 \text{ kg} = 2,600 \text{ g} : x \text{ kg}$$

$$\frac{1,000x}{1,000} = \frac{2,600}{1,000}$$

$$\text{Infant's weight} = 2.6 \text{ kg}$$

Decimal movement: $2600 = 2.6 \text{ kg}$

Step 2: Calculate the safe q12h dose for this infant.

$$30 \text{ mg} \times 2.6 \text{ kg} = 78 \text{ mg/day}$$

The safe dose for this infant is 78 mg dose q12h.

 Critical Thinking

Remember: To avoid medication errors it is imperative to calculate a safe dose for a child and compare it with the dose that has been ordered. Question doses that are significantly low and unusually high; there may be a reason.

When information concerning a pediatric dose is not present on the drug label, refer to the package insert, the PDR, or other reference text. Now try the following practice problems. Labels or portions of package inserts have been included for some problems.

 PRACTICE PROBLEMS

Round weights and doses to the nearest tenth where indicated. Use labels where provided to answer the questions.

22. A child weighs 35 lb and has an order for Keflex 150 mg p.o. q6h.

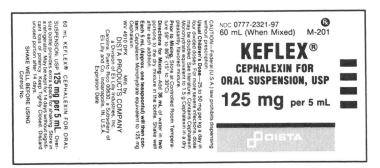

a) What is the recommended dosage in mg/kg/day? _____

b) What is the child's weight in kg to nearest tenth? _____

c) What is the safe dose range for this child? _____

d) Is the dose ordered safe? (Prove mathematically.) _____

e) How many mL will you administer for each dose? _____

23. Refer to the label. The PDR indicates 15 mg/kg/day q8h of kanamycin. Kanamycin 200 mg I.V. q8h is ordered for a child weighing 35 kg.

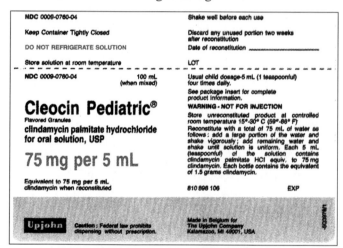

a) What is the safe dosage for this child for 24 hours? _____

b) What is the divided dose? _____

c) Is the dose ordered safe? (Prove mathematically.) _____

24. The recommended dose of clindamycin oral suspension is 8-25 mg/kg/day in four divided doses. A child weighs 40 kg.

a) What is the maximum dosage for this child in 24 hours? _____

b) What is the divided dose range? _____

25. Phenobarbital 10 mg q12h is ordered for a child weighing 9 lb. The recommended maintenance dosage is 3-5 mg/kg/day q12h.

a) What is the child's weight in kg to the nearest tenth? _____

b) What are the safe dose ranges for this child? _____

c) Is the dose ordered safe? (Prove mathematically.) _____

d) Phenobarbital elixer is available in a dose strength of 20 mg per 5 mL. What will you administer for one dose? _____

Notes

26. Morphine sulfate 7.5 mg s.c. q4h p.r.n. is ordered for a child weighing 84 lb. The recommended maximum dose for a child is 0.1-0.2 mg/kg/dose.

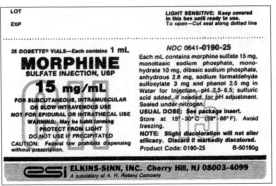

a) What is the child's weight in kg to the nearest tenth?   _____

b) What are the safe dose ranges for this child?   _____

c) Is the dose ordered safe? (Prove mathematically.)   _____

d) How many mL will you administer for one dose?   _____

27. The recommended dose of Dilantin is 4-8 mg/kg/day q12h. Dilantin 15 mg p.o. q12h is ordered for a child weighing 11 lb.

a) What is the child's weight in kg?   _____

b) What are the safe dose ranges for this child?   _____

c) Is the dose ordered safe? (Prove mathematically.)   _____

d) Dilantin suspension is available in a dose strength of 30 mg/5 mL. What would you administer for one dose?   _____

28. The recommended initial dose of mercaptopurine is 2.5 mg/kg/day p.o. The child weighs 44 lb.

a) What is the child's weight in kg?   _____

b) What is the safe daily dosage for this child?   _____

29. For a child the recommended dosage of I.V. vancomycin is 40 mg/kg/day. Vancomycin 200 mg I.V. q6h is ordered for a child weighing 38 lb.

a) What is the child's weight in kg to the nearest tenth?   _____

b) What is the safe dosage for this child in 24 hours?   _____

c) What is the divided dose?   _____

d) Is the dose ordered safe? (Prove mathematically.)   _____

30. A 16 lb child has an order for amoxicillin 125 mg p.o. q8h.

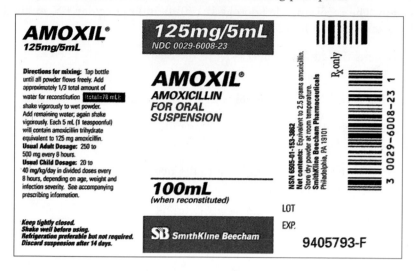

a) What is the recommended dosage in mg/kg/day? _____

b) What is the child's weight in kg to the nearest tenth? _____

c) What is the safe range of doses for this child in 24 hours. _____

d) Is the dose ordered safe? _____

31. A 44-lb child has an order for Ilosone oral suspension 250 mg p.o. q6h. The usual dosage for children under 50 lb is 30-50 mg/kg/day in divided doses q6h, and for children over 20 lb is 250 mg q6h.

a) What is thc child's wcight in kg? _____

b) What is the range of doses safe for this child in 24 hours? _____

c) Is the dose ordered safe? (Prove mathematically.) _____

32. Refer to the Fungizone insert to calculate the dose for an adult weighing 66.3 kg with good cardiorenal function. _____

1 vial   NDC 0003-0437-30
NSN 6505-01-084-9453

50 mg
FUNGIZONE®
INTRAVENOUS
Amphotericin B
for Injection USP

FOR INTRAVENOUS INFUSION
IN HOSPITALS ONLY

Caution: Federal law prohibits dispensing without prescription

Read all sides

□APOTHECON®
A BRISTOL-MYERS SQUIBB COMPANY

Partial Insert for Fungizone (Amphotericin B)

DOSAGE AND ADMINISTRATION
CAUTION: Under no circumstances should a total daily dose of 1.5 mg/kg be exceeded. Amphotericin B overdoses can result in cardio-respiratory arrest (see OVERDOSAGE).
  FUNGIZONE Intravenous should be administered by *slow* Intravenous Infusion. Intravenous Infusion should be given over a period of approximately 2 to 6 hours (depending on the dose) observing the usual precautions for intravenous therapy (see PRECAUTIONS, General). The recommended concentration for intravenous infusion is 0.1 mg/mL (1 mg/10 mL).
  Since patient tolerance varies greatly, the dosage of amphotericin B must be individualized and adjusted according to the patient's clinical status (e.g., site and severity of infection, etiologic agent, cardio-renal function, etc.).
  A single intravenous test dose (1 mg in 20 mL of 5% dextrose solution) administered over 20-30 minutes may be preferred. The patient's temperature, pulse, respiration, and blood pressure should be recorded every 30 minutes for 2 to 4 hours.
  In patients with **good cardio-renal function** and a well tolerated test dose, therapy is usually initiated with a daily dose of 0.25 mg/kg of body weight. However, in those patients having **severe and rapidly progressive fungal infection**, therapy may be initiated with a daily dose of 0.3 mg/kg of body weight. In patients with **impaired cardio-renal function** or a **severe reaction to the test dose**, therapy should be initiated with smaller daily doses (i.e., 5 to 10 mg).

Notes

33. A 200-lb adult is to be treated with Ticar for a complicated urinary tract infection. The recommended dosage is 150 to 200 mg/kg/day I.V. in divided doses every 4 or 6 hours.

    a) What is the adult's weight in kg to the nearest tenth? _____

    b) What is the daily dosage range in g for this client? _____

34. A child weighs 12 lb, 6 oz. The recommended dosage for a child of V-Cillin oral solution is 15 to 50 mg/kg/day in four divided doses.

    a) What is the child's weight in kg to the nearest tenth? _____

    b) What is the safe dose range for this child? _____

Answers on pp. 547-549

POINTS TO REMEMBER

- To convert lb to kg divide by 2.2; express answer to nearest tenth.
- To convert kg to lb multiply by 2.2; express answer to nearest pound.
- To convert g to kg divide by 1,000; round to the nearest tenth as indicated.
- To calculate doses the child's weight must be converted to the reference.
- To calculate the dose based on weight, do the following:
    1. Determine the child's weight in kg if needed.
    2. Multiply the child's weight in kg by the dose stated.
    3. Divide the total daily dose by the number of doses needed to administer.
    4. Calculate the number of tablets or volume to administer for each dose by use of ratio-proportion or the formula method.
- When the recommended dose is given as a range, calculate based on the low and high values for each dose.
- Question any discrepancies in doses ordered and remember that factors such as age, weight, and medical conditions can cause the differences. Ask the doctor to clarify the order when a discrepancy exists. Small discrepancies can be significant.
- Use appropriate resources to determine the safe range for a child's dose. Compare the safe dose with the dose ordered.

CALCULATION OF PEDIATRIC DOSES USING BODY SURFACE AREA (BSA)

A child's BSA is determined by comparing a child's weight and height with what is considered average or the norm. Many pediatric doses are prescribed based on the child's BSA. The BSA is determined from the height and weight of a child and the use of the West nomogram (Figure 20-1).

This information is then applied to a formula for dose calculation. Remember, all children are not the same size at the same age; therefore, the West nomogram

Notes

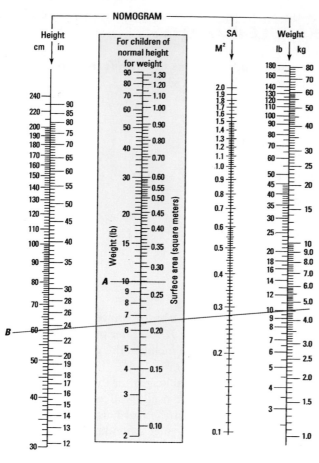

Figure 20-1   West nomogram for estimation of body surface area. (Nomogram modified with date from Behrman RE, Kleigman R, Jenson HB, editors: *Nelson textbook of pediatrics,* ed 16, Philadelphia, 2000, WB Saunders.)

can be used to determine the BSA of a child. The West nomogram is not easy to use, although it is still employed in some institutions. The nomogram can be used to calculate the BSA for both children and adults for heights up to 240 cm (95 inches) and weights up to 80 kg (180 lb). The west nomogram is the most well known BSA chart (see Figure 20-1). It is possible to determine the BSA from weight alone, if the child is of normal height and weight.

READING THE WEST NOMOGRAM CHART

Refer to the chart in Figure 20-1. It is important to notice that the increments of measurement and the spaces on the BSA nomogram are not consistent. **Always read the numbers to determine what the calibrations are measuring.** For example, refer to the column for children of normal height and weight (second column from left); notice that the calibrations between 15 and 20 lb are 1-lb increments. However, if you look at the bottom of the scale representing surface area in square meters there are four calibrations between 0.10 and 0.15. Each line, therefore, is read as 0.11, 0.12, 0.13, etc. If the child is of a normal height and weight for his or her age, the BSA can be determined from weight alone. Notice the boxed column listing weight on the left and surface in square meters on the right; this is used when a child is of normal height for his or her weight. For example, a child weighing 70 lb has a BSA of 1.10 m². Looking on the nomogram for a child who weighs 10 lb, using the nomogram column of normal height for weight, a 10-lb child has a BSA of 0.27 m². Using the nomogram for a child weighing 70 lb and having a normal height for weight, the child would have a BSA of 1.10 m².

PRACTICE PROBLEMS

Refer to the nomogram and determine the BSA (expressed in m²) for the following children of normal height and weight.

35. For a child weighing 30 lb   _____

36. For a child weighing 10 lb   _____

37. For a child weighing 52 lb   _____

38. For a child weighing 44 lb   _____

39. For a child weighing 11 lb   _____

40. For a child weighing 20 lb   _____

Answers on p. 549

In addition to determining the BSA based on weight, the BSA can also be calculated using both height and weight. If you refer to the chart, notice the columns for height and weight. This chart also includes the weight in lb and kg. Notice the column for height (in cm and inches).

For children who are not of normal height for their weight, the scales at the far left (height) and far right (weight) are used. Notice that both of these scales have two measurements: centimeters and inches for height, and pounds and kilograms for weight. To find the BSA, place a ruler extending from the height column on the left to the weight column on the far right. The estimated BSA for the child is where the line intersects the SA column. For example, using the far right and left scales, a child who weighs 50 lbs and is 36 in tall has a BSA of 0.8 m².

Note:

Remember, if the ruler is slightly off the height or weight, the BSA will be incorrect.

 PRACTICE PROBLEMS

Using the nomogram, calculate the following BSAs.

41. A child who is 90 cm long and weighs 50 lb.   _____

42. A child who is 60 cm long and weighs 10 lb.   _____

43. A child who is 100 cm long and weighs 10 kg.   _____

44. A child who is 30 inches long and weighs 20 lb.   _____

45. A child who weighs 60 lb and is 39 inches tall.   _____

46. A baby who weighs 13 lb and is 19 inches long.   _____

47. A child who weighs 30 lb and is 32 inches tall.   _____

48. A child who weighs 13 kg and is 65 cm tall.   _____

49. A child who is 90 cm long and weighs 40 lb.   _____

50. A child who is 19 inches long and weighs 5 lb.   _____

Answers on p. 549

DOSE CALCULATION BASED ON BSA

If you know the child's BSA, the dose is calculated by multiplying the recommended dose by the child's BSA (m²).

Example 1:   The recommended dose is 3 mg per m². The child has a BSA of 1.2 m².

$$1.2 \times 3 \text{ mg} = 3.6 \text{ mg}$$

Example 2:   The recommended dose is 30 mg per m². The child has a BSA of 0.75 m².

$$0.75 \times 30 = 22.5 \text{ mg.}$$

Note:

The average dose per m² is written.

CALCULATING USING THE FORMULA

The BSA is expressed in square meters (m²). The child's BSA is then inserted into the formula below.

Formula

$$\frac{\text{BSA of child (m}^2)}{1.7 \text{ (m}^2)} \times \text{Adult dose} = \text{Estimated child's dose}$$

If only the recommended dose for an adult is cited, then the formula is used to calculate the child's dose. The formula uses the average adult dose, the average adult BSA (1.7 m²), and the child's BSA in m².

Example 1:   The doctor has ordered a medication for which the average adult dose is 125 mg. What will the dose be for a child with a BSA of 1.4 m²?

$$\frac{1.4}{1.7} \times 125 \text{ mg} = 102.94 \text{ mg} = 102.9 \text{ mg}$$

Example 2:   The adult dose for a medication is 100 to 300 mg. What will the dose range be for a child with a BSA of 0.5 m²?

$$\frac{0.5}{1.7} \times 100 = 29.4 \text{ mg}$$

$$\frac{0.5}{1.7} \times 300 = 88.2 \text{ mg}$$

The dose range is 29.4-88.2 mg.

Notes

PRACTICE PROBLEMS: DETERMINING THE DOSE USING THE FORMULA

Using the West nomogram chart when indicated, calculate the child's dose for the following drugs. Express your answer to the nearest tenth.

51. The child's height is 32 inches and weight is 25 lb. The recommended adult dose is 25 mg.

    a) What is the child's BSA? _____

    b) What is the child's dose? _____

52. The child's height is 100 cm and weight is 10 kg. The adult dose is 200-400 mg.

    a) What is the child's BSA? _____

    b) What is the child's dose range? _____

53. The normal adult dose of a drug is 5-15 mg. What will the dose range be for a child whose BSA is 1.5 m²? _____

54. 5 mg of a drug is ordered for a child with a BSA of 0.8 m². The average adult dose is 20 mg. Is this a correct dose? (Prove mathematically.) _____

55. 7 mg of a drug is ordered for a child with a BSA of 0.9 m². The average adult dose is 25 mg. Is this correct? (Prove mathematically.) _____

56. An antibiotic for which the average adult dose is 250 mg is ordered for a child with a BSA of 1.5 m². What will the child's dose be? _____

57. The recommended dose of a drug is 20 to 30 mg per m². The child has a BSA of 0.74 m². What will the child's dose range be? _____

58. 8 mg of a drug is ordered for a child who has a BSA of 0.67 m². The average adult dose is 20 mg. Is the dose correct? (Prove mathematically.) _____

59. The child has a BSA of 0.94 m². The recommended adult dose of a drug is 10 to 20 mg. What will the child's dose range be? _____

60. The child's weight is 20 lb and height is 30 inches. The adult dose of a drug is 500 mg.

    a) What is the child's BSA? _____

    b) What is the child's dose? _____

61. The recommended adult dose for an antibiotic is 500 mg 4 times a day. The child's BSA is 1.3 m². What will the child's dose be? _____

62. The child's weight is 30 lb and height is 28 inches. The adult dose of a drug is 25 mg.

    a) What is the child's BSA? _____

    b) What is the child's dose? _____

63. The child's BSA is 0.52 m². The average adult dose for a medication is 15 mg. What will the child's dose be? _____

64. The recommended adult dose for a drug is 150 mg. The child's BSA is 1.10 m². What will the child's dose be? _____

Answers on p. 550

POINTS TO REMEMBER

- BSA is determined from the West nomogram using the child's height and weight and expressed as m².

- The normal height and weight column on the West nomogram is used only when the child's height and weight are within normal limits.

- When you know the child's BSA, the dose is determined by multiplying the BSA by the recommended dose. (This is used when the recommended dose is written using the average dose per m².)

- To determine whether a child's dose is safe, a comparison must be made between what is ordered and the calculation of the dose based on BSA.

- The formula for calculating a child's dosage when the average adult dose per adult mean body surface area (1.7) is written as

$$\frac{\text{BSA of child (m}^2)}{1.7\text{m}^2} \times \text{adult dose} = \text{estimated child's dose}$$

CALCULATING BSA WITH THE USE OF A FORMULA

BSA is used a great deal in calculating doses for children and adults, often to determine doses for medications such as chemotherapeutic agents that are used in the treatment of cancer. As already shown, BSA can be calculated using the tool called the West nomogram; however, it is a tool that requires learning to use and can result in an error if the ruler is just slightly off line.

To calculate BSA the client's height and weight are used (adults and children). Instead of using the West nomogram one can calculate the BSA with two tools:
1. Calculator
2. Formula

Calculators are increasingly being used for calculation of critical care doses and in pediatric units where extensive mathematics may be required. It has been determined that the safest way to calculate a BSA is to use a formula and a calculator that can perform square roots ($\sqrt{\ }$). The formula used is based on the units in which the measurements are obtained (e.g., kg, cm, lb, and inches).

Formula for Calculating BSA from kg and cm

Steps
1. Multiply the weight in kg by height in cm.
2. Divide the product obtained in Step 1 by 3,600.
3. Enter the square root sign into the calculator.
4. Round the final m² BSA to the nearest hundredth.

Note:

This formula uses metric measures.

Formula

$$BSA = \sqrt{\frac{\text{Weight (kg)} \times \text{Height (cm)}}{3,600}}$$

Example 1:   Calculate the BSA for a child who weighs 23 kg and whose height is 128 cm. Express BSA to the nearest hundredth

$$\sqrt{\frac{23 \text{ (kg)} \times 128 \text{ (cm)}}{3,600}} = \sqrt{0.817}$$

$$\sqrt{0.817} = 0.903 = 0.90 \text{ m}^2$$

The BSA was calculated as follows: $23 \times 128 \div 3,600 = 0.817$, then the square root ($\sqrt{\ }$) was entered. The final m² BSA was rounded to the nearest hundredth.

Example 2:   Calculate the BSA for an adult who weighs 100 kg and whose height is 180 cm. Express BSA to the nearest hundredth.

$$\sqrt{\frac{100 \text{ (kg)} \times 180 \text{ (cm)}}{3,600}} = \sqrt{5}$$

$$\sqrt{5} = 2.236 = 2.24 \text{ m}^2$$

Formula for Calculating BSA from lb and inches

The formula is the same with the exception of the number used in the denominator, which is 3,131, and the measurements used are household.

Formula

$$BSA = \sqrt{\frac{\text{Weight (lb)} \times \text{Height (in)}}{3,131}}$$

Example 1:   Calculate the BSA for child who weighs 25 lb and is 32 inches tall. Express the BSA to nearest hundredth.

$$\sqrt{\frac{25 \text{ (lb)} \times 32 \text{ (in)}}{3,131}} = \sqrt{0.255}$$

$$\sqrt{0.255} = 0.504 = 0.50 \text{ m}^2$$

Example 2: Calculate the BSA for an adult who weighs 143.7 lb and is 61.2 inches tall. Express the BSA to the nearest hundredth.

$$\sqrt{\frac{143.7 \text{ (lb)} \times 61.2 \text{ (in)}}{3{,}131}} = \sqrt{2.808}$$

$$\sqrt{2.808} = 1.675 = 1.68 \text{ m}^2$$

 PRACTICE PROBLEMS

Determine the BSA for the following clients using a formula. Express the BSA to the nearest hundredth.

65. An adult whose weight is 95.5 kg and height is 180 cm. _____

66. A child whose weight is 10 kg and height is 70 cm. _____

67. A child whose weight is 4.8 lb and height is 21 inches. _____

68. An adult whose weight is 170 lb and height is 67 inches. _____

69. A child whose weight is 92 lb and height is 35 inches. _____

70. A child whose weight is 24 kg and height is 92 cm. _____

Answers on pp. 550-551

Example: The recommended dose is 40 mg/m². The child's BSA is 0.55 m². Express your answer to the nearest whole number.
0.55 × 40 mg = 22 mg

Note:

As already covered in the chapter, once you know the BSA, the dose calculation involves just multiplication.

Remember: Always check a dose against m² recommendations using appropriate resources, for example, PDR, drug inserts.

Medications, particularly chemotherapy agents, often provide the recommended dose according to m² (BSA).

Example: Cisplatin is an antineoplastic agent. The recommended pediatric/adult I.V. dose for bladder cancer is 50-70 mg/m² every 3-4 weeks. For carmustine, which is used in Hodgkin's disease, and for brain tumors, the recommended I.V. dose for an adult is 150-200 mg/m².

Notes

POINTS TO REMEMBER

- The formula method to calculate BSA is more accurate than use of the nomogram.
- The formulas used to calculate BSA are:

$$BSA = \frac{wt\ (kg) \times ht\ (cm)}{3,600}$$

$$BSA = \frac{wt\ (lb) \times ht\ (in)}{3,131}$$

Calculating BSA with a formula requires the use of a calculator. The steps are as follows:

- Multiply height × weight (cm × kg, or lb × inches)
- Divide by 3,600 or 3,131 depending on the units of measure (divide by 3,600 if measures are in metric units [cm, kg], and by 3,131 if measures are in household units [in, lb]).
- Enter the $\sqrt{\ }$ (square root sign) to arrive at m².
- Round m² to hundredths (two decimal places).

PEDIATRIC ORAL AND PARENTERAL MEDICATIONS

Several methods have been presented to determine doses for children in this chapter. It is important, however, to bear in mind that while the dose may be determined according to weight, BSA, etc., the dose to administer is calculated using the same methods as for adults (ratio-proportion, formula). It is important to remember the following differences with children's doses.

Remember
1. Doses are smaller for children than for adults.
2. Most oral drugs for infants and small children come in liquid form to facilitate easy swallowing.
3. The oral route is preferred; however, when necessary, medications are administered by parenteral route.
4. Not more than 1 mL is injected I.M.
5. Parenteral doses are frequently administered using a tuberculin syringe.

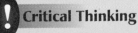 **Critical Thinking**

When in doubt, always double check pediatric doses to decrease the chance of an error. Never assume! Think before administering.

✓ CHAPTER REVIEW

Notes

Read the dose information or label given for the following problems. Express body weight conversion to the nearest tenth where indicated and doses to the nearest tenth.

1. Lasix 10 mg I.V. stat is ordered for a child weighing
   22 lb. The recommended initial dose is 1 mg/kg.
   Is the dose ordered safe? (Prove mathematically.) _____

2. Amoxicillin 150 mg p.o. q8h is ordered for an infant weighing 23 lb. The maximum daily dosage for an infant is amoxicillin p.o. 20 to 40 mg/kg/day divided q8h.

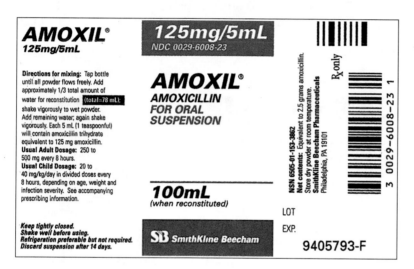

   a) What is the child's weight in kg to the nearest tenth? _____

   b) What is the recommended dosage range? _____

   c) What is the divided dose range? _____

   d) Is the dose ordered safe? (Prove mathematically.) _____

3. Furadantin oral suspension 25 mg p.o. q6h is ordered for a child weighing 17 kg. Recommended dose is 2.2-3.2 mg/lb/day.

   Available:

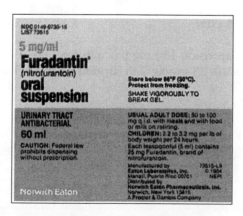

   a) What is the child's weight in lb to the nearest
      tenth? _____

Notes

    b) What is the dose range for this child? _____

    c) Is the dose ordered safe? (Prove mathematically.) _____

    d) How many mL must be given per dose to administer the ordered dose? _____

4. Dicloxacillin 100 mg p.o. q6h is ordered for a child weighing 35 kg. The recommended dosage is 12.5 mg/kg/day for children weighing less than 40 kg in equally divided doses q6h. Is the dosage ordered safe? (Prove mathematically.)

_____

5. Vibramycin 75 mg p.o. q12h is ordered for a child weighing 30 lb. Refer to the label below and determine if this is a safe dosage. (Prove mathematically.)

_____

6. Oxacillin oral solution 250 mg p.o. q6h is ordered for a child weighing 42 lb. The recommended dosage is 50 mg/kg/day in equally divided doses q6h. Is the dosage ordered safe? (Prove mathematically.) _____

7. Cleocin suspension 150 mg p.o. q8h is ordered for a child weighing 36 lb. The recommended dosage is 10-25 mg/kg/day divided q6-8h. Is the dosage ordered safe? (Prove mathematically.) _____

8. Keflex suspension 250 mg p.o. q6h is ordered for a child weighing 66 lb. The usual child dosage is 25-50 mg/kg/day in four divided doses. Available: Keflex suspension 125 mg/5 mL.

   a) Is the dosage ordered safe? (Prove mathematically.) _____

   b) How many mL would you give to administer one dose?   _____

9. Streptomycin sulfate 400 mg I.M. q12h is ordered for a child weighing 35 kg. The recommended dosage is 20-40 mg/kg/day divided q12h I.M.

   a) Is the dosage ordered safe? (Prove mathematically.) _____

   b) A 1-g vial of streptomycin sulfate is available in powdered form with the following instructions: Dilution with 1.8 mL of sterile water will yield 400 mg per mL. How many mL will you give to administer the ordered dose?

   _____

10. A child weighs 46 lb and has a mild infection. Gantrisin oral suspension 250 mg p.o. q6h is ordered. The recommended dosage is 120 mg/kg/day in four equally divided doses. Is the dosage ordered safe? (Prove mathematically.)

    _____

11. The recommended dosage for neonates receiving ceftazidime (Tazidime) is 30 mg/kg q12h.

    a) What is the child's weight in kg to the nearest tenth?   _____

    b) What is the safe dose for this neonate?   _____

12. A child weighs 14 kg. The usual dosage range of Velosef is 50-100 mg/kg/day in equally divided doses four times a day.

    a) What will the daily dosage range be for a child weighing 14 kg?   _____

    b) What are the divided dose ranges for this child?   _____

    c) Velosef 250 mg I.V. q6h has been ordered. Is this a safe dosage? (Prove mathematically.)

    _____

13. The recommended dose for Mithracin for the treatment of testicular tumors is 25-30 mcg/kg. A client weighs 190 lb.

    a) What is the client's weight in kg to the nearest tenth?   _____

    b) What is the dose range in mg for this client? (round to nearest tenth)   _____

Notes

Using the nomogram on p. 357, determine the BSA and calculate the child's dose by using the formula. Express doses to the nearest tenth.

14. The child's height is 30 inches and weight is 20 lb. The adult dose of an antibiotic is 500 mg.

   a) What is the BSA? _____

   b) What is the child's dose? _____

15. The child's height is 32 inches and weight is 27 lb. The adult dose for a medication is 25 mg.

   a) What is the BSA? _____

   b) What is the child's dose? _____

16. The child's height is 120 cm and weight is 40 kg. The adult dose for a medication is 250 mg.

   a) What is the BSA? _____

   b) What is the child's dose? _____

17. The child's height is 50 inches and weight is 75 lb. The adult dose for a medication is 30 mg.

   a) What is the BSA? _____

   b) What is the child's dose? _____

18. The child height is 50 inches and weight is 70 lb. The adult dose for a medication is 150 mg.

   a) What is the BSA? _____

   b) What is the child's dose? _____

Determine the child's dose for the following drugs. Express answers to the nearest tenth.

19. The adult dose of a drug is 50 mg. What will the dose be for a child with a BSA of 0.70 m²? _____

20. The adult dose of a drug is 10-20 mg. What will the dose range be for a child whose BSA is 0.66 m²? _____

21. The adult dose of a drug is 2,000 U. What will the dose be for a child with a BSA of 0.55 m²? _____

22. The adult dose of a drug is 200-250 mg. What will the dose range be for a child with a BSA of 0.55 m²? _____

23. The adult dose of a drug is 150 mg. What will the dose be for a child with a BSA of 0.22 m²? _____

Calculate the child's dose in the following problems. Determine if the doctor's order is correct. If the order is incorrect, give the correct dose. Express answers to the nearest tenth.

24. A child with a BSA of 0.49 m² has an order of 25 mg for a drug. The adult dose is 60 mg. _____

25. A child with a BSA of 0.32 m² has an order of 4 mg for a drug. The adult dose is 10 mg. _____

26. A child with a BSA of 0.68 m² has an order of 50 mg for a drug. The adult dose is 125-150 mg. _____

27. A child with a BSA of 0.55 m² has an order of 5 mg for a drug. The adult dose is 25 mg. _____

28. A child with a BSA of 1.2 m² has an order for 60 mg of a drug. The adult dose is 75-100 mg. _____

Using the formula method for calculating BSA, determine the BSA in the following clients and express answers to the nearest hundredth.

29. A 15-year-old who weighs 100 lb and is 55 inches tall. _____

30. An adult who weighs 60.9 kg and is 130 cm tall. _____

31. A child who weighs 55 lb and is 45 inches tall. _____

32. A child who weighs 60 lb and is 35 inches tall. _____

33. An adult who weighs 65 kg and 132 cm tall. _____

34. A child who weighs 24 lb and is 28 inches tall. _____

35. An infant who weighs 6 kg and is 55 cm tall. _____

36. A child who weighs 42 lb and is 45 inches tall. _____

37. An infant who weighs 8 kg and is 70 cm tall. _____

38. An adult who weighs 74 kg and is 160 cm tall. _____

Calculate the doses to be given. Use labels where provided.

39. Order: Azidothymidine (AZT) 7 mg p.o. q6h × LOS. _____

    Available: Azidothymidine (AZT) 10 mg/mL.

Notes

40. Order: Epivir 150 mg p.o. b.i.d.

    Available: _____

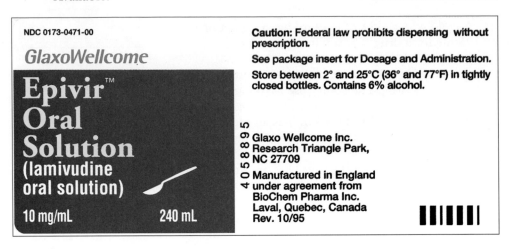

NDC 0173-0471-00

GlaxoWellcome

Epivir™ Oral Solution
(lamivudine oral solution)

10 mg/mL   240 mL

Caution: Federal law prohibits dispensing without prescription.

See package insert for Dosage and Administration.

Store between 2° and 25°C (36° and 77°F) in tightly closed bottles. Contains 6% alcohol.

4058895

Glaxo Wellcome Inc. Research Triangle Park, NC 27709

Manufactured in England under agreement from BioChem Pharma Inc. Laval, Quebec, Canada Rev. 10/95

41. Order: Digoxin 0.1 mg p.o. o.d.

    Available: _____

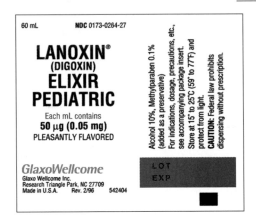

60 mL   NDC 0173-0264-27

LANOXIN®
(DIGOXIN)
ELIXIR PEDIATRIC

Each mL contains
50 μg (0.05 mg)
PLEASANTLY FLAVORED

GlaxoWellcome
Glaxo Wellcome Inc.
Research Triangle Park, NC 27709
Made in U.S.A.   Rev. 2/96   542404

Alcohol 10%, Methylparaben 0.1% (added as a preservative)
For indications, dosage, precautions, etc., see accompanying package insert.
Store at 15° to 25°C (59° to 77°F) and protect from light.
CAUTION: Federal law prohibits dispensing without prescription.

LOT
EXP

42. Order: Retrovir 80 mg p.o. q8h.

    Available: _____

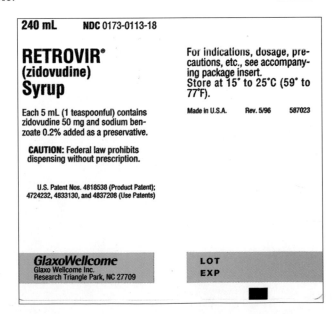

240 mL   NDC 0173-0113-18

RETROVIR®
(zidovudine)
Syrup

Each 5 mL (1 teaspoonful) contains zidovudine 50 mg and sodium benzoate 0.2% added as a preservative.

CAUTION: Federal law prohibits dispensing without prescription.

U.S. Patent Nos. 4818538 (Product Patent); 4724232, 4833130, and 4837208 (Use Patents)

For indications, dosage, precautions, etc., see accompanying package insert.
Store at 15° to 25°C (59° to 77°F).

Made in U.S.A.   Rev. 5/96   587023

GlaxoWellcome
Glaxo Wellcome Inc.
Research Triangle Park, NC 27709

LOT
EXP

43. Order: Augmentin 250 mg p.o. q6h.

    Available: _____

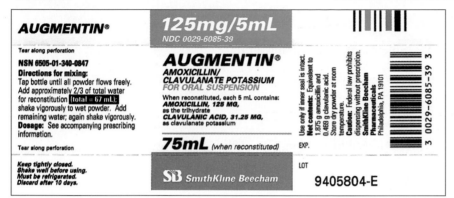

44. Order: Tegretol 0.25 g p.o. t.i.d.

    Available: _____

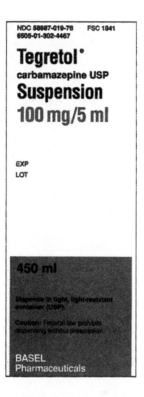

45. Order: Amoxicillin 100 mg p.o. t.i.d.

    Available: _____

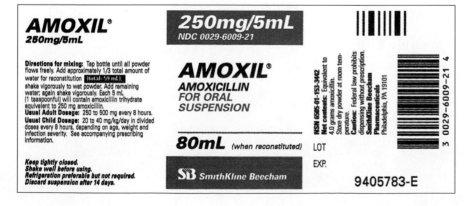

Calculate the doses below. Use the labels where provided. Calculate to the nearest hundredths where necessary.

46. Order: Gentamicin 7.3 mg I.M. q12h.

    Available: Gentamicin 20 mg/2 mL.   _____

47. Order: Atropine 0.1 mg s.c. stat.

    Available: Atropine 400 mcg/mL.   _____

48. Order: Ampicillin 160 mg I.M. q12h.

    Available: Ampicillin 250 mg/mL.   _____

49. Order: Morphine 3.5 mg s.c. q6h p.r.n. for pain.

    Available: Morphine sulfate 15 mg/mL.   _____

50. Order: Nebcin (tobramycin sulfate) 60 mg I.V. q8h.

    Available: _____

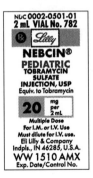

Calculate the doses to be given. Round answers to the nearest tenth as indicated (express answers in mL).

51. Order: Tylenol 0.4 g p.o. q4h prn for temp >101° F.

    Available: Tylenol elixir labeled 160 mg/5 mL.   _____

52. Order: Methotrexate 35 mg I.M. once a week.

    Available: Methotrexate 25 mg/mL.   _____

53. Order: Cleocin 100 mg I.V. q6h.

    Available: Cleocin 150 mg/mL.   _____

54. Order: Procaine penicillin 150,000 U I.M. q12h.

    Available: Procaine penicillin 300,000 U/mL.   _____

55. Order: Amikacin 150 mg I.V. q8h.

    Available: _____

    ```
    NDC 0015-3015-20
    Amikin®
    AMIKACIN SULFATE
    INJECTION For I.M. or I.V. Use
    EQUIVALENT TO
    100 mg  AMIKACIN
            Per 2 mL
    CAUTION: Federal law prohibits
    dispensing without prescription.
    ©Bristol-Myers Company
    ```

56. Order: Dilantin 62.5 mg p.o. b.i.d.

    Available: Dilantin oral suspension
    labeled 125 mg/5 mL.   _____

57. Order: Meperidine 20 mg I.M. q4h p.r.n.

    Available: Proventil syrup 2 mg/mL.   _____

58. Order: Erythromycin 300 mg p.o. q6h.

    Available: Erythromycin oral suspension labeled
    200 mg/5 mL.   _____

59. Order: Proventil 3 mg. p.o. b.i.d.

    Available: 2 mg/5 mL.   _____

60. Order: Tetracycline 250 mg p.o. q6h.

    Available: Tetracycline oral suspension labeled
    125 mg/5 mL.   _____

61. Order: Theophyline 40 mg p.o. q.i.d.

    Available: Theophyline elixir labeled 80 mg/15 mL. _____

Answers on pp. 551-556

UNIT FIVE

Basic I.V., Heparin, and Critical Care Calculations

The ability to accurately calculate flow rates for I.V. medications is essential to both heparin administration and critical care calculations.

Chapter 21
Basic I.V. Calculations

Chapter 22
Heparin Calculations

Chapter 23
Critical Care Calculations

Basic I.V. Calculations

When clients are receiving intravenous (I.V.) therapy, it is important to make sure they are receiving the correct amount at the correct rate of administration. The prescriber is responsible for writing the I.V. order, which **must** specify the following:

1. The name of the I.V. solution.
2. The name of any medication to be added if any.
3. The amount (volume) to be administered.
4. The time period the I.V. is to infuse.

For example, an I.V. order might read:

1,000 mL 5 % D/W I.V. in 8 hours.

> **Critical Thinking**
>
> If a client receives an I.V. infusion too rapidly and is not monitored closely, client reactions can vary from mild to severe (death). Administration of I.V. fluids at a proper rate is a priority and an essential nursing responsibility.

The nurse often has to perform calculations associated with I.V. therapy. The nursing responsibility includes administration of I.V. fluids at the correct rate and monitoring the client during the therapy. Before beginning the calculation aspects of I.V. therapy, let's begin with a general discussion. **I.V. therapy** is the method used to instill fluids or medications directly into the bloodstream. The advantages of administering medications by this route are the immediate availability of the medication to the body and the rapidity of action. The I.V. route is also used to meet nutritional requirements of a client, to replace electrolytes (for example, sodium, potassium), and to administer blood and blood products. Regardless of the purpose of the I.V. therapy, the nurse's primary responsibility is to administer the therapy correctly and at the correct rate.

METHODS OF INFUSION

I.V. fluids are administered by an I.V. infusion set, which includes a sealed bag or bottle containing the fluids. A drip chamber is connected to the I.V. bottle or bag. The flow rate is adjusted to drops per minute by use of a roller clamp. Some I.V. tubing has a sliding clamp attached that can be used to temporarily stop the I.V. infusion. Injection ports are located on the I.V. tubing and on most I.V. solution bags. Injection ports allow for injection of medications directly into the bag of solution or line. The injection ports also allow for attachment of secondary I.V. lines containing fluids or medications to the primary line. Figure 21-1 shows a primary line infusion set. I.V. fluids infuse by gravity flow. This means that for the I.V. solution to infuse it must be hung above the level of the client's heart, which will allow for adequate pressure to be exerted for the I.V. to infuse. The height of the I.V. bag therefore has a relationship to the rate of flow. The higher the I.V. bag is hung, the greater the pressure, therefore the I.V. will infuse at a more rapid rate.

I.V. lines are referred to as either *peripheral* or *central lines,* terms used in relation to the primary line. The infusion site of a **peripheral line** is an area such as the arm or hand, and on rare occasions, the leg. For a **central line,** a special catheter is used to access a large vein such as the subclavian or jugular. The special catheter is threaded through a large vein into the right atrium.

Medications may be added to a primary line either before starting or after it has been infusing. Medications that are often added include electrolytes, such as potassium chloride, and vitamins, such as multivitamins (MVI). These medications are usually diluted in a large volume of fluid (1,000 mL), particularly potassium chloride due to the side effects and untoward reactions that can occur. In some institutions I.V. solutions containing potassium chloride are stocked by the pharmacy and obtained on request by the unit, therefore eliminating the need to add this additive to an I.V. bag. **Secondary lines** attach to the primary line at an injection port. The main purpose of secondary lines is to infuse medications on an intermittent basis (for example, antibiotics q6hr). They can also be used to infuse other I.V. fluids as long as they are compatible with the fluid on the primary line. A secondary line is referred to as an I.V. piggyback (IVPB). Notice that the IVPB is hanging higher than the primary line (Figure 21-2).

Notes

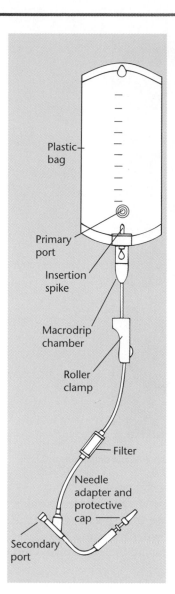

Figure 21-1 Intravenous infusion set. (From Clayton, BD, Stock YN: *Basic pharmacology for nurses,* ed 12, St Louis, 2001, Mosby.)

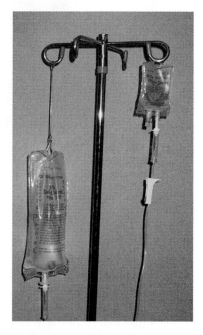

Figure 21-2 I.V. piggyback (gravity flow). (From Brown M, Mulholland JL: *Drug calculations: process and problems for clinical practice,* ed 6, St Louis, 2000, Mosby.)

The IVPB is hanging higher than the primary line because it gives it greater pressure than the primary, thereby allowing it to infuse first. Most secondary administration sets come with an extender that allows the nurse to lower the primary bag. Notice the secondary bags are smaller than the primary (50-100 mL are seen most often). The amount of solution used for the IVPB is determined by the medication being added. Some medications may have to be mixed in 250 mL of fluid for administration. IVPB medications can come premixed by the manufacturer or pharmacist, depending on the institution, or the nurse may have to prepare them.

An order for an IVPB infusion will not always include an infusion time. The Tandem piggyback setup is a small I.V. bag connected to the port of a primary infusion line or to an intermittent venous access. Unlike the piggyback setup, however, the small I.V. bag that is to infuse is placed at the same height as the primary infusion bag or bottle. In this setup the tandem and the main line infuse simultaneously (Figure 21-3).

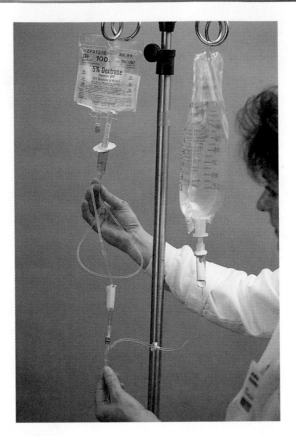

Note:

The nurse must monitor this type of setup closely and clamp the tandem setup immediately once the medication has infused to prevent the I.V. solution from the primary line from backing up into the tandem line.

Figure 21-3 Tandem/piggyback setup. (From Potter PA, Perry AG: *Fundamentals of nursing,* ed 5, St Louis, 2001, Mosby.)

Another type of secondary medication setup used in some institutions is called the **Add-Vantage System.** This system requires the use of a special type of I.V. bag that has a port for inserting the drug (usually in powder form and mixed, using the I.V. solution as a diluent). The contents of the vial are therefore mixed into the total solution and then infused (Figure 21-4, *A*).

The Baxter Mini-Bag Plus is also used to administer piggyback medication. The mini-bag, which is dispensed by the pharmacy, has a vial of unreconstituted medication attached to a special port (Figure 21-4, *B*).

Volume control devices are used for accurate measurement of small-volume medications and fluids. Most volume control devices have a capacity of 100 to 150 mL, and can be used with secondary or primary lines. They are also used intermittently for medication purposes. They have a port that allows medication to be injected and a certain amount of I.V. fluid added as a diluent (Figure 21-5). Volume control devices are referred to by their trade names: Volutrol, Soluset, or Buretrol, depending on the institution. They are used mostly in pediatric and critical care settings. These devices allow for precise control of the infusion and the medication.

Critical Thinking

When an infusion time is not stated for IVPB, check appropriate resources, such as a medication book or the hospital pharmacy. The nurse is responsible for any error that occurs in reference to I.V. administration, including incorrect rate of administration.

Step 1

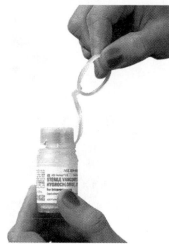

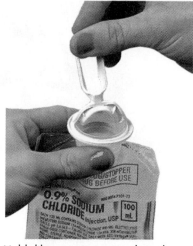

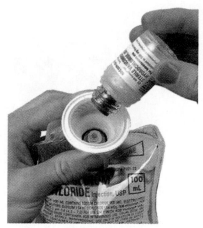

Swing the pull ring over the top of the vial and pull down far enough to start the opening. Then pull straight up to remove the cap. Avoid touching the rubber stopper and vial threads.

Hold diluent container and gently grasp the tab on the pull ring. Pull up to break the tie membrane. Pull back to remove the cover. Avoid touching the inside of the vial port.

Screw the vial into the vial port until it will go no further. Recheck the vial to assure that it is tight. Label appropriately.

Step 2

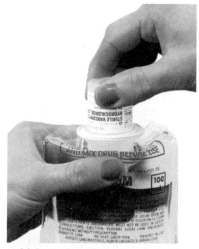

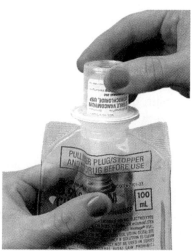

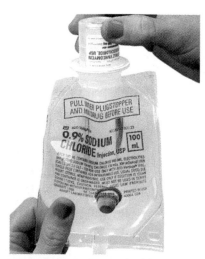

Hold the vial as shown. Push the drug vial down into container and grasp the inner cap of the vial through the walls of the container.

Pull the inner cap from the drug vial: allow drug to fall into diluent container for fast mixing. Do not force stopper by pushing on one side of inner cap at a time.

Verify that the plug and rubber stopper have been removed from the vial. The floating stopper is an indication that the system has been activated.

Figure 21-4   Assembling and administering medication with the ADD-Vantage system. Step 1: Assemble using aseptic technique. Step 2: Activate by pulling the plug/stopper to mix drug with diluent. (ADD-Vantage® is a registered trademark of Abbott Laboratories. Courtesy Abbott Laboratories, Abbott Park, Illinois.)

Continued

Step 3

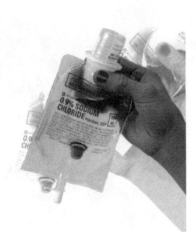

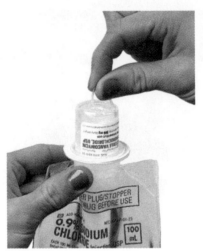

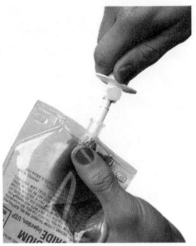

Mix container contents thoroughly to assure complete dissolution. Look through bottom of vial to verify complete mixing. Check for leaks by squeezing container firmly. If leaks are found, discard unit.

Pull up hanger on the vial.

Remove the white administration port cover and spike (pierce) the container with the piercing pin. Administer within the specified time.

Figure 21-4, cont'd   Step 3: Mix and administer within the specified time. (ADD-Vantage® is a registered trademark of Abbott Laboratories. Courtesy Abbott Laboratories, Abbott Park, Illinois.)

Indwelling infusion ports (Figure 21-6) are used for the purpose of administering I.V. medication intermittently or for access to a vein in an emergency situation. Infusion ports are referred to as *medlocks*, *saline locks*, or *heplocks*. The line is usually kept free from blockage or clotting by irrigating the line with heparin (anticoagulant) or sterile saline. The solution used and the amount of solution vary from institution to institution.

Recently various institutions have purchased a needleless system (Figure 21-7) for administration of medications through the primary line and for access devices such as saline locks. The needleless system doesn't require attachment of a needle by the nurse. The system allows for administration by I.V. push or bolus or via piggyback.

When medications are administered through indwelling infusion ports (also called access devices), they must be periodically flushed to maintain patency. Due to the bolusing of clients with heparin (a potent anticoagulant despite the use of dilute forms of heparin), heparin is now used only on the initial insertion of the catheter. For subsequent flushings of the port, normal saline is used (1 to 3 mL, depending on institution policy).

When medications are administered through the infusion port, the port must be flushed before and after medication is given. The letters used in most institutions to remember the technique for medication administration are S, I, S (saline, I.V. medications, saline). With early discharge and an increased number of home care clients discharged with infusion ports in place, it is imperative that clients be taught about the care of the infusion port.

Medications can be administered through a port used for direct injection of medication by syringe or directly into the vein by venipuncture. This is referred to as I.V. **push** or **bolus**. I.V. *push* indicates that a syringe is attached to the lock and the medication is pushed in. I.V. *bolus* indicates a volume of I.V. fluid is infused over a specific period of time through an I.V. administration set attached to the lock. There are guidelines, however, relating to the acceptable rate for I.V. push administration. **Check appropriate references for the rate (per minute) for**

Note:

Always refer to the policy at your institution or health care agency regarding the frequency, volume, and concentration of saline or heparin to be used to maintain the I.V. lock.

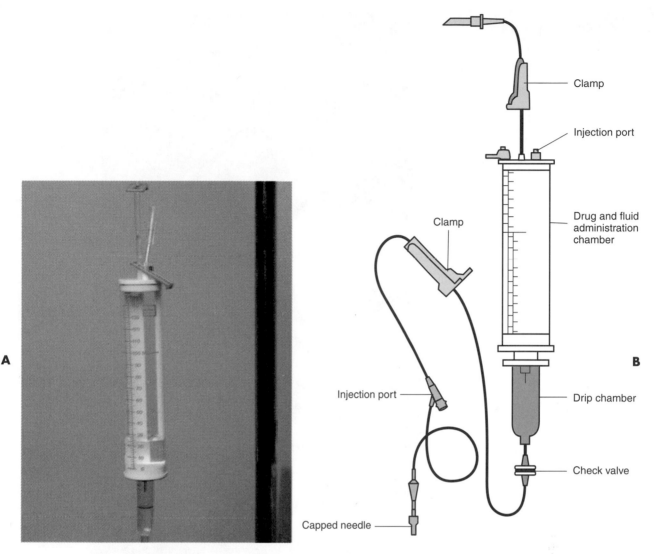

Clamp

Injection port

Clamp

Drug and fluid
administration
chamber

Injection port

Drip chamber

Check valve

Capped needle

Figure 21-5 **A,** Volume-controlled device. **B,** Parts of a volume control set. (**A** from Elkin M, Perry A, Potter P: *Nursing interventions and clinical skills,* ed 2, St Louis, 2000, Mosby. **B** redrawn from Pickar GD: *Dosage calculations,* ed 6, Albany, 1999, Delmar.)

I.V. push drug administration. Also check the institution's policy and a pharmacology reference regarding administration by I.V. push or bolus.

Electronic Infusion Devices

There are several electronic infusion devices on the market today (Figure 21-8). Special tubing is supplied by the manufacturers of these electronic devices. Each device can be set for a specific flow rate and generally emits an alarm if the rate is interrupted. The use of electronic infusion devices is based on the need to strictly regulate the I.V. Electronic infusion devices are essential in pediatrics and the critical care setting, where they provide for infusion of small amounts of fluids or medications with precise accuracy.

Electronic Rate Controllers

The rate of flow of the I.V. solution is monitored by a drop sensor attached to the tubing's drip chamber. The sensor monitors the flow rate. The controller depends on gravity to maintain the desired flow rate by a compression/decompression mechanism that pinches the I.V. tubing. The controller monitors the selected infusion rate

Notes

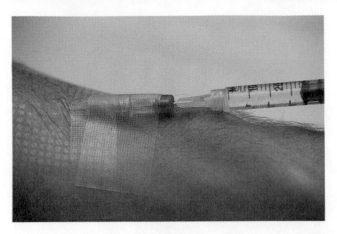

Figure 21-6   Example of an infusion indwelling port. (From Potter PA, Perry AG: *Fundamentals of nursing,* ed 5, St Louis, 2001, Mosby.)

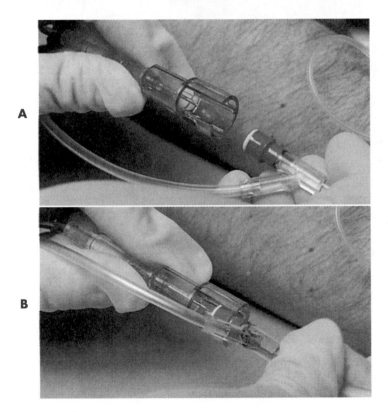

Figure 21-7   **A,** Needleless infusion system. **B,** Connection into an injection port. (From Elkin M, Perry A, Potter P: *Nursing interventions and clinical skills,* ed 2, St Louis, 2000, Mosby.)

by either drop counting (drops per minute) or volumetric delivery (milliliters per hour). This device is still seen in some institutions; however, more institutions are discontinuing their use in favor of electronic volumetric pumps (Figure 21-9).

Electronic Volumetric Pumps

These pumps infuse fluids into the vein under pressure and against resistance, and don't rely on gravity. The pumps are programmed to deliver a set amount of fluid per hr (see Figure 21-8). There is a wide range of electronic pumps. Because these pumps deliver mL/hr, any mL calculation that results in a decimal fraction must be rounded to a whole mL. Recently we have seen the advent of more sophisti-

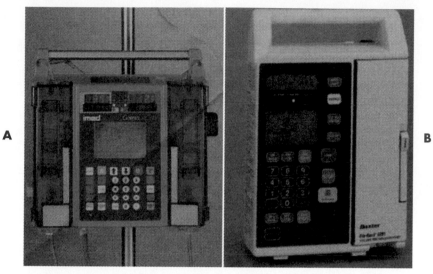

Figure 21-8 A, Dual-channel infusion pump. **B,** Single infusion pump. (From Kee J, Marshall SM: *Clinical calculations: with applications to general and specialty areas,* ed 4, Philadelphia, 2000, WB Saunders. **A,** Courtesy IMED Corp., San Diego, Calif. **B,** Courtesy Baxter Healthcare Corp.)

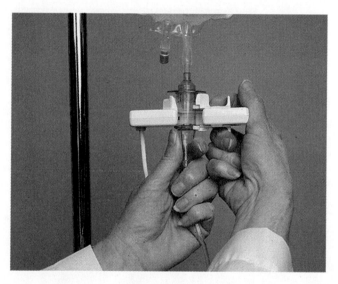

Figure 21-9 Sensor (electronic eye) connected to drip chamber to regulate drops. (From Elkin M, Perry A, Potter P: *Nursing interventions and clinical skills,* ed 2, St Louis, 2000, Mosby.)

cated pumps that allow infusions to be set by pump rate and the drug dosage to be administered.

Syringe Pumps

These are electronic devices that deliver medications or fluids by use of a syringe. The drug is measured in a syringe and attached to the special pump, and the medication is infused at the rate set (Figure 21-10). These pumps are useful in pediatrics and intensive care units, as well as labor and delivery areas.

Patient-Controlled Analgesia (PCA) Devices

This form of pain management allows the client to self-administer I.V. analgesics. This is accomplished by using a computerized infuser pump attached to the I.V. line (Figure 21-11). The PCA pump is programmed to allow doses of narcotics

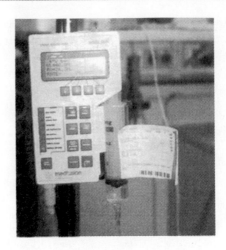

Figure 21-10 Syringe pump. (From Kee J, Marshall SM: *Clinical calculations: with applications to general and specialty areas,* ed 4, Philadelphia, 2000, WB Saunders.)

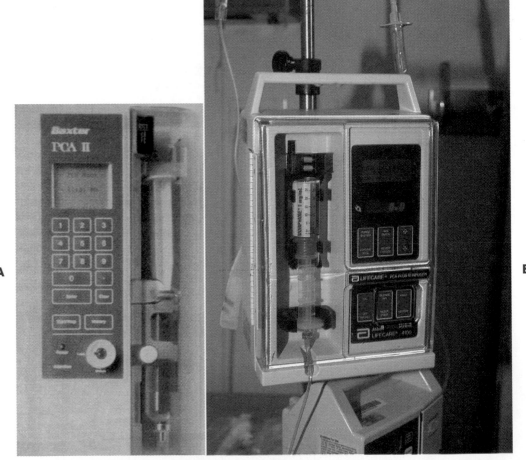

Figure 21-11 Patient-controlled analgesia (PCA) pumps. (**A** from Kee J, Marshall SM: *Clinical calculations: with applications to general and specialty areas,* ed 4, Philadelphia, 2000, WB Saunders. **B** from Elkin M, Perry A, Potter P: *Nursing interventions and clinical skills,* ed 2, St Louis, 2000, Mosby.)

only within specific limits to prevent overdosage. The dose and frequency of administration are ordered by the doctor and set on the pump. The patient self-medicates by use of a control button. The pump also keeps a record of the number of times the client uses it. The display on the pump lets clients know when they are able to medicate themselves and when it is impossible to give themselves another dose. The pump therefore has what is called a lockout interval. This is an interval during which no medications are delivered. A drug commonly administered by PCA is morphine (30 mg morphine per 30 mL).

Infusion Devices for the Home Care Setting

Another type of infusion device is the balloon device. These devices are used mainly on outpatient and home care settings to administer single-dose infusion therapies. One such device is the elastometric balloon device, which is made of soft, rubberized, disposable material that inflates to a predetermined volume to hold and dispense a single dose of I.V. medication. Baxter is a manufacturer of this type of I.V. system. Med Flow II, an ambulatory infusion device, is another system developed for ambulatory use. This device can be placed in a pocket to conceal it (Figure 21-12). Other infusion sets available include battery-operated pumps.

I.V. FLUIDS

There are several types of I.V. fluids. The type of fluid used is individualized according to the client and the reason for its use. I.V. solutions come prepared in plastic bags or glass bottles ranging from 50 mL (bags only) to 1,000 mL. I.V. solutions are clearly labeled with the exact components and amount of solution. When I.V. solutions are written in orders and charts, abbreviations are used. Ex-

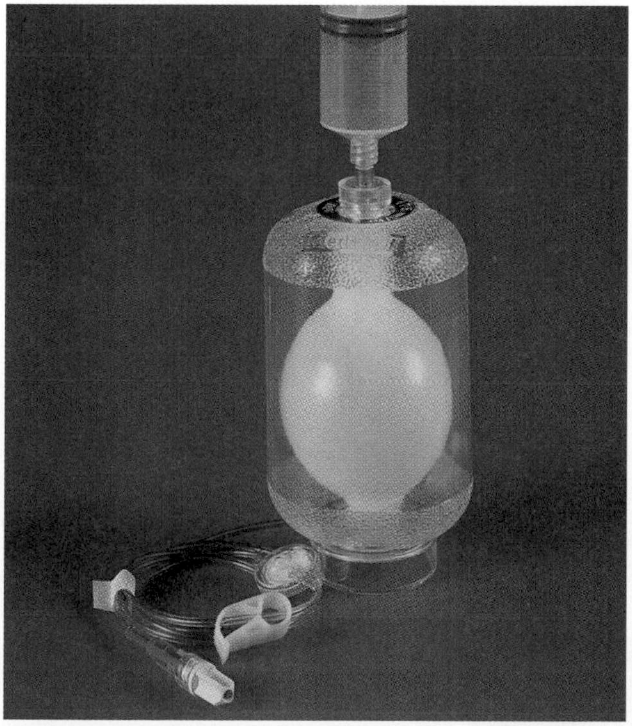

Note:

Regardless of the electronic device, clients need to be educated about them, the devices must be monitored to ascertain proper functioning, and the client must be monitored.

Figure 21-12 MedFlo II™ ambulatory infusion device. (From Brown M, Mulholland JL: *Drug calculations: process and problems for clinical practice,* ed 6, St Louis, 2000, Mosby. Courtesy MPS Acacia, Brea, Calif.)

<u>*Note:*</u>

The abbreviation letters indicate the solution components, and the numbers identify the percentage (%) strengths.

ample: D5W means Dextrose 5% in water. You may encounter various abbreviations; however, the percentage and initials, regardless of how written, have the same meaning: "D" is for dextrose, "W" is for water, "S" is for saline, and "NS" is for normal saline. Ringer's Lactate (Lactated Ringer's), a commonly used electrolyte solution, is abbreviated "RL" or "LR," and occasionally "RLS." As already discussed, potassium chloride (KCl) is commonly added to I.V. solutions. Potassium chloride is measured in milliequivalents (mEq). Saline (sodium chloride or NaCl) is also found in I.V. fluids. Refer to Box 21-1 and learn the common abbreviations for I.V. solutions. Figures 21-13 to 21-15 show various I.V. solutions.

Remember: Solutions of I.V. administration are individualized and determined by client needs.

BOX 21-1   Abbreviations for Common Intravenous Solutions

NS	Normal saline 0.9%
$\frac{1}{2}$ NS	Normal saline 0.45%
D5W or 5% D/W	Dextrose 5% in water
D5RL	Dextrose 5% and Lactated Ringer's (Ringer's Lactate)
RL or RLS	Lactated Ringer's solution (electrolytes)
D5NS	Dextrose 5% in normal saline
D5 and $\frac{1}{2}$ NS (0.45%)	Dextrose 5% in $\frac{1}{2}$ normal saline (0.45%)

From Brown M, Mulholland J: *Drug calculations: process and problems for clinical practice,* ed 6, St Louis, 2000, Mosby.

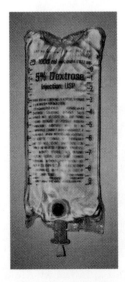

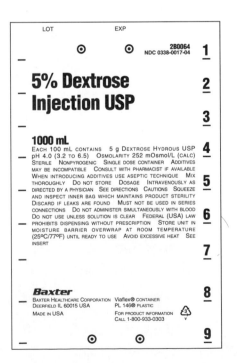

Figure 21-13   5% Dextrose. (From Brown M, Mulholland JL: *Drug calculations: process and problems for clinical practice,* ed 6, St Louis, 2000, Mosby.)

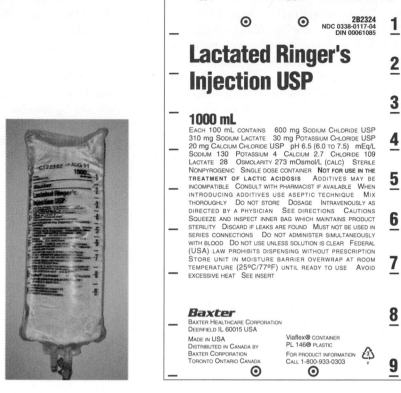

LOT   EXP

2B2324
NDC 0338-0117-04
DIN 00061085

Lactated Ringer's Injection USP

1000 mL

EACH 100 mL CONTAINS   600 mg SODIUM CHLORIDE USP
310 mg SODIUM LACTATE   30 mg POTASSIUM CHLORIDE USP
20 mg CALCIUM CHLORIDE USP   pH 6.5 (6.0 TO 7.5)   mEq/L
SODIUM 130   POTASSIUM 4   CALCIUM 2.7   CHLORIDE 109
LACTATE 28   OSMOLARITY 273 mOsmol/L (CALC)   STERILE
NONPYROGENIC   SINGLE DOSE CONTAINER   **NOT FOR USE IN THE
TREATMENT OF LACTIC ACIDOSIS**   ADDITIVES MAY BE
INCOMPATIBLE   CONSULT WITH PHARMACIST IF AVAILABLE   WHEN
INTRODUCING ADDITIVES USE ASEPTIC TECHNIQUE   MIX
THOROUGHLY   DO NOT STORE   DOSAGE   INTRAVENOUSLY AS
DIRECTED BY A PHYSICIAN   SEE DIRECTIONS   CAUTIONS
SQUEEZE AND INSPECT INNER BAG WHICH MAINTAINS PRODUCT
STERILITY   DISCARD IF LEAKS ARE FOUND   MUST NOT BE USED IN
SERIES CONNECTIONS   DO NOT ADMINISTER SIMULTANEOUSLY
WITH BLOOD   DO NOT USE UNLESS SOLUTION IS CLEAR   FEDERAL
(USA) LAW PROHIBITS DISPENSING WITHOUT PRESCRIPTION
STORE UNIT IN MOISTURE BARRIER OVERWRAP AT ROOM
TEMPERATURE (25°C/77°F) UNTIL READY TO USE   AVOID
EXCESSIVE HEAT   SEE INSERT

Baxter
BAXTER HEALTHCARE CORPORATION
DEERFIELD IL 60015 USA

MADE IN USA   Viaflex® CONTAINER
DISTRIBUTED IN CANADA BY   PL 146® PLASTIC
BAXTER CORPORATION   FOR PRODUCT INFORMATION
TORONTO ONTARIO CANADA   CALL 1-800-933-0303

1 2 3 4 5 6 7 8 9

Figure 21-14   Lactated Ringer's solution. (From Brown M, Mulholland JL: *Drug calculations: process and problems for clinical practice,* ed 6, St Louis, 2000, Mosby.)

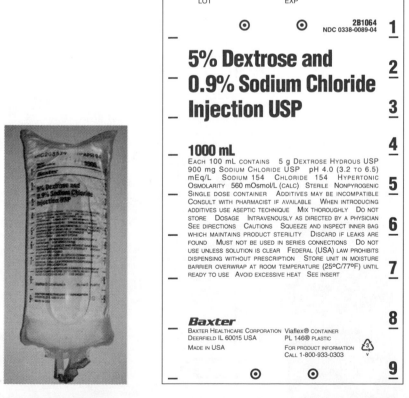

LOT   EXP

2B1064
NDC 0338-0089-04

5% Dextrose and 0.9% Sodium Chloride Injection USP

1000 mL

EACH 100 mL CONTAINS   5 g DEXTROSE HYDROUS USP
900 mg SODIUM CHLORIDE USP   pH 4.0 (3.2 TO 6.5)
mEq/L   SODIUM 154   CHLORIDE 154   HYPERTONIC
OSMOLARITY 560 mOsmol/L (CALC)   STERILE   NONPYROGENIC
SINGLE DOSE CONTAINER   ADDITIVES MAY BE INCOMPATIBLE
CONSULT WITH PHARMACIST IF AVAILABLE   WHEN INTRODUCING
ADDITIVES USE ASEPTIC TECHNIQUE   MIX THOROUGHLY   DO NOT
STORE   DOSAGE   INTRAVENOUSLY AS DIRECTED BY A PHYSICIAN
SEE DIRECTIONS   CAUTIONS   SQUEEZE AND INSPECT INNER BAG
WHICH MAINTAINS PRODUCT STERILITY   DISCARD IF LEAKS ARE
FOUND   MUST NOT BE USED IN SERIES CONNECTIONS   DO NOT
USE UNLESS SOLUTION IS CLEAR   FEDERAL (USA) LAW PROHIBITS
DISPENSING WITHOUT PRESCRIPTION   STORE UNIT IN MOISTURE
BARRIER OVERWRAP AT ROOM TEMPERATURE (25°C/77°F) UNTIL
READY TO USE   AVOID EXCESSIVE HEAT   SEE INSERT

Baxter
BAXTER HEALTHCARE CORPORATION Viaflex® CONTAINER
DEERFIELD IL 60015 USA   PL 146® PLASTIC
MADE IN USA   FOR PRODUCT INFORMATION
                               CALL 1-800-933-0303

1 2 3 4 5 6 7 8 9

Figure 21-15   5% Dextrose in normal saline (0.9%). (From Brown M, Mulholland JL: *Drug calculations: process and problems for clinical practice,* ed 6, St Louis, 2000, Mosby.)

Notes

Normal saline solutions are often written with 0.9 or % sign included (e.g., D5 0.9% NS). NS is the abbreviation used for normal saline. Normal saline is also referred to as sodium chloride (NaCl). Saline is available in different percentages. Normal saline is the common term used for 0.9% sodium chloride. Another common saline I.V. concentration is 0.45% NaCl, often written as "1/2 NS" (0.45% is 1/2 of 0.9%). Other saline solution strengths include 0.33% NaCl, also abbreviated as "1/3 NS," and 0.225% NaCl, also abbreviated as "1/4 NS." Some orders for I.V. fluids may therefore be written as D5 $^1/_2$ NS, D5 $^1/_4$ NS. Note: I.V. fluids can contain saline only or saline mixed with dextrose, which would be indicated with the percentage of dextrose (e.g., D5 0.9% NS). Figure 21-16 and 21-17 show saline solution and saline mixed with dextrose.

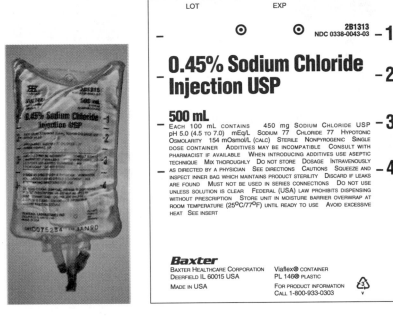

Figure 21-16 Normal saline 0.45%. (From Brown M, Mulholland JL: *Drug calculations: process and problems for clinical practice,* ed 6, St Louis, 2000, Mosby.)

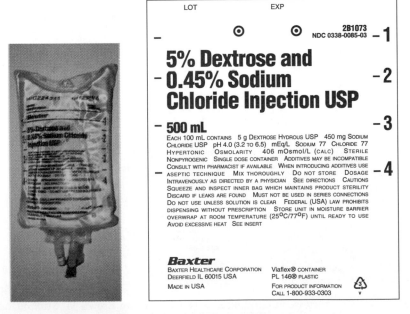

Figure 21-17 5% Dextrose in 1/2 (0.45%) normal saline. (From Brown M, Mulholland JL: *Drug calculations: process and problems for clinical practice,* ed 6, St Louis, 2000, Mosby.)

Juice glass – 180 mL   Small water cup – 120 mL
Water glass – 210 mL   Jello cup – 150 mL
Coffee cup – 240 mL   Ice cream – 120 mL
Soup bowl – 180 mL   Creamer – 30 mL

Client information

Date: 8/17/01

INTAKE					OUTPUT				
Time	Type	Amt	Time	IV/ Blood type	Amount absorbed	Time	Urine	Stool	Other
			7A	1000 mL D5W	800 mL	9A	400 mL		
			12P	IVPB	100 mL	1P	500 mL		
8 hr total					900 mL		900 mL		

Figure 21-18   Sample of charting I.V. fluids on I&O record.

I.V. fluids are charted on the I&O sheet; in some institutions they are also charted on the MAR. Figure 21-18 is a sample I&O charting record.

Calculating Percentage in I.V. Fluids

The amount of each ingredient in an I.V. fluid can be calculated; however, it is not necessary because the label on the I.V. solution indicates the amount of each ingredient. Calculation of the percentage of solutions was presented in Chapter 5, which deals with percentages.

As you may recall, it is possible to determine the percentage of substances such as dextrose in I.V. solutions. It is important to remember that **solution strength expressed as a percent means gram of drug per 100 mL of fluid.** Therefore, 5% dextrose solution will have 5 g of dextrose in each 100 mL. In addition to determining the amount of dextrose in the solution, other components such as sodium chloride can be determined. To calculate the amount of a specific component in an I.V. solution, a ratio-proportion can be used.

Note:

Percent means grams of drug per 100 mL of fluid.

Example 1:   Calculate the amount of dextrose in 500 mL D5W. Remember % = g per 100 mL, therefore 5% dextrose = 5 g dextrose per 100 mL.

$$5 \text{ g} : 100 \text{ mL} = x \text{ g} : 500 \text{ mL}$$

$$\frac{100x}{100} = \frac{2,500}{100}$$

$$x = 25 \text{ g}$$

500 mL D5W contains 25 g of dextrose.

Remember, ratio-proportions can be stated in various ways. This ratio-proportion could also be stated as follows:

$$\frac{5 \text{ g}}{100 \text{ mL}} = \frac{x \text{ g}}{500 \text{ mL}}$$

Notes

Example 2:   Calculate the amount of sodium chloride (NaCl) in 1,000 mL NS.

$$0.9\% = 0.9 \text{ g NaCl per } 100 \text{ mL}$$

$$0.9 \text{ g} : 100 \text{ mL} = x \text{ g} : 1,000 \text{ mL} \quad \text{or} \quad \frac{0.9 \text{ g}}{100 \text{ mL}} = \frac{x \text{ g}}{1,000 \text{ mL}}$$

$$\frac{100x}{100} = \frac{900}{100}$$

$$x = 9 \text{ g NaCl}$$

1,000 mL of NS contains 9 g of sodium chloride.

Example 3:   Calculate the amount of dextrose in 1,000 mL of 5% dextrose

and 0.45% normal saline (D5 and $\frac{1}{2}$ NS).

$$D5 = \text{dextrose } 5\% = 5 \text{ g dextrose per } 100 \text{ mL.}$$

$$NS = 0.45 \text{ g NaCl per } 100 \text{ mL}$$

$$\text{dextrose: } 5 \text{ g} : 100 \text{ mL} = x \text{ g} : 1,000 \text{ mL} \quad \text{or} \quad \frac{5 \text{ g}}{100 \text{ mL}} = \frac{x \text{ g}}{1,000 \text{ mL}}$$

$$\frac{100x}{100} = \frac{5,000}{100}$$

$$x = 50 \text{ g dextrose}$$

$$NaCl: 0.45 \text{ g} : 100 \text{ mL} = x \text{ g} : 1,000 \text{ mL}$$

$$\frac{100x}{100} = \frac{450}{100}$$

$$x = 4.5 \text{ g NaCl}$$

1,000 mL D5 0.45% NS contains 50 g dextrose and 4.5 g of NaCl.

Example 4:   Calculate the amount of dextrose and sodium chloride in
1,000 mL of D5 NS.

$$D5 = \text{dextrose } 5\% = 5 \text{ g dextrose per } 100 \text{ mL.}$$

$$NS = 0.9 \text{ g NaCl per } 100 \text{ mL}$$

$$\text{dextrose: } 5 \text{ g} : 100 \text{ mL} = x \text{ g} : 1,000 \text{ mL} \quad \text{or} \quad \frac{5 \text{ g}}{100 \text{ mL}} = \frac{x \text{ g}}{1,000 \text{ mL}}$$

$$\frac{100x}{100} = \frac{5,000}{100}$$

$$x = 50 \text{ g dextrose}$$

$$NaCl: 0.9 \text{ g} : 100 \text{ mL} = x \text{ g} : 1,000 \text{ mL} \quad \text{or} \quad \frac{0.9 \text{ g}}{100 \text{ mL}} = \frac{x \text{ g}}{1,000 \text{ mL}}$$

$$\frac{100x}{100} = \frac{5,000}{100}$$

$$x = 9 \text{ g NaCl}$$

1,000 mL D5NS contains 50 g of dextrose and 9 g of NaCl.

As demonstrated with the calculation of percentages in I.V. solutions, I.V. fluids contain certain amounts of dextrose, salts, and electrolytes. The composition

of I.V. fluids is indicated on I.V. labels; however, as shown, it can also be calculated with a ratio-proportion.

Parenteral nutrition is a form of nutritional support in which the nutrients are provided by the intravenous route. Parenteral nutrition solutions consist of glucose, amino acids, minerals, vitamins, and/or fat emulsions. The nutrients are infused by a peripheral or central line. Solutions less than 10% dextrose may be given by a peripheral vein; parenteral nutrition with greater than 10% dextrose requires administration by a central venous catheter. A central venous catheter is placed into a high-flow central vein, such as the superior vena cava, by the health care provider. Lipid emulsions are also given when the client is receiving parenteral nutrition. They provide supplemental kilocalories and prevent fatty acid deficiencies. These emulsions can be administered through a separate peripheral line, through a central line by a "y" connector tubing, or as mixtures to parenteral nutrition solution.

Clients who are unable to digest or absorb enteral nutrition are candidates for parenteral nutrition. Parenteral nutrition is referred to as TPN (total parenteral nutrition) and hyperalimentation. The same principles relating to I.V. therapy are applicable to parenteral nutrition, but more emphasis is placed on care for the site to prevent infection. Further discussion of parenteral nutrition can be found in nursing reference books. Flow rate and calculation of infusion times, which will be discussed in this chapter, is also applicable to parenteral nutrition solutions.

I.V. medication protocols are valuable references often posted in the medication room of an institution. They provide nurses with specifics about usual medication dosage, dilution for I.V. administration, compatibility, and specific observations that need to be made of a client during medication administration.

Note:

Always adhere to the protocol for administering I.V. drugs.

 PRACTICE PROBLEMS

Answer the following questions as briefly as possible.

1. What does PCA stand for? _____

2. If an I.V. is initiated in a client's lower arm, this is called what type of line?

    _____

3. IVPB means _____

4. A client has an I.V. of 1,000 mL 0.9% NS. The initials identify what type of

    solution? _____

5. A secondary line is hung _____, then the primary
    line.

6. Volumetric pumps force fluids into the vein by _____.

Identify the components and percentage strength of the following I.V. solutions.

7. D20W _____

8. D5W 10 mEq KCl _____

9. How many grams of dextrose does 500 mL D10W contain? _____

Notes

Calculate the amount of dextrose and/or sodium chloride in the following I.V. solutions.

10. 750 mL D5 NS

dextrose   _____

NaCl   _____

11. 250 mL D10W

dextrose   _____

12. 1,000 mL D5 0.33% NS

dextrose   _____

NaCl   _____

13. 500 mL D5 $\frac{1}{2}$ NS

dextrose   _____

NaCl   _____

Answers on p. 556

POINTS TO REMEMBER

- I.V. orders are written by the doctor or other prescriber certified to do so (e.g., nurse practitioner, physician's assistant, etc.).

- I.V. orders must specify the name of the solution, medications (if any are to be added), the amount to be administered, and the infusion time.

- There are several electronic devices on the market for infusing intravenous solutions. Always familiarize yourself with the equipment before use.

- Follow the institution's protocol for I.V. administration.

- Nurses have the primary responsibility for monitoring the client while receiving intravenous therapy.

- Nurses are responsible for any errors that occur in administration of I.V. fluids (e.g., inadequate dilution, too rapid infusion).

- Pay close attention to I.V. abbreviations. The letters indicate the solution components and the numbers indicate the solution strength.

- Solution strength expressed as a percent (%) indicates grams of solute per 100 mL of fluid.

- Principles relating to flow rate and infusion times are also applicable to parenteral nutrition solutions.

I.V. FLOW RATE CALCULATION

I.V. fluids are usually ordered on the basis of mL/hr. Example: 3,000 mL/24 hr, 1,000 mL in 8 hr. Small volumes of fluid are often used when the I.V. contains medications such as antibiotics. Rates for I.V. fluids are usually determined in gtt/min when an infusion device is not used. When an infusion device is used, the rate must be determined in mL/hr.

Calculating Flow Rates for Volumetric Pumps in mL/hr

When a client is using an electronic infuser such as a volumetric pump, the prescriber orders the volume and the nurse is responsible for programming the pump to deliver the ordered volume. The prescriber may order the I.V. volume in mL/hr; however, if not, the nurse must calculate it and program the pump.

Remember that the pump delivers volume in mL/hr, so if a decimal fraction is obtained, it must be rounded to the whole number.

$$\frac{\text{Amount of solution (mL)}}{\text{Time in hours}} = x \text{ mL/hr (whole number)}$$

Example 1:   Client on infusion pump has an order for 3,000 mL D5W over 24 hours.

1. Think: pump is regulated in mL/hr.
2. Set up in formula:

$$\frac{3,000 \text{ mL}}{24 \text{ hr}} = x \text{ mL/hr}$$

$$x = 125 \text{ mL/hr}$$

Answer: The pump would be set to deliver 125 mL/hr.

An alternative to the above formula would be to set up a ratio-proportion as follows:

$$3,000 \text{ mL} : 24 \text{ hr} = x \text{ mL} : 1 \text{ hr}$$

$$\frac{24 \, x}{24} = \frac{3,000}{24}$$

$$x = 125 \text{ mL/hr}$$

Remember, as stated in the chapter on ratio-proportion, a ratio-proportion can be set up in several formats. This could have been set up with the desired time for the infusion (usually 1 hr) over the total time ordered in hrs, and the other side would be the hourly amount in mL labeled "x" over the total volume to be infused in mL:

Note:

The terms in the ratio-proportion must be in the same sequence.

$$\frac{1 \text{ hr}}{24 \text{ hrs}} = \frac{x \text{ mL}}{3,000 \text{ mL}} \quad \text{or} \quad 1 \text{ hr} : 24 \text{ hrs} = x \text{ mL} : 3,000 \text{ mL}$$

Example 2:   A client on an infusion pump is to receive an antibiotic in 50 mL 0.9% NS over 30 minutes.

1. Think: The pump infuses in mL/hr. When the infusion time is less than an hr, which often occurs when administering antibiotics, use a ratio-proportion to determine mL/hr. Remember: 1 hr = 60 min.

Notes

2. Set up proportion:

$$50 \text{ mL} : 30 \text{ min} = x \text{ mL} : 60 \text{ min}$$

$$30 \, x = 50 \times 60$$

$$\frac{30x}{30} = \frac{3,000}{30}$$

$$x = 100 \text{ mL/hr}$$

Answer: The pump must be set to deliver 100 mL/hr for 50 mL to infuse within 30 minutes.

Note: The ratio-proportion could have been set up as follows:

$$\frac{50 \text{ mL}}{30 \text{ min}} = \frac{x \text{ mL}}{60 \text{ min}}$$

 PRACTICE PROBLEMS

Calculate the flow rate in mL/hr.

14. 1,800 mL of D5W in 24 hr by infusion pump. _____

15. 2,000 mL D5W in 24 hr by infusion pump. _____

16. 500 mL R/L in 12 hr by infusion pump. _____

17. 100 mL 0.45% NS in 45 min by infusion pump. _____

18. 1,500 mL D5RL in 24 hr by infusion pump. _____

19. 750 mL D5W in 16 hr by infusion pump. _____

20. 30 mL of antibiotic in 0.9 NS in 20 min by infusion pump. _____

Answers on p. 556

CALCULATING I.V. FLOW RATES IN gtt/min

When an electronic infusion device is *not* used, the nurse manually regulates the I.V. rate. To manually regulate an I.V. the nurse must determine gtt/min.

I.V. flow rates in gtt/min are determined by the type of I.V. administration tubing. The drop size is regulated by the size of the tubing. (The larger the tubing, the larger the drops.) The first step in calculating I.V. flow rates is to identify the type of tubing and its calibration. The calibration of the tubing is printed on each I.V. administration package (Figure 21-19).

I.V. TUBING

I.V. tubing has a drip chamber. The nurse determines the flow rate by adjusting the clamp and observing the drip chamber to count the drops per minute (Figure 21-20). The size of the drop depends on the type of I.V. tubing used. The calibration of I.V. tubing in gtt/mL is known as the *drop factor* and is indicated on the box in which the I.V. tubing is packaged. This calibration, which is necessary to calculate flow rates, is shown on the packaging of I.V. administration sets (see Figure 21-19).

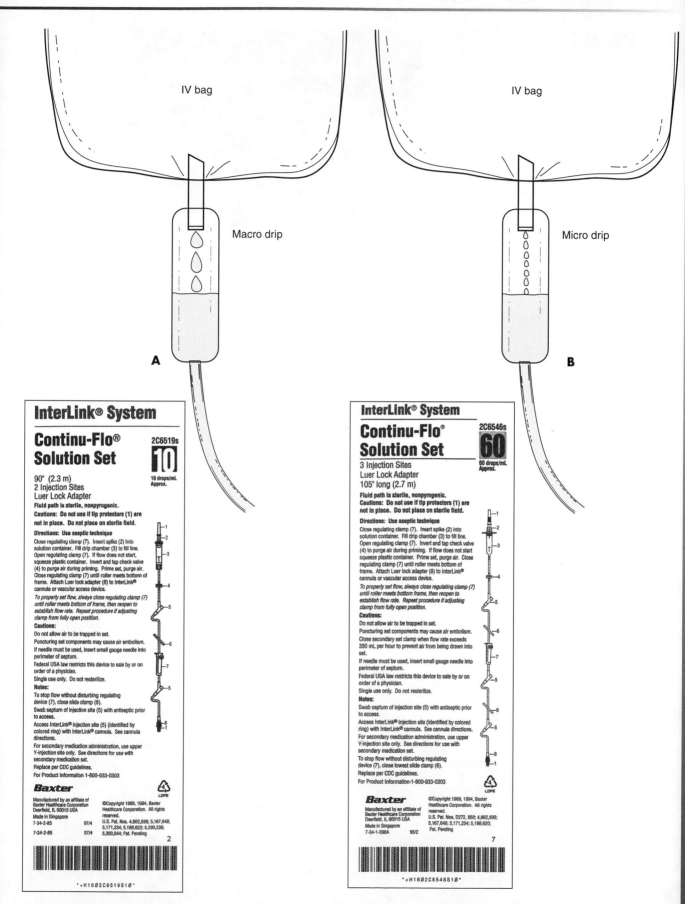

Figure 21-19   Administration sets. **A,** Set with drip factor of 10 (10 gtt = 1 mL). **B,** Set with drip factor of 60. (60 gtt = 1 mL).

Notes

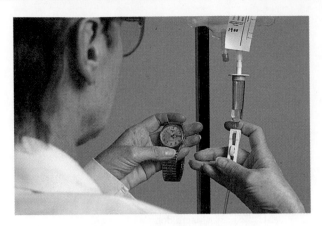

Figure 21-20 Observing the drip chamber to count drops per minute. (From Potter PA, Perry AG: *Fundamentals of nursing,* ed 5, St Louis, 2001, Mosby.)

The two common types of tubing used to administer I.V. fluids are as follows:

Macrodrop tubing

This is the standard type of tubing used for general I.V. administration. This type of tubing delivers a certain number of gtt/mL, as specified by the manufacturer. Macrodrop tubing delivers 10, 15, or 20 gtts equal to 1 mL. Macrodrops are large drops; therefore, large amounts of fluid are administered in macrodrops (Figure 21-21, *A*).

Microdrip tubing

Microdrip tubing delivers tiny drops, which can be inferred from micro. It is used when small amounts and more exact measurements are needed, for example, in pediatrics, for the elderly, and in critical care settings. Microdrip tubing delivers 60 gtt equal to 1 mL. Because there are 60 minutes in an hour, the number of microdrops per minute is equal to the number of mL/hr. For example, if clients are receiving 100 mL/hr, they are receiving 100 microdrops/min (Figure 21-21, *B*).

Figure 21-22 shows a comparison of calibrated drops.

Remember: The nurse must be aware of the drop factor to accurately administer I.V. fluids to a client.

Macrodrip Chamber   Microdrip Chamber

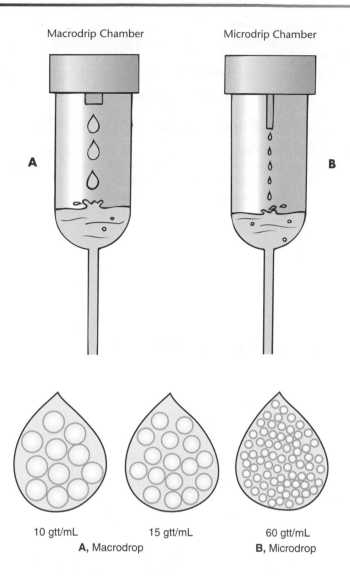

Figure 21-21 **A,** Macrodrip chamber. **B,** Microdrip chamber. (From Clayton BD, Stock YN: *Basic pharmacology for nurses,* ed 12, St Louis, 2001, Mosby.

10 gtt/mL   15 gtt/mL   60 gtt/mL

A, Macrodrop   **B,** Microdrop

Figure 21-22 Comparison of calibrated drop factors. **A,** Macrodrop. **B,** Microdrop.

 PRACTICE PROBLEMS

Identify the drop factor and type of tubing for the I.V. tubing pictured below.

21. _____

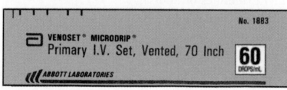

2C5419 s

Baxter-Travenol **10**

Vented Basic Set
10 drops/mL

22. _____

No. 1883

VENOSET® MICRODRIP®
Primary I.V. Set, Vented, 70 Inch   **60** DROPS/mL

ABBOTT LABORATORIES

Notes

23. _____

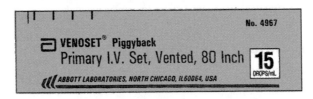

24. _____

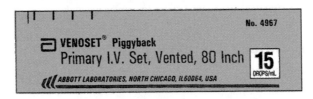

Answers on p. 557

POINTS TO REMEMBER

- Knowing the drop factor is the *FIRST* step to accurately administering I.V. fluids.
- The drop factor always appears on the package of the I.V. tubing.
- Macrodrops are large and deliver 10, 15, or 20 gtt/mL.
- Microdrops are small and deliver 60 gtt/mL.
- Drop factor = gtt/mL.

There are several formulas for calculating flow rates in relation to I.V. therapy. This book will present two formulas; however, the *focus* will be on Formula A. The most common calculation necessary when an infusion device is not used involves solving to determine gtt/min.

FORMULA METHOD FOR CALCULATING I.V. FLOW RATE

To calculate the flow rate at which an I.V. is to infuse, regardless of the formula used the nurse needs to know the following:
1. The volume or number of mL to infuse.
2. The drop factor (gtt/mL).
3. The time element (minutes or hours).
The information is then placed into a formula. Let's examine two formulas that might be used.

Formula A: This formula is the most popular when calculating flow rate when the rate can be expressed as 60 minutes or less.

$$x \text{ gtt/min} = \frac{\text{amount of solution (mL)} \times \text{drop factor}}{\text{time in min}}$$

Formula B:

$$\frac{V_1}{T_1} \times \frac{V_2}{T_2} = x \text{ gtt/min}$$

Note: Numbers have been placed in the formula for the purpose of explanation.

$$\frac{\text{Volume}}{\text{Time}} \times \frac{\text{Volume}}{\text{Time}} = x \text{ gtt/min}$$

Explanation of Formula B

V_1 = Volume (the total number of mL to infuse)
T_1 = Time in hours (the number of hours the I.V. is to infuse)
V_2 = Drop factor of the tubing used (for example, 10 gtt = 1 mL; 60 gtt = 1 mL)
T_2 = Time in minutes (since there are 60 minutes in an hour, the number is always 60, unless the I.V. is to infuse for a time period less than an hour, in which case you can place the number of minutes in this position)

Note:

To place the number of minutes in the T_1 position, the number of minutes must be expressed in hours by dividing the number of minutes by 60. It is easier to place the number of minutes directly into the formula in the T_2 position to avoid extra calculation.

Before calculating, let's review some basic principles:
1. Drops per minute are always expressed in whole numbers. You cannot regulate something at a half of a drop. Because drops are expressed in whole numbers, principles of rounding off are applied; for example, 19.5 gtt = 20 gtt.
2. Carry division of the problem one decimal place to round to a whole number of drops.
3. Answers must be labeled. The label is usually drops per minute, unless otherwise specified. Example: 100 gtt/min or 17 gtt/min. To reinforce the differences in gtt factor, the type of tubing is sometimes included as part of the label. Example: 100 microgtt/min or 17 macrogtt/min.

Let's look at some sample problems and step-by-step methods of using the formulas to obtain answers.

Example 1: Order: D5W to infuse at 100 mL/hr. Drop factor: 10 gtt/mL. How many gtt/min should the I.V. be regulated at?

➡ **Solution Using Formula A:**

1. Set up the problem, placing the information given in the correct position.

$$x \text{ gtt/min} = \frac{100 \text{ mL} \times 10 \text{ gtt/mL}}{60 \text{ min}}$$

2. Reduce where possible to make numbers smaller and easier to manage. Note that the labels are dropped when starting to perform mathematical steps.

$$x = \frac{100 \times 10}{60} = \frac{100 \times 1}{6} = \frac{100}{6}$$

3. Divide $\frac{100}{6}$ to obtain gtt/min.

Carry division one decimal place and round off to the nearest whole number.

$$x = \frac{100}{6} = 16.6$$

$$x = 17 \text{ gtt/min}$$

Answer: $x = 17$ gtt/min; 17 macrogtt/min

To deliver 100 mL/hr with a drop factor of 10 gtt/mL, the I.V. rate should be adjusted to 17 gtt/min. This answer can also be expressed with the type of tubing as part of the label, for example: 17 macrogtt/min.

▶ **Solution Using Formula B:**

1. Set up the problem, placing the information given in the correct position.

$$\frac{100 \text{ mL}}{1 \text{ hr}} \times \frac{10 \text{ gtt/mL}}{60 \text{ min}} = x \text{ gtt/min}$$

2. Reduce where possible to make numbers smaller and easier to manage. Note that the labels are dropped when starting to perform mathematical steps.

$$\frac{100}{1} \times \frac{10}{60} = \frac{100}{1} \times \frac{1}{6} = \frac{100}{6}$$

3. Divide $\dfrac{100}{6}$ to obtain gtt/min.

Carry division at least one decimal place and round off to the nearest whole number.

$$\frac{100}{6} = 16.6$$

$$x = 17 \text{ gtt/min}$$

Answer: $x = 17$ gtt/min; 17 macrogtt/min

Example 2:   Order: I.V. medication in 50 mL NS in 20 minutes. Drop factor: microdrip (60 gtt/mL). How many gtt/min should the I.V. be regulated at?

▶ **Solution Using Formula A:**

$$x \text{ gtt/min} = \frac{50 \text{ mL} \times 60 \text{ gtt/mL}}{20 \text{ min}}$$

$$x = \frac{50 \times 3}{1} = \frac{150}{1}$$

$$x = 150 \text{ gtt/min}$$

Answer: $x = 150$ gtt/min; 150 microgtt/min

To deliver 50 mL in 20 min with a drop factor of 60 gtt/mL, the I.V. should be adjusted to 150 gtt/min. This may sound like a lot; however, remember the tubing used is a microdrip.

▶ **Solution Using Formula B:**

1. $50 \text{ mL} \times \dfrac{60 \text{ gtt/mL}}{20 \text{ min}} = x \text{ gtt/min}$

Note: Here the 20 minutes is placed in the T_2 position because it represents the time in minutes. The time period is less than an hour. A (1) could also be placed under 50, not to denote 1 hr, but because 50/1 is the same as 50.

$$\frac{50 \text{ mL}}{1} \times \frac{60 \text{ gtt/mL}}{20 \text{ min}} = x \text{ gtt/min}$$

2. $50 \times \dfrac{3}{1}$ or $\dfrac{50}{1} \times \dfrac{3}{1} = 150$ gtt/min

$$x = 150 \text{ gtt/min}; \ 150 \text{ microgtt/min}$$

The formula method may also be used to calculate gtt/min for a volume of fluid to be administered in more than 1 hour. However, one way to keep the numbers smaller before beginning is to determine the mL/hr. This is done by dividing the amount of solution to infuse (mL) by the number of hours, then proceed to calculate gtt/min.

$$\frac{\text{amount of solution (mL)}}{\text{time in hours}} = x \text{ mL/hr}$$

Now let's look at some examples where the volume of fluid will infuse over more than 1 hour.

Example 1: Order 1,000 mL D5W to infuse in 8 hr. Drop factor: 10 gtt/mL. How many gtt/min should I.V. be regulated at?

1. Calculate the mL/hr.

$$x \text{ mL/hr} = \frac{1,000 \text{ mL}}{8 \text{ hr}}$$

$$x = 125 \text{ mL/hr}$$

2. Calculate the gtt/min.

$$x \text{ gtt/min} = \frac{125 \text{ mL} \times 10 \text{ gtt/mL}}{60 \text{ min}}$$

3. Reduce:

$$\frac{125 \times 10}{60} = \frac{125 \times 1}{6} = \frac{125}{6}$$

$$x = \frac{125}{6} = 20.8$$

$$x = 21 \text{ gtt/min}$$

Answer: $x = 21$ gtt/min or 21 macrogtt/min

Example 2: Order: 1,500 mL 0.9% NS in 10 hours. Drop factor: 20 gtt/mL. How many gtt/min should the I.V. infuse at?

1. Calculate mL/hr.

$$x \text{ mL/hr} = \frac{1,500 \text{ mL}}{10 \text{ hr}}$$

$$x = 150 \text{ mL/hr}$$

2. Calculate gtt/min.

$$x \text{ gtt/min} = \frac{150 \text{ mL} \times 20 \text{ gtt/mL}}{60 \text{ min}}$$

3. $x = \dfrac{150 \times 1}{3} = \dfrac{150}{3}$

4. $x = \dfrac{150}{3} = 50$ gtt/min

Answer: $x = 50$ gtt/min; 50 macrogtt/min

Note:

Formula A has been found easiest to use and will be used in the remainder of this text. Formula B can be used and will net the same answers; however, because it involves more, the student is encouraged to use the *easier formula*.

Notes

PRACTICE PROBLEMS

Calculate the flow rate in gtt/min using the formula method.

25. Administer D5R/L at 75 mL/hr. The drop
    factor is 10 gtt/mL.   _____

26. Administer D5 $\frac{1}{2}$ NS at 30 mL/hr. The drop

    factor is a microdrip.   _____

27. Administer R/L at 125 mL/hr. The drop
    factor is 15 gtt/mL.   _____

28. Administer 1,000 mL D5 0.33% NS in 6 hr.
    The drop factor is 15 gtt/mL.   _____

29. An I.V. medication in 60 mL of 0.9% NS is
    to be administered in 45 minutes. The drop
    factor is a microdrip.   _____

30. 1,000 mL of Ringer's lactate solution (RL) is to
    infuse in 16 hr. The drop factor is 15 gtt/mL. _____

31. Infuse 150 mL of D5W in 2 hr. The drop
    factor is 20 gtt/mL.   _____

32. Administer 3,000 mL D5 and $\frac{1}{2}$ NS in 24 hr.

    The drop factor is 10 gtt/mL.   _____

33. Infuse 2,000 mL D5W in 12 hr. The drop
    factor is 15 gtt/mL.   _____

34. An I.V. medication in 60 mL D5W is to be
    administered in 30 minutes. The drop factor
    is a microdrip.   _____

Answers on pp. 557-558

Calculation of I.V. Rates by Using a Shortcut Method

This shortcut method can be used only in settings where the I.V. sets have the same drop factor. Example: An institution where all the macrodrip sets deliver 10 gtt/mL. This method can also be used with microdrip sets (60 gtt/mL). It is important to note that this method can be used only if the rate of the I.V. infusion is expressed in mL/hr (mL/60 min). It is imperative that nurses become very familiar with the administration equipment at the institution where they work.

To use this method you must know the drop factor constant for the administration set you're using. The drop factor constant is sometimes referred to as the *division factor*.

To obtain the drop factor constant (division factor) for the I.V. administration set being used, divide 60 by the drop factor calibration.

Example: The drop factor for an I.V. administration set is 15 gtt/mL. To obtain the drop factor constant:

$$\frac{60}{15} = 4 \ (\text{drop factor constant} = 4)$$

After determining the drop factor constant, the gtt/min can be calculated in one step:

$$\frac{\text{mL/hr}}{\text{gtt/factor constant}} = \text{gtt/min}$$

 PRACTICE PROBLEMS

Calculate the drop factor constant for the following I.V. sets.

35. 20 gtt/mL   _____

36. 10 gtt/mL   _____

37. 60 gtt/mL   _____

Answers on p. 558

Note:

Now that you know how to determine the drop factor constant, let's look at examples of using a shortcut method to calculate gtt/min.

Example 1:   Administer 0.9% NS at 100 mL/hr. The drop factor is 20 gtt/mL.

$$x \ \text{gtt/min} = \frac{100 \ \text{mL} \times 20 \ \text{gtt/mL}}{60 \ \text{min}} = 33.3 = 33 \ \text{gtt/min}$$

$$x = 33 \ \text{gtt/min}$$

Notice in the example that because the time is 60 minutes, the administration set calibration (20) will be divided into 60 minutes to obtain a constant drop factor of 3. The constant drop factor for an I.V. set that delivers 20 gtt/mL is 3. Therefore, the above problem could be done using the shortcut method once you know the constant drop factor (division factor).

$$\text{gtt/min} = \frac{100 \ \text{mL/hr}}{3} = 33.3 = 33 \ \text{gtt/min}$$

Notice the 100 mL/hr rate divided by the drop factor constant gives the same answer.

Answer: 33 gtt/min; 33 macrodrop/min.

Example 2:   Administer D5W at 125 mL/hr. The drop factor is 15 gtt/mL.
1. Determine the drop factor constant.

$$60 \div 15 = 4$$

2. Calculate the gtt/min.

$$\text{gtt/min} = \frac{125 \ \text{mL/hr}}{4} = 31.2 = 31 \ \text{gtt/min}$$

Answer: 31 gtt/min; 31 macrogtt/min

Example 3:   Administer 0.9% NS at 75 mL/hr. The drop factor is 60 gtt/mL.

Note:

It is important to realize that with a microdrop, which delivers 60 gtt/mL, the gtt/min will be the same as mL/hr. This is because the set calibration is 60, and the drop factor constant is based on 60 minutes (1 hr) time, the drop factor constant is 1.

1. Determine the drop factor constant.

$$60 \div 60 = 1$$

2. Calculate the gtt/min.

$$\text{gtt/min} = \frac{75 \text{ mL/hr}}{1} = 75 \text{ gtt/min}$$

Answer: 75 gtt/min; 75 microgtt/min.

 PRACTICE PROBLEMS

Calculate the gtt/min using the shortcut method.

38. Order: D5W 200 mL/hr.
    Drop factor: 10 gtt/mL. _____

39. Order: RL 50 mL/hr.
    Drop factor: 15 gtt/mL. _____

40. Order: 0.45% NS 80 mL/hr.
    Drop factor: 60 gtt/mL. _____

41. Order: 0.9% NS 140 mL/hr.
    Drop factor: 20 gtt/min. _____

Answers on p. 558

Remember, the shortcut method discussed (using the constant drop factor) can be used to calculate the gtt/min for any volume of fluid that can be stated in mL/hr.

The shortcut method can be used if the *volume is large; however, an additional step* of changing mL/hr first must be done, then proceed to calculate the gtt/min using the shortcut method.

Example 1: Order: R/L 1,500 mL in 12 hr. Drop factor: 15 gtt/mL.

$$1,500 \text{ mL} \div 12 = 125 \text{ mL/hr.}$$

Now that you have mL/hr you can proceed with the shortcut method, using the drop factor constant.

$$\text{gtt/min} = \frac{125 \text{ mL}}{4} = 31.2 = 31 \text{ gtt/min}$$

Answer: 31 gtt/min; 31 macrogtt/min

If the volume of fluid to be infused is small, the volume must be multiplied and the time to get mL/hr.

Example 2: Order: 20 mL D5W in 30 minutes. Drop factor: 15 gtt/mL.

To express this in mL/hr you multiply by 2.

$$20 \text{ mL/30 min} = (20 \times 2)/(2 \times 30 \text{ min}) = 40 \text{ mL/hr}$$

$$\text{gtt/min} = \frac{40 \text{ mL}}{4} = 10 \text{ gtt/min}$$

Answer: 10 gtt/min; 10 macrogtt/min

PRACTICE PROBLEMS

Calculate the gtt/min using the shortcut method.

42. Order: 1,000 mL D5W in 10 hr.
    Drop factor: 10 gtt/mL. _____

43. Order: 1,500 mL R/L in 12 hr.
    Drop factor: 15 gtt/mL. _____

44. Order: 40 mL D5W in 20 minutes.
    Drop factor: 10 gtt/mL. _____

Answers on p. 558

CALCULATING I.V. FLOW RATES WHEN SEVERAL SOLUTIONS ARE ORDERED

I.V. orders are often written for different amounts or types of fluid to be given in a certain time period. These orders are frequently written for a 24-hr interval and usually are split over three shifts. I.V. solutions may have medications added, such as potassium chloride or multivitamins.

Steps to calculating:
1. Add up the total amount of fluid.
2. Proceed as with other I.V. problem calculations.

Note: When medications such as potassium chloride and vitamins are added to I.V. solutions, they are generally not considered in the total volume.

Example 1:   Order: The following I.V.s for 24 hours. Drop factor: 15 gtt/mL.

a) 1,000 mL D5W with 10 mEq potassium chloride (KCl)

b) 500 mL dextrose 5% in normal saline (D5NS) $\bar{c}$ 1 ampule multivitamin (MVI)

c) 500 mL D5W

1. Calculate mL/hr:

$$\frac{2,000 \text{ mL}}{24 \text{ hr}} = 83.3 = 83 \text{ mL/hr}$$

2. Calculate gtt/min:

$$x \text{ gtt/min} = \frac{83 \text{ mL} \times 15 \text{ gtt/mL}}{60 \text{ min}}$$

3. Reduce:

$$x = \frac{83 \times 15}{60} = \frac{83 \times 1}{4} = 20.7 = 21 \text{ gtt/min}$$

$$x = 21 \text{ gtt/min}$$

Answer: 21 gtt/min; 21 macrogtt/min.

Example 2:   I.V. orders are as follows:

a) 1,000 mL D5W

b) 1,000 mL normal saline (NS)

c) 500 mL D5 and $\frac{1}{2}$ NS

Note:

This could have been done using the shortcut method by determining the constant drop factor. Calculating the I.V. flow rate where indicated eliminates the step of adding up the solution volumes. The hourly rate becomes the total vol-ume. Example 2 could also have been done using the shortcut method by determining the constant drop factor.

Notes

Drop factor: 10 gtt/mL to infuse at 150 mL/hr.

The hourly rate is 150 mL/hr. Calculation is done based on this:

$$x \text{ gtt/min} = \frac{150 \text{ mL} \times 10 \text{ gtt/mL}}{60 \text{ min}}$$

$$x = \frac{150 \times 10}{60} = \frac{150 \times 1}{6} = 25 \text{ gtt/min}$$

$$x = 25 \text{ gtt/min}$$

Answer: 25 gtt/min; 25 macrogtt/min

 PRACTICE PROBLEMS

Calculate the flow rate in gtt/min.

45. Order: Dextrose 5% with Ringer's Lactate solution (D5RL) c̄ 20 U Pitocin × 2 L at 125 mL/hr. Drop factor: 15 gtt/mL.

   _____

46. Order: To infuse in 16 hr. Drop factor: 10 gtt/mL.

   a) D5W 500 mL c̄ 10 mEq KCl   _____

   b) D5W 1,000 mL   _____

   c) D5W 1,000 mL c̄ 1 ampule MVI   _____

47. Order: 1,000 mL D5 0.9% NS × 3 L at 100 mL/hr. Drop factor: microdrip.

   _____

48. Order: D5W 1,000 mL + 20 mEq KCl × 2 L to infuse in 10 hr. Drop factor: 15 gtt/mL.

   _____

Answers on pp. 558-559

I.V. MEDICATIONS

As previously discussed in the section on calculating I.V. flow rates, medications can be added directly to the I.V. solution.

Medications such as antibiotics can also be given by adding a secondary container of solution that contains the medication. The administration of medication by attaching it to a port on the primary line is referred to as *piggyback*.

The volume of the piggyback container is usually 50 to 100 mL and should infuse over 20, 30, or 60 minutes, depending on the type and amount of medication added. The same formula used to calculate I.V. infusion times is used to calculate the gtt/min.

Sample Problem:

Keflin 2 g is ordered IVPB (piggyback) over 30 minutes. The Keflin is placed in 100 mL of fluid after it is dissolved. The drop factor is 15 gtt/mL. How many gtt/min should the I.V. be regulated at?

To calculate: The 100 mL of fluid the medication is placed in is used as the volume.

$$x \text{ gtt/min} = \frac{100 \text{ (mL)} \times 15 \text{ (gtt/mL)}}{30 \text{ min}}$$

$$x = \frac{100 \times 15}{30} = \frac{100 \times 1}{2} = \frac{100}{2}$$

$$x = \frac{100}{2}$$

$$x = 50 \text{ gtt/min}$$

Answer: 50 gtt/min; 50 macrogtt/min

The I.V. would be regulated at 50 gtt/min; 50 macrogtt/min.

As shown earlier in the chapter, the smaller bag (piggyback) is hung higher than the larger (primary) bag. Because infusion flow is controlled by gravity, the primary bag will resume infusion after the piggyback is empty. The drops per minute will then have to be reset to the correct amount calculated for the primary I.V.

 PRACTICE PROBLEMS

Calculate the gtt/min for the following medications being administered IVPB. Use the labels where provided.

49. Order: Mezlocillin 3 g IVPB in 130 mL NS over 1 hr. Drop factor: 15 gtt/mL.

    _____

50. Order: Erythromycin 200 mg in 250 mL D5W to infuse over 1 hr. Drop factor: 10 gtt/mL.

    _____

51. Order: Ampicillin 1 g in 50 mL D5W over 45 minutes. Drop factor: 10 gtt/mL.

    _____

52. Order: Clindamycin 900 mg in 75 mL D5W over 30 minutes. Drop factor: 10 gtt/mL.

    _____

53. Order: Tagamet 300 mg IVPB q8hr. The medication has been added to 50 mL D5W to infuse over 30 minutes. Drop factor: 10 gtt/mL.

    _____

Notes

54. Order: Vancomycin 500 mg IVPB q24hr. The vancomycin reconstituted provides 50 mg/mL. The medication is placed in 100 mL of D5W to infuse over 60 minutes. Drop factor: 15 gtt/mL.

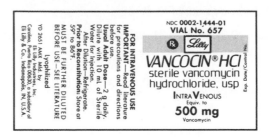

a) How many mL of medication must be added to the solution? _____

b) Calculate the gtt/min the I.V. should infuse at. _____

55. Order: Fungizone (amphotericin B) 20 mg I.V. Soluset (IVSS) in 300 mL D5W over 6 hr. The reconstituted material contains 50 mg/10 mL. Drop factor: 60 gtt/mL.

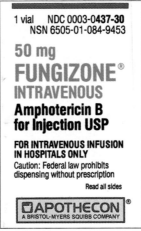

a) How many mL will you add to the I.V. solution? _____

b) How many gtt/min should the I.V. infuse at? _____

56. Order: Septra 300 mg in 300 mL D5W over 1 hr q6h. Drop factor: 10 gtt/mL.

Available: Septra in 20-mL vial labeled 320 mg trimethoprim (16 mg/mL) and 1,600 mg sulfamethoxazole (80 mg/mL). (Calculate the dose using trimethoprim.)

a) How many mL of medication will be added to the I.V.? (Round answer to nearest tenth.) _____

b) Calculate the gtt/min the I.V. should infuse at. _____

57. Order: Retrovir 100 mg I.V. q4h over 1 hr.

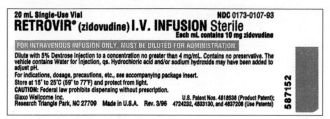

The medication is placed in 100 mL of D5W.
Drop factor: 10 gtt/min.

_____

Answers on pp. 559-560

DETERMINING THE AMOUNT OF DRUG IN A SPECIFIC AMOUNT OF SOLUTION

Sometimes medications are added to I.V. solutions, and the doctor orders a certain amount of the drug to be given in a certain time period.

Example 1:   The doctor may order 20 mEq of potassium to be placed in 1,000 mL of fluid to be administered at a rate of 2 mEq of potassium per hour. The flow rate (gtt/min) can be determined using the same formula as for other I.V.s, but first the volume to be infused must be calculated by use of ratio-proportion.

➤ Solution:

Step 1:   Calculate the number of mL of solution needed to deliver 2 mEq of potassium chloride.

What doctor ordered
↓

$$20 \text{ mEq} : 1{,}000 \text{ mL} = 2 \text{ mEq} : x \text{ mL}$$

↑   ↑   ↑

Total amount of drug Desired volume
in volume of solution   of solution

$$20 \text{ mEq} : 1{,}000 \text{ mL} = 2 \text{ mEq} : x \text{ mL}$$

$$20x = 1{,}000 \times 2$$

$$20x = 2{,}000$$

$$x = \frac{2{,}000}{20}$$

$$x = 100 \text{ mL}$$

Therefore 100 mL of fluid would be needed to administer 2 mEq of potassium chloride per hour.

Step 2:   Determine the rate of flow by substituting this information into the formula if 100 mL of solution (containing 2 mEq of potassium chloride) is to be administered over 1 hr using 15 gtt = 1 mL. The rate of flow is determined by the following:

$$x \text{ gtt/min} = \frac{100 \text{ mL} \times 15 \text{ gtt/mL}}{60 \text{ min}}$$

Notes

Notes

$$x = \frac{100 \times 15}{60} = \frac{100 \times 1}{4} = \frac{100}{4}$$

$$x = \frac{100}{4}$$

$$x = 25 \text{ gtt/min}$$

Answer: x = 25 gtt/min; 25 macrogtt/min
25 gtt/min would deliver 2 mEq of potassium chloride each hour from this solution.

Example 2: The doctor orders 100 U of regular insulin to be added to 500 mL of 0.45% saline (1/2 NS) to infuse at 10 U per hour. The I.V. flow rate should be how many mL per hour?

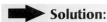 **Solution:**

Step 1: Set up a proportion with the known on one side and the unknown on the other.

$$100 \text{ U} : 500 \text{ mL} = 10 \text{ U} : x \text{ mL}$$

$$100x = 500 \times 10$$

$$100x = 5,000$$

$$x = \frac{5,000}{100}$$

$$x = 50 \text{ mL/hr}$$

For the client to receive 10 U of insulin per hour, 50 mL/hr must be administered.

Step 2: Determine the flow rate in gtt/min using the drop factor 20 gtt/mL.

$$x \text{ gtt/min} = \frac{50 \text{ mL} \times 20 \text{ gtt/mL}}{60 \text{ min}}$$

$$x = \frac{50 \times 20}{60} = \frac{50 \times 1}{3}$$

$$x = \frac{50}{3} = 16.6 = 17 \text{ gtt/min}$$

$$x = 17 \text{ gtt/min}; 17 \text{ macrogtt/min}$$ 16.6 → 17

 PRACTICE PROBLEMS

Solve the following problems using the steps indicated.

58. Order: 15 mEq of potassium chloride in 1,000 mL of D5 and $\frac{1}{2}$ NS to be administered at a rate of 4 mEq/hr.

a) How many mL of solution are needed to administer 4 mEq/hr? _____

b) Drop factor: 10 gtt/mL; calculate the gtt/min to deliver 4 mEq/hr. _____

Notes

59. Order: 10 U of regular insulin per hour. 50 U of insulin is placed in 250 mL NS.

    a) How many mL/hr should the I.V. infuse at? _____

    b) Drop factor: 15 gtt/mL. Calculate
       the gtt/min.   _____

60. Order: 15 U of regular insulin per hour. 40 U of insulin is placed in 250 mL of NS.

    a) How many mL/hr should the I.V. infuse at? _____

    b) Drop factor: 60 gtt/mL. Calculate
       the gtt/min.   _____

Answers on p. 560

DETERMINING INFUSION TIMES AND VOLUMES

You may need to calculate the following:
   a) Time in hours—How long it will take a certain amount of fluid to infuse or how long it may last
   b) Volume—The total number of mL a client will receive in a certain time period
These unknown elements can be determined by use of the same formula and simple mathematics.

Remember the formula:

$$x \text{ gtt/min} = \frac{\text{amount of solution (mL)} \times \text{drop factor}}{\text{time in minutes}}$$

STEPS TO CALCULATING A PROBLEM WITH AN UNKNOWN

1. Take information given in the problem and place it in the formula.
2. Place an x in the formula in the position of the unknown. If you're trying to determine time in hours, place x in the position for minutes; once you find the minutes, divide the number of minutes by 60 (60 minutes = 1 hr) to get the number of hours. If you're trying to determine the volume the client would receive, place an x in the position for amount of solution, and label x mL.
3. Obtain an algebraic equation so that you can solve for x.
4. Solve the equation.
5. Label the answer in hours or mL for volume.

Sample Problem

An I.V. is regulated at 20 microgtt/min. How many hours will it take for 100 mL to infuse?

Note:

If it is regulated at 20 microdrops, then the drop factor is a micro-drip (60 gtt/mL). You cannot convert macro-drip into a microdrip and vice versa.

Note:

In the sample problem you are being asked the number of hours. How-ever, in this formula time is in minutes, so place an x in the position for minutes, 60 gtt/mL is drop factor, and place the number of gtt/min in the formula. Let's now examine the problem set up in the formula.

Note:

The label is hours be-cause that's what you were asked.

 Problem Setup in Formula:

1. $20 \text{ microgtt/min} = \dfrac{100 \text{ mL} \times 60 \text{ gtt/mL}}{x \text{ time in min}}$

2. Reduce: $\dfrac{20x}{20} = \dfrac{100 \times 60}{20}$

$$x = 100 \times 3$$

$$x = 300 \text{ min}$$

3. Change minutes into hours:

$$60 \text{ minutes} = 1 \text{ hr}$$

$$\text{Therefore } \dfrac{300 \text{ min}}{60} = 5 \text{ hrs}$$

$$x = 5 \text{ hrs}$$

Note: Placing 20 gtt/min over 1 doesn't alter the value.

$$\dfrac{20 \text{ microgtt/min}}{1} = \dfrac{100 \text{ mL} \times 60 \text{ gtt/mL}}{x \text{ time in min}}$$

When calculating time intervals and the time or the answer comes out in hours and minutes, express the entire time in hours. For example 1 hour and 30 minutes = 1.5 hr or 1 1/2 hr; 1 1/2 hr is the preferred term.

When calculating volume, proceed with the problem in the same way as calcu-lating time interval except x is placed in a different position and labeled mL.

Sample Problem

An I.V. is regulated at 17 macrogtt/min. The drop factor is 15 gtt/mL. How much fluid volume in mL will the client receive in 8 hr?

Note:

Because this formula uses minutes, 8 hrs was changed to minutes by multiplying 8 × 60 (60 minutes = 1 hr).

 Problem Setup in Formula

1. $17 \text{ macrogtt/min} = \dfrac{x \text{ mL} \times 15 \text{ gtt/mL}}{480 \text{ min}}$

2. Reduce: $17 = \dfrac{x \times \overset{1}{\cancel{15}}}{\underset{32}{\cancel{480}}}$

$$17 = \dfrac{x}{32}$$

3. $x = 17 \times 32 = 544 \text{ mL}$

$$x = 544 \text{ mL}$$

Note:

Label on this answer is mL.

Some of the problems illustrated in calculating an unknown may be solved without the formula; however, using the formula is recommended.

 ## PRACTICE PROBLEMS

Solve for the unknown in the following problems as indicated.

61. You find that there is 150 mL of D5W left in an I.V. The I.V. is infusing at 60 microgtt/min. How many hours will the fluid last? _____

62. 0.9% NS is infusing at 35 macrogtt/min. The drop factor is 15 gtt/mL. How many mL of fluid will the client receive in 5 hr? _____

63. 180 mL of D5 R/L is left in an I.V. that is infusing at 45 macrogtt/min. The drop factor is 15 gtt/mL. How many hours will the fluid last? _____

64. D5 1/2 NS is infusing at 45 macrogtt/min. The drop factor is 15 gtt/mL. How many mL will the client receive in 8 hr? _____

65. There is 90 mL of D5 0.33% NS left in an I.V. The drop factor is 60 gtt/mL. How many hours will the fluid last? _____

Answers on pp. 560-561

RECALCULATING AN I.V. FLOW RATE

Flow rates on I.V.s change when a client stands, sits, or is repositioned in bed. Therefore nurses must frequently check the flow rates. I.V.s generally are labeled with a start and finish time, as well as markings with specific time periods. Sometimes I.V.s infuse ahead of schedule or they are behind schedule if not monitored closely. When this happens, the I.V. flow rate must be recalculated. To recalculate the flow rate the nurse uses the volume remaining and time remaining.

The recalculated flow rate should not vary from the original rate by more than 25%. It is recommended that if the recalculated rate varies more than 25% from the original, the prescriber should be notified. The order may have to be revised.

When an I.V. is significantly ahead or behind schedule, you may need to notify the prescriber, depending on the client's condition and the use of appropriate nursing judgment. **Always assess the client** before making any change in an I.V. rate. Changes depend on the client's condition. Check the institution's policy regarding the percentage of adjustment that can be made.

To determine whether the new rate calculation is > (greater) or < (less) than 25%, use the amount of increase or decrease divided by the original rate.

$$\frac{\text{Amount of} \uparrow \text{or} \downarrow}{\text{original rate}} = \% \text{ of variation of original rate}$$

To recalculate the I.V. rate, use the remaining volume and remaining time, then proceed with calculating the gtt/min. Let's look at some examples:

Example: 1,000 mL of D5 R/L was to infuse in 8 hr at 31 gtt/min (31 macrogtt/min). The drop factor is 15 gtt/mL. After 4 hr you notice 700 mL of fluid left in the I.V. Recalculate the flow rate for the remaining solution. Note: The infusion is behind schedule. After 4 hrs, 1/2 of the volume (or 500 mL) should have infused.

Notes

➡️ Solution:

Using shortcut method

$$\text{Time remaining} = 4 \text{ hr.}$$

$$\text{Volume remaining} = 700 \text{ mL.}$$

$$700 \text{ mL} \div 4 = 175 \text{ mL/hr}$$

Drop factor is 15 gtt/mL.

Drop factor constant therefore is 4.

$$\frac{175 \text{ mL/hr}}{4} = 43.7 = 44 \text{ gtt/min}$$

Answer: 44 gtt/min; 44 macrogtt/min (recalculated rate). To determine the percentage of the change:

$$\frac{44 - 31}{31} = \frac{13}{31} = 0.419 = 42\%$$

Course of Action: Assess the client, notify the prescriber. This increase could result in serious consequences to the client if seriously ill or a child. The increase is >25%.

In this situation the flow rate has to be increased from 31 gtt/min to 44 gtt/min, which is more than 25% of the original. Always assess the client first to determine the client's ability to tolerate an increase in fluid. In addition to assessing the client's status, the prescriber should be notified. This same method can be used if an I.V. is ahead of schedule.

Example of I.V. Ahead of Schedule. An I.V. of 1,000 mL D5W is to infuse from 8 AM to 4 PM (8 hr). The drop factor is 10 gtt/mL. The rate is set at 20 gtt/min (20 macrogtt/min). In 5 hr you notice 700 mL has infused. Recalculate the flow rate for the remaining solution.

➡️ Solution:

$$300 \text{ mL} \div 3 = 100 \text{ mL/hr.}$$

Drop factor is 10 gtt/mL, therefore the drop factor constant is 6.

$$\frac{100 \text{ mL}}{6} = 16.6 = 17 \text{ gtt/min}$$

Answer: 17 gtt/min; 17 macrogtt/min
Determine the % of change:

$$\frac{17 - 20}{20} = \frac{-3}{20} = -0.15 = -15\%$$

In this situation the flow rate has to be decreased from 20 gtt/min (20 macrogtt/min) to 17 gtt/min (17 macrogtt/min), but this is not a change greater than 25% of the original; −15% is within the acceptable 25% of change. However, the client's condition must still be assessed to determine the ability to tolerate the change, and the prescriber may still require notification.

 Critical Thinking

Never arbitrarily increase or decrease an I.V. rate without assessing a client and informing the prescriber. Increasing or decreasing the rate without thought can result in serious harm to a client.

Course of Action: This is an acceptable decrease; it's less than 25%. Adjust the rate if client can tolerate it, and assess during the remainder of the infusion.

 PRACTICE PROBLEMS

For each of the problems, recalculate the I.V. flow rates in gtt/min rates, determine the % of change, and state your course of action.

66. 500 mL of 0.9% NS was ordered to infuse in 8 hr at the rate of 16 gtt/min (16 macrogtt/min). The drop factor is 15 gtt/mL. After 5 hr you find 250 mL of fluid left.

     a) _____ gtt/min

     b) _____ %

67. 250 mL of D5W was to infuse in 3 hr. Drop factor: 15 gtt/mL. With 1 1/2 hr remaining, you find 200 mL left.

     a) _____ gtt/min

     b) _____ %

68. 1,500 mL D5 R/L to infuse in 12 hrs at 42 gtt/min (42 macrogtt/min). After 6 hr, 650 mL has infused. Drop factor: 20 gtt/mL.

     a) _____ gtt/min

     b) _____ %

69. 1,000 mL D5 0.33% NS was to infuse in 12 hrs at 28 gtt/min (28 macrogtt/min). After 4 hr 250 mL has infused. Drop factor: 20 gtt/mL.

     a) _____ gtt/min

     b) _____ %

70. 500 mL D5 0.9% NS to infuse in 5 hr at 33 gtt/min (33 microgtt/min). After 2 hr, 250 mL has infused. Drop factor: 60 gtt/mL.

     a) _____ gtt/min

     b) _____ %

Answers on p. 561-562

CALCULATING TOTAL INFUSION TIMES

I.V. fluids are ordered by the prescriber for administration at a certain mL/hr, such as 1,000 mL D5W to infuse at 100 mL/hr. **The nurse needs to be able to determine the number of hours that an I.V. solution takes to infuse.** When the nurse calculates the total time for a certain volume of solution to infuse I.V., this is referred to as **determining total infusion time.** To calculate infusion time it is necessary for the nurse to have knowledge of the following:
a) Amount (volume) to infuse
b) Drop rate (gtt/mL)
c) Set calibration

Knowing the length of time for an infusion helps the nurse monitor I.V. therapy and prepare for the hanging of a new solution as the one infusing is being completed. Determining infusion times helps avoid such things as a line clotting off due to not knowing when an I.V. was to be completed. A nurse who knows the infusion time can anticipate when to hang a new IV infusion and when to determine lab values that may have to be obtained after certain amount of fluid has infused.

Calculating Infusion Time

Infusion time is determined by taking the total number of mL to infuse and dividing it by the number of mL/hr the solution is infusing at. This can also be done by using a ratio-proportion, which would be the ratio for ordered rate in mL/hr on one side and the ratio for total mL to infuse to x hr.

Formula

$$\frac{\text{Total number of mL to infuse}}{\text{mL/hr infusing at}} = \text{total infusion time}$$

Example 1:   Calculate the infusion time for an I.V. of 1,000 mL D5W that is infusing at a rate of 125 mL/hr.

1,000 mL (total number of mL to infuse)

125 mL/hr (mL/hr to infuse)

$$\frac{1,000}{125} = 1,000 \div 125 = 8 \text{ hr}$$

Infusion time = 8 hr

Example 2:   1,000 mL of D5 and $\dfrac{1}{2}$ NS is ordered to infuse at 150 mL/hr.

Calculate the infusion time to the nearest hundredth.

$$\frac{1,000 \text{ mL}}{150 \text{ mL/hr}} = 6.66$$

Fractions of hours can be changed to minutes: 6 represents the total number of hours; 0.66 represents a fraction of an hour and can be converted to minutes. This is done by multiplying 0.66 by 60 and then rounding off to the nearest whole number.

$$0.66 \times 60 = 39.6 = 40$$

Infusion time = 6 hr and 40 minutes

Once infusion time has been calculated, the nurse can use this information to determine the time an I.V. would be completed. For Example 2 this would be determined as follows: add the calculated infusion time to the time the infusion was started. If the I.V. in Example 2 was hung at 7:00 AM, add the 6 hr and 40 minutes to that time. The I.V. would be completed at 1:40 PM.

An easy way to do this is by using military time to determine the time it would be completed.

Example: 7:00 AM = 0700

After converting 7:00 AM to military time add 6 hr and 40 minutes to arrive at your answer—1340.

Note: Converting traditional time to military time is covered in Chapter 12. Refer to that chapter to refresh your memory on how to do this.

CHARTING I.V. THERAPY

At some institutions, continuous I.V. therapy may be charted on a special I.V. record or I.V. flow sheet. Medications that are administered intermittently by piggyback are charted on other medication sheets according to the order (e.g., standing medication sheet, prn, or single, stat medication record). Forms used to chart I.V. therapy (whether a client is receiving I.V. solution that contains medications or solution without medications) vary from institution to institution.

 PRACTICE PROBLEMS

Determine infusion time for the following I.V.s. State time in traditional and military time.

71. An I.V. of 500 mL NS is to infuse at 60 mL/hr.

   a) Determine the infusion time. _____

   b) The I.V. was started at 10:00 PM. When would the I.V. totally infuse? _____

72. An I.V. of 250 mL D5W is to infuse at 80 mL/hr.

   a) Determine the infusion time. _____

   b) The I.V. was started at 2:00 AM. When would the I.V. totally infuse? _____

73. 1,000 mL of D5W is to infuse at 40 mL/hr.

   a) Determine the infusion time. _____

   b) The I.V. was started at 2:10 PM on August 26. When would the I.V. totally infuse? _____

74. An I.V. of 1,000 mL D5 R/L is to infuse at 60 mL/hr.

   a) Determine the infusion time. _____

   b) The I.V. was started at 6:00 AM. At what time would this I.V. be complete? _____

75. An I.V. of 500 mL D5W is to infuse at 75 mL/hr.

   a) Determine the infusion time. _____

   b) The I.V. was started at 2:00 PM. At what time would the I.V. be complete? _____

Answers on p. 562

Notes

CALCULATING INFUSION TIME WHEN mL/hr IS NOT INDICATED

There are situations where the prescriber may order the I.V. solution and not indicate mL/hr. The only information may be the total number of mL to infuse, the flow rate (gtt/min) of the I.V., and the number of gtt/mL that the tubing delivers. In this situation, before calculating the infusion time, the following must be done:

1. Convert gtt/min to mL/min.
2. Convert mL/min to mL/hr.

After completing these steps, you are ready to calculate the infusion time for the I.V. using the same formula: $\dfrac{\text{Total number of mL to infuse}}{\text{mL/hr infusing at}}$

Example 1:   A client is receiving 1,000 mL of RL. The I.V. is infusing at 21 macrogtt/min (21 gtt/min). The administration set delivers 10 gtt/mL. Calculate the infusion time.

Step 1:   Use a ratio-proportion stated in any format as discussed in previous chapters to change gtt/min to mL/min.

$$10 \text{ gtt} : 1 \text{ mL} = 21 \text{ gtt} : x \text{ mL}$$

$$10x = 21$$

$$x = 21 \div 10 = 2.1 \text{ mL/min}$$

Step 2:   Convert mL/min to mL/hr.

$$2.1 \text{ mL/min} \times (60 \text{ min}) = 126 \text{ mL/hr}$$

Step 3:   Determine infusion time as already shown.

a) $\dfrac{1,000 \text{ mL}}{126 \text{ mL/hr}} = 7.93 \text{ hr}$

b) $0.93 \times 60 = 55.8 = 56$ minutes

Infusion time = 7 hr and 56 minutes

Note: To determine the time the infusion would be completed you would add the infusion time to the time the I.V. was started.

 PRACTICE PROBLEMS

Determine the infusion time for following I.V.s.

76. A client is receiving 1,000 mL D5W at 25 microgtt/min. Drop factor is microdrip.   _____

77. A client is receiving 250 mL of NS at 17 macrogtt/min. Drop factor: 15 gtt/mL.   _____

78. A client is receiving 1,000 mL D5W. The I.V. is infusing at 30 macrogtt/min. Drop factor: 20 gtt/mL.   _____

79. A client is receiving 1,000 mL D5W at 20 macrogtt/min. Drop factor: 10 gtt/mL.   _____

80. A client is receiving 100 mL at 10 macrogtt/min.
Drop factor: 15 gtt/mL.   _____

Answers on pp. 562-563

There may be times when it is necessary for the nurse to determine the infusion time for small volumes of fluid that will infuse in less than an hr. To do this the nurse must first do the following:
1. Calculate the mL/min.
2. Divide the total volume by the mL/min to obtain the infusion time.

Example 1:   An I.V. antibiotic of 30 mL is infusing at 20 macrogtt/min. Drop factor 10 gtt/mL. Determine the infusion time.

Step 1:   Calculate the mL/min.

$$10 \text{ gtt} : 1 \text{ mL} = 20 \text{ gtt} : x \text{ mL}$$

$$\frac{10x}{10} = \frac{20}{10}$$

$$x = 2 \text{ mL/min}$$

Step 2:   Divide the total volume by mL/min.

$$30 \text{ mL} \div 2 \text{ mL/min} = 15 \text{ minutes}$$

The infusion time is 15 minutes

Note:

A ratio-proportion may be stated in any format discussed in previous chapters.

 PRACTICE PROBLEMS

Determine the infusion times for the following:

81. An I.V. medication of 35 mL is infusing at 30 macrogtt/min. Drop factor: 15 gtt/mL.   _____

82. An I.V. medication of 20 mL is infusing at 35 microgtt/min. Drop factor: 60 gtt/mL.   _____

Answers on p. 563

LABELING SOLUTION BAGS

The markings on I.V. solution bags are not as precise as, for example, those on a syringe. Most I.V. bags are marked in increments of 50 to 100 mL. After calculating the amount of solution to infuse in 1 hr, the nurse may mark the bag to indicate where the level of fluid should be at each hour. Marking the I.V. bag allows the nurse to check that the fluid is infusing on time. Many institutions have commercially prepared labels for this purpose. In institutions where the commercially prepared labels are not available, regular white surgical tape may be attached to the side of the bag to serve the same purpose (Figure 21-23 shows an I.V. with timing tape for visualizing the amount infused each hour). The tape should indicate the start and finish time.

Notes

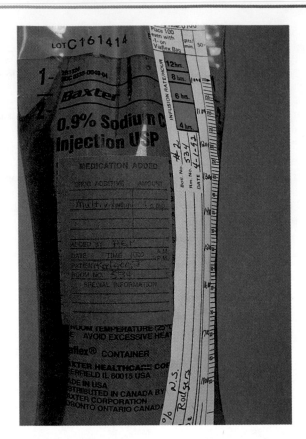

Figure 21-23   I.V. solution with time taping. (From Potter PA, Perry AG: *Fundamentals of nursing,* ed 5, St Louis, 2001, Mosby.)

I.V. THERAPY AND CHILDREN

Pediatric Intravenous Administration

Administration of I.V. fluids to children is very specific due to their physiological development. Microdrop sets are used for infants and small children; electronic devices are used to control the rate of delivery. The rate of infusion for infants and children must be carefully monitored. The intravenous drop rate must be slow for small children to prevent complications such as cardiac failure because of fluid overload. There are various intravenous devices that decrease the size of the drop to "mini" or "micro" drop or 1/60 mL, therefore delivering 60 minidrops or microdrops per mL. Intravenous medications may be administered to a child over a period of time (several hours) or on an intermittent basis. For intermittent medication administration, several methods of delivery are used, including the following:

Small-volume I.V. bags—These may be used if the child has a primary I.V. line in place. A secondary tubing set is attached to a small-volume I.V. bag and the piggyback method is used.

Calibrated burettes—These are often referred to by their trade names: Buretrol, Volutrol, or Soluset. (Figure 21-24 shows a typical system that consists of a calibrated chamber that can hold a capacity of 100 to 150 mL of fluid.) The burette is calibrated in small increments that allow accuracy and exact measurements of small volume. The fluid chamber holds 100 to 150 mL of fluid. The fluid in the fluid chamber of the burette is infused in a specific time period, usually 60 minutes or less. Medication is added to the I.V. fluid in the chamber for a prescribed dilution of volume (see Figure 21-24).

An electronic controller or pump may also be used to administer intermittent I.V. medications. When used, the electronic device alarms when the buretrol

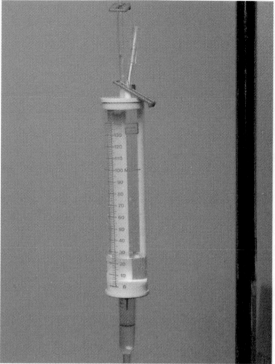

Figure 21-24 Volume-controlled device (burette). (From Potter PA, Perry AG: *Fundamentals of nursing,* ed 5, St Louis, 2001, Mosby.)

chamber is empty. Buretrols may also be used in the adult setting for clients with fluid restrictions.

Intravenous infusions should be monitored as frequently as every hour, and a solution to flush the I.V. tubing is administered after the medication.

Regardless of the method used for medication administration in children, **a solution to flush the I.V. tubing is administered after medication.** The purpose of the flush is to make sure the medication has cleared the tubing and the total dose is administered. Most institutions flush with normal saline solution as opposed to heparin. The amount of fluid used varies according to the length of the tubing from the medication source to the infusion site. **When I.V. medications are diluted for administration, the policy for including medication volume as part of the volume specified for dilution varies from institution to institution, as does the amount of flush. When calculating flow rates (gtt/min, mL/hr), it varies from institution to institution as to whether the flush is included. The nurse has the responsibility for checking the protocol at the institution to ensure correct procedure is followed.**

Note: In the sample calculations that follow, a 15-mL volume will be used as a flush unless otherwise specified, and the drug volume will be considered as part of the total dilution volume. The flush will not be considered in the total volume.

CALCULATING I.V. MEDICATIONS BY BURETTE

A calibrated burette can be used to administer medications by using a roller clamp rather than a pump. In this case it is necessary to use the formula presented ear-

Note:

In doing the calculations, the total volume will include adding the medication to the diluent to calculate the gtt/min.

lier in this chapter and calculate gtt/min. Remember, burettes are volume control devices and have a drop factor of 60 gtt/mL.

$$\text{gtt/min} = \frac{\text{total volume (mL)} \times \text{drop factor (gtt/mL)}}{\text{time in minutes}}$$

Example 1: An antibiotic dose of 100 mg diluted in 20 mL of D5W to infuse over 30 minutes. A 15 mL flush follows. The administration set is a microdrip (burette).

Step 1: Read the drug label and determine what volume the 100 mg is contained in. This is 2 mL.

Step 2: Allow 18 mL D5W to run into the burette and then add the 2 mL containing the 100 mg of medication. Roll the burette between your hands to allow medication to mix thoroughly.

Note:

Reducing numbers can make them smaller and easier to deal with. If the flush is considered with the intermittent medication, note the total volume will be diluted drug + flush, and then proceed with calculation (gtt/min, mL/hr).

Step 3: Determine the flow rate necessary to deliver the medication plus the flush in 30 minutes.

Total volume is 20 mL. Infusion time 30 minutes.

$$x \text{ gtt/min} = \frac{20 \text{ mL (diluted drug)} \times 60 \text{ gtt/mL}}{30 \text{ min}}$$

$$x = \frac{20 \times 60}{30} = 40 \text{ gtt/min}$$

Answer: $x = 40$ gtt/min; 40 microgtt/min

Step 4: Adjust the I.V. flow rate to deliver 40 microgtt/min (40 gtt/min).

Step 5: Label the burette with the drug name, dosage, and medication infusing label.

Step 6: When the medication is completed, add the 15 mL flush, and continue to infuse at 40 microgtt/min. Replace the label with a "flush infusing" label.

Step 7: When the flush is completed, restart the primary line, and remove the flush infusing label. Document the medication on the MAR and the volume of fluid on the I&O according to agency policy.

Note:

Always think and remember, volume control sets are microdrip and mL/hr = gtt/min when drop factor is 60 gtt/mL.

To express the volume of gtt/min in mL/hr, remember that a microdrip administration set delivers 60 gtt/mL; therefore gtt/min = mL/hr. In this case if the gtt/min = 40, then the mL/hr = 40.

As already mentioned, the burette can be used along with an electronic controller or pump. When used as previously stated, the electronic device will alarm each time the burette empties. Let's examine the calculation necessary if the burette is used along with the pump or a controller. Calculations where the burette is used with a pump or controller are done in mL/hr. Let's use the same example shown previously to illustrate the difference in calculation steps.

Example 1: An antibiotic dose of 100 mg diluted in 20 mL of D5W is to infuse over 30 minutes. A 15 mL flush follows. An infusion controller is used, and the tubing is a microdrip burette.

The same steps 1 and 2 are followed as shown in previous example for burette only.

Step 1: Calculate the flow rate for this microdrip.

Total volume is 20 mL, the flush is not considered in the volume.

Step 2: Total volume is 20 mL. Infusion time is 30 minutes. Use a ratio-proportion to calculate the rate in mL/hr.

$$20 \text{ mL} : 30 \text{ minutes} = x \text{ mL} : 60 \text{ minutes}$$

$$30x = 60 \times 20$$

$$\frac{30x}{30} = \frac{1,200}{30} = 40 \text{ mL/hr.}$$

$$x = 40 \text{ mL/hr}$$

Answer: Set the controller to infuse at 40 mL/hr.

Example 2: An antibiotic dose of 150 mg in 1 mL is to be diluted in 35 mL NS to infuse over 45 minutes. A 15 mL flush follows. A volumetric pump will be used.

Total volume is 35 mL. Infusion time is 45 minutes. Calculate mL/hr rate.

$$35 \text{ mL} : 45 \text{ minutes} = x \text{ mL} : 60 \text{ minutes}$$

$$45x = 35 \times 60$$

$$\frac{45 x}{45} = \frac{2,100}{45} = 46.6 = 47 \text{ mL/hr}$$

$$x = 47 \text{ mL/hr.}$$

Answer: Set the pump to infuse at 47 mL/hr.

> **Note:**
>
> When medication has infused, add the 15 mL flush and continue to infuse at 40 mL/hr; replace the label with a "flush infusing label." Once the flush is finished, restart the primary I.V. or disconnect from lock. Remove the "flush infusing label. Document the medication on the MAR and the volume of fluid on the I&O according to the institution's policy.

> **Note:**
>
> As shown earlier in chapter, the shortcut method using the drop factor constant could be used. Ratio-proportion can be stated using several formats.

 PRACTICE PROBLEMS

Determine the volume of solution that must be added to the burette in the following problems. Then determine the flow rate in gtt/min for each I.V. using a microdrip, then indicate mL/hr for a controller.

83. An I.V. medication dose of 500 mg is ordered to be diluted to 30 mL and infuse over 50 minutes. The dose of medication is contained in 3 mL. Determine the following:

a) Dilution volume _____

b) gtt/min _____

c) mL/hr _____

84. The volume of a 20-mg dose of medication is 2 mL. Dilute to 15 mL and administer over 45 minutes with a 15 mL flush to follow. The administration set is a microdrip. Determine the following:

a) Dilution volume _____

b) gtt/min _____

c) mL/hr _____

Answers on p. 563

Notes

As seen in the chapter on pediatric doses, medications can be calculated based on mg/kg or BSA—I.V. doses for children are calculated on that basis as well. The I.V. medication can be assessed to determine if it is within normal range as well. The safe daily dose is calculated and then compared to the order.

To determine whether an I.V. dose for a child is safe, consult an appropriate drug resource for the recommended dose. Remember to carefully read the reference to determine if the drug is calculated according to BSA in m^2 (common with chemotherapy drugs), mcg, or U per day or per hour. When a dose is within the normal limits, calculate and administer the dose. If a dose is not within the normal limits, consult the prescriber before administering the drug. Note: if the order is based on the child's BSA and the BSA is not known, you will need to use the West nomogram or the formula presented and determine the BSA. Let's look at some examples.

Example 1: A child's BSA is 0.8 m^2 and the order is for 1.8 mg of a medication in 100 mL D5W at 10 AM. The recommended dose is 2 mg/m^2.

Step 1: As previously shown in Chapter 20, if BSA is known calculate the dose for the child by multiplying the recommended dose by the BSA. The recommended dose is 2 mg/m^2, and the child's BSA is 0.8 m^2.

$$0.8 \ (m^2) \times 2 \ mg = 1.6 \ mg$$

Step 2: Determine if dose is within the normal range.

The safe dose is 1.6 mg for this child, but 1.8 mg is ordered. Notify the prescriber before administering the dose.

Example 2: A child weighing 10 kg has an order for I.V. Solumedrol 125 mg I.V. q6h for 48 hours. The recommended dose is 30 mg/kg.

Step 1: Determine the dose for the child.

$$10 \ kg \times 30 \ mg = 300 \ mg$$

Step 2: Determine if dose ordered is within normal range.

The dose: 125 mg q6h (4 doses).

$$125 \ mg \times 4 = 500 \ mg$$

Check with the prescriber; the dose is more than what child should receive.

 PRACTICE PROBLEMS

Determine the normal dose range for the following problems to the nearest tenth. State your course of action.

85. A child weighing 17 kg has an I.V. of 250 mL D5W containing 2,500 U of medication, which is to infuse at 50 mL/hr. The recommended dosage for the medication is 10-25 U/kg/hr. Determine whether the dose ordered is within normal limits. _____

86. A child with a BSA of 0.75 m^2 has an order for 84 mg I.V. of a drug in 100 mL D5W q12h. The recommended dosage is 100-250 mg/m^2/day in two divided doses. Determine whether the dose ordered is within normal limits. _____

Answers on pp. 563-564

ENTERAL FEEDINGS

Enteral nutrition involves the provision of nutrients to the gastrointestinal tract. This nutrition is provided to clients who are unable to ingest food safely or have eating difficulties. Enteral nutrition may be provided with nasogastric, jejunal, or gastric tube. It may be blended foods or tube feeding formulas (Figure 21-25). Tube feedings can be administered in several ways. Depending on the client's needs, they may be given as a bolus amount via gravity several times a day using a large-volume syringe, as a continuous gravity drip over a period of 1/2 to 1 hour several times a day using a pouch to hang the feeding, or as a continuous drip per infusion pump. When clients are receiving a continuous feeding, the feeding is placed in a special pouch or container and attached to a feeding pump. A common feeding pump is the Kangaroo pump (Figure 21-26). When the feeding pump is used the feeding to be delivered is in mL/hr. For the purpose of this chapter we will focus on administering a feeding by the continuous drip method using an enteral infusion pump.

When an order is written for feedings by continuous infusion, the nurse attaches the feeding to a special pump and administers it at the prescribed rate in mL/hr. A sample order is Jevity at 65 mL/hr via PEG (percutaneous endoscopic gastrostomy), or by NG (nasogastric). The feeding order also includes a certain volume of water with feeding (100-250 mL). Some orders may be written as follows: Pulmo Care 400 mL q8hr followed by 100 mL of water after each feed. When the prescriber does not indicate mL per hour, the nurse uses the same formula as with I.V. calculation to determine mL/hr. In pediatrics the order often specifies the formula and mL/hr. Example: Similac 24 at 20 mL/hr continuously by NG tube.

Example 1: Order: Pulmo Care 400 mL q8hr followed by 100 mL of water after each feed. Determine mL/hr.

$$\frac{400 \text{ mL}}{8 \text{ hr}} = 50 \text{ mL/hr}$$

The pump would be set at 50 mL/hr.

Example 2: Order: Nepro 1,200 mL over 16 hours. Determine mL/hr.

$$\frac{1,200 \text{ mL}}{16 \text{ hr}} = 75 \text{ mL/hr}$$

The pump would be set to deliver 75 mL/hr.

Note:

The amount of water given with a tube feeding and how it is administered varies from one institution to the next. Check the institution's policy relating to administering enteral feedings.

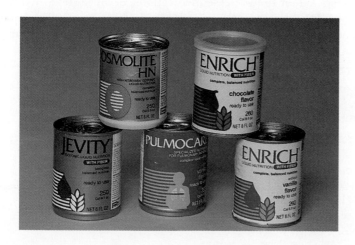

Figure 21-25 Sample formula preparations. (From Elkin M, Perry A, Potter P: *Nursing interventions and clinical skills*, ed 2, St Louis, 2000, Mosby.)

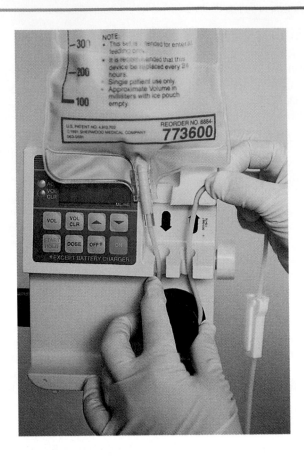

Figure 21-26   Kangaroo pump. (From Elkin M, Perry A, Potter P: *Nursing interventions and clinical skills, ed 2, St Louis, 2000, Mosby.)*

In addition to nutrients, medications may be given through a tube as well. Liquid medications are preferred; however, some tablets may be crushed, dissolved in water, and administered.

Never assume. Not all medications are designed for administration via tube, so check with the pharmacist. A medication's effectiveness could be dependent on the location of the tube (e.g., stomach or jejunum).

 Critical Thinking

> Always verify that the medications to be administered are not sublingual, enteric-coated, or time-release medications, because such medications are absorbed differently and the effects of a medication may be altered. Consult the pharmacist before tablets are crushed, and before capsules are opened and dissolved for the tube feeding administration.

 PRACTICE PROBLEMS

Determine mL/hr for the following continuous feedings:

87. Ensure 480 mL via NG tube over 8 hr. Follow with 100 mL of water after each feeding.   _____

88. Periative 1,600 mL over 24 hr via gastrostomy.
    Follow with 250 mL of water.

_____

Answers on p. 564

Notes

Calculations of Solutions

Due to special circumstances in adults and children, nutritional liquids may require dilution before they are used. Nutritional formulas may be diluted with sterile or tap water. **Always consult a reference regarding what to reconstitute a nutritional formula with.**

To prepare a prescribed solution of a certain strength from a solute, first let's review some basic terms.

Solute—a concentrated or solid substance to be dissolved or diluted.

Solvent—a liquid substance that dissolves another substance.

Solution—a solute plus a solvent.

To prepare a solution of a specific strength, use the following steps:

1. Desired solution strength $\times$ $\dfrac{\text{amount of}}{\text{desired solution}}$ = $\dfrac{\text{solute}}{\text{(solution to be dissolved)}}$

Note: The strength of the desired solution is written as a fraction; the amount of desired solution is expressed as mL or ounces, depending on problem. This will give you the amount of solute you will need to add to the solvent to prepare the desired solution.

2. Amount of desired solution−solute = amount of liquid needed to dissolve substance (solvent).

Example 1: Order: 1/3-strength Ensure 900 mL via NG tube over 8 hr.

Solution:

Step 1:

$$\underset{\substack{\text{desired} \\ \text{strength}}}{1/3} \times \underset{\substack{\text{amount of} \\ \text{solution}}}{900 \text{ mL}} = x \text{ (solute)}$$

$$\frac{900}{3} = x$$

$$x = 300 \text{ mL}$$

You need 300 mL of the formula (solute).

Step 2:

$$\underset{\substack{\text{amount of} \\ \text{solution}}}{900 \text{ mL}} - \underset{\text{(solute)}}{300 \text{ mL}} = \underset{\substack{\text{amount needed} \\ \text{to dissolve}}}{600 \text{ mL}}$$

Therefore you would add 600 mL water to 300 mL Ensure to make 900 mL 1/3-strength Ensure.

Notes

Example 2:   3/4-strength Isomil 4 oz po q4h for 24 hr.

[Note] 4 oz q4h = 6 feedings 4 oz × 6 = 24 oz

1 oz = 30 mL; therefore 24 oz = 720 mL

$$\frac{3}{4} \times 720 \text{ mL} = x \text{ mL}$$

$$\frac{2,160}{4} = x$$

x = 540 mL of the formula (solute)

720 mL   −   540 mL =   180 mL
amount of   solute   amount needed
solution   to dissolve

Therefore you would add 180 mL water to 540 mL Isomil to make 720 mL 3/4-strength Isomil.

 PRACTICE PROBLEMS

Prepare the following strength solutions.

89. 2/3-strength Sustacal 300 mL po qid.

90. 3/4-strength Ensure 16 oz via NG tube over 8 hr.

91. 1/2-strength Ensure 20 oz via gt over 5 hr.

Answers on p. 564

POINTS TO REMEMBER

- To determine flow rates for an electronic infusion device (pump or controller), determine mL/hr by using the following:

$$\frac{\text{Total mL ordered}}{\text{Total hr ordered}} = \text{mL/hr (rounded to the nearest whole number)}$$

- Drop factor = gtt/mL

- Calculation of gtt/min can be done using two formulas:

    A) x gtt/min = $\dfrac{\text{amount of (mL)} \times \text{gtt factor (gtt/mL)}}{\text{time in minutes}}$

    B) $\dfrac{V_1}{T_1} \times \dfrac{V_2}{T_2} = x$ gtt/min

    Formula A is used most often, and is easiest to use.

- To calculate the I.V. flow rate, the nurse must have the volume of solution, the time factor, and the drop factor of the I.V. tubing.

- Microdrops always deliver 60 gtt/mL.

- Macrodrops differ according to the manufacturer. They can deliver 10, 15, or 20 gtt/mL.

Notes

POINTS TO REMEMBER—cont'd

- A shortcut method can be used to calculate flow rates infusing in 1 hr or less, and for more than one hour, by determining mL/hr and determining the constant drop factor for the I.V. set.

- To determine the constant drop factor for any I.V. set, divide 60 by the calibration of the set.

- I.V. flow rates must be monitored by the nurse. When I.V. solutions are behind or ahead of schedule, the flow rate must be recalculated using

$$\frac{\text{volume (mL) remaining}}{\text{time remaining}}$$

- Never increase or decrease an I.V. flow rate without recalculating and assessing a client to determine if the change can be tolerated.

- I.V. flow rates should not be increased or decreased more than 25% of their original rate. Know the policy of the institution regarding recalculating I.V. flow rates. Check with the prescriber regarding an I.V. increase > to 25%. To determine the percent of increase and decrease, divide the amount of ↑ or ↓ by the original rate.

- Read I.V. labels carefully to determine whether the correct solution is being administered.

- Infusion time is calculated by dividing the total volume to infuse by the mL/hr the solution is infusing at. To obtain the completion time for an I.V., add the infusion time calculated to the time the I.V. was started. (Time can be stated in traditional or military time.)

- Commercial labeling for I.V. bags is used to assess the volume a client is receiving per hr.

- Pediatric I.V. medications are diluted for administration. It is important to know the institution's policy as to whether the medication volume is included as part of the total dilution volume.

- A flush is used following administration of I.V. medications in children. The volume of the flush will vary depending on the length of the I.V. tubing from the medication source. Check the institution's policy as to whether the volume of the flush is added to the diluted medication volume.

- Use an appropriate reference to calculate normal dosage range for I.V. administration, and compare it to the dosage ordered to determine whether it's within the normal range.

- Pediatric I.V. medication administration requires frequent assessment.

- Enteral feedings (continuous) are placed on an infusion pump and administered in mL/hr. Doctors usually prescribe feeding in mL/hr. If not, the nurse must calculate mL/hr to deliver the feeding.

- To prepare a solution of a specific strength write the desired solution strength as a fraction and multiply it by the amount of desired solution. This will give you the amount of solute needed.

- The amount of desired solution − solute = amount of liquid needed to dissolve the substance (solvent).

Notes

CHAPTER REVIEW

Calculate the I.V. flow rate in gtt/min for the following I.V. administrations, unless another unit of measure is stated.

1. 1,000 mL D5RL to infuse in 8 hr.
   Drop factor: 20 gtt/mL.   _____

2. 2,500 mL D5NS to infuse in 24 hr.
   Drop factor: 10 gtt/mL.   _____

3. 500 mL D5W to infuse in 4 hr.
   Drop factor: 15 gtt/mL.   _____

4. 300 mL NS to infuse in 6 hr.
   Drop factor 60 gtt/mL microdrop.   _____

5. 1,000 mL D5W for 24 hr KVO (keep vein open).
   Drop factor 60 gtt/mL (microdrop).   _____

6. 1,000 mL D5 and 1/2 NS with 20 mEq KCl over
   12 hr. Drop factor: 10 gtt/mL.   _____

7. 1,000 mL RL to infuse in 10 hr.
   Drop factor: 20 gtt/mL.   _____

8. 1,500 mL NS to infuse in 12 hr.
   Drop factor: 10 gtt/mL.   _____

9. A unit of whole blood (500 mL) to infuse in 4 hr.
   Drop factor: 20 gtt/mL.   _____

10. A unit of packed cells (250 mL) to infuse in 4 hr.
    Drop factor: 20 gtt/mL.   _____

11. 1,500 mL D5W in 8 hr.
    Drop factor: 20 gtt/mL.   _____

12. 3,000 mL RL in 24 hr.
    Drop factor: 15 gtt/mL.   _____

13. Infuse 2 L RL in 24 hr.
    Drop factor: 15 gtt/mL.   _____

14. 1,000 mL D5W with 10 mEq KCl to infuse in 7 hr.
    Drop factor: 10 gtt/mL.   _____

15. 500 mL D5W in 4 hr.
    Drop factor: 60 gtt/mL (microdrop).   _____

16. 1,000 mL D5 0.45% NS in 6 hr.
    Drop factor: 20 gtt/mL.   _____

17. 250 mL D5W in 8 hr.
    Drop factor: 60 gtt/mL (microdrop).   _____

18. 1 L of D5W to infuse at 50 mL/hr.
    Drop factor: 60 gtt/mL (microdrop). _____

19. 2 L D5RL at 150 mL/hr.
    Drop factor: 15 gtt/mL. _____

20. 500 mL D5W in 6 hr.
    Drop factor: 15 gtt/mL. _____

21. 1,500 mL NS in 12 hr.
    Drop factor: 10 gtt/mL. _____

22. 1,500 mL D5W in 24 hr.
    Drop factor: 15 gtt/mL. _____

23. 2,000 mL D5W in 16 hr.
    Drop factor: 20 gtt/mL. _____

24. 500 mL D5W in 8 hr.
    Drop factor: 15 gtt/mL. _____

25. 250 mL D5W in 10 hr.
    Drop factor: 60 gtt/mL (microdrop). _____

26. Infuse 300 mL of D5W at 75 mL/hr.
    Drop factor: 60 gtt/mL (microdrop). _____

27. Infuse 125 mL/hr of D5RL.
    Drop factor: 20 gtt/mL. _____

28. Infuse 40 mL/hr of D5W.
    Drop factor: 60 gtt/mL (microdrop). _____

29. Infuse an I.V. medication with a volume
    of 50 mL in 45 minutes.
    Drop factor: 60 gtt/mL (microdrop). _____

30. Infuse 90 mL/hr of NS.
    Drop factor: 15 gtt/mL. _____

31. Infuse 150 mL/hr of D5RL.
    Drop factor: 10 gtt/mL. _____

32. Infuse 2,500 mL of D5W in 24 hr.
    Drop factor: 15 gtt/mL. _____

33. Infuse an I.V. medication in 50 mL
    of 0.9% NS in 40 minutes.
    Drop factor: 10 gtt/mL. _____

34. Infuse an I.V. medication in 100 mL D5W
    in 30 minutes. Drop factor: 20 gtt/mL. _____

35. Infuse 250 mL 0.45% NS in 5 hr.
    Drop factor: 20 gtt/mL. _____

Notes

Notes

36. Infuse 1,000 mL of D5W at 80 mL/hr.
    Drop factor: 20 gtt/mL.   _____

37. Infuse 150 mL of D5RL in 30 minutes.
    Drop factor: 10 gtt/mL.   _____

38. Infuse Kefzol 0.5 g in 50 mL D5W in
    30 minutes.
    Drop factor: 60 gtt/mL (microdrop).   _____

39. Infuse Plasmanate 500 mL over 3 hr.
    Drop factor: 10 gtt/mL.   _____

40. Infuse albumin 250 mL over 2 hr.
    Drop factor: 15 gtt/mL.   _____

41. The prescriber orders the following I.V.s for 24 hr.
    Drop factor: 10 gtt/mL.

    a) 1,000 mL D5W with 1 ampule MVI (multivitamin)
    b) 500 mL D5W
    c) 250 mL D5W   _____

42. Infuse vancomycin 1 g IVPB in 150 mL D5W
    in 1.5 hr. Drop factor: 60 gtt/mL (microdrop).   _____

43. If 2 L D5W is to infuse in 16 hr, how many mL
    are to be administered per hour?   _____

44. If 500 mL of RL is to infuse in 4 hr, how
    many mL are to be administered per hour?   _____

45. If 200 mL of NS is to infuse in 2 hr, how
    many mL are to be administered per hour?   _____

46. If 500 mL of D5W is to infuse in 8 hr, how
    many mL are to be administered per hour?   _____

47. Infuse a hyperalimentation solution of 1,100 mL
    in 12 hr. How many mL are to be
    administered per hour?   _____

48. Infuse 500 mL Intralipids I.V. in 6 hr.
    Drop factor: 10 gtt/mL.   _____

49. Infuse 3,000 mL D5W in 20 hr.
    Drop factor: 20 gtt/mL.   _____

50. An I.V. of 500 mL D5W with 200 mg
    of minocycline is to infuse in 6 hr.
    Drop factor: 15 gtt/mL.   _____

51. An I.V. of D5W 500 mL was ordered to infuse
    over 10 hr at a rate of 13 gtt/min (13 macrogtt/min).
    Drop factor: 15 gtt/mL. After 3 hr you notice
    that 300 mL of I.V. solution is left. Recalculate
    the gtt/min for the remaining solution.   _____ gtt/min

    Determine the % of change in I.V. rate and state
    your course of action.   _____ %

52. An I.V. of D5W 1,000 mL was ordered to infuse over 8 hr at a rate of 42 gtt/min (42 macrogtt/min). Drop factor: 20 gtt/mL. After 4 hr you notice only 400 mL has infused. Recalculate the gtt/min for the remaining solution. _____ gtt/min

    Determine the % of change and state your course of action. _____ %

53. An I.V. of 1,000 mL D5 and 1/2 NS has been ordered to infuse at 125 mL/hr. Drop factor: 15 gtt/mL. The I.V. was hung at 7 AM. At 11 AM you check the I.V., and there is 400 mL left. Recalculate the gtt/min for the remaining solution. _____ gtt/min

    Determine the % of change and state your course of action. _____ %

54. An I.V. of 500 mL of 0.9% NS is to infuse in 6 hr at a rate of 14 gtt/min (14 macrogtt/min). Drop factor: 10 gtt/mL. The I.V. was started at 7 AM. You check the I.V. at 8 AM, and 250 mL has infused. Recalculate the gtt/min for the remaining solution. _____ gtt/min

    Determine the % of change and state your course of action. _____ %

55. An I.V. of 1,000 mL D5W is to infuse in 10 hr. Drop factor: 15 gtt/mL. The I.V. was started at 4 AM. At 10 AM 600 mL remains in the bag. Is the I.V. on schedule? If not, recalculate the gtt/min for the remaining solution. _____ gtt/min

    Determine the % of change and state your course of action. _____ %

56. 900 mL of RL is infusing at a rate of 80 gtt/min (80 macrodrops/min). Drop factor: 15 gtt/mL. How long will it take for the I.V. to infuse? (Express time in hours and minutes.) _____

57. A client is receiving 1,000 mL of D5W at 100 mL/hr. How many hours will it take for the I.V. to infuse? _____

58. 1,000 mL of D5W is infusing at 20 gtt/min (20 macrogtt/min). Drop factor: 10 gtt/mL. How long will it take for the I.V. to infuse? (Express time in hours and minutes.) _____

59. 450 mL of NS is infusing at 25 gtt/min (25 macrogtt/min). Drop factor: 20 gtt/mL. How many hours will it take for the I.V. to infuse? _____

60. 100 mL of D5W is infusing at 10 gtt/min (10 macrogtt/min). The administration set delivers 15 gtt/mL. How many hours will it take for the I.V. to infuse? _____

61. An I.V. is regulated at 25 gtt/min (25 macrogtt/min). Drop factor: 15 gtt/mL. How many mL of fluid will the client receive in 8 hr?   _____

62. An I.V. is regulated at 40 gtt/min (40 microdrop/min). Drop factor: 60 gtt/mL. How many mL of fluid will the client receive in 10 hr?   _____

63. An I.V. is regulated at 30 gtt/min (30 macrogtt/min). Drop factor: 15 gtt/mL. How many mL of fluid will the client receive in 5 hr?   _____

64. 10 mEq of potassium chloride is placed in 500 mL of D5W to be administered at the rate of 2 mEq/hr.

    a) How many mL of solution is needed to administer 2 mEq?   _____

    b) Calculate the gtt/min to deliver 2 mEq/hr. Drop factor: 20 gtt/mL.   _____

65. 30 mEq of potassium chloride is added to 1,000 mL of D5W to be administered at the rate of 4 mEq/hr.

    a) How many mL of solution is needed to administer 4 mEq?   _____

    b) Calculate the gtt/min to deliver 4 mEq/hr. Drop factor: 15 gtt/mL.   _____

66. Order: Humulin regular U 100 7 U/hr. The I.V. solution contains 50 U of Humulin regular insulin in 250 mL of 0.9% NS. How many mL/hr should the I.V. infuse at?   _____

67. Order: Humulin regular U 100 18 U/hr. The I.V. solution contains 100 U of Humulin regular insulin in 250 mL of 0.9% NS. How many mL/hr should the I.V. infuse at?   _____

68. Order: Humulin regular U 100 11 U/hr. The I.V. solution contains 100 U of Humulin regular insulin in 100 mL of 0.9% NS. How many mL/hr should the I.V. infuse at?   _____

69. Infuse gentamicin 65 mg in 150 mL 0.9% NS IVPB over 1 hr. Drop factor: 10 gtt/mL. How many gtt/min should the I.V. infuse at?   _____

70. Infuse ampicillin 1 g that has been diluted in 40 mL 0.9% NS in 40 minutes. Drop factor: 60 gtt/mL (microdrop). How many gtt/min should the I.V. infuse at?   _____

71. Administer I.V. medication with a volume
of 35 mL in 30 minutes.
Drop factor: 60 gtt/mL (microdrop).
How many gtt/min should the I.V. infuse at? _____

72. Administer I.V. medication with a volume
of 80 mL in 40 minutes.
Drop factor: 15 gtt/mL.
How many gtt/min should the I.V. infuse at? _____

73. Administer 50 mL of an antibiotic in 25 minutes.
Drop factor: 10 gtt/mL. How many gtt/min would
you regulate the I.V. at? _____

74. An I.V. is to infuse at 65 mL/hr.
Drop factor: 15 gtt/mL. How many gtt/min
should the I.V. infuse at? _____

75. 50 mL of 0.9% NS with 1 g ampicillin is infusing
at 50 microgtt/min (50 gtt/min).
Drop factor: 60 gtt/mL (microdrop). Determine
the infusion time. (Express time in hours
and minutes.) _____

76. 500 mL RL is to infuse at a rate of 80 mL/hr.
If the I.V. was started at 7 PM, what time will
the I.V. be completed? _____

State time in military and traditional time. _____

77. A volume of 150 mL of NS is to infuse at
25 mL/hr. _____

a) Calculate the infusion time. _____

b) The I.V. was started at 3:10 AM. What time
will the I.V. be completed? _____

State time in traditional and military time. _____

78. The doctor orders 2.5 L of D5W to inf
at 150 mL/hr. Determine the infusion t. _____

79. A child is to receive 10 U of a medication. The dose of 10 U is contained in
1 mL. Dilute to 30 mL and infuse in 20 minutes. A 5 mL flush is to follow.
Medication is placed in a burette.

a) gtt/min _____

b) mL/hr _____

80. A child is to receive 80 mg of a medication. The dose of 80 mg is contained
in 2 mL. Dilute to 80 mL and infuse in 60 minutes. A 15 mL flush is to
follow. Medication is placed in a burette.

a) gtt/min _____

b) mL/hr _____

Notes

81. A dose of 250 mg in 5 mL has been ordered diluted to 40 mL and infused in 45 minutes. A 15 mL flush follows. Medication is placed in a burette.

    a) gtt/min   _____

    b) mL/hr   _____

82. A child weighing 23 kg has an order for 500 mg of a medication in 100 mL D5W q12h. The normal daily dosage range is 40-50 mg/kg/day. Determine if the dosage ordered is within normal range and state your course of action. _____

83. A child weighing 20 kg has an order for 2 mg I.V. of a medication at 10 AM in 100 mL D5W. The normal daily dosage is 0.05 mg/kg/day. Determine if the dosage ordered is within normal range and state your course of action. _____

84. A child weighing 15 kg has an order for 55 mcg of a medication I.V. q12h. The dosage range is 6-8 mcg/kg/day q12h. Determine if the dosage ordered is within normal range and state your course of action. _____

85. A client has an order for Jevity 1,200 mL by continuous feeding through a gastrostomy tube over 16 hours, followed by 250 mL of free water. The feeding is placed on an infusion pump. Calculate the mL/hr to set the pump at. _____ mL/hr

Calculate the amount of dextrose and/or sodium chloride in each of the following I.V. solutions.

86. 0.5 L D5 $\frac{1}{4}$ NS

    dextrose   _____ g

    NaCl   _____ g

87. 750 mL D5 $\frac{1}{2}$ NS

    dextrose   _____ g

    NaCl   _____ g

Prepare the following solution strength.

88. 1/8-strength Ensure 4 oz via nasogastric tube q4h for 24 hr.

Answers on pp. 564-572

Chapter 22

Heparin Calculations

Objectives

After reviewing this chapter, you should be able to:

1. State the importance of calculating heparin doses accurately
2. Calculate heparin doses being administered I.V. (mL/hr, U/hr, gtt/min)
3. Calculate s.c. doses of heparin
4. Calculate and determine whether the client is receiving a heparin dose within the normal heparinizing range

Heparin is a potent anticoagulant that prevents clot formation and blood coagulation. Heparin dosages are expressed in USP units (U). The therapeutic range for heparin is determined individually by monitoring the client's partial thromboplastin time (PTT). **However, the normal adult heparin dosage is 20,000 to 40,000 U every 24 hours.** Heparin can be administered I.V. or s.c. When administered I.V., heparin is ordered in U/hr, or mL/hr. Usually, however, heparin is ordered on the basis of the units/hr or per day when ordered intravenously. Heparin is available in single and multidose vials, as well as in commercially prepared I.V. solutions. Heparin sodium for injection is available in several strengths (e.g., 100 units per mL; 5,000 units per mL; 20,000 units per mL). Heparin lock fluid solution, which is used for flushing), is available in 10 and 100 units per mL. **It is extremely important that the nurse is aware that heparin sodium for injection and heparin lock solution are different drugs and can never be used interchangeably.**

Figure 22-1 shows the various heparin dose strengths. Heparin is administered using an electronic infusion device, and the client requires continuous monitoring. The nurse's primary responsibility is to administer the correct dose and ensure the dosage is safe.

When in doubt regarding a dose a client is receiving, check it with the prescriber before administering it.

Critical Thinking

Heparin comes in different strengths; read labels carefully before administering to ensure the client's safety. Verify the dose, vial, and amount to be given.

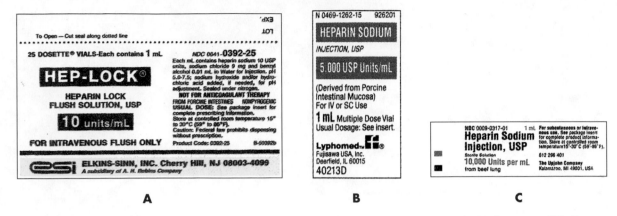

Figure 22-1 Heparin labels. **A,** Hep-Lock flush solution 10 U/mL; **B,** 5,000 U/mL; **C,** 10,000 U/mL.

Doses of heparin are highly individualized and based on a client's coagulation time. Lovenox (Enoxaprin) and fragmin (Dalteparin) are also injectable anticoagulants prescribed for prevention and treatment of deep vein thrombosis (DVT) and pulmonary emboli (PE) after knee and hip surgery.

CALCULATION OF s.c. DOSES

Because of its inherent dangers and to ensure an accurate and exact dose, heparin is administered s.c. A tuberculin syringe is used. Heparin is also available for use in pre-packaged syringes. Institutional policies differ regarding the administration of heparin and the nurse is responsible for knowing and following the policies. The methods of calculating presented in previous chapters are used to calculate s.c. heparin, except the dose is never rounded and is administered using a tuberculin syringe. The prescriber will order heparin in units, and an order written in any other unit of measure should be questioned before administration. If the desired dose is not available in a commercially prepared heparin, the nurse will be responsible for preparing the solution. **Always read labels and the prescribed dosage carefully.**

Example 1:   Order: Heparin 7,500 U s.c.

Available: Heparin labeled 10,000 U/mL.

What will you administer to the client?

Setup:
1. No conversion is necessary. There is no conversion for units.
2. Think—what would be a logical dose?
3. Set up in ratio-proportion or formula and solve.

▶ Solution Using Ratio-Proportion:

$$10,000 \text{ U} : 1 \text{ mL} = 7,500 \text{ U} : x \text{ mL}$$

$$10,000x = 7,500$$

$$x = \frac{7,500}{10,000}$$

$$x = 0.75 \text{ mL}$$

▶ Solution Using Formula:

$$\frac{7,500 \text{ U}}{10,000 \text{ U}} \times 1 \text{ mL} = x \text{ mL}; \quad \frac{7,500 \text{ U}}{10,000 \text{ U}} = \frac{x \text{ mL}}{1 \text{ mL}}$$

$$x = 0.75 \text{ mL}$$

The dose of 0.75 mL is reasonable because the ordered dose is less than what is available. Therefore less than 1 mL will be needed to administer the dose. This dose can be measured accurately only with a tuberculin syringe (calibrated in tenths and hundredths of a mL). This dose would not be rounded to the nearest tenth of a mL. A tuberculin syringe is shown below illustrating the dose to be administered (Figure 22-2).

CALCULATION OF I.V. HEPARIN SOLUTIONS

Using Ratio-Proportion to Calculate U/hr

Calculating U/hr of heparin can be done by using ratio-proportion.

Example: An I.V. solution of heparin is ordered for a client. D5W 1,000 mL containing 20,000 U of heparin is to infuse at 30 mL/hr. Calculate the dose of heparin the client is to receive per hour.

Set up a proportion:

$$20,000 \text{ U} : 1,000 \text{ mL} = x \text{ U} : 30 \text{ mL}$$

$$1,000x = 20,000 \times 30$$

$$\frac{1,000x}{1,000} = \frac{600,000}{1,000} = 600 \text{ U/hr}$$

$$x = 600 \text{ U/hr}$$

or

$$\frac{20,000 \text{ U}}{1,000 \text{ mL}} = \frac{x \text{ U}}{30 \text{ mL}} = 600 \text{ U/hr}$$

$$x = 600 \text{ U/hr}$$

Note:

Ratio-proportions can be stated in several formats.

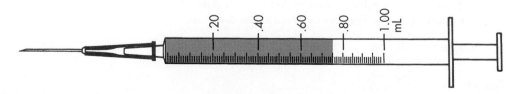

Figure 22-2   Tuberculin syringe illustrating 0.75 mL drawn up.

Using the Set Calibration and Flow Rate

Calculating mL/hr from U/hr

Because heparin is ordered in U/hr and infused using an electronic infusion device, it is necessary to do calculations in mL/hr.

Example: Order: Infuse heparin 850 U/hr from a solution containing D5W 500 mL with heparin 25,000 U I.V.

Set up proportion:

$$25{,}000 \text{ U} : 500 \text{ mL} = 850 \text{ U} = x \text{ mL} \quad \text{or} \quad \frac{25{,}000 \text{ U}}{500 \text{ mL}} = \frac{850 \text{ U}}{x \text{ mL}} = 17 \text{ mL/hr}$$

$$25{,}000 \, x = 500 \times 850$$

$$\frac{250{,}000 x}{25{,}000} = \frac{425{,}000}{25{,}000}$$

$$x = 17 \text{ mL/hr}$$

To infuse 850 U/hr from a solution of 25,000 U in D5W 500 mL, the flow rate would be 17 mL/hr.

Hourly doses can be calculated when the set calibration and flow rate are given. Remember, these problems in gtt/mL are for practice only. Heparin is given as I.V., usually in mL/hr.

Example: A client is receiving 12,500 U of heparin in 250 mL of D5W, infusing at 30 gtt/min (30 macrogtt/min) Drop factor: 15 gtt/mL. Calculate the hourly dose the client is receiving. This is solved using a series of steps.

First—Convert the gtt/min to mL/min.

$$15 \text{ gtt} : 1 \text{ mL} = 30 \text{ gtt} : x \text{ mL}$$

$$\frac{15x}{15} = \frac{30}{15}$$

$$x = 2 \text{ mL/min}$$

Then—Convert mL/min to mL/hr.

$$2 \text{ mL/min} \times 60 \text{ min} = 120 \text{ mL/hr}$$

After doing these steps, the proportion can be set up to calculate the units per hour.

$$12{,}500 \text{ U} : 250 \text{ mL} = x \text{ U} : 120 \text{ mL}$$

$$\frac{250x}{250} = \frac{1{,}500{,}000}{250}$$

$$x = 6{,}000 \text{ U/hr}$$

The client is receiving 6,000 U of heparin per hour

Calculating gtt/min from Units/hr ordered

Since I.V. heparin is ordered in units per hour, after calculating the mL/hr another calculation must be done to determine the flow rate.

Example 1: Infuse 8,000 U/hr of heparin from a solution containing 20,000 U in 250 mL D5W. Drop factor: 10 gtt/mL.

First calculate mL/hr to be administered:

$$20,000 \text{ U} : 250 \text{ mL} = 8,000 \text{ U} : x \text{ mL}$$

$$20,000x = 8,000 \times 250$$

$$\frac{20,000x}{20,000} = \frac{2,000,000}{20,000} = 100 \text{ mL/hr}$$

$$x = 100 \text{ mL/hr}$$

Then calculate the flow rate in gtt/min:

$$x \text{ gtt/min} = \frac{100 \text{ mL} \times 10 \text{ gtt/mL}}{60 \text{ min}}$$

$$x = 100 \times \frac{1}{6} = \frac{100}{6} = 17 \text{ gtt/min}$$

(17 macrogtt/min)

Note:

This could have also been done by using the constant drop factor (shortcut).

Answer: 17 gtt/min; 17 macrogtt/min

The constant drop factor for a 10 gtt/mL set is 6 (60 ÷ 10).

$$100 \div 6 = 17 \text{ gtt/min}$$

(17 macrogtt/min)

DETERMINING IF A DOSE IS WITHIN THE SAFE HEPARINIZING RANGE

To determine whether a client is receiving a safe heparinizing dose remember the normal adult heparinizing range is 20,000 to 40,000 units I.V. per 24 hours. Because heparin is ordered in U/hr, calculate the U/hr the client is receiving then analyze the order in relation to the normal heparinizing range.

Example 1: Order: Infuse a solution of heparin 40,000 U in 1,000 mL 0.9% NS to infuse at 40 mL/hr. Calculate the U/hr infusing and determine if the dosage is within the normal daily range. If not, state what your course of action is.

Step 1: Calculate the U/hr infusing.

$$1,000 \text{ mL} : 40,000 \text{ U} = 40 \text{ mL} : x \text{ U}$$

$$1,000x = 40,000 \times 40$$

$$\frac{1,000x}{1,000} = \frac{1,600,000}{1,000}$$

$$x = 1,600 \text{ U/hr}$$

Step 2: Determine the heparinizing dosage.

$$1,600 \text{ U/hr} \times 24 \text{ hr} = 38,400 \text{ U/24 hr.}$$

The dosage is safe, it is within the 20,000-40,000 U in 24 hr heparinizing range.

Example 2: Order: Infuse a solution of Heparin 20,000 U in 1,000 mL D5W

To infuse at 25 mL/hr, calculate the U/hr infusing and determine if the dosage is within the normal daily range.

Notes

Step 1: Calculate the U/hr infusing.

$$1{,}000 \text{ mL} : 20{,}000 \text{ U} = 25 \text{ mL} : x \text{ U}$$

$$1{,}000x = 20{,}000 \times 25$$

$$\frac{1{,}000x}{1{,}000} = \frac{500{,}000}{1{,}000}$$

$$x = 500 \text{ U/hr}$$

Step 2: Determine the heparinizing dosage.

$$500 \text{ U/hr} \times 24 \text{ hr} = 12{,}000 \text{ U/24 hr}$$

The dosage is less than the heparinizing range of 20,000-40,000 U in 24 hr; notify the prescriber.

 PRACTICE PROBLEMS

Calculate the units indicated by problem.

1. Order: Infuse 1,000 U/hr of heparin from a solution of 1,000 mL 0.45% NS with 25,000 U heparin. Calculate the mL/hr. _____

2. Order: Infuse 500 mL 0.45% NS with 30,000 U heparin at 600 U/hr. Drop factor: 10 gtt/mL. Calculate the gtt/min. _____

3. Order: Infuse D5 0.9% N.S. 500 mL with 25,000 U heparin at 40 gtt/min (40 macrogtt/min). Drop factor: 20 gtt/mL. Calculate U/hr. _____

4. Order: Infuse 750 mL D5W with 30,000 U heparin at 25 mL/hr. Calculate the U/hr. _____

5. Order: Infuse D5W 1,000 mL with 25,000 U heparin at 100 mL/hr. Determine the following: If not within normal range, state your course of action.

_____ U/hr _____ U/24hr _____ within normal range?

Answers on pg. 573

POINTS TO REMEMBER

- Heparin is a potent anticoagulant; it is often administered I.V., but can be administered s.c.

- Heparin is measured in USP units, abbreviated U.

- The normal heparinizing dosage is 20,000-40,000 U/day.

- Heparin doses must be accurately calculated to prevent inherent dangers associated with the medication.

- When administering s.c. heparin a tuberculin syringe is used (calibrated in tenths and hundredths of a mL). Answers are *not* rounded off.

- Read heparin labels carefully; it comes in several strengths.

- There are several I.V. calculations that can be done (mL/hr, gtt/min, U/hr).

- Heparin is commonly ordered in U/hr and infused using an electronic infusion device.

- Heparin sodium for injection and heparin lock solution cannot be used interchangeably.

- Based on the normal heparinizing dose, the nurse can determine whether an order is within the normal range.

- The method of calculating I.V. heparin doses can also be used to calculate I.V. doses for other medications. Ratio-proportion is the best method.

- Heparin doses are individualized.

- Monitoring the client's coagulation times while receiving heparin is a **must.**

Notes

✓ **CHAPTER REVIEW**

For questions 1 through 12, calculate the dose of heparin you will administer, and shade the dose on the syringe provided. For questions 13 through 47, calculate the units as indicated by the problem. Use labels where provided to calculate doses.

1. Order: Heparin 3,500 U s.c. o.d.

   Available:

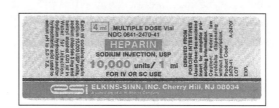

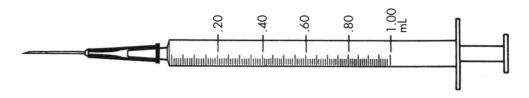

2. Order: Heparin 16,000 U s.c. stat.

   Available:

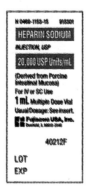

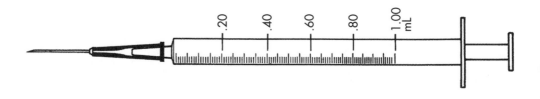

3. Order: Heparin 2,000 U s.c. o.d.

   Available: Heparin labeled 2,500 U/ml.

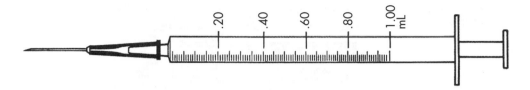

4. Order: Heparin 2,000 U s.c. o.d.

   Available: Heparin labeled 5,000 U/ml.

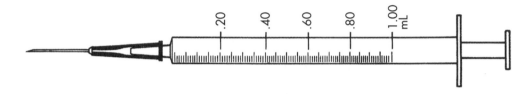

5. Order: Heparin 500 U s.c. q4h.

   Available:

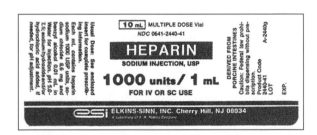

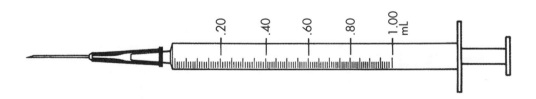

6. Order: Heparin flush 10 U q shift to flush a heparin lock.

   Available:

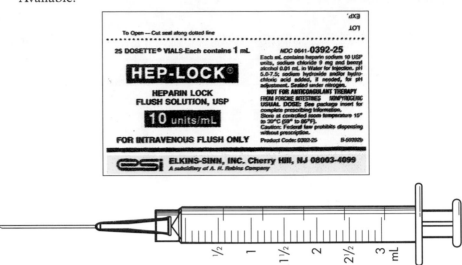

7. Order: Heparin 50,000 U I.V. in D5W 500 mL.

   Available: 10,000 U/mL.

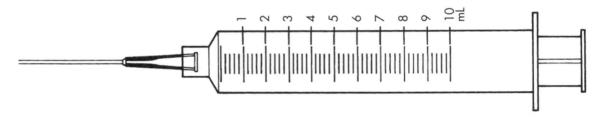

8. Order: Heparin 15,000 U s.c. o.d.

   Available: Heparin labeled 20,000 U/mL.

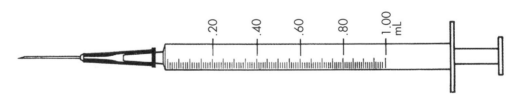

9. Order: 3,000 U of heparin to a liter of I.V. solution.

   Available: 2,500 U/mL.

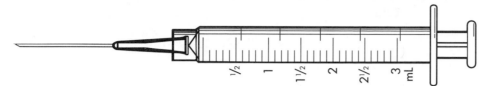

10 Order: Heparin 17,000 U s.c. o.d.

   Available: Heparin labeled 20,000 U/mL.

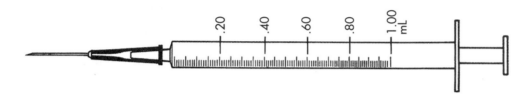

11. Order: Heparin bolus of 8,500 U I.V. stat.

   Available: 10,000 U/mL.

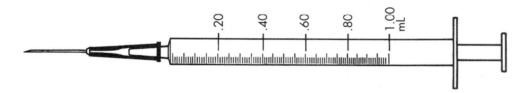

12. Order: Heparin 2,500 U s.c. q12h.

   Available: Heparin labeled 10,000 U/mL.

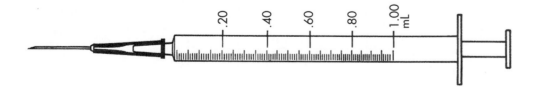

13. Order: Heparin 2,000 U/hr I.V. You have 25,000 U of heparin in 1,000 mL of 0.9% NS.

    a) How many mL/hr will deliver
    2,000 U/hr?   _____

14. Order: Heparin 1,500 U/hr I.V. Available: 25,000 U of heparin in 500 mL D5W.

    a) How many mL/hr will deliver
    1,500 U/hr?   _____

15. Order: Heparin 1,800 U/hr I.V. Available: 25,000 U heparin in 250 mL D5W.

    a) How many mL/hr will deliver
    1,800 U/hr?   _____

16. Order: 40,000 U heparin in 1 L 0.9% NS and infuse at 25 mL/hr.

    a) Calculate the hourly heparin dose (U/hr).   _____

17. Order: Heparin 25,000 U in 250 mL D5W and infuse at 11 mL/hr.

    a) Calculate the hourly heparin dose (U/hr).   _____

18. Order: Heparin 40,000 U in 500 mL D5W and infuse at 30 mL/hr.

    a) Calculate the hourly heparin dose (U/hr).   _____

19. Order: Heparin 20,000 U in 500 mL D5W to infuse at 12 mL/hr.

    a) Calculate the hourly heparin dose (U/hr).   _____

20. Order: Heparin 25,000 U in 500 mL D5W to infuse at 15 mL/hr.

    a) Calculate the hourly heparin dose (U/hr).   _____

21. Order: 1 L of 0.9% NS with 40,000 U heparin over 24 hr. Drop factor: 15 gtt/mL.

    a) Calculate the hourly dose of heparin (U/hr). _____

    b) Calculate the gtt/min.   _____

22. Order: 1 L of D5W with 15,000 U heparin over 10 hr. Calculate the following:

    a) mL/hr   _____

    b) U/hr   _____

23. Order: 1 L D5W with 35,000 U of heparin at 20 mL/hr. Calculate the following using a microdrop administration set:

    a) hourly dose (U/hr)   _____

    b) gtt/min   _____

24. Order: 500 mL of 0.9% NS with 10,000 U heparin at 20 gtt/min. (20 macrogtt/min). Drop factor: 10 gtt/mL. Calculate the following:

    a) mL/hr   _____

    b) hourly unit dose (U/hr)   _____

25. 500 mL of D5W with 25,000 U heparin at 25 mL/hr.

    a) Calculate the hourly unit dose
       of heparin (U/hr).   _____

26. Order: 500 mL of D5W with 20,000 U heparin at 40 mL/hr.

    a) Calculate the hourly unit dose (U/hr).   _____

27. Order: Infuse 1,400 U/hr of heparin I.V. Heparin 40,000 U in 1,000 mL of D5W. The administration set delivers 15 gtt/mL. Calculate the following:

    a) mL/hr   _____

    b) gtt/min   _____

28. Order: Heparin 40,000 U I.V. in IL 0.9% NS at 1,000 U/hr. Drop factor: 15 gtt/mL. Calculate the following:

    a) mL/hr   _____

    b) gtt/min   _____

29. Order: 1,000 U heparin I.V. qh. Solution available is 25,000 U of heparin in 500 mL D5W. The administration set is a microdrop.

    a) Calculate the gtt/min.   _____

30. Order: Administer 2,000 U heparin I.V. every hour. Solution available is 25,000 U of heparin in 1 L 0.9% NS. Drop factor: 15 gtt/mL.

    a) Calculate the gtt/min.   _____

31. A client is receiving an I.V. of 1,000 mL of D5W with 50,000 U heparin infusing at 15 gtt/min (15 macrogtt/min). Drop factor: 15 gtt/mL.

    a) Calculate the hourly dose of heparin the
       client is receiving (U/hr).   _____

32. A client is receiving an I.V. of 250 mL 0.45% NS with 25,000 U heparin at 20 gtt/min (20 macrogtt/min). Drop factor: 10 gtt/mL.

    a) Calculate the hourly dose of heparin (U/hr). _____

Notes

33. A client is receiving 500 mL of D5W with 20,000 U of heparin at 20 gtt/min (20 macrogtt/min). Drop factor: 60 gtt/mL (microdrop).

   a) Calculate the hourly dose of heparin (U/hr). _____

34. A client is receiving an I.V. of 25,000 U heparin in 1 L of D5W infusing at 14 gtt/min (14 macrogtt/min). Drop factor: 15 gtt/mL.

   a) Calculate the hourly dose of heparin (U/hr). _____

35. A client is receiving an I.V. of 1,000 mL D5W with 20,000 U heparin infusing at 24 gtt/min (24 macrogtt/min). Drop factor: 10 gtt/mL.

   a) Calculate the hourly dose of heparin (U/hr). _____

Calculate the following hourly doses of heparin (U/hr).

36. Order: 30,000 U of heparin in 500 mL of D5W
    to infuse at 25 mL/hr.   _____

37. Order: 20,000 U of heparin in 1 L of D5W
    to infuse at 40 mL/hr.   _____

38. Order: 40,000 U of heparin in
    500 mL 0.45% NS to infuse at 25 mL/hr.   _____

39. Order: 35,000 U of heparin in 1 L of D5W
    to infuse at 20 mL/hr.   _____

40. Order: 25,000 U of heparin in 1 L of D5W
    to infuse at 30 mL/hr.   _____

41. Order: 40,000 U of heparin in 1 L of D5W
    to infuse at 30 mL/hr.   _____

42. Order: 20,000 U of heparin in 1 L of D5W
    to infuse at 80 mL/hr.   _____

43. Order: 50,000 U of heparin in 1 L of D5W
    to infuse at 70 mL/hr.   _____

44. Order: 20,000 U of heparin in
    500 mL 0.45% NS to infuse at 30 mL/hr.   _____

45. Order: 30,000 U of heparin in 1 L of D5W
    at 25 mL/hr.   _____

Calculate the following U/hr, and determine if within the normal daily range (heparinizing). If not, state your course of action.

46. Order: 1 L D5 0.9% N.S. with heparin 50,000 U to infuse at 40 mL/hr.

    a) _____ U/hr

    b) _____ U/24hr

    c) _____ Within normal range?

47. Order: 500 mL D5W with heparin 30,000 U to infuse at 15 mL/hr.

    a) _____ U/hr

    b) _____ U/24hr

    c) _____ Within normal range?

Answers on pp. 573-579

Critical Care Calculations

The content in this chapter may not be required as part of the nursing curriculum. It is included as a reference for nurses working in specialty areas.

This chapter will provide basic information on medicated I.V. drips and titration. Critically ill clients receive medications that are potent and require close monitoring. Because of the potency of the medications and their tendency to induce changes in blood pressure and heart rate, accurate calculation of doses is essential. Medications in the critical care area can be ordered by mL/hr, gtt/min, mcg/kg/min, or mg/hr. Infusion pumps and volume control devices are usually used to administer these medications. The process of administering calculated doses of potent drugs is referred to as *titration*. Examples of medicated I.V. drips that require titration are Aramine, nitroprusside, Levophed, and epinephrine.

Titrated medications are added to a specific volume of fluid and then adjusted to infuse at the rate at which the desired effect is obtained. **The drugs that are titrated are potent antiarrhythmic, vasopressor, and vasodilator medications; they must be monitored very carefully by the nurse.** Due to the potency of medications used, minute changes in the infusion can cause an effect on the client. Infusion pumps are used for titration; when one is not available, a microdrip set calibrated at 60 gtt/mL must be used.

An example of an order that involves titration of medication is "Titrate sodium nitroprusside (Nipride) to maintain the client's blood pressure below 140 mm Hg." The nurse may start, for example, at 3 mcg/kg/min and gradually increase the rate until the systolic blood pressure is maintained below 140 mm Hg. Each time there is a change in rate, the dose of medication the client receives is changed; therefore it is essential that the dose be recalculated each time the nurse changes the rate.

Remember: Because electronic devices are routinely used or a microdrip set (60 gtt/mL), if one is not available it is important to remember that mL/hr is the same as gtt/min.

CALCULATING mL/hr RATE

Calculating mL/hr from a drug dosage ordered I.V. is one of the most common calculations the nurse encounters. Let's look at some examples illustrating this before getting into other calculations that may be done.

Example 1: A solution of trandate (Labetalol) 100 mg/100 mL D5W is to infuse at a rate of 25 mg/hr. Calculate the mL/hr.

Calculate the mL/hr using the solution strength available.

$$100 \text{ mg} : 100 \text{ mL} = 25 \text{ mg} : x \text{ mL}$$

$$100x = 100 \times 25$$

$$\frac{100x}{100} = \frac{2{,}500}{100}$$

$$x = 25 \text{ mg/hr}$$

To infuse 25 mg/hr, set the I.V. rate at 25 mL/hr.

Example 2: A solution of Isuprel 2 mg/250 mL D5W is to infuse at a rate of 5 mcg/min.

Step 1: Calculate the dose per hr.

$$60 \text{ minutes} = 1 \text{ hr}$$

$$5 \text{ mcg/min} \times 60 \text{ min} = 300 \text{ mcg/hr}$$

Step 2: Convert 300 mcg to mg to match the available strength.

$$1000 \text{ mcg} = 1 \text{ mg}$$

$$300 \text{ mcg} = 0.3 \text{ mg}$$

Step 3: Calculate the mL/hr

$$2 \text{mg} : 250 \text{ mL} = 0.3 \text{ mg} : x \text{ mL}$$

$$2x = 250 \times 0.3$$

$$\frac{2x}{2} = \frac{75}{2}$$

$$x = 37.5 = 38 \text{ mL/hr}$$

Note:

Conversions may be made from solution strength to dosage ordered, or the opposite.

To infuse 5 mcg/min, set the I.V. rate at 38 mL/hr.

❙ Remember: Ratio–proportions can be set up using several formats.

Now that you've seen examples of calculating mL/hr rate, let's look at some other calculations.

CALCULATING CRITICAL CARE DOSES PER HOUR OR PER MINUTE

Example 1: Infuse dopamine 400 mg in 500 mL D5W at 30 mL/hr. Calculate the dose in mcg/min and mcg/hr.

→ Solution:

1. Use ratio-proportion to determine the dose per hour first.

$$400 \text{ mg} : 500 \text{ mL} = x \text{ mg} : 30 \text{ mL}$$

$$\underbrace{\phantom{400 \text{ mg} : 500 \text{ mL}}}_{\text{known}} \qquad \underbrace{\phantom{x \text{ mg} : 30 \text{ mL}}}_{\text{unknown}}$$

$$500x = 400 \times 30$$

$$500x = 12,000$$

$$x = \frac{12,000}{500}$$

$$x = 24 \text{ mg/hr}$$

2. The next step is to convert 24 mg to mcg, because the question asked for mcg/min and mcg/hr. Change mg to mcg by using the equivalent 1,000 mcg = 1 mg. To change mg to mcg multiply by 1,000 or, because it's a metric measure, move the decimal point three places to the right.

$$24 \text{ mg} = 24,000 \text{ mcg/hr}$$

3. Now that you have the mcg per hour, the next step is to change mcg/hr to mcg/min. This is done by dividing the number of mcg/hr by 60 (60 minutes = 1 hour).

$$24,000 \text{ mcg/hr} \div 60 = 400 \text{ mcg/min}$$

Remember, accurate math is essential because these medications are extremely potent.

DRUGS ORDERED IN MILLIGRAMS PER MINUTE

Drugs such as lidocaine and Pronestyl are ordered in mg/min.

Example 2: A client is receiving Pronestyl at 60 mL/hr. The solution available is Pronestyl 2 g in 500 mL D5W. Calculate the mg/hr and the mg/min the client will receive.

1. A conversion is necessary; g has to be converted to mg. This is what you are being asked for (mg/min, mg/hr).

$$\text{Equivalent: } 1 \text{ g} = 1,000 \text{ mg}$$

Therefore 2 g = 2,000 mg (1,000 × 2)

2. Now determine the mg/hr by setting up a proportion.

$$2,000 \text{ mg} : 500 \text{ mL} = x \text{ mg} : 60 \text{ mL}$$

$$500x = 2,000 \times 60$$

$$\frac{500x}{500} = \frac{120,000}{500}$$

$$x = 240 \text{ mg/hr}$$

3. Convert mg/hr to mg/min.

$$240 \text{ mg/hr} \div 60 = 4 \text{ mg/min}$$

CALCULATING DOSES BASED ON mcg/kg/min

Drugs are also ordered for clients based on dose per kg per minute. These drugs include Nipride, dopamine, and dobutamine, for example.

Example 3:   Order: Dopamine 2 mcg/kg/min. The solution available is 400 mg in 250 mL D5W. The client weighs 150 lb.

1. Convert the client's weight in lb to kg.

$$2.2 \text{ lb} = 1 \text{ kg}$$

To convert the client's weight divide 150 lb by 2.2.

$$150 \text{ lb} \div 2.2 = 68.18 \text{ kg} = 68 \text{ kg}$$

2. Now that you have the client's weight in kg, determine the dose per minute.

$$68 \text{ kg} \times 2 \text{ mcg} = 136 \text{ mcg/min}$$

TITIRATION OF INFUSIONS

As already mentioned, critical care medications are ordered within parameters to obtain a desirable response in a client. When a solution is titrated, **the lowest dose of the medication is set first** and increased or decreased as necessary. **The higher dose should not be exceeded without a new order.**

Example: Nipride has been ordered to titrate at 3-6 mcg/kg/min to maintain a client's systolic blood pressure below 140 mm Hg. The solution contains 50 mg Nipride in 250 mL D5W. The client weighs 56 kg. Determine the flow rate setting for a volumetric pump.

1. Convert to **like units.**
    Equivalent: 1,000 mcg = 1 mg
    Therefore 50 mg = 50,000 mcg

2. Calculate the concentration of solution in mcg/mL.

$$50,000 \text{ mcg} : 250 \text{ mL} = x \text{ mcg} : 1 \text{ mL}$$

$$\frac{250x}{250} = \frac{50,000}{250}$$

$$x = 200 \text{ mcg/mL}$$

The concentration of solution is 200 mcg/mL.

3. Calculate the dose range using the upper and lower doses.

$$(\text{Lower dose}) \ 3 \text{ mcg} \times 56 \text{ kg} = 168 \text{ mcg/min}$$

$$(\text{Upper dose}) \ 6 \text{ mcg} \times 56 \text{ kg} = 336 \text{ mcg/min}$$

4. Convert dose range to mL/min.

$$(\text{Lower dose}) \ 200 \text{ mcg} : 1 \text{ mL} = 168 \text{ mcg} : x \text{ mL}$$

$$\frac{200x}{200} = \frac{168}{200}$$

$$x = 0.84 \text{ mL/min}$$

$$(\text{Upper dose}) \ 200 \text{ mcg} : 1 \text{ mL} = 336 \text{ mcg} : x \text{ mL}$$

$$\frac{200x}{200} = \frac{336}{200}$$

$$x = 1.68 \text{ mL/min}$$

5. Convert mL/min to mL/hr.

$$(\text{Lower dose}) \ 0.84 \text{ mL} \times 60 \text{ min} = 50.4 = 50 \text{ mL/hr (gtt/min)}$$

$$(\text{Upper dose}) \ 1.68 \text{ mL} \times 60 \text{ min} = 100.8 = 101 \text{ mL/hr (gtt/min)}$$

A dose range of 3 to 6 mcg/kg/min is equal to a flow rate of 50 to 101 mL/hr (gtt/min). The client has stabilized and is now maintained at 60 mL/hr. What dose will be infusing per minute?

$$200 \text{ mcg} : 1 \text{ mL} = x \text{ mcg} : 60 \text{ mL}$$

$$x = 12{,}000 \text{ mcg/hr}$$

$$12{,}000 \text{ mcg} \div 60 \text{ min} = 200 \text{ mcg/min}$$

PRACTICE PROBLEMS

1. A client weighing 50 kg is to receive a Dobutrex solution of 250 mg in 500 mL D5W ordered to titrate between 2.5-5 mcg/kg/min

   a) Determine the flow rate setting
   for a volumetric pump.   _____

   b) If the client's rate is being maintained
   at 25 mL/hr after several titrations,
   what is the dose infusing per minute?   _____

2. Order: Epinephrine at 30 mL/hr. The solution available is 2 mg of epinephrine in 250 mL D5W. Calculate the following:

   a) mg/hr   _____

   b) mcg/hr   _____

   c) mcg/min   _____

3. Aminophylline 0.25 g is added to 500 mL D5W to infuse in 8 hrs. Calculate the following:

   a) mg/hr   _____

   b) mg/min   _____

4. Order: Pitocin at 15 microgtts/min. The solution contains 10 U Pitocin in 1,000 mL D5W.

   a) Calculate the number of units per hour
   the client is receiving.   _____

5. Order: 3 mcg/kg/min of Nipride.
   Available: 50 mg of Nipride in 250 mL D5W. Client's weight is 60 kg.

   a) Calculate the flow rate in mL/hr that
   will deliver this dose.   _____

6. A nitroglycerin drip is infusing at 3 mL/hr. The solution available is 50 mg of nitroglycerin in 250 mL D5W. Calculate the following:

   a) mcg/hr   _____

   b) mcg/min   _____

Answers on pp. 579-580

Notes

POINTS TO REMEMBER

- When calculating doses to be administered without any type of electronic infusion pump, always use microgtt tubing (60 gtt = 1 mL). This is preferred because the drops are smaller, so more accurate titration is possible.

- The safest way to administer medications is by an infusion device.

- Calculate doses accurately. Double checking math calculations helps ensure a proper dose.

- Obtain an accurate weight of your client.

- Before determining mL/hr or gtt/min, calculate the dose first.

- Use a calculator whenever possible.

- Use an infusion pump for titration of I.V. drugs in mL/hr.

 ## CHAPTER REVIEW

Calculate the doses as indicated. Use the labels where provided.

1. Client is receiving Isuprel at 30 mL/hr. The solution available is 2 mg of Isuprel in 250 mL D5W. Calculate the following:

   a) mg/hr   _____

   b) mcg/hr   _____

   c) mcg/min   _____

2. Client is receiving epinephrine at 40 mL/hr. The solution available is 4 mg of epinephrine in 500 mL D5W. Calculate the following:

   a) mg/hr   _____

   b) mcg/hr   _____

   c) mcg/min   _____

3. Infuse dopamine 800 mg in 500 mL D5W at 30 mL/hr. Calculate the dose in mcg/hr and mcg/min.

a) mcg/hr   _____

b) mcg/min   _____

c) Calculate the number of mL you will add
to the I.V. for this dose.   _____

```
EXP.  LOT   NDC 0641-0112-25      POTENT DRUG: MUST DILUTE BEFORE USING
            25 x 5 mL Single Use Vials   Each mL contains dopamine hydrochloride 40 mg (equivalent
            DOPAMINE                 to 32.3 mg dopamine base) and sodium bisulfite 10 mg in
            HCl INJECTION, USP       Water for Injection.  pH 2.5-5.0.  Sealed under nitrogen.
            200 mg/5 mL              USUAL DOSE:  See package insert.
                                     Do not use if solution is discolored.
            (40 mg/mL)               Store at 15° - 30° C (59° - 86° F).
            FOR IV INFUSION ONLY     Caution:  Federal  law  prohibits  dispensing  without
                                     prescription.                          B-50112c
            eSi  ELKINS-SINN, INC. Cherry Hill, NJ 08003-4099
                 A subsidiary of A. H. Robins Company
```

4. Infuse Nipride at 30 mL/hr. The solution available is 50 mg sodium nitroprusside in D5W 250 mL. Calculate the following:

a) mcg/hr   _____

b) mcg/min   _____

```
Protect from light.     a  2 mL Single-dose Fliptop Vial  NDC 0074-3024-01
Exp.                    NITROPRESS®
                        Sodium Nitroprusside Injection
Lot                     50 mg / 2 mL Vial  (25 mg/mL)
                        FOR I.V. INFUSION ONLY.
                        Monitor blood pressure before and during
                        administration.   06-7378-2/R2-12/93
                        ABBOTT LABS, NORTH CHICAGO, IL 60064, USA
```

5. Order: 100 mg Aramine in 250 mL D5W to infuse at 25 mL/hr. Calculate the following:

a) mcg/hr   _____

b) mcg/min   _____

```
                        MSD     NDC 0006-3222-10
                              10 mL INJECTION
                              ARAMINE®
                              (METARAMINOL
                              BITARTRATE, MSD)
                              1% Metaraminol Equivalent
                                 10 mg per mL
                              MERCK SHARP & DOHME
                              DIVISION OF MERCK & CO., INC.
                              WEST POINT, PA 19486, USA
                                                          MULTIPLE DOSE VIAL   Lot   Exp.
```

6. Order: Lidocaine 2 g in 250 mL D5W to infuse at 60 mL/hr. Calculate the following:

a) mg/hr   _____

b) mg/min   _____

7. Order: Aminophylline 0.25 g to be added to 250 mL of D5W. The order is to infuse over 6 hrs.

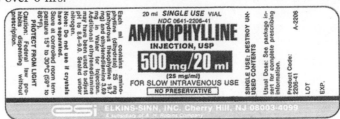

  a) Calculate the mg/hr the client will receive. _____

8. A client is receiving Pronestyl at 30 mL/hr. The solution available is 2 g Pronestyl in 250 mL D5W. Calculate the following:

  a) mg/hr   _____

  b) mg/min   _____

9. Order: Pitocin (oxytocin) drip at 45 microgtts/min. The solution available is 20 U Pitocin in 1,000 mL D5W. Calculate the following:

  Available:

  a) U/min   _____

  b) U/hr   _____

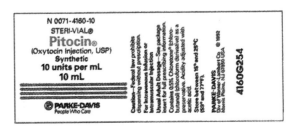

10. Order: 30 U Pitocin (oxytocin) in 1,000 mL D5W. Client is receiving oxytocin 40 mL/hr.

  a) How many U/hr of oxytocin is the
     client receiving?   _____

11. 30 units of Pitocin are added to 500 mL D5RL for an induction. The client is receiving 45 mL/hr.

  a) How many U/hr of Pitocin is the
     client receiving?   _____

12. A client is receiving bretylium at 30 microgtt/min. The solution available is 2 g bretylium in 500 mL D5W. Calculate the following:

  a) mg/hr   _____

  b) mg/min   _____

13. A client is receiving bretylium at 45 microgtts/min. The solution available is 2 g bretylium in 500 mL D5W. Calculate the following:

    a) mg/hr   _____

    b) mg/min   _____

14. A client is receiving nitroglycerin 50 mg in 250 mL D5W. The order is to infuse 500 mcg/min.

    a) How many mL/hr would be needed
       to deliver this amount?   _____

15. Dopamine has been ordered to maintain a client's b/p; 400 mg dopamine has been placed in 500 mL D5W to infuse at 35 mL/hr.

    a) How many mg are being administered
       per hour?   _____

16. Order: A client is receiving Isuprel 2 mg in 250 mL D5W. The order is to infuse at 30 mL/hr. Calculate the following:

    a) mg/hr   _____

    b) mcg/hr   _____

    c) mcg/min   _____

17. Order: 1 g of aminophylline in 1,000 mL D5W to infuse over 10 hrs.

    a) Calculate the mg/hr the client will receive.   _____

18. Ritodrine (Yutopar) 150 mg is placed in 500 mL D5W to infuse at 30 mL/hr.

    a) Calculate the mg/hr the client is receiving.   _____

19. A client is receiving Lidocaine 2 g in 250 mL D5W. The solution is infusing at 22 mL/hr. Calculate the following:

    a) mg/hr   _____

    b) mg/min   _____

20. Order: Epinephrine 4 mg in 250 mL D5W at 8 mL/hr. Calculate the following:

    a) mcg/hr   _____

21. Order: Afronad 500 mg in 250 mL 0.9% NS at 30 mL/hr. Calculate the following:

    a) mg/hr   _____

    b) mg/min   _____

Notes

Notes

22. Order: Dobutamine 500 mg to infuse at 30 mL/hr in 500 mL D5W. Calculate the following:

    Available:

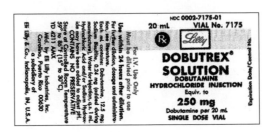

    a) mcg/hr   _____

    b) mcg/min   _____

23. Order: 2 g/hr of magnesium sulfate.

    Available: 25 g of 50% magnesium sulfate in 300 mL D5W.

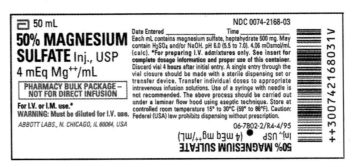

    a) How many mL/hr would be needed
       to administer the required dose?   _____

24. Order: Dopamine 400 mg in 500 mL 0.9% NS to infuse at 200 mcg/min. A volumetric pump is being used.

    a) Calculate the mL/hr.   _____

25. Order: 3 g/hr of magnesium sulfate.

    Available: 25 g of 50% magnesium sulfate in 300 mL D5W.

    a) How many mL/hr would be needed to
       administer the required dose?   _____

26. A client with chest pain has an order for nitroglycerin 50 mg in 250 mL D5W at 10 mcg/min.

    a) Calculate the I.V. rate in gtt/min using
       a microdrop administration set.   _____

27. Order: Nipride 50 mg in 250 mL D5W to infuse at 2 mcg/kg/min. Client's weight is 120 lb.

    a) Calculate the dose per minute.   _____

28. Order: Dobutrex 250 mg in 500 mL of D5W at 3 mcg/kg/min. The client weighs 80 kg.

    a) How many mcg/min should the
       client receive?   _____

29. Order: Infuse 500 mL D5W with 800 mg theophylline at 0.7 mg/kg/hr. The client weighs 73.5 kg.

    a) How many mg should this patient
       receive per hour?   _____

30. Order: Infuse 1 g of aminophylline in 1,000 mL of D5W at 0.7 mg/kg/hr. The client weighs 110 lb.

    a) Calculate the dose in mg/hr.   _____

    b) Calculate the dose in mg/min.   _____

    c) Reference states no more than 20 mg/min.
       Is the order safe?   _____

31. Norepinephrine (Levophed) 2-6 mcg/min has been ordered to maintain a client's systolic blood pressure at 100. The solution is titrated at 2 mg in 500 mL D5W.

    a) Determine the flow rate setting for
       a volumetric pump.   _____

32. Ritodrine (Yutopar) 150 mg is diluted in 500 mL of D5W. The order is to infuse at 0.15 mg/min.

    a) Calculate the flow rate to deliver this dose
       by volumetric pump.   _____

33. Esmolol is to titrate between 50 and 75 mcg/kg/min. The client weighs 60 kg. The solution strength is 5,000 mg of Esmolol in 500 mL D5W.

    a) Determine the flow rate for a volumetric
       pump.   _____

    b) The titration rate is at 30 mL/hr. What is
       the dose infusing per minute?   _____

34. Order: Dobutamine 500 mg in 250 mL D5W to infuse at 10 mcg/kg/min. The client weighs 65 kg.

    a) Calculate the flow rate in mL/hr (gtt/min).   _____

35. Aminophylline 0.25g is added to 250 mL D5W. The order is to infuse over 6 hr.

    a) Calculate the mg/hr the client will receive.   _____

Notes

36. A client is receiving Lidocaine 1 g in 500 mL D5W at a rate of 20 mL/hr. Calculate the following:

    a) mg/hr   _____

    b) mg/min   _____

37. A client is receiving Septra 300 mg in 500 mL D5W (based on trimethoprim) at a rate of 15 gtt/min (15 microgtt/min). The tubing is a microdrop (60 gtt/mL). Calculate the following:

    a) mg/min   _____

    b) mg/hr   _____

38. Esmolol 1.5 g in 250 mL D5W has been ordered at a rate of 100 mcg/kg/min for a client weighing 102.4 kg. Determine the following:

    a) mcg/min dosage   _____

    b) mL/hr   _____

39. Dopamine 400 mg in 500 mL D5W to infuse at 20 mL/hr. Determine the following:

    a) mg/min   _____

    b) mcg/min   _____

40. A client has an order for Amrinone 250 mg in 250 mL 0.9% NS at 3 mcg/kg/min. Client's weight is 59.1 kg. Determine the flow rate in mL/hr.

                                      _____

41. Inocar 250 mg in 250 mL of 0.9% NS to infuse at a rate of 5 mcg/kg/min is ordered for a client weighing 165 lb. Calculate the following:

    a) mcg/min   _____

    b) mcg/hr   _____

    c) mL/hr   _____

Answers on pp. 580-585

Dimensional Analysis

Objectives

After reviewing this chapter, you should be able to:

1. **Define dimensional analysis**
2. **Implement unit cancellation in dimensional analysis**
3. **Perform conversions using dimensional analysis**
4. **Use dimensional analysis to calculate doses**
5. **Calculate I.V. flow rates using dimensional analysis (gtt/min)**

UNDERSTANDING DIMENSIONAL ANALYSIS

Dimensional analysis is the use of a simple technique with a fancy name for the process of manipulating units. By manipulating units you are able to eliminate or cancel unwanted units. It is considered to be a common-sense approach that eliminates the need to memorize a formula.

Dimensional analysis is also referred to as the *factor-label method* or the *unit factor method.* Dimensional analysis can be viewed as a problem-solving method. The advantage of dimensional analysis is that because only one equation is needed, it eliminates memorization of formulas. Dimensional analysis can be used for all calculations you may encounter once you become comfortable with the process. This chapter will discuss dimensional analysis and provide examples of how it might be used in calculations. Although some may find the formalism of the term *dimensional analysis* intimidating at first, you will find it's quite simple once you have worked a few problems. This chapter will demonstrate the use of dimensional analysis in making conversions and calculating doses. This method as stated can be used for all calculations, including I.V. calculations. Note: Remember, as stated in the discussion of calculation methods, it is important that you understand that you as the learner must choose a method of calculation you're comfortable with and use it consistently.

UNDERSTANDING THE BASICS OF DIMENSIONAL ANALYSIS

To introduce the basics relating to dimensional analysis, let's begin by looking at how the process works in making conversions before we look at its use in calculating doses. As you recall from previous chapters, you learned what was referred to as *equivalents* or *conversion factors.* For example 1 g = 1,000 mg, 1 grain = 60 mg. When we begin using this process for dosage calculations, you will quickly see how dimensional analysis allows multiple factors to be entered in one equation. This method is particularly useful when you have a medication ordered in one unit and it's available in another. Although multiple factors can be placed in a dimensional analysis equation, you can decide to do the conversion before you set up the equation using one of the methods learned in earlier chapters, or by using dimensional analysis to perform the conversion before calculating the dose.

Performing Conversions Using Dimensional Analysis

The equivalents or conversion factors you learned can be written in a fraction format, which is important to understand in using dimensional analysis. Let's look at the equivalent 1 kg = 1,000 mg.

This can be written as:

$$\frac{1 \text{ kg}}{1,000 \text{ g}} \quad \text{or} \quad \frac{1,000 \text{ g}}{1 \text{ kg}}$$

Now let's look at the basics in using dimensional analysis for converting units of measure. It is necessary to state the equivalent (conversion factor) in fraction format maintaining the desired unit in the numerator.

An equivalent (conversion factor) will give you two fractions:

Example: $2.2 \text{ lb} = 1 \text{ kg} = \dfrac{2.2 \text{ lb}}{1 \text{ kg}} \quad \text{or} \quad \dfrac{1 \text{ kg}}{2.2 \text{ lb}}$

$1,000 \text{ mcg} = 1 \text{ mg} = \dfrac{1,000 \text{ mcg}}{1 \text{ mg}} \quad \text{or} \quad \dfrac{1 \text{ mg}}{1,000 \text{ mcg}}$

To Make Conversions Using Dimensional Analysis:

1. Identify the desired unit.
2. Identify the equivalent needed.
3. Write the equivalent in fraction format, keeping the desired unit in the numerator of the fraction. This is written first in the equation.
4. Label all factors in the equation and label what you desire x (unit desired).
5. Identify unwanted or undesired units and cancel them.
6. If all the labels but the answer label are not eliminated, recheck the equation.
7. Perform the mathematical process indicated.

> ## ❗ Critical Thinking
>
> Stating the equivalent incorrectly will not allow you to eliminate desired units. Knowing when the equation is set up correctly is an important part of the concept of dimensional analysis.

Let's look at examples to demonstrate the dimensional analysis process.

Example 1:   1.5 g = _____ mg

1. The desired unit is mg.
2. Equivalent: 1,000 mg = 1 g
3. Write the equivalent keeping mg in the numerator to allow you to cancel the unwanted unit kg.
4. Write the equivalent first stated as a fraction followed by a multiplication sign (×).
5. Perform the indicated mathematical operations.

Note:

You have not changed the value of the unit, you have simply rewritten the equivalency or conversion factor in a fraction format.

Note:

How the fraction is written depends on the unit you want to cancel or eliminate to get the unit desired.

Setup:

$$x \text{ mg} = \frac{1{,}000 \text{ mg}}{1 \cancel{g}} \times 1.5 \cancel{g} \text{ OR } x \text{ mg} = \frac{1{,}000}{1\cancel{g}} = \frac{1.5 \cancel{g}}{1}$$

$$1{,}000 \times 1.5 = 1{,}500 \text{ mg}$$

$$x = 1{,}500 \text{ mg}$$

The above problem could be done by decimal movement. It is shown in this format to illustrate dimensional analysis.

Example 2:   110 lb = _____ kg
1. The desired unit is kg.
2. Equivalent: 2.2 lb = 1 kg
3. Proceed to set up the problem as outlined.

Setup:

$$x \text{ kg} = \frac{1 \text{ kg}}{2.2 \cancel{lb}} \times 110 \cancel{lb} \text{ OR } x \text{ kg} = \frac{1 \text{ kg}}{2.2 \cancel{lb}} \times \frac{110 \cancel{lb}}{1}$$

$$x = \frac{110}{2.2}$$

$$x = 50 \text{ kg}$$

Note:

Placing a one under a value doesn't alter the value of the number. What you desire or are looking for is labeled *x.*

Remember: State all answers following the rules of the system. When there is more then one equivalent for a unit of measure, use the conversion factor used most often.

 PRACTICE PROBLEMS

Set up the following problems using the dimensional analysis format, cancel the units. Do not solve.

1. 15 mg = gr   _____

2. grv =   _____ mg

3. 400 mcg =   _____ mg

4. 2 tbs =   _____ mL

5. 0.007 g =   _____ mg

6. 0.5 L =   _____ mL

7. 529 mg =   _____ g

8. 1,600 mL = _____ L

9. 46.4 kg =   _____ lb

10. 5 cm =   _____ inches

Answers on p. 585

POINTS TO REMEMBER

- Identify the desired unit and label it *x*.
- State the equivalent (conversion factor) in fraction format with the desired unit in the numerator.
- Label all factors in the equation.
- State the equivalent first in the equation followed by a × sign.
- Remember the rules relating to conversions.
- Cancel the undesired units.

DOSE CALCULATION USING DIMENSIONAL ANALYSIS

As stated previously, dimensional analysis can be used to calculate doses with the use of a single equation. A single equation can also be used to calculate a dose when the dose desired is in units that differ from the available. When using dimensional analysis to calculate doses, it is important to extract the essential information needed from the problem.

In earlier chapters relating to calculating doses you learned how to read medication labels. Remember, doses are always expressed in relation to the form or unit of measure (mL) that contains them.

Examples: 100 mg/tab, 500 mg/cap, 40 mg/2 mL.

When using dimensional analysis to calculate doses, the above examples become crucial factors in the equation and are entered as a fraction with a numerator and denominator.

Steps in Calculating Doses Using Dimensional Analysis

1. Identify the unit of measure desired in the calculation. With oral (solid) forms the unit will be tab or cap. For parenteral and oral liquids the unit is mL.
2. On the left side of the equation, place the name or appropriate abbreviation for *x*, what you desire or are looking for.
3. On the right side of the equation, place the available information from the problem in a fraction format. The abbreviation or unit matching the desired unit must be placed in the numerator.
4. Enter the additional factors from the problem, usually what is ordered. Set up the numerator so that it matches the unit in the previous denominator.
5. Cancel out the like units or abbreviations on the right side of the equation. The remaining unit should match the unit on the left side of the equation and be the unit desired.
6. Solve for the unknown *x*.

Let's look at an example using the above steps.

Example: Order: Lasix 40 mg p.o. q.d.

Available: Tablets labeled 20 mg.

1. Place the unit of measure desired in the calculation on the left side of the equation and label it *x*.

$$x \text{ tab} =$$

2. Place the information from the problem on the right side of the equation in a fraction format with the unit matching the desired unit in the numerator. (In this problem each tab contains 20 mg.)

$$x \text{ tab} = \frac{1 \text{ tab}}{20 \text{ mg}}$$

3. Enter the additional factors from the problem, what is ordered, matching the numerator in the previous denominator (in the problem the order is 40 mg). Placing a 1 under it doesn't change the value.

$$x \text{ tab} = \frac{1 \text{ tab}}{20 \text{ mg}} \times \frac{40 \text{ mg}}{1}$$

4. Cancel the like units on the right side of the equation. The remaining unit should be what is desired, and match the unit on the left side.

$$x \text{ tab} = \frac{1 \text{ tab}}{20 \text{ m\!g}} \times \frac{40 \text{ m\!g}}{1}$$

$$x = \frac{1 \times 40}{20}$$

$$x = \frac{40}{20}$$

$$x = 2 \text{ tabs}$$

Note:

When mg was canceled you were left with tabs.

Now let's look at an example with parenteral medications. You would follow the same steps illustrated in Example 1.

Example 2: Order: Gentamicin 55 mg I.M. q8h

Available: Gentamicin 80 mg/2mL

1. On the left side of the equation place the unit desired in this problem (mL).

$$x \text{ mL} =$$

2. On the right side place the available information from the problem in fraction format, placing the unit matching the desired in the numerator.

$$x \text{ mL} = \frac{2 \text{ mL}}{80 \text{ mg}}$$

3. Enter the additional factors from the problem, what is ordered matching the numerator in the previous denominator (in this problem the order is 55 mg).

$$x \text{ mL} = \frac{2 \text{ mL}}{80 \text{ mg}} \times \frac{55 \text{ mg}}{1}$$

4. Cancel out the like units on the right side of the equation. The remaining unit should match the unit on the left side of the equation and be the unit desired.

$$x \text{ mL} = \frac{2 \text{ mL}}{80 \text{ mg}} \times \frac{55 \text{ mg}}{1}$$

$$x = \frac{2 \times 55}{80}$$

$$x = \frac{110}{80} = 1.37$$

$$x = 1.4 \text{ mL}$$

As previously mentioned, dimensional analysis can be used when a drug is ordered in one unit and available in another, thereby necessitating a conversion. However, the same steps are followed as previously shown.

- An additional fraction is entered into the equation as the second fraction. This fraction is the equivalent or the conversion factor needed. The numerator has to match the unit of the previous denominator.
- The last fraction is the drug ordered. This is written so that the numerator of the fraction matches the unit in the denominator of the fraction immediately before.

Let's look at an example:

Example 3: Order: Ampicillin 0.5 g I.M. q6h

Available: Ampicillin labeled 250 mg/mL

1. On the left side of the equation, place the unit of measure desired in the calculation and label it *x*.

$$x \text{ mL} =$$

2. Place the information from the problem on the right side of the equation in a fraction format, placing the unit matching the desired in the numerator.

$$x \text{ mL} = \frac{1 \text{ mL}}{250 \text{ mg}}$$

3. The order is for 0.5 g and the medication is available in 250 mg; a conversion is therefore needed.

From previous chapters we know 1 g = 1,000 mg; this fraction is placed next in the form of a fraction (the numerator of the fraction must match the denominator of the immediate previous fraction).

$$x \text{ mL} = \frac{1 \text{ mL}}{250 \text{ mg}} \times \frac{1,000 \text{ mg}}{1 \text{ g}}$$

4. Next place the amount of drug ordered in the equation. This will match the denominator of the fraction immediately before. In this problem it's 0.5 g.

$$x \text{ mL} = \frac{1 \text{ mL}}{250 \text{ mg}} \times \frac{1,000 \text{ mg}}{1 \text{ g}} \times \frac{0.5 \text{ g}}{1}$$

5. Cancel out like units on the right side of the equation; the remaining unit should match the unit on the left side of equation and be the desired unit.

Notes

$$x \text{ mL} = \frac{1 \text{ mL}}{250 \text{ mg}} \times \frac{1{,}000 \text{ mg}}{1 \text{ g}} \times \frac{0.5 \text{ g}}{1}$$

$$x = \frac{1{,}000 \times 0.5}{250}$$

$$x = \frac{500}{250}$$

$$x = 2 \text{ mL}$$

POINTS TO REMEMBER

- Incorrect placement of units can give an incorrect answer. Even when calculating with dimensional analysis, thinking and reasoning are essential. Follow guidelines presented relating to dosage calculation.

- Use one method consistently, depending on the method that makes sense to you.

PRACTICE PROBLEMS

Set up the following problems using dimensional analysis. Do not solve.

11. A dose strength of 0.3 g has been ordered.

    Available: 0.4 g/1.5 mL.

12. A dose strength of gr $^1/_4$ is ordered.

    Available: 15 mg/mL.

13. Order: Ampicillin 1 g p.o. stat.

    Available: Ampicillin capsules labeled 500 mg.

14. Order: Augmentin 400 mg p.o. q8h.

    Available: Augmentin oral suspension 400 mg/5 mL.

15. Order: Zantac 150 mg I.V. qd.

    Available: Zantac 25 mg/mL.

16. Order: Aldomet 250 mg p.o. b.i.d.

    Available: Tabs labeled 125 mg.

17. Order: Digoxin 0.125 mg p.o. qd.

    Available: Scored tabs labeled 0.25 mg.

18. Order: Dilantin 300 mg p.o. t.i.d.

    Available: Dilantin oral suspension labeled 125 mg/5 mL.

19. Order: Keflex 1 g p.o. q6h.

    Available: Keflex oral suspension labeled 125 mg/5 mL.

20. Order: Clindamycin 0.3 g I.V. q6h.

    Available: Clindamycin 150 mg/mL.

Answers on p. 586

POINTS TO REMEMBER

- To avoid error, follow the steps outlined when setting up an equation to calculate a dose.
- Thinking and reasoning are necessary, even when using dimensional analysis.
- In dimensional analysis the unit desired is always written first, to the left of the equation followed by an equal sign (=).
- Conversions are made by incorporating a conversion factor stated as a fraction directly into the dimensional analysis equation.
- All factors entered in the equation must include the quantity and label.
- Apply principles learned in relation to dose calculations.

USING DIMENSIONAL ANALYSIS TO CALCULATE I.V. FLOW RATES

As you've already learned in Chapter 21 relating to calculation of intravenous solutions, there are several calculations that can be done relating to I.V. fluids. As previously stated, dimensional analysis is a process that can be used for any calculations encountered in the clinical situation. This section will focus on using dimensional analysis to calculate I.V. flow rates. Remember, it can also be used for other calculations related to I.V. therapy. Using dimensional analysis to calculate I.V. flow rates will require that you remember concepts already presented in this chapter. Let's look at calculating gtt/min using the process of dimensional analysis. Remember, I.V. fluids are ordered using small volumes of fluid that usually contain medication, or in large volumes to infuse over several hours.

Calculating Small Volumes of I.V. Fluid in gtt/min

Example 1: An I.V. medication of 50 mL is to infuse in 30 min.
Drop factor: 15 gtt/mL.

1. You are calculating gtt/min, so write gtt/min to the left of the equation followed by the equal sign (=), label gtt/min *x,* since that is what you're looking for:

$$\frac{x \text{ gtt}}{\text{min}} =$$

2. Extract the information that contains gtt from the problem; the drop factor is 15 gtt/1 mL.

   Write this factor into the equation, placing gtt in the numerator.

$$\frac{x\ \text{gtt}}{\text{min}} = \frac{15\ \text{gtt}}{1\ \text{mL}}$$

3. The next fraction is written so that the denominator matches the previous fraction. Go back to the problem and you'll see that the order is to infuse 50 mL in 30 minutes. Enter third fraction so 50 mL is in the numerator and 30 minutes is in the denominator.

$$\frac{x\ \text{gtt}}{\text{min}} = \frac{15\ \text{gtt}}{1\ \text{mL}} \times \frac{50\ \text{mL}}{30\ \text{min}}$$

4. Now that you have the completed equation, cancel the units and notice you're left with the desired gtt/min.

$$\frac{x\ \text{gtt}}{\text{min}} = \frac{15\ \text{gtt}}{1\ \text{mL}} \times \frac{50\ \text{mL}}{30\ \text{min}}$$

$$x = \frac{15 \times 50}{40} = \frac{750}{30} = 25$$

$$x = 25\ \text{gtt/min};\ 25\ \text{macrogtt/min}$$

Remember: Reducing can make numbers smaller, and you could have set this up using the shortcut method with the constant drop factor as shown in the I.V. chapter.

Calculating gtt/min Using Large Volumes of I.V. Fluid

Remember, I.V.s can be ordered in large volumes to infuse over several hours, or the large volume can be ordered by total volume to infuse and the mL/hr rate of infusion. Example: 1,000 mL D5W at a rate of 125 mL/hr. Remember that when a large volume to infuse is ordered over several hours, a preliminary step can be done to change it to mL/hr. Example: 1,000 mL D5W to infuse in 8 hr. Divide the total volume by the number of hours and get mL/hr. In this case 1,000 mL ÷ 8 = 125 mL/hr. Let's look at a calculation involving large volumes of fluid.

Example 2: Order: 1,000 mL D5W to infuse at 125 mL/hr.

  Drop factor: 20 gtt/mL.

▶ **Solution:**

Begin by converting the time in hr to minutes. 1 hr = 60 minutes. Now proceed to set up the problem in the dimensional analysis equation.

1. Enter the gtt/min being calculated first, followed by the equal sign (=).

$$\frac{x\ \text{gtt}}{\text{min}} =$$

2. Enter the drop factor (20 gtt/mL) with gtt in the numerator.

$$\frac{x\ \text{gtt}}{\text{min}} = \frac{20\ \text{gtt}}{1\ \text{mL}}$$

Notes

3. Take from the problem the amount to be administered over 1 hr (60 minutes) and write the fraction so that it matches the denominator of the fraction immediately before it.

$$\frac{x \text{ gtt}}{\text{min}} = \frac{20 \text{ gtt}}{1 \text{ mL}} \times \frac{125 \text{ mL}}{60 \text{ min}}$$

4. Now that you have the completed equation, cancel the units and proceed with the mathematical process to obtain the answer.

$$\frac{x \text{ gtt}}{\text{min}} = \frac{20 \text{ gtt}}{1 \text{ mL}} \times \frac{125 \text{ mL}}{60 \text{ min}}$$

$$x = \frac{20 \times 125}{60} = 41.6 = 42 \text{ gtt/min}$$

$$x = 42 \text{ gtt/min}; 42 \text{ macrogtt/min}$$

Note: The above problem could have been done without changing 1 hr to 60 minutes; however, if it is left as 1 hr you will need to add the additional fraction (1 hr = 60 minutes). Using the same problem the equation would be stated as follows:

$$\frac{x \text{ gtt}}{\text{min}} = \frac{20 \text{ gtt}}{1 \text{ mL}} \times \frac{125 \text{ mL}}{1 \text{ hr}} \times \frac{1 \text{ hr}}{60 \text{ min}}$$

Notice the conversion factor 1 hr = 60 minutes is written so the numerator matches the denominator of the fraction immediately before it. To solve the equation cancel units and proceed as follows:

$$\frac{x \text{ gtt}}{\text{min}} = \frac{20 \text{ gtt}}{1 \text{ mL}} \times \frac{125 \text{ mL}}{1 \text{ hr}} \times \frac{1 \text{ hr}}{60 \text{ min}}$$

$$x = \frac{20 \times 125 \times 1}{60} = 41.6 = 42 \text{ gtt/min}$$

$$x = 42 \text{ gtt/min}; 42 \text{ macrogtt/min}$$

 PRACTICE PROBLEMS

Calculate the following rates in gtt/min. Set problem up and solve using dimensional analysis.

21. D5W 100 mL to infuse in 40 minutes.

Drop factor: 15 gtt/mL. _____

22. 0.9% NS 40 mL to infuse in 30 minutes.

Drop factor: 60 gtt/mL. _____

23. D5 0.33% NS 20 mL to infuse in 1 hr.

Drop factor: 60 gtt/mL (microdrop). _____

24. R/L 150 mL/hr.

Drop factor: 15 gtt/mL. _____

25. D5W 1,500 mL/12 hr.

Drop factor: 10 gtt/mL.

_____

Notes

Answers on p. 586

POINTS TO REMEMBER

- Apply principles learned relating to I.V. therapy when using dimensional analysis to calculate.

- Reduction can be done to make numbers smaller.

- Large volumes and small volumes can be calculated in gtt/min.

- Shortcut methods learned can be used to calculate flow rates using dimensional analysis.

 ## CHAPTER REVIEW

Calculate the following drug doses using the dimensional analysis method. For injectables express your answer to the nearest tenth, as indicated.

1. Order: Antivert 25 mg p.o. o.d.

   Available: Tablets labeled 12.5 mg.   _____

2. Order: Potassium chloride 20 mEq in 1 L of D5W.

   Available: Potassium chloride 30 mEq/15 mL.   _____

3. Order: Morphine sulfate 20 mg I.M. stat.

   Available: Morphine sulfate 15 mg/mL.   _____

4. Order: Kefzol 0.5 g I.V. q6h.

   Available: Kefzol labeled 225 mg/mL.   _____

5. Order: Capoten 18.75 mg p.o. o.d.

   Available: Tablet scored in fourths labeled 25 mg.   _____

6. Order: Thiamine 80 mg I.M. stat.

   Available: Thiamine 100 mg/mL.   _____

7. Order: Heparin 6,500 U s.c. q12h.

   Available: 10,000 U/mL. (Express answer in hundredths.)   _____

8. Order: Cleocin 300 mg I.V. q6h.

    Available: Cleocin 0.6 g/4 mL.   _____

9. Order: Trandate 300 mg p.o. b.i.d.

    Available: Trandate tablets labeled 150 mg.   _____

10. Order: Solumedrol 175 mg I.V. qd.

    Available: Solumedrol labeled 62.5 mg/mL.   _____

For questions 11-15, set up the problem using dimensional analysis and make the conversion as indicated.

11. 3 qt =   _____ mL

12. 79 lb =   _____ kg

13. 5 mcg =   _____ mg

14. 2,400 mL =   _____ L

15. 8 inches =   _____ cm

Calculate the gtt/min for the following using dimensional analysis. Round gtt/min to the nearest whole number.

16. D5 R/L 75 mL/hr.

    Drop factor: 10 gtt/mL.   _____

17. D5 R/L 1,500 mL over 10 hr.

    Drop factor: 15 gtt/mL.   _____

18. D5W 100 mL/hr.

    Drop factor: 60 gtt/mL (microdrop).   _____

19. D5 0.33% NS 200 mL over 12 hr.

    Drop factor: 60 gtt/mL (microdrop).   _____

20. D5W 500 mL in 8 hr.

    Drop factor: 15 gtt/mL.   _____

Answers on pp. 586-588

Comprehensive Posttest

Solve the following calculation problems. Remember to apply the principles learned in the text relating to doses. Use labels where provided. Shade in the dose on the syringe where indicated.

1. Order: Augmentin 300 mg p.o. q8h.

   Available: _____

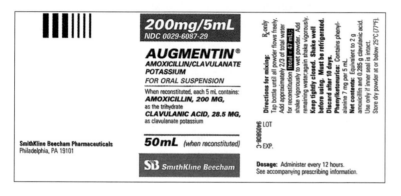

2. Order: Procan SR 1 g p.o. q6h for a client with atrial fibrillation.

   Available: Procan SR tablets 500 mg. _____

3. Order: Lanoxicaps 0.2 mg p.o. q.d.

   Available: _____

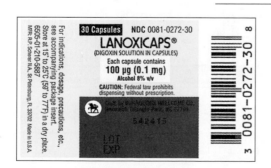

4. Order: Septra DS 1 tab p.o. q12h × 14 days.

Available:

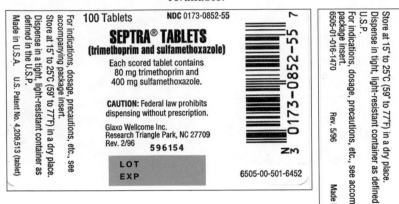

A

B

a) Indicate by letter which tablets you would
   choose to administer to the client based
   on the order and why.   _____

5. Order: Corvert 1 mg I.V. stat for a client with atrial arrhythmia; repeat in 10
   minutes if arrhythmia does not terminate.

Available: _____

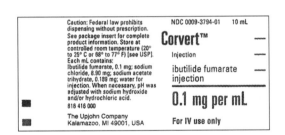

6. Order: Heparin 6,500 U s.c.o.d. (Express your answer in hundredths.)

Available: _____

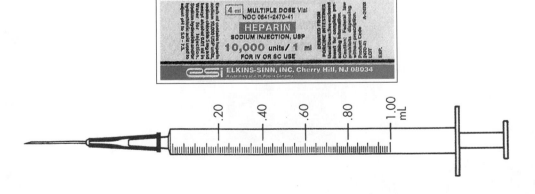

7. Order: Cipro 0.75 g I.V. q12h × 7 days.

Available: _____

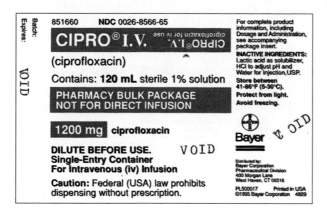

8. Order: Amphotericin B 75 mg in 1,000 mL D5W to infuse over 6 hr o.d. The reconstituted solution contains 50 mg/10 mL.

Available:

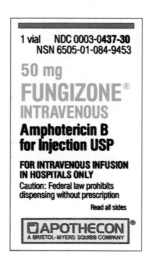

a) How many mL will you add to the I.V. solution? _____

b) The I.V. is to infuse in 6 hr. The administration set delivers 10 gtt/mL. How many gtt/min should the I.V. infuse at? _____

9. The recommended dose of Retrovir for adults with symptomatic HIV infection is 1 mg/kg infused over 1 hour q4h. Determine dose for a client weighing 110 lb.

Available: _____

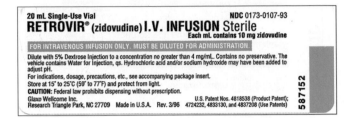

10. Order: Epivir 0.3 g p.o. q.d.

Available: _____

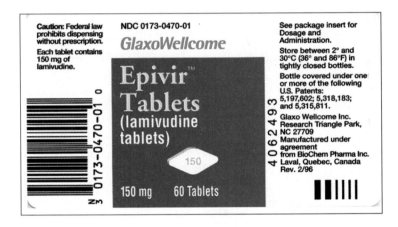

11. Order: Tazicef 0.25 g I.V. q12h.

Available:

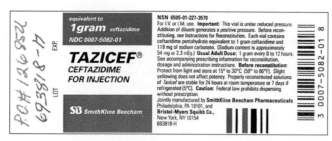

Directions for reconstitution state the following for I.V. infusion: 1-g vial, add 10 mL sterile water to provide 95 mg/mL; 2-g vial, add 10 mL sterile water to provide 180 mg/mL.

a) Using the label provided, what concentration will you prepare?   _____

b) How many mL will you administer?   _____

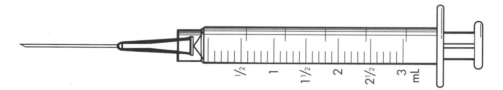

12. Order: Thorazine 75 mg p.o. b.i.d.

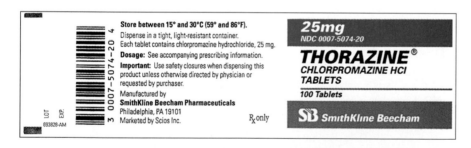

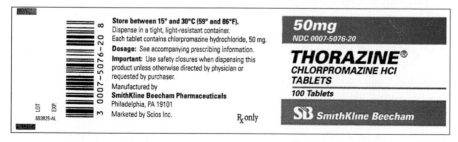

a) How many of which tablets would be best to administer to the client?   _____

13. Order: Transfuse 1 U packaged red blood
    cells (250 mL) over 3 hr. The administration
    set delivers 20 gtt/mL. How many gtt/min
    should the I.V. infuse at?   _____

14. Order: Lactated Ringer's solution 1,000 mL
    to infuse at 80 mL/hr. The administration set
    delivers 15 gtt/mL. How many gtt/min should
    the I.V. infuse at?   _____

15. A client is receiving 500 mg of Flagyl IVPB q8h.
    The Flagyl has been placed in 100 mL D5W
    to infuse over 45 minutes. The administration
    set delivers 10 gtt/mL. How many gtt/min
    should the I.V. infuse at?   _____

16. Calculate the infusion time for an I.V. of 1,000 mL
    of D5NS infusing at 60 mL/hr. Express time in
    hours and minutes.   _____

17. The doctor orders Septra Suspension 60 mg
    p.o. q12h for a child weighing 12 kg. The
    pediatric drug reference states that Septra
    Suspension contains trimethoprim (TMP)
    40 mg and sulfamethoxazole (SMZ) 200 mg
    in 5 mL oral suspension, and the safe dose
    of the medication is based on trimethorpim.
    The safe dose is 6 to 12 mg/kg/day of TMP
    given q12h. Is the dose ordered safe?   _____

18. A medicated I.V. of 100 mL is to infuse at a rate of 50 mL/hr.

    a) Determine the infusion time.   _____

    b) The I.V. was started at 10:00 AM. When
       will it be completed? (State time in military
       and traditional time.)   _____

19. A client is to receive 10 mcg/min of nitroglycerin
    I.V. The concentration of solution is 50 mg in
    250 mL D5W. What should the flow rate be
    (in mL/hr) to deliver 10 mcg/min?   _____

20. Order: Humulin Regular U-100 6 U and Humulin NPH U-100 16 U s.c. at 7:30 AM.

    What is the total volume you will administer? _____

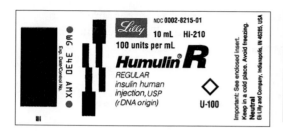 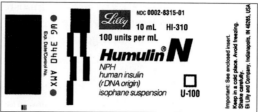

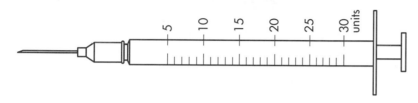

21. A dose of 500 mg in a volume of 3 mL is ordered to dilute 55 mL to infuse over 50 minutes. A 20-mL flush is to follow.

    a) What is the dilution volume? _____

    b) How many gtt/min should the I.V. infuse at? (Administration set is a microdrop.) _____

    c) Indicate the mL/hr. _____

22. Order: Zocor 40 mg p.o. q.d.

    Available:

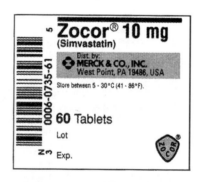

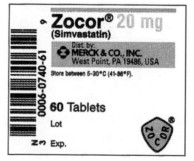

    Which strength of Zocor would you give and why? _____

23. Calculate the BSA using the formula for a child who weighs 102 lb and is 51 inches tall. Calculate the BSA to the nearest hundredth.

    _____

24. Zovirax I.V. is to be administered to a child who has herpes simplex encephalitis. The child weighs 13.6 kg and is 60 cm tall. The recommended dose is 500 mg/m². Use the formula to calculate the BSA.

Available:

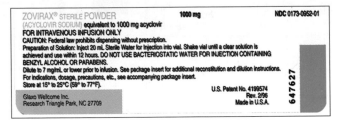

a) What is the BSA? (Express your answer to the nearest hundredth.)

    _____

b) What will the dose be? (Express your answer to the nearest tenth and whole number.)

    _____

c) The reconstituted material provides 50 mg/mL. Calculate the number of mL to administer.

    _____

25. Order: Capoten 50 mg p.o. t.i.d. Hold if systolic blood pressure (SBP) ≤ 100.

Available:

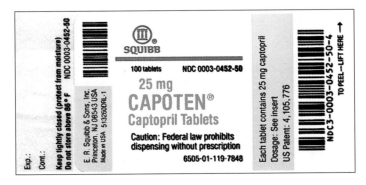

a) How many tabs will you give?

    _____

b) The client's blood pressure is 90/60. What should the nurse do?

    _____

26. Prepare the following strength solution: 2/5 strength Ensure Plus 250 mL.

    _____

27. 400 mL of Pulmocare over 6 hr via NG tube. The feeding is placed in an enteral infusion pump. Determine mL/hr. (Express your answer to nearest whole number.)

    _____

28. A medication of 1 g in 4 mL is to be diluted to 70 mL and infused over 50 minutes. A 15 mL flush follows. Medication is placed in a burette.

   a) gtt/min   _____

   b) mL/hr   _____

29. A child weighing 21.4 kg has an order for 500 mg of a medication in 100 mL D5W q12h. The normal daily dosage range is 40-50 mg/kg/day. Determine if the dose is within normal range, and state your course of action.   _____

30. Calculate the amount of dextrose and NaCl in the following I.V. solution:

   2 L of D5 1/4 NS.

   Dextrose   _____ g

   Sodium chloride   _____ g

31. 500 mL D5W was to infuse in 3 hours at 28 gtt/min (28 macrogtt/min). The drop factor is 10 gtt/mL. After 1 1/2 hours you notice 175 mL has infused. Recalculate the I.V. flow rate, determine the percentage of change, and state your course of action.   _____

32. 1,000 mL D5R/L was to infuse in 8 hours at 31 gtt/min (31 macrogtt/min). After 4 hours you notice 600 mL has infused. The administration set delivers 15 gtt/mL. Recalculate the I.V. flow rate, determine the percentage of change, and state your course of action.   _____

33. Order: Infuse D5W 500 mL with 20,000 U heparin at 25 mL/hr. Determine the following. If not within normal range, state your course of action.

   _____ U/hr

   _____ U/24 hr

   Within normal range?   _____

Answers on pp. 588-592

Answer Key

ANSWERS TO PRETEST FOR UNIT ONE

1. ix, i̅x̅, IX
2. xvi, x̅v̅i̅, XVI
3. xxiii, x̅x̅i̅i̅i̅, XXIII
4. xss, x̅s̅s̅
5. xxii, x̅x̅i̅i̅, XXII
6. $11\frac{1}{2}$
7. 12
8. 18
9. 24
10. 6
11. $\frac{2}{3}$
12. $\frac{1}{4}$
13. $\frac{1}{75}$
14. $\frac{4}{5}$
15. $\frac{4}{6} = \frac{2}{3}$

16. 2
17. $5\frac{1}{3}$
18. $\frac{23}{45}$
19. $4\frac{13}{42}$
20. $18\frac{2}{3}$
21. 0.9
22. 0.3
23. 0.7
24. 0.9
25. $\frac{7}{8}$
26. $\frac{11}{12}$
27. 87.45
28. 5.008
29. 40.112
30. 47.77

31. 1,875
32. 23.7
33. 36.8
34. 0.674
35. 0.375
36. 0.6
37. $x = 12$
38. $x = 2$
39. $x = 3$
40. $x = 0.5$ or $\frac{1}{2}$
41. 0.4
42. 0.7
43. 1.5
44. 0.74
45. 0.83
46. 1.23

	Percent	Decimal	Ratio	Fraction
47.	6%	0.06	3 : 50	$\frac{3}{50}$
48.	35%	0.35	7 : 20	$\frac{7}{20}$
49.	525%	5.25	21 : 4	$5\frac{1}{4}$
50.	1.5%	0.015	3 : 200	$\frac{3}{200}$

51. 4.75
52. 5
53. $0.3\frac{1}{3}\%$

54. 20%
55. 18.3%

CHAPTER 1

Answers to Practice Problems

1. xv, x̄v, XV
2. xiii, x̄iii, XIII
3. xxviii, x̄xviii, XXVIII
4. xi, x̄i, XI
5. xvii, x̄vii, XVII
6. xiv, x̄iv, XIV
7. xxix, x̄xix, XXIX
8. iv, īv, IV
9. xix, x̄ix, XIX
10. xxxiv, x̄xxiv, XXXIV

Answers to Chapter Review

1. vi, v̄i, VI
2. xxx, x̄xx, XXX
3. iss, īss, iss
4. xxvii, x̄xvii, XXVII
5. xii, x̄ii, XII
6. xviii, x̄viii, XVIII
7. xx, x̄x, XX
8. iii, īii, III
9. xxi, x̄xi, XXI
10. xxvi, x̄xvi, XXVI

11. $7\frac{1}{2}$
12. 19
13. 15
14. 30
15. $\frac{1}{2}$
16. 3
17. 22
18. 16
19. 5
20. 27

CHAPTER 2

Answers to Practice Problems

1. LCD = 30; therefore $\frac{6}{30}$ has the lesser value.

2. LCD = 8; therefore $\frac{6}{8}$ has the lesser value.

3. $\frac{1}{150}$ has the lesser value; the denominator (150) is larger.

4. $\frac{6}{18}$ has the lesser value; the numerator (6) is smaller.

5. $\frac{3}{5}$ has the lesser value; the numerator (3) is smaller.

6. $\frac{1}{8}$ has the lesser value; the numerator (1) is smaller.

7. $\frac{1}{40}$ has the lesser value; the denominator (40) is larger.

8. $\frac{1}{300}$ has the lesser value; the denominator (300) is larger.

9. $\frac{4}{24}$ has the lesser value; the numerator (4) is smaller.

10. LCD = 6; therefore $\frac{1}{6}$ has the lesser value.

11. LCD = 72; therefore $\frac{6}{8}$ has the higher value.

12. LCD = 6; therefore $\frac{7}{6}$ has the higher value.

13. LCD = 72; therefore $\frac{6}{12}$ has the higher value.

14. LCD = 120; therefore $\frac{1}{6}$ has the higher value.

15. $\frac{1}{75}$ has the higher value; the denominator (75) is smaller.

16. $\frac{6}{5}$ has the higher value; the numerator (6) is larger.

17. LCD $= 24$; therefore $\frac{4}{6}$ has the higher value.

18. $\frac{8}{9}$ has the higher value; the numerator (8) is larger.

19. $\frac{1}{10}$ has the higher value; the denominator (10) is smaller.

20. $\frac{6}{15}$ has the higher value; the numerator (6) is larger.

21. $\frac{10 \div 5}{15 \div 5} = \frac{2}{3}$

22. $\frac{7 \div 7}{49 \div 7} = \frac{1}{7}$

23. $\frac{64 \div 2}{128 \div 2} = \frac{32}{64} = \frac{1}{2}$

24. $\frac{100 \div 2}{150 \div 2} = \frac{50}{75} = \frac{2}{3}$

25. $\frac{20 \div 4}{28 \div 4} = \frac{5}{7}$

26. $\frac{14 \div 2}{98 \div 2} = \frac{7}{49} = \frac{1}{7}$

27. $\frac{10 \div 2}{18 \div 2} = \frac{5}{9}$

28. $\frac{24 \div 12}{36 \div 12} = \frac{2}{3}$

29. $\frac{10 \div 10}{50 \div 10} = \frac{1}{5}$

30. $\frac{9 \div 9}{27 \div 9} = \frac{1}{3}$

31. $\frac{9 \div 9}{9 \div 9} = \frac{1}{1} = 1$

32. $\frac{15 \div 15}{45 \div 15} = \frac{1}{3}$

33. $\frac{124 \div 31}{155 \div 31} = \frac{4}{5}$

34. $\frac{12 \div 6}{18 \div 6} = \frac{2}{3}$

35. $\frac{36 \div 4}{64 \div 4} = \frac{9}{16}$

36. $3\frac{3}{5}$

37. $4\frac{2}{7}$

38. $1\frac{5}{8}$

39. $2\frac{11}{12}$

40. $1\frac{3}{25}$

41. $\frac{29}{25}$

42. $\frac{34}{8}$

43. $\frac{9}{2}$

44. $\frac{27}{8}$

45. $\frac{79}{5}$

46. $1\frac{1}{2}$

47. $2\frac{19}{24}$

48. $7\frac{1}{6}$

49. $8\frac{1}{15}$

50. $22\frac{5}{6}$

51. $\frac{19}{21}$

52. $1\frac{31}{40}$

53. $\frac{11}{16}$

54. $\frac{1}{12}$

55. $\frac{1}{24}$

56. $\frac{8}{15}$

57. $\frac{18}{125}$

58. $\frac{3}{50}$

59. $7\frac{7}{32}$

60. $\frac{5}{27}$

61. $1\frac{13}{20}$

62. $\frac{1}{30}$

63. 15

64. 1

65. $2\frac{2}{19}$

Answers to Chapter Review

1. $1\frac{2}{8} = 1\frac{1}{4}$

2. $7\frac{2}{4} = 7\frac{1}{2}$

3. $3\frac{4}{6} = 3\frac{2}{3}$

4. $2\frac{3}{4}$

5. $4\frac{3}{14}$

6. $6\frac{7}{10}$

7. $4\frac{1}{2}$

8. $2\frac{1}{5}$

9. $4\frac{4}{15}$

10. $7\frac{9}{13}$

11. $\frac{5}{2}$

12. $\frac{59}{8}$

13. $\frac{43}{5}$

14. $\frac{65}{4}$

15. $\frac{16}{5}$

16. $\frac{13}{5}$

17. $\frac{84}{10}$

18. $\frac{37}{4}$

19. $\frac{51}{4}$

20. $\frac{47}{7}$

21. LCD $= 30.\ 1\frac{13}{30}$

22. LCD $= 24.\ \frac{13}{24}$

23. LCD $= 4.\ \frac{88}{4} = 22$

24. LCD $= 10.\ \frac{7}{10}$

25. LCD $= 36.\ \frac{234}{36} = 6\frac{18}{36} = 6\frac{1}{2}$

26. $\frac{1}{9}$

27. LCD $= 4.\ \frac{3}{4}$

28. $2\frac{2}{4} = 2\frac{1}{2}$

29. LCD $= 30.\ \frac{19}{30}$

30. LCD $= 4.\ 1$

31. LCD $= 20.\ \frac{11}{20}$

32. LCD $= 24.\ \frac{7}{24}$

33. LCD $= 6.\ \frac{17}{6} = 2\frac{5}{6}$

34. LCD $= 15.\ \frac{19}{15} = 1\frac{4}{15}$

35. LCD $= 21.\ \frac{5}{21}$

36. $\frac{4}{36} = \frac{1}{9}$

37. $9\frac{11}{32}$

38. 14

39. 10

40. 27

41. $\frac{10}{16} = \frac{5}{8}$

42. $\frac{2}{30} = \frac{1}{15}$

43. $\frac{12}{120} = \frac{1}{10}$

44. $\frac{7}{27}$

45. $\frac{50}{75} = \frac{2}{3}$

46. $\frac{42}{75} = \frac{14}{25}$

47. $\frac{2}{3}$

48. 2

49. $\frac{28}{72} = \frac{7}{18}$

50. $\frac{24}{6} = 4$

51. $\frac{8}{6} = \frac{4}{3} = 1\frac{1}{3}$

52. $1\frac{25}{50} = 1\frac{1}{2}$

53. $7\frac{1}{2}$

54. $\frac{15}{300} = \frac{1}{20}$

55. 1

CHAPTER 3

Answers to Practice Problems

1. eight and thirty-five hundredths
2. eleven and one thousandth
3. four and fifty-seven hundredths
4. five and seven ten thousandths
5. ten and five tenths
6. one hundred sixty-three thousandths

7. 0.4
8. 84.07
9. 0.07
10. 2.23
11. 0.05
12. 0.009
13. 0.5
14. 2.87
15. 0.375
16. 0.175

17. 7.35
18. 0.087
19. 18.4
20. 40.449
21. 3.95
22. 3.87
23. 2.92
24. 43.1
25. 0.035
26. 5.88
27. 0.04725
28. 0.9125
29. 9,650
30. 1.78
31. 100.8072
32. 4
33. 1.16
34. 70.88
35. 30.46
36. 0.59

37. 3.6
38. 1
39. 2
40. 3.55
41. 0.61
42. 0.74
43. 0.0005
44. 0.00004
45. 584
46. 500
47. 0.75
48. 0.555
49. 0.5
50. $\dfrac{3}{4}$
51. $\dfrac{1}{2,000}$
52. $\dfrac{1}{25}$

Answers to Chapter Review

1. 0.444
2. 0.8
3. 1.5
4. 0.2
5. 0.725
6. 9.783
7. 28.9
8. 2.743
9. 5.12
10. 2.5
11. 6.33
12. 1.5
13. 1.5
14. 15
15. 31.2
16. 0.9448
17. 1.8
18. 0.1

19. 1.43
20. 0.15
21. 0.125
22. 0.06
23. 6.5
24. $1\dfrac{1}{100}$
25. $\dfrac{13}{200}$
26. 0.175 mg
27. 0.08 mg
28. 0.125 mg
29. 4.5 mg
30. 1.2 mg
31. 0.8
32. 565
33. 849
34. 23.4

35. 0.2
36. 0.65
37. 0.38
38. 0.52
39. 0.98
40. 0.35
41. 4.248
42. 0.567
43. 2.325
44. 7.839
45. 5.833

CHAPTER 4

Answers to Practice Problems

1. $\dfrac{15}{2}$, 15 : 2

2. 100 mg; 0.5 mL, 0.5 mL : 100 mg, 100 mg/0.5 mL, 0.5 mL/100 mg

3. 0.2 mg : 1 tab, 1 tab : 0.2 mg, 0.2 mg/1 tab, 1 tab/0.2 mg

4. 1 g : 10 mL, 10 mL : 1 g, 1 g/10 mL, 10 mL/1 g

5. 500 mg : 1 cap, 1 cap : 500 mg, 500 mg/1 cap, 1 cap/500 mg

6. $x = 9.6$

7. $x = 3$

8. $x = 2.4$

9. $x = 7.5$

10. $x = 18$

Answers to Chapter Review

1. 2 : 3
2. 1 : 9
3. 3 : 4
4. 1 : 5
5. 1 : 2
6. 1 : 5
7. $\dfrac{3}{7}$
8. $\dfrac{2}{3}$
9. $\dfrac{1}{7}$
10. $1\dfrac{1}{3}$
11. $\dfrac{3}{4}$
12. $x = 5$
13. $x = 2$

14. $x = 4$
15. $x = 3.33$
16. $x = 4.5$
17. $x = 0.8$
18. $x = 1.33$
19. $x = 0.16$
20. $x = 0.1$
21. 1,000 U : 1 mL OR 1 mL : 1,000 U

$$\dfrac{1 \text{ mL}}{1,000 \text{ U}} \quad \text{OR} \quad \dfrac{1,000 \text{ U}}{1 \text{ mL}}$$

22. 1 tab : 0.2 mg OR 0.2 mg : 1 tab

$$\dfrac{0.2 \text{ mg}}{1 \text{ tab}} \quad \text{OR} \quad \dfrac{1 \text{ tab}}{0.2 \text{ mg}}$$

23. 1 cap : 250 mg OR 250 mg : 1 cap

$$\dfrac{250 \text{ mg}}{1 \text{ cap}} \quad \text{OR} \quad \dfrac{1 \text{ cap}}{250 \text{ mg}}$$

24. 125 mg : 5 mL OR 5 mL : 125 mg

$$\dfrac{5 \text{ mL}}{125 \text{ mg}} \quad \text{OR} \quad \dfrac{125 \text{ mg}}{5 \text{ mL}}$$

25. 40 mg : 1 mL OR 1 mL : 40 mg

$$\dfrac{1 \text{ mL}}{40 \text{ mg}} \quad \text{OR} \quad \dfrac{40 \text{ mg}}{1 \text{ mL}}$$

CHAPTER 5

Answers to Practice Problems

1. 50 grams
2. 100 grams
3. 12.5 grams
4. 50 grams
5. 7.5 grams
6. $\dfrac{1}{100}$
7. $\dfrac{1}{50}$
8. $\dfrac{1}{2}$
9. $\dfrac{4}{5}$
10. $\dfrac{3}{100}$
11. 0.1
12. 0.35

13. 0.5
14. 0.142
15. 0.0025
16. 1 : 4
17. 11 : 100
18. 3 : 4
19. 9 : 200
20. 1 : 250

21. 40%
22. 275%
23. 50%
24. 25%
25. 70%
26. 4%
27. 75%
28. 10%

29. 1%
30. 50%
31. 18
32. 15
33. 1%
34. 10%
35. 4%

Answers to Chapter Review

Percent	Ratio	Fraction	Decimal
1. 0.25%	1 : 400	$\dfrac{1}{400}$	0.0025
2. 71%	71 : 100	$\dfrac{71}{100}$	0.71
3. 7%	7 : 100	$\dfrac{7}{100}$	0.07
4. 2%	1 : 50	$\dfrac{1}{50}$	0.02
5. 6%	3 : 50	$\dfrac{3}{50}$	0.06
6. 3.3%	1 : 30	$\dfrac{1}{30}$	0.033
7. 61%	61 : 100	$\dfrac{61}{100}$	0.61
8. 0.7%	7 : 1,000	$\dfrac{7}{1,000}$	0.007
9. 5%	1 : 20	$\dfrac{1}{20}$	0.05
10. 2.5%	1 : 40	$\dfrac{1}{40}$	0.025

11. 4.8 ounces
12. 56

13. 0.83%
14. 13.3%

15. 37.5

ANSWERS TO POSTTEST FOR UNIT ONE

1. v, v̄, V
2. xvii, x̄vii, XVII
3. xxvii, x̄xvii, XXVII
4. xxix, x̄xix, XXIX
5. xxx, x̄xx, XXX
6. $6\dfrac{1}{2}$
7. 24
8. 19
9. 25

10. 15
11. $1\dfrac{1}{3}$
12. $\dfrac{2}{3}$
13. $\dfrac{3}{7}$
14. $\dfrac{2}{3}$
15. $1\dfrac{3}{5}$

16. $1\dfrac{4}{21}$
17. $1\dfrac{2}{9}$
18. $25\dfrac{1}{3}$
19. $1\dfrac{22}{35}$
20. $1\dfrac{17}{36}$
21. 1.1

22. 0.1

23. 0.1

24. 0.9

25. $\dfrac{2}{3}$

26. $\dfrac{3}{4}$

27. 37.7

28. 17.407

29. 105.7

30. 32.94

31. 84.8

32. 22.5

33. 0.5

34. 0.850

35. 3.002

36. 0.493

37. $x = 4$

38. $x = 2.5$ or $2\dfrac{1}{2}$

39. $x = 0.1$ or $\dfrac{1}{10}$

40. $x = 4$

41. 0.6

42. 1

43. 1.4

44. 0.68

45. 0.83

46. 1.22

	Percent	Decimal	Ratio	Fraction
47.	10%	0.1	1 : 10	$\dfrac{1}{10}$
48.	60%	0.6	3 : 5	$\dfrac{3}{5}$
49.	$66\dfrac{2}{3}\%$	0.67	2 : 3	$\dfrac{2}{3}$
50.	25%	0.25	1 : 4	$\dfrac{1}{4}$
51.	18			
52.	18.75			
53.	66 2/3%			
54.	0.25%			
55.	38.46%			

CHAPTER 6

Answers to Practice Problems

1. 0.3 g

2. 6,000 mcg

3. 700 mL

4. 0.18 mg

5. 20 mcg

6. 4,500 mL

7. 4,200 mg

8. 900 mg

9. 3.25 L

10. 0.042 kg

11. 0.529 g

12. 0.645 mg

13. 347,000 mL

14. 238,000,000 mcg

15. 3.5 L

16. 40 g

17. 658,000 g

18. 0.051 L

19. 1,600 mcg

20. 0.028 L

Answers to Chapter Review

1. gram (g), liter (L), meter (m)

2. kilogram (kg)

3. 0.001 L

4. a) L (liter), mL (milliliter), cc (cubic centimeter)

   b) g (gram), mg (milligram), mcg (microgram), kg (kilogram)

5. 1 g

6. 1,000 mL

7. 1 mg

8. 1 L

9. L

10. mcg or μg

11. mL

12. g

13. kg

14. thousand times

15. the thousandth part of

16. 0.6 g

17. 50 kg

18. 0.4 mg

19. 0.04 L

20. 4.2 mcg

21. 0.005 g

22. 0.06 g

23. 2.6 mL

24. 100 mL

25. 0.03 mL

26. 0.95 mg

27. 58,500 mL

28. 130 mL

29. 276,000 mg

30. 0.55 L

31. 56,500 mL

32. 0.205 kg

33. 25 g

34. 1,000 mL

35. 15 mg

36. 0.25 mg

37. 8,000 g

38. 2,000 L

39. 5,000 mL

40. 750 mL

41. 330 mg

42. 0.75 g

43. 6,280 g

44. 0.0365 g

45. 0.0022 g

46. 0.4 kg

47. 24 mL

48. 0.1 g

49. 150,000 mg

50. 0.085 mg

CHAPTER 7
Answers to Practice Problems

1. m
2. oz, ℥
3. gr
4. dr, ℥
5. pt

6. 15 mL
7. 10 mL
8. ℥ 2 ½, ℥ iiss, ℥ iiss
9. ℥ 8, ℥ viii, ℥ viii
10. oz 1

11. ℥ x, ℥ 10, 10 oz, oz 10
12. gr ½, gr ss, grss
13. m16, mxiv
14. 1 T, 1 tbs (varies)
15. 5 glassfuls

Answers to Chapter Review

1. gr 8$\frac{1}{2}$, gr viiiss
2. m 3, m iii
3. dr 5, ℥ v
4. oz 8, ℥ viii, 8 oz (varies)
5. qt
6. pt
7. gr $\frac{1}{125}$
8. f℥ viss, f℥ viss, f℥ 6$\frac{1}{2}$
9. f℥ ii, f℥ ii, f℥ 2

10. oz 5, ℥ v, ℥ 5
11. m i, m i, m1
12. m60, mlx
13. f℥ viii, f℥8
14. f℥ xvi, f℥16
15. f℥ xxxii, f℥32
16. f℥ $\frac{1}{2}$, f℥ss, f℥ss
17. gtt
18. tablespoon

19. teaspoon
20. 5 mL
21. 4 mL
22. 8 ounces
23. 15 mL
24. 16 ounces
25. 32 ounces

CHAPTER 8
Answers to Practice Problems

1. 0.6 L
2. 16 mg
3. 4,000 g
4. 0.003 mg
5. 0.0003 g
6. 10 g
7. 1,900 mL
8. 0.0005 kg
9. 70 mcg
10. 0.65 L
11. 40 mg
12. 0.00012 kg
13. 0.18 g
14. 1.7 L
15. 15,000 g
16. 3,500 mg
17. 160 g
18. 4 mL
19. 0.001 L

20. 0.008 g
21. 0.5 L
22. 4,000 g
23. 1,400 mL
24. ℥ 3/4
25. 4,500 mcg
26. ℥ iv, ℥4, ℥ iv
27. 6,500 mL
28. 0.06 kg
29. 0.6 g
30. 736 mcg
31. 1.6 L
32. 15 mL
33. 180 mg
34. 0.025 mg
35. 0.0052 kg
36. 27.27 kg
37. gr 1/4
38. 150 mL

39. 300 mg
40. 210 mL
41. 1/4 qt
42. 3 tbs
43. 3 g
44. 90 mg
45. 4 tsp
46. 330 mg
47. 4,000 mL
48. 158.4 lb or 158$\frac{2}{5}$ lb
49. 0.48 mg
50. 2,400 mL
51. 700 mL
52. 550 mL
53. 900 mL
54. 81 mL/hr
55. 31 mL/hr
56. 42 mL/hr

Answers to Chapter Review

1. 7 mg
2. 0.001 g
3. 6 kg
4. 0.005 L
5. 450 mL
6. $\overline{3}$ ii or $\overline{3}$ 2
7. 0.2 mg
8. gr $\dfrac{1}{60}$
9. $\overline{3}$3, $\overline{3}$iii, $\overline{3}$iii
10. 120 mg
11. 1,500 mL
12. grss, gr$\overline{ss}$, gr $\dfrac{1}{2}$
13. 1,600 mL
14. 103.4 lb or 103$\dfrac{2}{5}$ lb
15. 0.003 L
16. 34.09 kg
17. 8 mg
18. 2,250 mL
19. 30 mg
20. 0.4 mg
21. 6.172 kg

22. 40 tsp
23. 46.36 kg
24. 0.204 kg
25. 1,500 mL
26. 0.2 mg
27. 48,600 mL
28. 700 mL
29. 165 mL
30. 20 mL
31. 240 mg (gri = 60 mg)
32. 30 mL
33. 8 mL
34. gr $\dfrac{3}{4}$
35. 3 g
36. 600 mL
37. 150 mg
38. 22.5 mg
39. 600 mg (gr i = 60 mg)
40. 8.8 lb or 8$\dfrac{4}{5}$ lb
41. 3,250 mcg
42. $\overline{3}$ iiss, $\overline{3}$ iiss, $\overline{3}$ 2$\dfrac{1}{2}$
43. 0.5 mg

44. 6,653 mg
45. 4,000 mg
46. 0.036 g
47. 800 mg
48. gr 135 or gr cxxxv
49. gr $\dfrac{1}{120}$
50. 2 L
51. 245 mL
52. 1,310 mL
53. 540 mL
54. 720 mL
55. 270 mL
56. 105 mL
57. 180 mL
58. 725 mL
59. 450 mL
60. 925 mL
61. 63 mL/hr
62. 27 mL/hr
63. 88 mL/hr
64. 375 mL
65. 275 mL

CHAPTER 9

Answers to Practice Problems

1. 39.2° F
2. 38.3° C
3. 100.6° F
4. 38.5° C
5. 99.5° F
6. 68° F to 77° F
7. 38.3° C
8. −13.9° C
9. 98.6° F
10. 7.8° C

11. 4 inches
12. 4.5 cm
13. 375 mm
14. 51.25 cm
15. 37 cm
16. 2.6 inches
17. 250 cm
18. 12.8 inches
19. 15.2 inches
20. 50 cm

21. 9.1 kg
22. 29.1 kg
23. 10 kg
24. 55 kg
25. 38.6 kg
26. 44 lb
27. 101 lb
28. 216 lb
29. 23 lb
30. 77 lb

Answers to Chapter Review

1. 38.6° C
2. 25° C
3. 59° F to 86° F
4. 97.7° F

5. 42.8° F
6. 14° F
7. −17.8° C
8. 39.3° C

9. 84.2° F
10. 222.8° F
11. 21.1° C
12. 103.3° F

13. 18° C

14. 45 cm

15. 12.4 inches

16. 445 mm

17. 80 cm

18. 30 mm

19. 79 mm

20. 10 cm

21. 28.6 kg

22. 68.2 kg

23. 35.5 kg

24. 36.8 kg

25. 12.3 kg

26. 170 lb

27. 15 lb

28. 10 lb

29. 20 lb

30. 123 lb

CHAPTER 10

Answers to Practice Problems

1. metric, apothecary, and household
2. elderly and children
3. route
4. smaller
5. souffle
6. topical

7. assessment, nursing diagnosis, planning, implementation, evaluation, teaching
8. critical thinking
9. calibrated
10. buccal

Answers to Chapter Review

1. drug, dose, client, route, time, documentation
2. identification band, asking the name, getting a staff member to help identify the client
3. three
4. after
5. parenteral, oral, inhalation, insertion, topical, percutaneous

6. 30 mL or 1 oz
7. False
8. oral syringe
9. milliliters (mL)
10. 30 mL

CHAPTER 11

Answers to Practice Problems

1. everyday
2. after meals
3. right ear
4. hour
5. every twelve hours, every 12 hours
6. Give or administer Zidovudine 200 milligrams orally (by mouth) every 4 hours.
7. Give or administer Procaine penicillin G 400,000 units by intravenous injection every 8 hours.
8. Give or administer Gentamicin Sulfate 45 milligrams by intravenous piggyback injection, every 12 hours.
9. Give or administer Regular Humulin insulin 5 units by subcutaneous injection before meals and at bedtime (hour of sleep).

10. Give or administer vitamin B_{12} 1,000 micrograms by intramuscular injection every other day.
11. Give or administer Prilosec 20 milligrams orally (by mouth) twice a day.
12. Give or administer Tofranil 75 milligrams orally (by mouth) at bedtime (hour of sleep).
13. Give or administer Restoril 30 milligrams orally (by mouth) at bedtime (hour of sleep).
14. Give or administer Mylanta 1 ounce orally (by mouth) every 4 hours when necessary (when required).
15. Give or administer Synthroid 200 micrograms orally (by mouth) every day.

Answers to Chapter Review

1. name of the client
2. date and time the order was written
3. name of the medication
4. dose of medication
5. route by which medication is to be administered
6. time and/or frequency of administration
7. signature of the person writing the order
8. twice a day
9. both eyes
10. as desired
11. subcutaneous
12. with
13. before meals
14. four times a day
15. twice a week
16. hour of sleep (bedtime)
17. once a day
18. elixir
19. left eye
20. syrup
21. nothing by mouth
22. sublingual
23. p.c. or pc
24. t.i.d. or tid
25. I.M. or IM
26. q.8.h. or q8h
27. supp
28. I.V. or IV
29. s.o.s. or sos
30. $\bar{s}$
31. stat or STAT
32. OD or O.D.
33. ung or oint
34. ss or $\overline{ss}$
35. mEq
36. q.h.s. or qhs
37. p.r. or pr
38. Give or administer Methergine 0.2 milligrams orally (by mouth) every 4 hours for (times) six doses.
39. Give or administer Digoxin 0.125 milligrams orally (by mouth) once a day.
40. Give or administer Regular Humulin insulin 14 units by subcutaneous injection every day at 7:30 AM.
41. Give or administer Demerol 50 milligrams by intramuscular injection and Atropine $\frac{1}{150}$ grains by intramuscular injection on call to the operating room.
42. Give or administer ampicillin 500 milligrams orally (by mouth) immediately and then 250 milligrams orally (by mouth) four times a day thereafter.
43. Give or administer Lasix 40 milligrams by intramuscular injection immediately.
44. Give or administer Librium 50 milligrams orally (by mouth) every 4 hours when necessary (when required) for agitation.
45. Give or administer potassium chloride 20 milliequivalents by intravenous injection times 2 liters. (Administer potassium chloride 20 mEq in each of the next 2 liters of intravenous fluid.)
46. Give or administer Tylenol 10 grains orally (by mouth) every 4 hours when necessary (when required) for pain.
47. Give or administer Mylicon 80 milligrams orally (by mouth) after meals and at bedtime (hour of sleep).
48. Give or administer folic acid 1 milligram orally (by mouth) once a day.
49. Give or administer Nembutal 100 milligrams orally (by mouth) at bedtime (hour of sleep) when necessary (when required).
50. Give or administer aspirin 10 grains orally (by mouth) every 4 hours when necessary (when required) for temperature greater than 101° F.
51. Give or administer Dilantin 100 milligrams orally (by mouth) three times a day.
52. Give or administer Minipress 2 milligrams orally (by mouth) two times a day. Hold for systolic blood pressure less than 120.
53. Give or administer Compazine 10 milligrams by intramuscular injection every 4 hours when necessary (when required) for nausea or vomiting.
54. Give or administer ampicillin 1 gram by intravenous piggyback injection every 6 hours for (times) 4 doses.
55. Give or administer heparin 5,000 units by subcutaneous injection every 12 hours.
56. Give or administer Dilantin suspension 200 milligrams every morning and 300 milligrams by nasogastric tube at bedtime (hour of sleep).

57. Give or administer Benadryl 50 milligrams orally (by mouth) immediately (at once).

58. Give or administer vitamin B$_{12}$ 1,000 micrograms by intramuscular injection three times a week.

59. Give or administer Milk of Magnesia 1 ounce orally (by mouth) at bedtime (hour of sleep) when necessary (when required) for constipation.

60. Give or administer Septra 1 double-strength tablet orally (by mouth) every day.

61. Give or administer Neomycin ophthalmic 1% ointment to the right eye three times a day.

62. Give or administer Carafate 1 gram by nasogastric tube four times a day.

63. Give or administer morphine sulfate 15 milligrams by subcutaneous injection immediately (at once) and 10 milligrams by subcutaneous injection every 4 hours when necessary (when required) for pain.

64. Give or administer ampicillin 120 milligrams by intravenous Soluset every 6 hours for (times) 7 days.

65. Give or administer prednisone 10 milligrams orally (by mouth) every other day.

66. route of administration

67. frequency/time interval of administration

68. dose of medication (drug)

69. name of medication (drug)

70. dose of medication (drug) and route of administration

CHAPTER 12

Answers to Practice Problems

1. 0730
2. 1030
3. 2010
4. 1745
5. 0016
6. 2:07 AM
7. 5:43 PM
8. 12:04 AM

Answers to Practice Exercise 1 (Reading of Medication Record, Figure 12-1)

Date 4/2/01

	Medication	Dosage	Route	Time
1.	Keflex	250 mg	p.o.	10 AM
2.	Keflex	250 mg	p.o.	2 PM
3.	MVI	1 tab	p.o.	10 AM
4.	Colace	100 mg	p.o.	10 AM

Date 4/3/01

1.	Keflex	250 mg	p.o.	6 PM
2.	Keflex	250 mg	p.o.	10 PM
3.	Colace	100 mg	p.o.	6 PM

Answers to Chapter Review

1. 12:32 AM
2. 2:20 AM
3. 4:50 PM
4. 1:45 PM
5. 9:22 PM
6. 0520
7. 2400 (0000 used in military)
8. 0005
9. 1630
10. 1335
11. AM
12. PM
13. 0300
14. Hospital, institution, or health care facility
15. No, b.i.d. means the order will be given two times in 24 hours, whereas a q2h order would be given twelve times in 24 hours.

Answers to Chapter Review Exercise 1 (Figure 12-4)

ST. BARNABAS HOSPITAL
BRONX, NY 10457

DEPARTMENT OF NURSING
MEDICATION ADMINISTRATION RECORD

DIAGNOSIS:
Pancreatitis

ALLERGIC TO: NKDA	DATE 4/9/01

Addkerograph or printed label with client identification.

LEGEND
Omitted doses (use red pen):
Document in Medication Omission Record

1. NPO   3. I.V. Out   5. Other
2. Off-unit   4. Pt. Refused

Page ____ of ____

ORDER DATE / EXP DATE	STANDING MEDICATION / MED-DOSE-FREQ-ROUTE	DATE 2001 / HOUR	4/9 INIT.	4/10 INIT.	4/11 INIT.	4/12 INIT.	4/13 INIT.	4/14 INIT.	4/15 INIT.	4/16 INIT.	4/17 INIT.
RN. INIT. 4/9/01 DM 5/9/01	Norvasc 5 mg PO daily hold for SBP <100	9A B/P									
RN. INIT. 4/9/01 DM 5/9/01	Thiamine 100 mg PO daily	9A									
RN. INIT. 4/9/01 DM 4/16/01	Heparin 5,000 units sq q12h	9A site 9P site									
RN. INIT. 4/9/01 DM 5/9/01	FeSO4 325 mg PO tid.	9A 1P 5P									
RN. INIT.											

INJECTION CODES:
RT = RIGHT THIGH   RA = RIGHT ARM   ▲ RAB = UPPER RIGHT ABDOMEN   ▲ LAB = UPPER LEFT ABDOMEN
LT = LEFT THIGH   LA = LEFT ARM   ▼ RAB = LOWER RIGHT ABDOMEN   ▼ LAB = LOWER LEFT ABDOMEN

Form 225   5/97

Used with permission of St. Barnabas Hospital, Bronx, New York.

Answers to Chapter Review Exercise 2 (Figure 12–5)

ST. BARNABAS HOSPITAL
BRONX, NY 10457

DEPARTMENT OF NURSING
MEDICATION ADMINISTRATION RECORD

DIAGNOSIS:
Pancreatitis

ALLERGIC TO:	NKDA	DATE 4/10/01

Addressograph or printed label with client identification.

	ORDER DATE / EXP DATE	REORDER DATE / EXP DATE	P.R.N. MEDICATION / MED-DOSE-FREQ-ROUTE										
DM R.N. INIT.	4/10/01		Percocet 2 tabs	DATE	4 10								
			PO q4h prn for	TIME	2p								
			pain X 3 days	SITE	PO								
REORD INIT.	4/13/01			INIT.	DM								
DM R.N. INIT.	4/10/01		Tylenol 650 mg	DATE									
			PO q4h prn for	TIME									
			Temp >101°F	SITE									
REORD INIT.	4/17/01			INIT.									
R.N. INIT.				DATE									
				TIME									
				SITE									
REORD INIT.				INIT.									
R.N. INIT.				DATE									
				TIME									
				SITE									
REORD INIT.				INIT.									
R.N. INIT.				DATE									
				TIME									
				SITE									
REORD INIT.				INIT.									

INITIAL IDENTIFICATION

	INITIAL	PRINT NAME, TITLE		INITIAL	PRINT NAME, TITLE		INITIAL	PRINT NAME, TITLE
1	DM	Deborah C Morris RN	1			1		
2			2			2		
3			3			3		
4			4			4		

Used with permission of St. Barnabas Hospital, Bronx, New York.

CHAPTER 13

Answers to Practice Problems

1. Trade name: Augmentin
   Generic name: amoxicillin clavulanate potassium
   Form: oral suspension
   Dose strength: 125 mg/5 mL
   Total volume: 100 mL (when reconstituted)
2. Trade name: Vistaril
   Generic name: hydroxyzine hydrochloride
   Dose strength: 50 mg/mL
   Total volume: 10 mL
   Form: injectable liquid

3. Dose strength: 100 mg per capsule (100 mg/cap)
   Total volume: 1,000 capsules
4. Generic name: enalapril maleate
   Dose strength: 2.5 mg per tablet (2.5 mg/tab)
   Total volume: 1,000 tablets
5. Trade name: Coumadin
   Form: tablets
   Dose strength: $2 \frac{1}{2}$ mg per tablet ($2 \frac{1}{2}$ mg/tab)
   NDC number: 0056-0176-90

Answers to Chapter Review

1. Generic name: prazosin hydrochloride
   Trade name: Minipress
   Form: capsules
   Dose strength: 1 mg per capsule (1 mg/cap)
2. Generic name: digoxin
   Trade name: Lanoxin
   Total volume: 2 mL
   Form: injectable liquid
   Dose strength: 0.25 mg/mL, 0.5 mg/2 mL
3. Generic name: dexamethasone, MSD
   Trade name: Decadron
   Form: tablets
   Dose strength: 0.25 mg per tablet (0.25 mg/tab)
4. Generic name: levothyroxine sodium
   Trade name: Synthroid
   Form: tablets
   Dose strength: 50 mcg per tablet (50 mcg/tab),
   0.05 mg per tablet (0.05 mg/tab)
5. Generic name: potassium chloride
   Trade name: none
   Form: injectable liquid
   Dose strength: 2 mEq/mL
6. Generic name: docusate calcium
   Trade name: Surfak
   Form: capsules
   Dose strength: 50 mg per capsule (50 mg/cap)
7. Generic name: streptomycin sulfate
   Trade name: none
   Form: injectable

   Directions for mixing: The dry powder is dissolved by adding 9 mL water, USP or sodium chloride for injection.
   Dose strength after reconstitution: 400 mg/mL.
   Storage instructions: In dry form store below 86° F (30° C). Protect reconstituted solution from light, may store at room temperature for 4 weeks.
8. Generic name: lamivudine
   Trade name: Epivir
   Total volume: 240 mL
   Form: oral solution
   Dose strength: 10 mg/mL
9. Generic name: acyclovir sodium
   Trade name: Zovirax
   Directions for mixing: Inject 20 mL sterile water for injection into vial. Shake vial until a clear solution is achieved and use within 12 hours. Do not use bacteriostatic water for injection containing benzyl alcohol or Parabens.
   Storage: Store at 15° C to 25° C (59° F to 77° F)
   Form: injectable (I.V. infusion only)
   Dose strength: 1,000 mg/20 mL
10. Generic name: ranitidine hydrochloride
    Trade name: Zantac
    NDC number: 0173-0363-00
    Form: injectable liquid
    Dose strength: 25 mg/mL
11. Generic name: ciprofloxacin hydrochloride
    Trade name: Cipro
    Amount: 50 tablets
    Form: tablets
    Dose strength: 750 mg per tablet (750 mg/tab)

12. Generic name: amphotericin B
    Trade name: Fungizone
    Form: injectable
    Drug manufacturer: Apothecon

13. Generic name: medroxyprogesterone acetate
    Trade name: Depo-Provera
    Form: injectable
    Dose strength: 150 mg/mL
    Use: contraceptive (intramuscular use only); shake vigorously before using

14. Generic name: medroxyprogesterone acetate
    Trade name: Depo-Provera
    Dose strength: 400 mg/mL
    Directions for use: for intramuscular use only; shake vigorously before using

15. Generic name: diltiazem hydrochloride (HCl)
    Trade name: Cardizem
    Amount: 100 tablets
    Form: tablets
    Dose strength: 120 mg per tablet (120 mg/tab)

16. Generic name: ibutilide fumarate
    Trade name: Corvert
    Directions for use: for I.V. use only
    Form: injectable liquid (intravenous infusion only)
    Dose strength: 0.1 mg/mL

17. Generic name: heparin sodium
    Trade name: none
    Directions for use: s.c. or I.V. use
    Dose strength: 1,000 U/mL
    Total volume: 30 mL

18. Trade name: Zocor
    Generic name: simvastatin
    Dose strength: 10 mg per tablet (10 mg/tab)
    NDC number: 0006-0735-61

19. Generic name: diltiazem HCl
    Form: sustained release capsules
    Dose strength: 60 mg per capsule (60 mg/tab)

20. Trade name: Ativan
    Dose strength: 0.5 mg per tablet (0.5 mg/tab)
    Total volume: 100 tablets

CHAPTER 14

Answers to Practice Problems

1. Less than 1 tab
2. More than 1 tab
3. Less than 1 tab
4. Less than 1 tab
5. More than 1 tab
6. 5 mg : 1 tab = 7.5 mg : x tab

$$\frac{5x}{5} = \frac{7.5}{5}$$

$$x = \frac{7.5}{5}$$

OR

$$\frac{5 \text{ mg}}{1 \text{ tab}} = \frac{7.5 \text{ mg}}{x \text{ tab}}$$

$$\frac{5x}{5} = \frac{7.5}{5}$$

$x = 1.5$ tabs or $1\frac{1}{2}$ tabs. 5 mg is less than 7.5 mg; therefore you will need more than 1 tab to administer the dose.

7. equivalent: 60 mg = gr 1 (gr $\frac{3}{4}$ = 45 mg)

30 mg : 1 tab = 45 mg : x tab

$$\frac{30x}{30} = \frac{45}{30}$$

$$x = \frac{45}{30}$$

OR

$$\frac{30 \text{ mg}}{1 \text{ tab}} = \frac{45 \text{ mg}}{x \text{ tab}}$$

$$\frac{30x}{30} = \frac{45}{30}$$

$$x = \frac{45}{30}$$

$x = 1.5$ tabs or $1\frac{1}{2}$ tabs. 45 mg is more than 30; therefore you need more than 1 tab to administer the dose.

8. equivalent: 60 mg = gr 1

$$\left(\text{gr } 1\frac{1}{2} = 90 \text{ mg}\right)$$

100 mg : 1 cap = 90 mg : x cap

$$\frac{100x}{100} = \frac{90}{100}$$

$$x = \frac{90}{100}$$

OR

$$\frac{100 \text{ mg}}{1 \text{ cap}} = \frac{90 \text{ mg}}{x \text{ cap}}$$

$$\frac{100x}{100} = \frac{90}{100}$$

$$x = \frac{90}{100}$$

x = 1 cap. It would be impossible to administer 0.9 of a capsule. A 10% margin of difference is allowed between what is ordered and what is administered. Using this 10% safety margin, no more than 110 mg and no less than 90 mg may be given. The doctor ordered gr1$\frac{1}{2}$ (90 mg). The capsules available are 100 mg. Capsules are not dividable. Administering 1 cap is within the 10% margin of difference allowed.

9. 0.5 mg : 1 mL = 0.25 mg : x mL

$$\frac{0.5x}{0.5} = \frac{0.25}{0.5}$$

$$x = \frac{0.25}{0.5}$$

OR

$$\frac{0.5 \text{ mg}}{1 \text{ mL}} = \frac{0.25 \text{ mg}}{x \text{ mL}}$$

$$\frac{0.5x}{0.5} = \frac{0.25}{0.5}$$

$$x = \frac{0.25}{0.5}$$

x = 0.5 mL, $\frac{1}{2}$ mL. 0.25 mg is less than 0.5 mg; you will need less than 1 mL to administer the dose.

10. 125 mg : 5 mL = 100 mg : x mL

$$\frac{125x}{125} = \frac{500}{125}$$

$$x = \frac{500}{125}$$

OR

$$\frac{125 \text{ mg}}{5 \text{ mL}} = \frac{100 \text{ mg}}{x \text{ mL}}$$

$$\frac{125x}{125} = \frac{500}{125}$$

$$x = \frac{500}{125}$$

x = 4 mL. 100 mg is less than 125 mg; therefore you will need less than 5 mL to administer the dose.

11. 40 mEq : 10 mL = 20 mEq : x mL

$$\frac{40x}{40} = \frac{200}{40}$$

$$x = \frac{200}{40}$$

OR

$$\frac{40 \text{ mEq}}{10 \text{ mL}} = \frac{20 \text{ mEq}}{x \text{ mL}}$$

$$\frac{40x}{40} = \frac{200}{40}$$

x = 5 mL. 20 mEq is less than 40 mEq; you will need less than 10 mL to administer the dose.

12. 10,000 U : 1 mL = 5,000 U : x mL

$$\frac{10,000x}{10,000} = \frac{5,000}{10,000}$$

$$x = \frac{5,000}{10,000}$$

OR

$$\frac{10,000 \text{ U}}{1 \text{ mL}} = \frac{5,000 \text{ U}}{x \text{ mL}}$$

$$\frac{10,000x}{10,000} = \frac{5,000}{10,000}$$

$$x = \frac{5,000}{10,000}$$

x = 0.5 mL, $\frac{1}{2}$ ml. 10,000 U is more than 5,000 U; therefore you will need less than 1 mL to administer the dose.

13. 80 mg : 2 mL = 50 mg : x mL

$$\frac{80x}{80} = \frac{100}{80}$$

$$x = \frac{100}{80}$$

OR

$$\frac{80 \text{ mg}}{2 \text{ mL}} = \frac{50 \text{ mg}}{x \text{ mL}}$$

$$\frac{80x}{80} = \frac{100}{80}$$

$$x = \frac{100}{80}$$

$x = 1.25 = 1.3$ mL. 50 mg is less than 80 mg; therefore you will need less than 2 mL to administer the dose.

14. Equivalent: 1,000 mg = 1 g (0.5 g = 500 mg)

250 mg : 1 cap = 500 mg : x cap

$$\frac{250x}{250} = \frac{500}{250}$$

$$x = \frac{500}{250}$$

OR

$$\frac{250 \text{ mg}}{1 \text{ cap}} = \frac{500 \text{ mg}}{x \text{ cap}}$$

$$\frac{250x}{250} = \frac{500}{250}$$

$x = 2$ caps. 500 mg is more than 250 mg; therefore you will need more than 1 cap to administer the dose.

15. 125 mg : 5 mL = 400 mg : x mL

$$\frac{125x}{125} = \frac{2,000}{125}$$

$$x = \frac{2,000}{125}$$

OR

$$\frac{125 \text{ mg}}{5 \text{ mL}} = \frac{400 \text{ mg}}{x \text{ mL}}$$

$$\frac{125x}{125} = \frac{2,000}{125}$$

$$x = \frac{2,000}{125}$$

$x = 16$ mL. 400 mg is larger than 125 mg; therefore you will need more than 5 mL to administer the dose.

16. 80 mg : 1 mL = 50 mg : x mL

$$\frac{80x}{80} = \frac{50}{80}$$

$$x = \frac{50}{80}$$

OR

$$\frac{80 \text{ mg}}{1 \text{ mL}} = \frac{50 \text{ mg}}{x \text{ mL}}$$

$$\frac{80x}{80} = \frac{50}{80}$$

$$x = \frac{50}{80}$$

$x = 0.62 = 0.6$ mL. 50 mg is less than 80 mg; therefore you will need less than 1 mL to administer the dose.

17. gr $\frac{1}{2}$: 1 mL = gr 1 : x mL

$$\frac{\frac{1}{2}x}{\frac{1}{2}} = \frac{1}{}$$

$$x = 1 \div \frac{1}{2} = 1 \times \frac{2}{1}$$

$$\frac{2}{1} = 2$$

OR

$$\frac{\text{gr } \frac{1}{2}}{1 \text{ mL}} = \frac{\text{gr } 1}{x \text{ mL}} \left(\frac{\text{gr } \frac{1}{2}}{1 \text{ mL}} = \frac{\text{gr } 1}{x \text{ mL}} \right)$$

$$\frac{\frac{1}{2}x}{\frac{1}{2}} = \frac{1}{}$$

$$x = \frac{1}{}$$

$$x = 1 \div \frac{1}{2} = 1 \times \frac{2}{1}$$

$$\frac{2}{1} = 2$$

$x = 2$ mL. gr $\frac{1}{2}$ is less than gr 1; therefore you will need more than 1 mL to administer the dose.

18. gr v : 1 tab = gr xv : x tab

gr 5 : 1 tab = gr 15 : x tab

$$\frac{5x}{5} = \frac{15}{5}$$

$$x = \frac{15}{5}$$

OR

$$\frac{\text{gr } 5}{1 \text{ tab}} = \frac{\text{gr } 15}{x \text{ tab}}$$

$$\frac{5x}{5} = \frac{15}{5}$$

$x = 3$ tabs. gr 15 is more than gr 5; therefore you will need more than 1 tab to administer the dose.

19. Equivalent: 1,000 mg = 1 g (0.24 g = 240 mg)

80 mg : 7.5 mL = 240 mg : x mL

$$\frac{80x}{80} = \frac{1,800}{80}$$

$$x = \frac{1,800}{80}$$

OR

$$\frac{80 \text{ mg}}{7.5 \text{ mL}} = \frac{240 \text{ mg}}{x \text{ mL}}$$

$$\frac{80x}{80} = \frac{1,800}{80}$$

$$x = \frac{1,800}{80}$$

$x = 22.5$ mL or $22\frac{1}{2}$ mL. 240 mg is more

than 80 mg; therefore you would need more than 7.5 mL to administer the dose.

20. 10 g : 15 mL = 20 g : x mL

$$\frac{10x}{10} = \frac{300}{10}$$

$$x = \frac{300}{10}$$

OR

$$\frac{10 \text{ g}}{15 \text{ mL}} = \frac{20 \text{ g}}{x \text{ mL}}$$

$$\frac{10 x}{10} = \frac{300}{10}$$

$$x = \frac{300}{10}$$

$x = 30$ mL. 20 g is more than 10 g; therefore you would need more than 15 mL to administer the dose.

21. 0.5 mg : 2 mL = 0.125 mg : x mL

$$\frac{0.5}{0.5} x = \frac{0.25}{0.5}$$

$$x = \frac{0.25}{0.5}$$

OR

$$\frac{0.5 \text{ mg}}{2 \text{ mL}} = \frac{0.125}{x \text{ mL}}$$

$$\frac{0.5 \, x}{0.5} = \frac{0.25}{0.5}$$

$x = 0.5$ mL, $\frac{1}{2}$ mL. 0.125 mg is less than

0.5 mg; therefore you will need less than 2 mL to administer the dose.

22. 0.25 mg : 1 mL = 0.75 mg : x mL

$$\frac{0.25x}{0.25} = \frac{0.75}{0.25}$$

$$x = \frac{0.75}{0.25}$$

OR

$$\frac{0.25 \text{ mg}}{1 \text{ mL}} = \frac{0.75 \text{ mg}}{x \text{ mL}}$$

$$\frac{0.25x}{0.25} = \frac{0.75}{0.25}$$

$x = 3$ mL. 0.75 mg is more than 0.25 mg; therefore you will need more than 1 mL to administer the dose.

23. 125 mg : 5 mL = 375 mg : x mL

$$\frac{125x}{125} = \frac{375 \times 5}{125}$$

$$x = \frac{1,875}{125}$$

OR

$$\frac{125 \text{ mg}}{5 \text{ mL}} = \frac{375 \text{ mg}}{x \text{ mL}}$$

$$\frac{125x}{125} = \frac{375 \times 5}{125}$$

$x = 15$ mL. 375 mg is more than 125 mg; therefore you will need more than 5 mL to administer the dose.

24. 7,500 U : 1 mL = 10,000 U : x mL

$$\frac{7,500x}{7,500} = \frac{10,000}{7,500}$$

$$x = \frac{10,000}{7,500}$$

OR

$$\frac{7,500 \text{ U}}{1 \text{ mL}} = \frac{10,000 \text{ U}}{x \text{ mL}}$$

$$\frac{7,500x}{7,500} = \frac{10,000}{7,500}$$

$x = 1.33 = 1.3$ mL. 10,000 U is more than 7,500 U; therefore you will need more than 1 mL to administer the dose.

25. 0.3 mg : 1 tab = 0.45 mg : x tab

$$\frac{0.3 \, x}{0.3} = \frac{0.45}{0.3}$$

$$x = \frac{0.45}{0.3}$$

OR

$$\frac{0.3 \text{ mg}}{1 \text{ tab}} = \frac{0.45 \text{ mg}}{x \text{ tab}}$$

$$\frac{0.3 \, x}{0.3} = \frac{0.45}{0.3}$$

$x = 1.5$ tabs or $1\frac{1}{2}$ tabs. 0.45 mg is more than 0.3 mg; therefore you will need more than 1 tab to administer the dose.

Note:

Questions 26–40 and Chapter Review Parts I and II: Answers only are provided. Refer to set-up for 1–25, if needed.

26. 1.2 mL	31. 1.7 mL	36. 0.8 mL
27. 1.9 mL	32. 2.2 mL	37. 5 mL
28. 0.7 mL	33. 2 mL	38. 3.3 mL
29. 2 mL	34. 2.2 mL	39. 0.9 mL
30. 1.1 mL	35. 0.6 mL	40. 1.6 mL

Answers to Chapter Review Part I

1. 1 tab	12. 1 tab	23. 2 tabs
2. 1 cap	13. 2 caps	24. 2 caps
3. 2 caps	14. 2 caps	25. 1 cap
4. 2 tabs	15. 2 tabs	26. 3 tabs
5. 2 tabs	16. 1 tab	27. 1 tab
6. 0.5 tab or $\frac{1}{2}$ tab	17. 2 caps	28. 2 tabs
	18. 2 caps	29. $1\frac{1}{2}$ tabs or 1.5 tabs
7. 1 tab	19. 1 tab	
8. 1 tab	20. 2 tabs	30. 2 tabs
9. 1 tab		31. 2 tabs
10. 1 tab	21. 0.5 tab or $\frac{1}{2}$ tab	32. 2 tabs
11. 2 caps	22. 1 tab	33. 2 tabs

Answers to Chapter Review Part II

34. 4 mL	39. 2.3 mL	44. 1 mL
35. 20 mL	40. 1 mL	45. 0.5 mL
36. 1.3 mL	41. 1 mL	46. 0.5 mL
37. 10 mL	42. 0.67 mL	47. 10 mL
38. 0.7 mL	43. 7.5 mL	48. 0.75 mL

49.	1.1 mL	55.	6.3 mL	61.	1 mL
50.	0.5 mL	56.	0.8 mL	62.	16.7 mL
51.	0.5 mL	57.	20 mL	63.	45 mL
52.	0.8 mL	58.	30 mL	64.	1.3 mL
53.	4 mL	59.	40 mL	65.	1.4 mL
54.	6 mL	60.	10 mL	66.	6.7 mL

CHAPTER 15

Answers to Practice Problems

1. $\dfrac{0.4 \text{ mg}}{0.2 \text{ mg}} \times 1 \text{ tab} = x \text{ tab}$

$$\frac{0.4}{0.2} = x$$

$x = 2$ tabs. 0.4 mg is greater than 0.2 mg; therefore you will need more than 1 tab to administer the dose.

OR

$$\frac{0.4 \text{ mg}}{0.2 \text{ mg}} = \frac{x \text{ tab}}{1 \text{ tab}}$$

$$\frac{0.2x}{0.2} = \frac{0.4}{0.2}$$

$$x = \frac{0.4}{0.2} = 2 \text{ tabs}$$

2. Equivalent: 1,000 mg = 1 g (0.75 g = 750 mg)

$$\frac{750 \text{ mg}}{250 \text{ mg}} \times 1 \text{ cap} = x \text{ cap}$$

$$\frac{750}{250} = x$$

$x = 3$ caps. 750 mg is larger than 250 mg; therefore you will need more than 1 cap to administer the dose.

OR

$$\frac{750 \text{ mg}}{250 \text{ mg}} = \frac{x \text{ cap}}{1 \text{ cap}}$$

$$\frac{250x}{250} = \frac{750}{250}$$

$$x = \frac{750}{250} = 3 \text{ caps}$$

3. $\dfrac{90 \text{ mg}}{60 \text{ mg}} \times 1 \text{ tab} = x \text{ tab}$

$$\frac{90}{60} = x$$

$x = 1.5$ or $1\dfrac{1}{2}$ tabs. 90 is larger than 60 mg; therefore you will need more than 1 tab to administer the dose.

OR

$$\frac{90 \text{ mg}}{60 \text{ mg}} = \frac{x \text{ tab}}{1 \text{ tab}}$$

$$\frac{60x}{60} = \frac{90}{60}$$

$$x = \frac{90}{60} = 1.5 \text{ or } 1\frac{1}{2} \text{ tabs}$$

4. $\dfrac{7.5 \text{ mg}}{2.5 \text{ mg}} \times 1 \text{ tab} = x \text{ tab}$

$$\frac{7.5}{2.5} = x$$

$x = 3$ tabs. 7.5 mg is larger than 2.5 mg; therefore you will need more than 1 tab to administer the dose.

OR

$$\frac{7.5 \text{ mg}}{2.5 \text{ mg}} = \frac{x \text{ tab}}{1 \text{ tab}}$$

$$\frac{2.5x}{2.5} = \frac{7.5}{2.5}$$

$$x = \frac{7.5}{2.5} = 3 \text{ tabs}$$

5. Equivalent: 1,000 mcg = 1 mg (0.05 mg = 50 mcg)

$$\frac{50 \text{ mcg}}{25 \text{ mcg}} \times 1 \text{ tab} = x \text{ tab}$$

$$\frac{50}{25} = x$$

$x = 2$ tabs. 50 mcg is larger than 25 mcg; therefore you will need more than 1 tab to administer the dose.

OR

$$\frac{50 \text{ mcg}}{25 \text{ mcg}} = \frac{x \text{ tab}}{1 \text{ tab}}$$

$$\frac{25x}{25} = \frac{50}{25}$$

$$x = \frac{50}{25} = 2 \text{ tabs}$$

6. Equivalent: 1,000 mcg = 1 mg
   (0.4 mg = 400 mcg)

$$\frac{400 \text{ mcg}}{200 \text{ mcg}} \times 1 \text{ tab} = x \text{ tab}$$

$$\frac{400}{200} = x$$

$x = 2$ tabs. 400 mg is more than the dose available; therefore you will need more than one tab to administer the dose.

OR

$$\frac{400 \text{ mcg}}{200 \text{ mcg}} = \frac{x \text{ tab}}{1 \text{ tab}}$$

$$\frac{200x}{200} = \frac{400}{200}$$

$$x = 2 \text{ tabs}$$

7. $$\frac{1,000 \text{ mg}}{500 \text{ mg}} \times 1 \text{ tab} = x \text{ tab}$$

$$\frac{1,000}{500} = x$$

$x = 2$ tabs. 1,000 mg is more than 500 mg; therefore you will need more than 1 tab to administer the dose.

OR

$$\frac{1,000 \text{ mg}}{500 \text{ mg}} = \frac{x \text{ tab}}{1 \text{ tab}}$$

$$\frac{500x}{500} = \frac{1,000}{500}$$

$$x = \frac{1,000}{500} = 2$$

8. Equivalent: 1,000 mg = 1 g (0.6 g = 600 mg)

$$\frac{600 \text{ mg}}{600 \text{ mg}} \times 1 \text{ cap} = x \text{ cap}$$

$$\frac{600}{600} = x$$

$x = 1$ cap. 0.6 g = 600 mg. 600 mg tabs are available; therefore give 1 cap to administer the dose.

OR

$$\frac{600 \text{ mg}}{600 \text{ mg}} = \frac{x \text{ cap}}{1 \text{ cap}}$$

$$\frac{600x}{600} = \frac{600}{600}$$

$$x = \frac{600}{600} = 1 \text{ cap}$$

9. Equivalent: 1,000 mcg = 1 mg
   (1.25 mg = 1,250 mcg)

$$\frac{1,250 \text{ mcg}}{625 \text{ mcg}} \times 1 \text{ tab} = x \text{ tab}$$

$$\frac{1,250}{625} = x$$

$x = 2$ tabs. 1,250 mcg is more than 625 mcg; therefore you will need more than one tab to administer the dose.

OR

$$\frac{1,250 \text{ mcg}}{625 \text{ mcg}} = \frac{x \text{ tab}}{1 \text{ tab}}$$

$$\frac{625x}{625} = \frac{1,250}{625}$$

$$x = \frac{1,250}{625} = 2 \text{ tabs}$$

10. $$\frac{10 \text{ mg}}{15 \text{ mg}} \times 1 \text{ mL} = x \text{ mL}$$

$$\frac{10}{15} = x$$

$x = 0.66 = 0.7$ mL. 10 mg is less than 15 mg; you will need less than 1 mL to administer the dose.

OR

$$\frac{10 \text{ mg}}{15 \text{ mg}} = \frac{x \text{ mL}}{1 \text{ mL}}$$

$$\frac{15x}{15} = \frac{10}{15}$$

$$x = \frac{10}{15} = 0.66 = 0.7 \text{ mL}$$

11. $$\frac{400 \text{ mg}}{200 \text{ mg}} \times 5 \text{ mL} = x \text{ mL}$$

$$\frac{2,000}{200} = x$$

$x = 10$ mL. 400 mg is more than 200 mg, therefore you will need more than 5 mL to administer the dose.

OR

$$\frac{400 \text{ mg}}{200 \text{ mg}} = \frac{x \text{ mL}}{5 \text{ mL}}$$

$$\frac{200x}{200} = \frac{2,000}{200}$$

$$x = \frac{2,000}{200} = 10 \text{ mL}$$

12. $\dfrac{15 \text{ mEq}}{20 \text{ mEq}} \times 10 \text{ mL} = x \text{ mL}$

$$\dfrac{150}{20} = x$$

$x = 7\dfrac{1}{2}$ or 7.5 mL. 15 mEq is less than

20 mEq; therefore you will need less than 10 mL to administer the dose.

OR

$$\dfrac{15 \text{ mEq}}{20 \text{ mEq}} = \dfrac{x \text{ mL}}{10 \text{ mL}}$$

$$\dfrac{20x}{20} = \dfrac{150}{20}$$

$$x = \dfrac{150}{20} = 7\dfrac{1}{2} \text{ or } 7.5 \text{ mL}$$

13. $\dfrac{125 \text{ mg}}{250 \text{ mg}} \times 5 \text{ mL} = x \text{ mL}$

$$\dfrac{625}{250} = x$$

$x = 2\dfrac{1}{2}$ or 2.5 mL. 125 mg is less than

250 mg; therefore you will need less than 5 mL to administer the dose.

OR

$$\dfrac{125 \text{ mg}}{250 \text{ mg}} = \dfrac{x \text{ mL}}{5 \text{ mL}}$$

$$\dfrac{250x}{250} = \dfrac{625}{250}$$

$$x = \dfrac{625}{250} = 2\dfrac{1}{2} \text{ or } 2.5 \text{ mL}$$

14. $\dfrac{0.025 \text{ mg}}{0.05 \text{ mg}} \times 5 \text{ mL} = x \text{ mL}$

$$\dfrac{0.125}{0.05} = x$$

$x = 2\dfrac{1}{2}$ or 2.5 mL. 0.025 mg is less than

0.05 mg; therefore you will need less than 5 mL to administer the dose.

OR

$$\dfrac{0.025 \text{ mg}}{0.05 \text{ mg}} = \dfrac{x \text{ mL}}{5 \text{ mL}}$$

$$\dfrac{0.05x}{0.05} = \dfrac{0.125}{0.05}$$

$$x = \dfrac{0.125}{0.05} = 2\dfrac{1}{2} \text{ or } 2.5 \text{ mL}$$

15. $\dfrac{375 \text{ mg}}{125 \text{ mg}} \times 5 \text{ mL} = x \text{ mL}$

$$\dfrac{1,875}{125} = x$$

$x = 15$ mL. 375 mg is more than 125 mg; therefore you will need more than 5 mL to administer the dose.

OR

$$\dfrac{375 \text{ mg}}{125 \text{ mg}} = \dfrac{x \text{ mL}}{5 \text{ mL}}$$

$$\dfrac{125x}{125} = \dfrac{1,875}{125}$$

$$x = \dfrac{1,875}{125} = 15 \text{ mL}$$

Answers to Chapter Review

Note:

For Chapter Review Problems, only answers are shown. If needed, review setup of problems in Practice Problems 1–15.

1.	1 tab	12.	2 caps	25.	10 mL	38.	2 caps (pulvules)
2.	1 tab	13.	1 tab	26.	0.8 mL	39.	5 mL
3.	2 caps	14.	3 tabs	27.	2 mL	40.	1 tab
4.	1 tab	15.	2 caps	28.	0.6 mL	41.	2 tabs
5.	2 tabs	16.	0.7 mL	29.	0.8 mL	42.	1.3 mL
6.	$1\frac{1}{2}$ tabs or 1.5 tabs	17.	1 mL	30.	0.5 mL	43.	2 mL
		18.	0.4 mL	31.	0.3 mL	44.	3 mL
7.	1 cap	19.	12 mL	32.	1 mL	45.	2 tabs
8.	1 cap	20.	10 mL	33.	2 mL	46.	2 tabs
9.	2 caps	21.	11.3 mL	34.	3.2 mL	47.	2 tabs
10.	2 tabs	22.	0.6 mL	35.	5 mL	48.	6 mL
11.	$1\frac{1}{2}$ tabs or 1.5 tabs	23.	2 mL	36.	1 tab	49.	12 mL
		24.	1.8 mL	37.	1 tab	50.	2.5 mL
						51.	1 tab

CHAPTER 16

Answers to Practice Problems

The answers to the practice problems include the rationale for the answer where indicated. Where necessary, the methods for calculation of the dose are shown as well.

Note:

Unless stated, no conversion is required to calculate dose. In problems that required a conversion before calculating the dose, the problem setup shown illustrates the problem after appropriate conversions have been made.

1. 0.025 mg = 25 mcg
    50 mcg : 1 tab = 25 mcg : x tab

    OR

    $\dfrac{25 \text{ mcg}}{50 \text{ mcg}} \times 1 \text{ tab} = x \text{ tab}$; $\dfrac{25 \text{ mcg}}{50 \text{ mcg}} = \dfrac{x \text{ tab}}{1 \text{ tab}}$

    Answer: 0.5 or $\dfrac{1}{2}$ tab. This is an acceptable answer since the tabs are scored. (For administration purposes state as $\dfrac{1}{2}$ tab.)

2. 25 mg : 1 tab = 6.25 mg : x tab

    OR

    $\dfrac{6.25 \text{ mg}}{25 \text{ mg}} \times 1 \text{ tab} = x \text{ tab}$; $\dfrac{6.25 \text{ mg}}{25 \text{ mg}} - \dfrac{x \text{ tab}}{1 \text{ tab}}$

    Answer: $\dfrac{1}{4}$ tab. This is logical since the tablets are scored in quarters; therefore you could accurately administer the dose.

3. Conversion is necessary: 1,000 mg = 1 g.
    Therefore 1.2 g = 1,200 mg
    400 mg : 1 tab = 1,200 mg : x tab

    OR

    $\dfrac{1,200 \text{ mg}}{400 \text{ mg}} \times 1 \text{ tab} = x \text{ tab}$; $\dfrac{1,200 \text{ mg}}{400 \text{ mg}} = \dfrac{x \text{ tab}}{1 \text{ tab}}$

    Answer: 3 tabs. The dose ordered is greater than what is available; therefore you will need more than 1 tab to administer the dose. The maximum number of tabs that can be given is 3.

4. It would be best to administer one of the 5-mg tablets and one of the 2.5-mg tablets (5 mg + 2.5 mg = 7.5 mg).

5. a) 125-mcg tablet is the appropriate strength to use (0.125 mg = 125 mcg).

    b) 1 tab. Even though the tablets are scored, $\frac{1}{2}$ of 500 mcg would still be twice the dose desired.

    125 mcg : 1 tab = 125 mcg : x tab

    OR

    $$\frac{125 \text{ mcg}}{125 \text{ mcg}} \times 1 \text{ tab} = x \text{ tab}; \quad \frac{125 \text{ mcg}}{125 \text{ mcg}} = \frac{x \text{ tab}}{1 \text{ tab}}$$

    Answer: 1 tab

6. a) 500-mg caps would be appropriate to use.
    b) 2 caps (500 mg each). 1,000 mg = 1 g; therefore 2 caps of 500 mg each would be the least number of capsules. Using the 250-mg strength capsules would require 4 caps.
    c) 2 caps q6h = 8 caps. Multiplying the number of caps needed by the number of days gives you the number of capsules required.

    8 (number of caps per day) $\times$ 7 (number of days) = 56 (total caps needed)

    500 mg : 1 cap = 1,000 mg : x cap

    $$\frac{1,000 \text{ mg}}{500 \text{ mg}} \times 1 \text{ cap} = x \text{ cap}; \quad \frac{1,000 \text{ mg}}{500 \text{ mg}} = \frac{x \text{ cap}}{1 \text{ cap}}$$

    $$x = 2 \text{ caps}$$

7. 5 mg : 1 tab = 10 mg : x tab

    $$\frac{10 \text{ mg}}{5 \text{ mg}} \times 1 \text{ tab} = x \text{ tab}; \quad \frac{10 \text{ mg}}{5 \text{ mg}} = \frac{x \text{ tab}}{1 \text{ tab}}$$

    Answer: 2 tabs. The dose ordered is greater than what is available; therefore you will need more than 1 tab to administer the dose.

8. a) $1\frac{1}{2}$ tabs; the tablets are scored. (State as $1\frac{1}{2}$ tabs for administration purposes.)

    10 mg : 1 tab = 15 mg : x tab

    $$\frac{15 \text{ mg}}{10 \text{ mg}} \times 1 \text{ tab} = x \text{ tab}; \quad \frac{15 \text{ mg}}{10 \text{ mg}} = \frac{x \text{ tab}}{1 \text{ tab}}$$

    $$x = 1\frac{1}{2} \text{ tab}$$

    b) 15 mg $\times$ 3 (t.i.d.) = 45 mg/day. The total number of mg received for 3 days = 135 mg.

    45 mg $\times$ 3 = 135 mg

9. 0.075 mg = 75 mcg

    50 mcg : 1 tab = 75 mcg : x tab

    OR

    $$\frac{75 \text{ mg}}{50 \text{ mg}} \times 1 \text{ tab} = x \text{ tab}; \quad \frac{75 \text{ mg}}{50 \text{ mg}} = \frac{x \text{ tab}}{1 \text{ tab}}$$

    Answer: 1.5 or $1\frac{1}{2}$ tabs, since the tabs are scored.

    (State as $1\frac{1}{2}$ for administration purposes.)

10. 1.3 g = 1,300 mg

    650 mg : 1 tab = 1,300 mg : x tab

    OR

    $$\frac{1,300 \text{ mg}}{650 \text{ mg}} \times 1 \text{ tab} = x \text{ tab}; \quad \frac{1,300 \text{ mg}}{650 \text{ mg}} = \frac{x \text{ tab}}{1 \text{ tab}}$$

    Answer: 2 tabs. The dose ordered is more than what is available; therefore, you will need more than 1 tab to administer the dose.

11. 30 mg : 1 cap = 90 mg : x cap

    OR

    $$\frac{90 \text{ mg}}{30 \text{ mg}} \times 1 \text{ cap} = x \text{ cap}; \quad \frac{90 \text{ mg}}{30 \text{ mg}} = \frac{x \text{ cap}}{1 \text{ cap}}$$

    Answer: 3 caps. The dose ordered is greater than what is available. You will need more than 1 cap to administer the dose.

12. 100 mg : 1 tab = 200 mg : x tab

    OR

    $$\frac{200 \text{ mg}}{100 \text{ mg}} \times 1 \text{ tab} = x \text{ tab}; \quad \frac{200 \text{ mg}}{100 \text{ mg}} = \frac{x \text{ tab}}{1 \text{ tab}}$$

    Answer: 2 tabs. The dose ordered is greater than what is available; therefore you will need more than 1 tab to administer the dose.

13. a) 2 caps (1 g = 1,000 mg)

    500 mg $\times$ 2 = 1,000 mg.

    Answer: 2 caps.

    b) 1 cap (500 mg = 0.5 g)

    1 cap of 500 mg

    Initial dose: 500 mg : 1 cap = 1,000 mg : x cap

    OR

    $$\frac{1,000 \text{ mg}}{500 \text{ mg}} \times 1 \text{ cap} = x \text{ cap};$$

    $$\frac{1,000 \text{ mg}}{500 \text{ mg}} = \frac{x \text{ cap}}{1 \text{ cap}}$$

    Daily dose: 500 mg : 1 cap = 500 mg : x cap

    OR

$$\frac{500 \text{ mg}}{500 \text{ mg}} \times 1 \text{ cap} = x \text{ cap}; \quad \frac{500 \text{ mg}}{500 \text{ mg}} = \frac{x \text{ cap}}{1 \text{ cap}}$$

Answer: 1 cap

14. 125 mg : 1 tab = 250 mg : x tab

OR

$$\frac{250 \text{ mg}}{125 \text{ mg}} \times 1 \text{ tab} = x \text{ tab} \quad \frac{250 \text{ mg}}{125 \text{ mg}} = \frac{x \text{ tab}}{1 \text{ tab}}$$

Answer: 2 tabs. The dose ordered is more than what is available; therefore you will need more than 1 tab to administer the dose.

15. Conversion is necessary.

$$\text{gr } 1\frac{1}{2} = 90 \text{ mg}$$

a) 30-mg tablets
b) three 30-mg tablets. This strength will allow the client to take 3 tabs to achieve the desired dose, as opposed to six 15-mg tabs. This dose is logical since the maximum number of tablets administered is three.

30 mg : 1 tab = 90 mg : x tab

OR

$$\frac{90 \text{ mg}}{30 \text{ mg}} \times 1 \text{ tab} = x \text{ tab}; \quad \frac{90 \text{ mg}}{30 \text{ mg}} = \frac{x \text{ tab}}{1 \text{ tab}}$$

Answer: 3 30-mg tabs

16. The best strength to use is 1.5 mg. This would allow the client to swallow the least amount.
1.5 mg : 1 tab = 3 mg : x tab

OR

$$\frac{3 \text{ mg}}{1.5 \text{ mg}} \times 1 \text{ tab} = x \text{ tab}; \quad \frac{3 \text{ mg}}{1.5 \text{ mg}} = \frac{x \text{ tab}}{1 \text{ tab}}$$

Answer: 2 1.5-mg tabs would be the least number of tablets; 0.75 mg would require the client to swallow 4 tabs to receive the dose (0.75 × 4 = 3).

17. 50 mg : 1 tab = 100 mg : x tab

OR

$$\frac{100 \text{ mg}}{50 \text{ mg}} \times 1 \text{ tab} = x \text{ tab}; \quad \frac{100 \text{ mg}}{50 \text{ mg}} = \frac{x \text{ tab}}{1 \text{ tab}}$$

Answer: You need 2 tabs to administer 100 mg. 2 tabs t.i.d. (3 times a day) = 6 tabs × 3 days = 18 tabs

18. It would be best to administer 1 80-mg tablet and 1 40-mg tablet (80 + 40 = 120 mg). This would be the least number of tablets.

19. Conversion is required. Equivalent: gr 1 = 65 mg.

$$\text{gr } x = 650 \text{ mg}$$

325 mg : 1 tab = 650 mg : x tab

OR

$$\frac{650 \text{ mg}}{325 \text{ mg}} \times 1 \text{ tab} = x \text{ tab}; \quad \frac{650 \text{ mg}}{325 \text{ mg}} = \frac{x \text{ tab}}{1 \text{ tab}}$$

Answer: 2 tabs. The dose ordered is larger than the required dose; therefore more than 1 tab will be required.

20. 0.5 mg : 1 tab = 1 mg : x tab

OR

$$\frac{1 \text{ mg}}{0.5 \text{ mg}} \times 1 \text{ tab} = x \text{ tab}; \quad \frac{1 \text{ mg}}{0.5 \text{ mg}} = \frac{x \text{ tab}}{1 \text{ tab}}$$

$$x = 2 \text{ tabs}$$

Answer: 2 tabs (0.5 × 2 = 1)

21. 1 mg : 1 cap = 3 mg : x cap

OR

$$\frac{3 \text{ mg}}{1 \text{ mg}} \times 1 \text{ cap} = x \text{ cap}; \quad \frac{3 \text{ mg}}{1 \text{ mg}} = \frac{x \text{ cap}}{1 \text{ cap}}$$

Answer: 3 caps. They are administered in whole numbers. The answer is logical. The maximum number of tablets or capsules administered is three.

22. Conversion is required. Equivalent: gr 1 = 60 mg. Therefore

$$\text{gr } \frac{1}{150} = 0.4 \text{ mg}$$

0.4 mg : 1 tab = 0.4 mg : x tab

OR

$$\frac{0.4 \text{ mg}}{0.4 \text{ mg}} \times 1 \text{ tab} = x \text{ tab}; \quad \frac{0.4 \text{ mg}}{0.4 \text{ mg}} = \frac{x \text{ tab}}{1 \text{ tab}}$$

Answer: 1 tab. The label indicates gr $\frac{1}{150}$ = 0.4 mg. Therefore only 1 tab is needed to administer the dose.

23. Choose the 6-mg tab and give 1 tab, which allows the client to swallow the least number of tabs without scoring.

6 mg : 1 tab = 6 mg : x tab

OR

$$\frac{6 \text{ mg}}{6 \text{ mg}} \times 1 \text{ tab} = x \text{ tab}; \quad \frac{6 \text{ mg}}{5 \text{ mg}} = \frac{x \text{ tab}}{1 \text{ tab}}$$

Answer: 1 6-mg tab

24. Conversion is required. Equivalent: 1,000 mg = 1 g; therefore 0.2 g = 200 mg

100 mg : 1 tab = 200 mg : x tab

OR

$$\frac{200 \text{ mg}}{100 \text{ mg}} \times 1 \text{ tab} = x \text{ tab}; \quad \frac{200 \text{ mg}}{100 \text{ mg}} = \frac{x \text{ tab}}{1 \text{ tab}}$$

Answer: 2 tabs. The dose ordered is larger than what is available; therefore more than 1 tab is needed.

25. $40 \text{ mg} : 1 \text{ tab} = 60 \text{ mg} : x \text{ tab}$

OR

$$\frac{60 \text{ mg}}{40 \text{ mg}} \times 1 \text{ tab} = x \text{ tab}; \quad \frac{60 \text{ mg}}{40 \text{ mg}} = \frac{x \text{ tab}}{1 \text{ tab}}$$

Answer: $1\frac{1}{2}$ tabs or 1.5 tabs. The tabs are scored, so 1 tab can be broken to administer the dose. (State as $1\frac{1}{2}$ tabs for administration purposes.)

26. $5 \text{ mg} : 1 \text{ tab} = 2.5 \text{ mg} : x \text{ tab}$

OR

$$\frac{2.5 \text{ mg}}{5 \text{ mg}} \times 1 \text{ tab} = x \text{ tab}; \quad \frac{2.5 \text{ mg}}{5 \text{ mg}} = \frac{x \text{ tab}}{1 \text{ tab}}$$

Answer: 0.5 tab or $\frac{1}{2}$ tab. This is an acceptable answer (0.5 tab or $\frac{1}{2}$ tab) since the tablets are scored. The dose ordered is less than what is available. You will need less than 1 tab to administer the required dose. (State as $\frac{1}{2}$ tab for administration purposes.)

27. $200 \text{ mg} : 1 \text{ tab} = 400 \text{ mg} : x \text{ tab}$

OR

$$\frac{400 \text{ mg}}{200 \text{ mg}} \times 1 \text{ tab} = x \text{ tab}; \quad \frac{400 \text{ mg}}{200 \text{ mg}} = \frac{x \text{ tab}}{1 \text{ tab}}$$

Answer: 2 tabs. The dose ordered is more than what is available. You will need more than 1 tab to administer the dose.

28. $75 \text{ mg} : 1 \text{ cap} = 150 \text{ mg} : x \text{ cap}$

OR

$$\frac{150 \text{ mg}}{75 \text{ mg}} \times 1 \text{ cap} = x \text{ cap}; \quad \frac{150 \text{ mg}}{75 \text{ mg}} = \frac{x \text{ cap}}{1 \text{ cap}}$$

Answer: 2 caps. The dose ordered is more than what is available. You will need more than 1 cap to administer the dose.

29. Change 1 g to 1,000 mg (1,000 mg = 1 g)

$$500 \text{ mg} : 1 \text{ tab} = 1,000 \text{ mg} : x \text{ tab}$$

OR

$$\frac{1,000 \text{ mg}}{500 \text{ mg}} \times 1 \text{ tab} = x \text{ tab}; \quad \frac{1,000 \text{ mg}}{500 \text{ mg}} = \frac{x \text{ tab}}{1 \text{ tab}}$$

Answer: 2 tabs. The dose ordered is greater than what is available. You will need more than 1 tab to administer the dose.

30. $25 \text{ mg} : 1 \text{ tab} = 12.5 \text{ mg} : x \text{ tab}$

OR

$$\frac{12.5 \text{ mg}}{25 \text{ mg}} \times 1 \text{ tab} = x \text{ tab}; \quad \frac{12.5 \text{ mg}}{25 \text{ mg}} = \frac{x \text{ tab}}{1 \text{ tab}}$$

Answer: 0.5 tab or $\frac{1}{2}$ tab (2 quarters). The dose ordered is less than what is available. You will need less than 1 tab to administer the dose.

(State as $\frac{1}{2}$ tab for administration purposes.)

31. It would be best to administer one 75-mcg tablet and one 25-mcg tablet for a total of 100 mcg. This would be the least number of tablets (75 mcg + 25 mcg = 100 mcg).

32. $12.5 \text{ mg} : 1 \text{ tab} = 25 \text{ mg} : x \text{ tab}$

OR

$$\frac{25 \text{ mg}}{12.5 \text{ mg}} \times 1 \text{ tab} = x \text{ tab}; \quad \frac{25 \text{ mg}}{12.5 \text{ mg}} = \frac{x \text{ tab}}{1 \text{ tab}}$$

Answer: 2 tabs. The dose ordered is more than what is available. You will need more than 1 tab to administer the dose.

33. $0.5 \text{ mg} : 1 \text{ tab} = 0.25 \text{ mg} : x \text{ tab}$

OR

$$\frac{0.25 \text{ mg}}{0.5 \text{ mg}} \times 1 \text{ tab} = x \text{ tab}; \quad \frac{0.25 \text{ mg}}{0.5 \text{ mg}} = \frac{x \text{ tab}}{1 \text{ tab}}$$

Answer: 0.5 tab or $\frac{1}{2}$ tab. This is an acceptable answer since the tablet is scored. (State answer as $\frac{1}{2}$ tab for administration purposes.)

34. Conversion is necessary: 1,000 mg = 1 g; therefore 0.25 g = 250 mg

$$250 \text{ mg} : 1 \text{ tab} = 250 \text{ mg} : x \text{ tab}$$

OR

$$\frac{250 \text{ mg}}{250 \text{ mg}} \times 1 \text{ tab} = x \text{ tab}; \quad \frac{250 \text{ mg}}{250 \text{ mg}} = \frac{x \text{ tab}}{1 \text{ tab}}$$

Answer: 1 tab. 0.25 g = 250 mg, which is equal to 1 tab.

35. Label indicates 0.025 mg = 25 mcg.

$$25 \text{ mcg} : 1 \text{ tab} = 25 \text{ mcg} : x \text{ tab}$$

OR

$$\frac{25 \text{ mcg}}{25 \text{ mcg}} \times 1 \text{ tab} = x \text{ tab}; \quad \frac{25 \text{ mcg}}{25 \text{ mcg}} = \frac{x \text{ tab}}{1 \text{ tab}}$$

Answer: 1 tab. 0.025 mg is equal to 25 mcg. Therefore only 1 tab is needed to administer the dose.

36. $325 \text{ mg} : 1 \text{ tab} = 650 \text{ mg} : x \text{ tab}$

OR

$$\frac{650 \text{ mg}}{325 \text{ mg}} \times 1 \text{ tab} = x \text{ tab}; \quad \frac{650 \text{ mg}}{325 \text{ mg}} = \frac{x \text{ tab}}{1 \text{ tab}}$$

Answer: 2 tabs. The dose ordered is greater than what is available; you will need more than 1 tab to administer the dose.

37. Conversion is necessary. 1,000 mg = 1 g; therefore 0.2 g = 200 mg

$$100 \text{ mg} : 1 \text{ cap} = 200 \text{ mg} : x \text{ cap}$$

OR

$$\frac{200 \text{ mg}}{100 \text{ mg}} \times 1 \text{ cap} = x \text{ cap}; \quad \frac{200 \text{ mg}}{100 \text{ mg}} = \frac{x \text{ cap}}{1 \text{ cap}}$$

Answer: 2 caps. The dose ordered is greater than what is available. You will need more than 1 cap to administer the dose.

38. $400 \text{ mg} : 1 \text{ tab} = 800 \text{ mg} : x \text{ tab}$

OR

Note:

The setup shown for problems that required conversions reflect converting of what the doctor ordered to what is available. Unless stated in Problems 42-70, no conversion is required to calculate the dose.

42. $50 \text{ mg} : 15 \text{ mL} = 100 \text{ mg} : x \text{ mL}$

OR

$$\frac{100 \text{ mg}}{50 \text{ mg}} \times 15 \text{ mL} = x \text{ mL}; \quad \frac{100 \text{ mg}}{50 \text{ mg}} = \frac{x \text{ mL}}{15 \text{ mL}}$$

Answer: 30 mL. In order to administer the dose required, more than 15 mL will be necessary. The dosage ordered is 2 times larger than what the available strength is.

$$\frac{800 \text{ mg}}{400 \text{ mg}} \times 1 \text{ tab} = x \text{ tab}; \quad \frac{800 \text{ mg}}{400 \text{ mg}} = \frac{x \text{ tab}}{1 \text{ tab}}$$

Answer: 2 tabs. The dose ordered is greater than what is available. You will need more than 1 tab to administer the dose.

39. $30 \text{ mg} : 1 \text{ tab} = 60 \text{ mg} : x \text{ tab}$

$$\frac{60 \text{ mg}}{30 \text{ mg}} \times 1 \text{ tab} = x \text{ tab}; \quad \frac{60 \text{ mg}}{30 \text{ mg}} = \frac{x \text{ tab}}{1 \text{ tab}}$$

Answer: 2 tabs. The dose ordered is greater than what is available. You will need more than 1 tab to administer the dose.

40. Conversion: 1,000 mg = 1 g. Therefore 0.3 g = 300 mg

$$100 \text{ mg} : 1 \text{ tab} = 300 \text{ mg} : x \text{ tab}$$

OR

$$\frac{300 \text{ mg}}{100 \text{ mg}} \times 1 \text{ tab} = x \text{ tab}; \quad \frac{300 \text{ mg}}{100 \text{ mg}} = \frac{x \text{ tab}}{1 \text{ tab}}$$

Answer: 3 tabs. The dose ordered is greater than what is available. You will need more than 1 tab to administer the dose. Three tablets is the maximum number of tablets that should be given.

41. $80 \text{ mg} : 1 \text{ cap} = 160 \text{ mg} : x \text{ cap}$

OR

$$\frac{160 \text{ mg}}{80 \text{ mg}} \times 1 \text{ cap} = x \text{ cap}; \quad \frac{160 \text{ mg}}{80 \text{ mg}} = \frac{x \text{ cap}}{1 \text{ cap}}$$

Answer: 2 caps. The dose ordered is greater than what is available. You will need more than 1 cap to administer the dose.

43. Conversion is required. Equivalent: 1 g = 1,000 mg

$$500 \text{ mg} : 10 \text{ mL} = 1,000 \text{ mg} : x \text{ mL}$$

OR

$$\frac{1,000 \text{ mg}}{500 \text{ mg}} \times 10 \text{ mL} = x \text{ mL}; \quad \frac{1,000 \text{ mg}}{500 \text{ mg}} = \frac{x \text{ mL}}{10 \text{ mL}}$$

Answer: 20 mL. To administer the required dose, which is 2 times larger than the strength it is available in, more than 10 mL is required.

44. 40 mEq : 15 mL = 40 mEq : x mL

    OR

    $\dfrac{40\ mEq}{40\ mEq} \times 15\ mL = x\ mL; \quad \dfrac{40\ mEq}{40\ mEq} = \dfrac{x\ mL}{15\ mL}$

    Answer: 15 mL. The dose ordered is contained in 15 mL of the medication.

45. 80 mg : 15 mL = 120 mg : x mL

    OR

    $\dfrac{120\ mg}{80\ mg} \times 15\ mL = x\ mL; \quad \dfrac{120\ mg}{80\ mg} = \dfrac{x\ mL}{15\ mL}$

    Answer: 22.5 mL. To administer the dose required, more than 15 mL will be necessary.

46. 200 mg : 5 mL = 250 mg : x mL

    OR

    $\dfrac{250\ mg}{200\ mg} \times 5\ mL = x\ mL; \quad \dfrac{250\ mg}{200\ mg} = \dfrac{x\ mL}{5\ mL}$

    Answer: 6.3 mL. The dose ordered is greater than what is available. The answer to the nearest tenth is 6.3 mL.

47. 125 mg : 5 mL = 100 mg : x mL

    OR

    $\dfrac{100\ mg}{125\ mg} \times 5\ mL = x\ mL; \quad \dfrac{100\ mg}{125\ mg} = \dfrac{x\ mL}{5\ mL}$

    Answer: 4 mL. The amount is ordered is less than what is available, so less than 5 mL will be needed to administer the required dose.

48. Use the mcg equivalent to calculate the dose.

    50 mcg : 1 mL = 125 mcg : x mL

    OR

    $\dfrac{125\ mcg}{50\ mcg} \times 1\ mL = x\ mL$

    Answer: 2.5 mL. or $2\frac{1}{2}$ mL. ($2\frac{1}{2}$ mL is preferred for administration purposes.) The dose ordered is larger than what is available so you will need more than 1 mL to administer the dose.

49. 125 mg : 5 mL = 250 mg : x mL

    OR

    $\dfrac{250\ mg}{125\ mg} \times 5\ mL = x\ mL; \quad \dfrac{250\ mg}{125\ mg} = \dfrac{x\ mL}{5\ mL}$

    Answer: 10 mL. The dose ordered is more than what is available. You will need more than 5 mL to administer the dose.

50. Conversion is required. Equivalent: 1,000 mg = 1 g.

    Therefore 0.5 g = 500 mg

    125 mg : 5 mL = 500 mg : x mL

    OR

    $\dfrac{500\ mg}{125\ mg} \times 5\ mL = x\ mL; \quad \dfrac{500\ mg}{125\ mg} = \dfrac{x\ mL}{5\ mL}$

    Answer: 20 mL. The dose ordered is 4 times larger than the available strength; therefore more than 5 mL will be needed to administer the dose.

51. 20 mg : 5 mL = 60 mg : x mL

    $\dfrac{20x}{20} = \dfrac{300}{20}$

    OR

    $\dfrac{60\ mg}{20\ mg} \times 5\ mL = x\ mL; \quad \dfrac{60\ mg}{20\ mg} = \dfrac{x\ mL}{5\ mL}$

    Answer: 15 mL. The dose ordered is more than what is available. You will need more than 5 mL to administer the dose.

52. 30 mg : 1 mL = 150 mg : x mL

    OR

    $\dfrac{150\ mg}{30\ mg} \times 1\ mL = x\ mL; \quad \dfrac{150\ mg}{30\ mg} = \dfrac{x\ mL}{1\ mL}$

    Answer: 5 mL. The dose ordered is 5 times larger than the available strength. You will need more than 1 mL to administer the required dose.

53. 12.5 mg : 5 mL = 25 mg : x mL

    OR

    $\dfrac{25\ mg}{12.5\ mg} \times 5\ mL = x\ mL; \quad \dfrac{25\ mg}{12.5\ mg} = \dfrac{x\ mL}{5\ mL}$

    Answer: 10 mL. The dose needed is 2 times more than the available strength, so you will need more than 5 mL to administer the required dose.

54. The label indicates that 5 mL = 300 mg of the medication.

    300 mg : 5 mL = 600 mg : x mL

    OR

    $\dfrac{600\ mg}{300\ mg} \times 5\ mL = x\ mL; \quad \dfrac{600\ mg}{300\ mg} = \dfrac{x\ mL}{5\ mL}$

a) 10 mL. The dose ordered is 2 times more than the available strength. You will need more than 5 mL to administer the required dose.

b) Two containers are needed. One container delivers 300 mg.

55. $2 \text{ mg} : 1 \text{ mL} = 10 \text{ mg} : x \text{ mL}$

    OR

    $$\frac{10 \text{ mg}}{2 \text{ mg}} \times 1 \text{ mL} = x \text{ mL}; \quad \frac{10 \text{ mg}}{2 \text{ mg}} = \frac{x \text{ mL}}{1 \text{ mL}}$$

    Answer: 5 mL. The dose ordered is 5 times greater than the available strength. More than 1 mL will be needed to administer the required dose.

56. Conversion is required. Equivalent: 1,000 mg = 1 g.

    Therefore 0.5 g = 500 mg.

    $62.5 \text{ mg} : 5 \text{ mL} = 500 \text{ mg} : x \text{ mL}$

    OR

    $$\frac{500 \text{ mg}}{62.5 \text{ mg}} \times 5 \text{ mL} = x \text{ mL}; \quad \frac{500 \text{ mg}}{62.5 \text{ mg}} = \frac{x \text{ mL}}{5 \text{ mL}}$$

    Answer: 40 mL. The dose ordered is larger than the available strength. You will need more than 5 mL to administer the required dose.

57. $200,000 \text{ U} : 5 \text{ mL} = 500,000 \text{ U} : x \text{ mL}$

    OR

    $$\frac{500,000 \text{ U}}{200,000 \text{ U}} \times 5 \text{ mL} = x \text{ mL}; \quad \frac{500,000 \text{ U}}{200,000 \text{ U}} = \frac{x \text{ mL}}{5 \text{ mL}}$$

    Answer: 12.5 mL or $12\frac{1}{2}$ mL. The amount ordered is greater than the strength available, you will need more than 5 mL to administer the required dose.

58. Conversion is required. Equivalent: 1 g = 1,000 mg.

    $125 \text{ mg} : 5 \text{ mL} = 1,000 \text{ mg} : x \text{ mL}$

    OR

    $$\frac{1,000 \text{ mg}}{125 \text{ mg}} \times 5 \text{ mL} = x \text{ mL}; \quad \frac{1,000 \text{ mg}}{125 \text{ mg}} = \frac{x \text{ mL}}{5 \text{ mL}}$$

    Answer: 40 mL. The dose ordered is more than the strength available. You will need more than 5 mL to administer the dose.

59. $16 \text{ mg} : 5 \text{ mL} = 24 \text{ mg} : x \text{ mL}$

    OR

$$\frac{24 \text{ mg}}{16 \text{ mg}} \times 5 \text{ mL} = x \text{ mL}; \quad \frac{24 \text{ mg}}{16 \text{ mg}} = \frac{x \text{ mL}}{5 \text{ mL}}$$

Answer: 7.5 mL or $7\frac{1}{2}$ mL. The dose ordered is greater than the available strength. You will need more than 5 mL to administer the required dose.

60. $500 \text{ mg} : 15 \text{ mL} = 650 \text{ mg} : x \text{ mL}$

    OR

    $$\frac{650 \text{ mg}}{500 \text{ mg}} \times 15 \text{ mL} = x \text{ mL};$$

    $$\frac{650 \text{ mg}}{500 \text{ mg}} = \frac{x \text{ mL}}{15 \text{ mL}}$$

    Answer: 19.5 mL or $19\frac{1}{2}$ mL. The dose ordered is more than the strength available. You will need more than 15 mL to administer the required dose.

61. $300 \text{ mg} : 5 \text{ mL} = 400 \text{ mg} : x \text{ mL}$

    OR

    $$\frac{400 \text{ mg}}{300 \text{ mg}} \times 5 \text{ mL} = x \text{ mL}; \quad \frac{400 \text{ mg}}{300 \text{ mg}} = \frac{x \text{ mL}}{5 \text{ mL}}$$

    Answer: 6.66 = 6.7 mL to the nearest tenth. The dose ordered is more than what is available. You will need more than 5 mL to administer the dose.

62. $10 \text{ mg} : 1 \text{ mL} = 150 \text{ mg} : x \text{ mL}$

    OR

    $$\frac{150 \text{ mg}}{10 \text{ mg}} \times 1 \text{ mL} = x \text{ mL}; \quad \frac{150 \text{ mg}}{10 \text{ mg}} = \frac{x \text{ mL}}{1 \text{ mL}}$$

    Answer: 15 mL. The dose ordered is greater than the available strength, so you will need more than 1 mL to administer the required dose.

63. Conversion is necessary. 1,000 mg = 1 g; therefore 0.3 g = 300 mg

    $50 \text{ mg} : 5 \text{ mL} = 300 \text{ mg} : x \text{ mL}$

    OR

    $$\frac{300 \text{ mg}}{50 \text{ mg}} \times 5 \text{ mL} = x \text{ mL}; \quad \frac{300 \text{ mg}}{50 \text{ mg}} = \frac{x \text{ mL}}{5 \text{ mL}}$$

    Answer: 30 mL. The dose ordered is greater than the available strength, so you will need more than 5 mL to administer the required dose.

64. $100{,}000 \text{ U} : 1 \text{ mL} = 200{,}000 \text{ U} : x \text{ mL}$

    OR

    $$\frac{200{,}000 \text{ U}}{100{,}000 \text{ U}} \times 1 \text{ mL} = x \text{ mL}; \quad \frac{200{,}000 \text{ U}}{100{,}000 \text{ U}} = \frac{x \text{ mL}}{1 \text{ mL}}$$

    Answer: 2 mL. The dose ordered is greater than the available strength, so you will need more than 1 mL to administer the required dose.

65. $100 \text{ mg} : 1 \text{ mL} = 150 \text{ mg} : x \text{ mL}$

    OR

    $$\frac{150 \text{ mg}}{100 \text{ mg}} \times 1 \text{ mL} = x \text{ mL}; \quad \frac{150 \text{ mg}}{100 \text{ mg}} = \frac{x \text{ mL}}{1 \text{ mL}}$$

    Answer: 1.5 mL or $1\frac{1}{2}$ mL. ($1\frac{1}{2}$ mL is the best answer for administration purposes.) The dose ordered is greater than the available strength, so you will need more than 1 mL to administer the required dose.

66. Conversion is necessary. $1{,}000 \text{ mg} = 1 \text{ g}$; therefore $0.25 \text{ g} = 250 \text{ mg}$

    $125 \text{ mg} : 5 \text{ mL} = 250 \text{ mg} : x \text{ mL}$

    OR

    $$\frac{250 \text{ mg}}{125 \text{ mg}} \times 5 \text{ mL} = x \text{ mL}; \quad \frac{250 \text{ mg}}{125 \text{ mg}} = \frac{x \text{ mL}}{5 \text{ mL}}$$

    Answer: 10 mL. The dose ordered is greater than the available strength; therefore you will need more than 5 mL to administer the dose.

67. $200 \text{ mg} : 5 \text{ mL} = 200 \text{ mg} : x \text{ mL}$

    OR

    $$\frac{200 \text{ mg}}{200 \text{ mg}} \times 5 \text{ mL} = x \text{ mL}; \quad \frac{200 \text{ mg}}{200 \text{ mg}} = \frac{x \text{ mL}}{5 \text{ mL}}$$

Answer: 5 mL. The dose ordered is equivalent to what is available. Label indicates 200 mg = 5 mL.

68. $20 \text{ mg} : 5 \text{ mL} = 30 \text{ mg} : x \text{ mL}$

    OR

    $$\frac{30 \text{ mg}}{20 \text{ mg}} \times 5 \text{ mL} = x \text{ mL}; \quad \frac{30 \text{ mg}}{20 \text{ mg}} = \frac{x \text{ mL}}{5 \text{ mL}}$$

Answer: 7.5 mL. The dose ordered is greater than the available strength, so you will need more than 5 mL to administer the required dose.

69. $15 \text{ mg} : 1 \text{ mL} = 150 \text{ mg} : x \text{ mL}$

    OR

    $$\frac{150 \text{ mg}}{15 \text{ mg}} \times 1 \text{ mL} = x \text{ mL}; \quad \frac{150 \text{ mg}}{15 \text{ mg}} = \frac{x \text{ mL}}{1 \text{ mL}}$$

Answer: 10 mL. The dose ordered is 10 times more than the available strength, so you will need more than 1 mL to administer the required dose.

70. $30 \text{ mg} : 1 \text{ mL} = 50 \text{ mg} : x \text{ mL}$

    OR

    $$\frac{50 \text{ mg}}{30 \text{ mg}} \times 1 \text{ mL} = x \text{ mL}; \quad \frac{50 \text{ mg}}{30 \text{ mg}} = \frac{x \text{ mL}}{1 \text{ mL}}$$

Answer: 1.7 mL (1.66 mL to the nearest tenth). The dose ordered is greater than the available strength, so you will need more than 1 mL to administer the required dose.

Answers to Chapter Review

Note:

Refer to Problems 1-67 for setup of problems, if needed.

1. 3 tabs
2. 3 caps
3. 2 tabs
4. 3 tabs
5. 2 tabs
6. $12\frac{1}{2}$ mL

    (12.5 mL)

7. 1 tab
8. 2 tabs
9. $\frac{1}{2}$ tab
10. 2 tabs
11. 2 mL
12. 30 mL

13. $\frac{1}{2}$ tab
14. 20.3 mL
15. 8 mL
16. 56.3 mL
17. 3 tabs
18. 2 tabs
19. 2 tabs

20. 6.3 mL
21. 1 0.3-mg tab and 1 0.2-mg tab
22. 1 tab
23. 1 tab
24. 30 mL
25. 2 caps

CHAPTER 17

Answers to Practice Problems

Note:

Problems requiring conversion reflect converting of what the doctor ordered to what is available.

1.

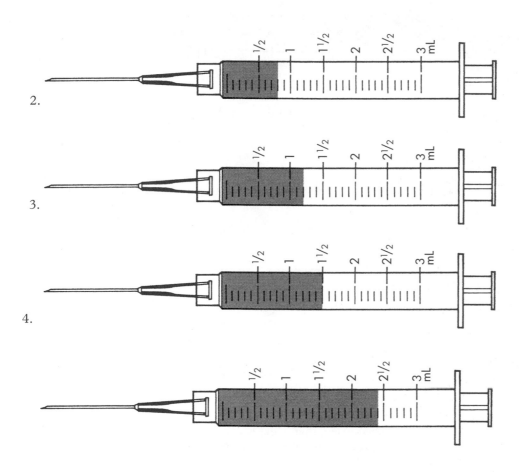

2.

3.

4.

5. 1.4 mL	14. 10 mL	24. 20 mL
6. 1 mL	15. 10 mL	25. 2 mEq/mL
7. 0.9 mL	16. 0.1 mg/mL	26. 50 mL
8. 0.4 mL	17. I.V. use only	27. 50 mEq/50 mL or
9. 4.4 mL	18. 10 mL	1 mEq/mL
10. 7 mL	19. 25 mg/mL	28. 10 mL
11. 3.2 mL	20. 2 mL	29. 1,000 U/mL
12. 20 mL	21. 2 mL	30. 10 mL
13. 25 mg/mL; 500 mg/20 mL	22. 2 mg/2 mL	31. 100 U/mL
is also correct.	23. 1 mL	32. 100 mL
		33. 125 mg/5 mL

34. 5 mg : 1 mL = 10 mg : x mL OR $\dfrac{10 \text{ mg}}{5 \text{ mg}} \times 1 \text{ mL} = x \text{ mL}$

$\dfrac{10 \text{ mg}}{5 \text{ mg}} = \dfrac{x \text{ mL}}{1 \text{ mL}}$

Answer: 2 mL. The dose ordered is more than what is available; therefore you will need more than 1 mL to administer the dose.

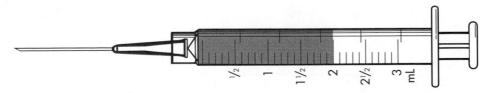

35. 10 mg : 1 mL = 5 mg : x mL OR $\dfrac{5 \text{ mg}}{10 \text{ mg}} \times 1 \text{ mL} = x \text{ mL}$

$\dfrac{5 \text{ mg}}{10 \text{ mg}} = \dfrac{x \text{ mL}}{1 \text{ mL}}$

Answer: 0.5 mL or $\dfrac{1}{2}$ mL. The dose ordered is less than what is available; therefore you will need

less than 1 mL to administer the dose. ($\dfrac{1}{2}$ mL is preferred for administration purposes.)

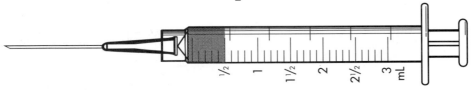

36. 2 mg : 1 mL = 1 mg : x mL OR $\dfrac{1 \text{ mg}}{2 \text{ mg}} \times 1 \text{ mL} = x \text{ mL}$

$\dfrac{1 \text{ mg}}{2 \text{ mg}} = \dfrac{x \text{ mL}}{1 \text{ mL}}$

Answer: 0.5 mL or 1/2 mL. The dose ordered is less than what is available, therefore, you will need less than 1 mL to administer the dose. (1/2 mL is preferred for administration purposes.)

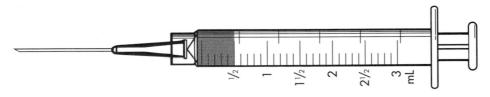

37. 5 mg : 1 mL = 8 mg : x mL OR $\dfrac{8 \text{ mg}}{5 \text{ mg}} \times 1 \text{ mL} = x \text{ mL}$

$\dfrac{8 \text{ mg}}{5 \text{ mg}} = \dfrac{x \text{ mL}}{1 \text{ mL}}$

Answer: 1.6 mL. The dose ordered is more than what is available, therefore, you will need more than 1 mL to administer the dose.

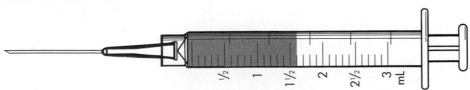

38. Conversion is required. Equivalent: 1,000 mcg = 1 mg

    Therefore 0.05 mg = 50 mcg

    $$100 \text{ mcg} : 1 \text{ mL} = 50 \text{ mcg} : x \text{ mL} \qquad \text{OR} \qquad \frac{50 \text{ mcg}}{100 \text{ mcg}} \times 1 \text{ mL} = x \text{ mL}; \frac{50 \text{ mcg}}{100 \text{ mcg}} = \frac{x \text{ mL}}{1 \text{ mL}}$$

    Answer: 0.5 mL or $\frac{1}{2}$ mL. The dose ordered is less than what is available. (Answer of $\frac{1}{2}$ mL

    is preferred for administration purposes.) Therefore you will need less than 1 mL to administer the dose.

    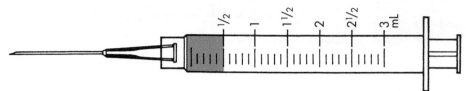

39. Demerol:

    $$75 \text{ mg} : 1 \text{ mL} = 50 \text{ mg} : x \text{ mL} \qquad \text{OR} \qquad \frac{50 \text{ mg}}{75 \text{ mg}} \times 1 \text{ mL} = x \text{ mL}; \frac{50 \text{ mg}}{75 \text{ mg}} = \frac{x \text{ mL}}{1 \text{ mL}}$$

    Answer: 0.66 mL = 0.7 mL. The dose ordered is less than what is available. Therefore less than 1 mL would be required to administer the dose.

    Vistaril:

    $$50 \text{ mg} : 1 \text{ mL} = 25 \text{ mg} : x \text{ mL} \qquad \text{OR} \qquad \frac{25 \text{ mg}}{50 \text{ mg}} \times 1 \text{ mL} = x \text{ mL}; \frac{25 \text{ mg}}{50 \text{ mg}} = \frac{x \text{ mL}}{1 \text{ mL}}$$

    Answer: 0.5 mL or $\frac{1}{2}$ mL. The dose ordered is less than what is available. Therefore you will need

    less than 1 mL to administer the dose. The total number of mL you will prepare to administer is 1.2 mL. This dose is measurable on the small hypodermics. These two medications are often administered in the same syringe. (0.7 mL + 0.5 mL = 1.2 mL)

    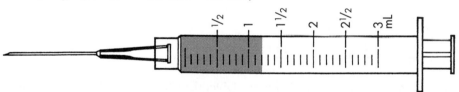

40. $$10 \text{ mg} : 2 \text{ mL} = 5 \text{ mg} : x \text{ mL} \qquad \text{OR} \qquad \frac{5 \text{ mg}}{10 \text{ mg}} \times 2 \text{ mL} = x \text{ mL}; \frac{5 \text{ mg}}{10 \text{ mg}} = \frac{x \text{ mL}}{2 \text{ mL}}$$

    $x = 1$ mL. The dose required is less than the dose available; therefore you will need less than 2 mL to administer the dose.

    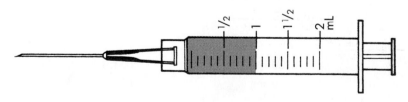

41. $20,000 \text{ U} : 1 \text{ mL} = 5,000 \text{ U} : x \text{ mL}$ OR $\dfrac{5,000 \text{ U}}{20,000 \text{ U}} \times 1 \text{ mL} = x \text{ mL}; \dfrac{5,000 \text{ U}}{20,000 \text{ U}} = \dfrac{x \text{ mL}}{1 \text{ mL}}$

Answer: 0.25 mL. The dose ordered is less than what is available; therefore you will need less than 1 mL to administer the dose. This dose can be measured accurately on the 1 mL (tuberculin) syringe since it is measured in hundredths of a mL. The dose you are administering is $\dfrac{25}{100}$.

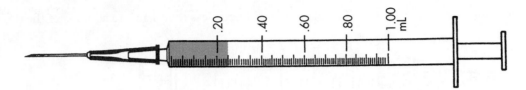

42. Conversion is required. Equivalent: 60 mg = gr 1

Therefore gr $\dfrac{1}{4}$ = 15 mg

$10 \text{ mg} : 1 \text{ mL} = 15 \text{ mg} : x \text{ mL}$ OR $\dfrac{15 \text{ mg}}{10 \text{ mg}} \times 1 \text{ mL} = x \text{ mL}; \dfrac{15 \text{ mg}}{10 \text{ mg}} = \dfrac{x \text{ mL}}{1 \text{ mL}}$

Answer: 1.5 mL or $1\dfrac{1}{2}$ mL. The dose ordered is more than what is available; therefore you will need more than 1 mL to administer the dose. The preferred answer is $1\dfrac{1}{2}$ mL for administration purposes, and the syringe has fraction markings.

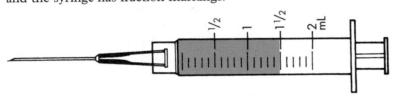

43. $10 \text{ mg} : 1 \text{ mL} = 20 \text{ mg} : x \text{ mL}$ OR $\dfrac{20 \text{ mg}}{10 \text{ mg}} \times 1 \text{ mL} = x \text{ mL}; \dfrac{20 \text{ mg}}{10 \text{ mg}} = \dfrac{x \text{ mL}}{1 \text{ mL}}$

Answer: 2 mL. The dose ordered is more than what is available; therefore you will need more than 1 mL to administer the required dose.

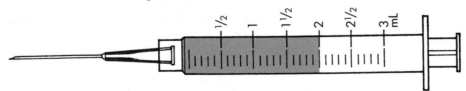

Alternate method for solving:

$40 \text{ mg} : 4 \text{ mL} = 20 \text{ mg} : x \text{ mL}$ OR $\dfrac{20 \text{ mg}}{40 \text{ mg}} \times 4 \text{ mL} = x \text{ mL}; \dfrac{20 \text{ mg}}{40 \text{ mg}} = \dfrac{x \text{ mL}}{4 \text{ mL}}$

This setup still gives an answer of 2 mL.

Answers to Chapter Review

1. Conversion is required. Equivalent: 1,000 mg = 1 g

   Therefore 0.3 g = 300 mg

   $$150 \text{ mg} : 1 \text{ mL} = 300 \text{ mg} : x \text{ mL} \qquad \text{OR} \qquad \frac{300 \text{ mg}}{150 \text{ mg}} \times 1 \text{ mL} = x \text{ mL}; \quad \frac{300 \text{ mg}}{150 \text{ mg}} = \frac{x \text{ mL}}{1 \text{ mL}}$$

   Answer: 2 mL. The dose ordered is more than the dose available, therefore you will need more than 1 mL to administer the dose.

   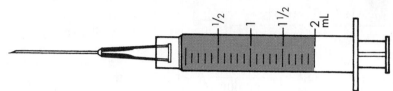

2. Conversion is required. Equivalent: 60 mg = gr 1.

   Therefore gr $\dfrac{1}{150}$ = 0.4 mg

   $$0.4 \text{ mg} : 1 \text{ mL} = 0.4 \text{ mg} : x \text{ mL} \qquad \text{OR} \qquad \frac{0.4 \text{ mg}}{0.4 \text{ mg}} \times 1 \text{ mL} = x \text{ mL}; \quad \frac{0.4 \text{ mg}}{0.4 \text{ mg}} = \frac{x \text{ mL}}{1 \text{ mL}}$$

   Answer: 1 mL. After making the conversion, you can see that, although the dose ordered was in gr, it is equivalent to the same number of mL as what is available.

   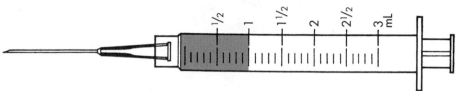

3. Conversion is required. Equivalent: 1,000 mg = 1 g

   Therefore 0.5 g = 500 mg

   $$225 \text{ mg} : 1 \text{ mL} = 500 \text{ mg} : x \text{ mL} \qquad \text{OR} \qquad \frac{500 \text{ mg}}{225 \text{ mg}} \times 1 \text{ mL} = x \text{ mL}; \quad \frac{500 \text{ mg}}{225 \text{ mg}} = \frac{x \text{ mL}}{1 \text{ mL}}$$

   Answer: 2.2 mL. The dose ordered is more than what is available; therefore you will need more than 1 mL. The dose here was rounded off to the nearest tenth of a mL. The small hypodermics are marked in tenths of a mL. To round to the nearest tenth, the math is carried to the hundredths place.

   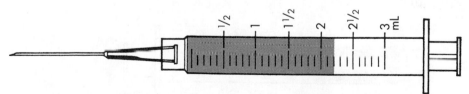

4. Conversion is required. Equivalent: 1,000 mcg = 1 mg

   Therefore 100 mcg = 0.1 mg

   $$0.5 \text{ mg} : 2 \text{ mL} = 0.1 \text{ mg} : x \text{ mL} \qquad \text{OR} \qquad \frac{0.1 \text{ mg}}{0.5 \text{ mg}} \times 2 \text{ mL} = x \text{ mL}; \quad \frac{0.1 \text{ mg}}{0.5 \text{ mg}} = \frac{x \text{ mL}}{2 \text{ mL}}$$

   Answer: 0.4 mL. The dose ordered is less than what is available. The dose required would be less than 2 mL.

   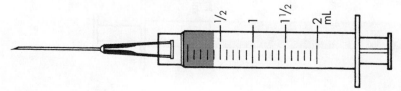

5. 4 mg : 1 mL = 2 mg : x mL   OR $\dfrac{2 \text{ mg}}{4 \text{ mg}} \times 1 \text{ mL} = x \text{ mL}; \dfrac{2 \text{ mg}}{4 \text{ mg}} = \dfrac{x \text{ mL}}{1 \text{ mL}}$

Answer: 0.5 mL or $\dfrac{1}{2}$ mL. The dose ordered is less than what is available; therefore less than 1 mL is required to administer the dose. (The preferred answer for administration purposes is $\dfrac{1}{2}$ mL.)

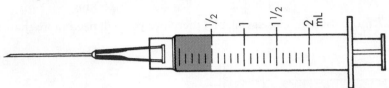

6. 300,000 U : 1 mL = 250,000 U : x mL   OR $\dfrac{250,000 \text{ U}}{300,000 \text{ U}} \times 1 \text{ mL} = x \text{ mL}; \dfrac{250,000 \text{ U}}{300,000 \text{ U}} = \dfrac{x \text{ mL}}{1 \text{ mL}}$

Answer: 0.8 mL. 0.83 mL is rounded to the nearest tenth. The dose ordered is less than what is available; therefore you will need less than 1 mL to administer the dose.

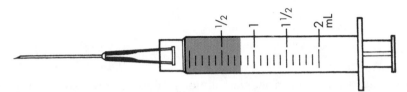

7. 125 mg : 2 mL = 100 mg : x mL   OR $\dfrac{100 \text{ mg}}{125 \text{ mg}} \times 2 \text{ mL} = x \text{ mL}; \dfrac{100 \text{ mg}}{125 \text{ mg}} = \dfrac{x \text{ mL}}{2 \text{ mL}}$

Answer: 1.6 mL. The amount ordered is less than what is available; therefore you will need less than 2 mL to administer the required dose.

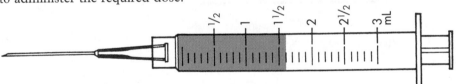

8. 0.2 mg : 1 mL = 0.4 mg : x mL   OR $\dfrac{0.4 \text{ mg}}{0.2 \text{ mg}} \times 1 \text{ mL} = x \text{ mL}; \dfrac{0.4 \text{ mg}}{0.2 \text{ mg}} = \dfrac{x \text{ mL}}{1 \text{ mL}}$

Answer: 2 mL. The dose ordered is more than what is available; therefore you will need more than 1 mL to administer the required dose.

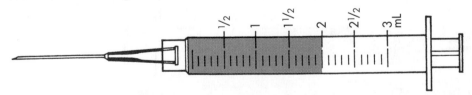

9. 10,000 U : 1 mL = 8,000 U : x mL   OR $\dfrac{8,000 \text{ U}}{10,000 \text{ U}} \times 1 \text{ mL} = x \text{ mL}; \dfrac{8,000 \text{ U}}{10,000 \text{ U}} = \dfrac{x \text{ mL}}{1 \text{ mL}}$

Answer: 0.8 mL. The dose ordered is less than what is available. You will need less than 1 mL to administer the dose.

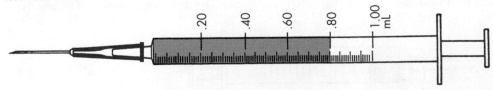

10. $10 \text{ mg} : 1 \text{ mL} = 4 \text{ mg} : x \text{ mL}$ **OR** $\dfrac{4 \text{ mg}}{10 \text{ mg}} \times 1 \text{ mL} = x \text{ mL}; \quad \dfrac{4 \text{ mg}}{10 \text{ mg}} = \dfrac{x \text{ mL}}{1 \text{ mL}}$

Answer: 0.4 mL. The dose ordered is less than what is available; therefore you will need less than 1 mL to administer the dose.

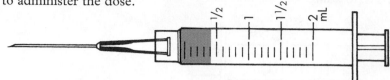

11. $5 \text{ mg} : 1 \text{ mL} = 10 \text{ mg} : x \text{ mL}$ **OR** $\dfrac{10 \text{ mg}}{5 \text{ mg}} \times 1 \text{ mL} = x \text{ mL}; \quad \dfrac{10 \text{ mg}}{5 \text{ mg}} = \dfrac{x \text{ mL}}{1 \text{ mL}}$

Answer: 2 mL. The dose ordered is more than what is available; therefore you will need more than 1 mL to administer the dose.

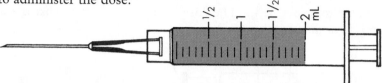

12. Conversion is required. Equivalent: 60 mg = gr 1

Therefore gr $\dfrac{1}{4}$ = 15 mg

     $30 \text{ mg} : 1 \text{ mL} = 15 \text{ mg} : x \text{ mL}$ **OR** $\dfrac{15 \text{ mg}}{30 \text{ mg}} \times 1 \text{ mL} = x \text{ mL}; \quad \dfrac{15 \text{ mg}}{30 \text{ mg}} = \dfrac{x \text{ mL}}{1 \text{ mL}}$

     gr $\dfrac{1}{2}$: 1 mL = gr $\dfrac{1}{4}$: x mL

If fractions are used:

$$\dfrac{\text{gr } \dfrac{1}{4}}{\text{gr } \dfrac{1}{2}} \times 1 \text{ mL} = x \text{ mL} \qquad \textbf{OR} \qquad \dfrac{\text{gr } \dfrac{1}{4}}{\text{gr } \dfrac{1}{2}} = \dfrac{x \text{ mL}}{1 \text{ mL}}$$

Answer: 0.5 mL or $\dfrac{1}{2}$ mL. The dose ordered is less than what is available; therefore you will need less than 1 mL to administer the dose. (The preferred answer is $\dfrac{1}{2}$ mL for administration purposes.)

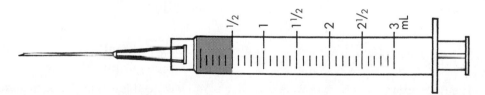

13. $50 \text{ mg} : 1 \text{ mL} = 25 \text{ mg} : x \text{ mL}$ **OR** $\dfrac{25 \text{ mg}}{50 \text{ mg}} \times 1 \text{ mL} = x \text{ mL}; \quad \dfrac{25 \text{ mg}}{50 \text{ mg}} = \dfrac{x \text{ mL}}{1 \text{ mL}}$

Answer: 0.5 mL or $\dfrac{1}{2}$ mL. The dose ordered is less than what is available; therefore you will need less than 1 mL to administer the dose. (The preferred answer is $\dfrac{1}{2}$ mL for administration purposes.)

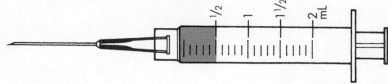

14. $2 \text{ mg} : 1 \text{ mL} = 1.5 \text{ mg} : x \text{ mL}$ OR $\dfrac{1.5 \text{ mg}}{2 \text{ mg}} \times 1 \text{ mL} = x \text{ mL}; \quad \dfrac{1.5 \text{ mg}}{2 \text{ mg}} = \dfrac{x \text{ mL}}{1 \text{ mL}}$

Answer: 0.8 mL. 0.75 mL is rounded to nearest tenth. The dose ordered is less than what is available. You will need less than 1 mL to administer the dose.

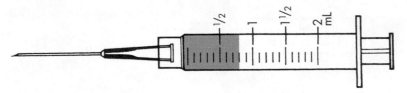

15. $4 \text{ mg} : 1 \text{ mL} = 3 \text{ mg} : x \text{ mL}$ OR $\dfrac{3 \text{ mg}}{4 \text{ mg}} \times 1 \text{ mL} = x \text{ mL}; \quad \dfrac{3 \text{ mg}}{4 \text{ mg}} = \dfrac{x \text{ mL}}{1 \text{ mL}}$

Answer: 0.8 mL. 0.75 mL is rounded to nearest tenth. The dose ordered is less than what is available. You will need less than 1 mL to administer the dose.

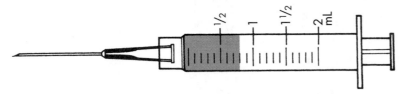

16. Conversion is required. Equivalent: gr 1 = 60 mg

Therefore gr $\dfrac{1}{300}$ = 0.2 mg

$0.4 \text{ mg} : 1 \text{ mL} = 0.2 \text{ mg} : x \text{ mL}$ OR $\dfrac{0.2 \text{ mg}}{0.4 \text{ mg}} \times 1 \text{ mL} = x \text{ mL}; \quad \dfrac{0.2 \text{ mg}}{0.4 \text{ mg}} = \dfrac{x \text{ mL}}{1 \text{ mL}}$

Answer: 0.5 mL or $\dfrac{1}{2}$ mL (The preferred answer is $\dfrac{1}{2}$ mL for administration purposes.) The dose ordered is one half of what is available. You will need less than 1 mL to administer the dose.

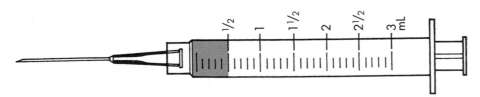

17. $5 \text{ mg} : 1 \text{ mL} = 3 \text{ mg} : x \text{ mL}$ OR $\dfrac{3 \text{ mg}}{5 \text{ mg}} \times 1 \text{ mL} = x \text{ mL}; \quad \dfrac{3 \text{ mg}}{5 \text{ mg}} = \dfrac{x \text{ mL}}{1 \text{ mL}}$

Answer: 0.6 mL. The dose ordered is less than what is available. You will need less than 1 mL to administer the dose.

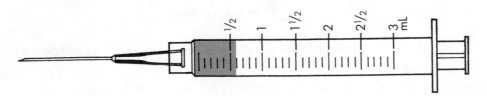

18. $250 \text{ mg} : 2 \text{ mL} = 400 \text{ mg} : x \text{ mL}$ OR $\dfrac{400 \text{ mg}}{250 \text{ mg}} \times 2 \text{ mL} = x \text{ mL}; \quad \dfrac{400 \text{ mg}}{250 \text{ mg}} = \dfrac{x \text{ mL}}{2 \text{ mL}}$

Answer: 3.2 mL. The dose ordered is more than what is available. You will need more than 2 mL to administer the dose.

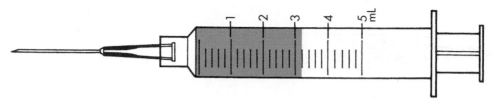

19. $125 \text{ mg} : 2 \text{ mL} = 40 \text{ mg} : x \text{ mL}$ OR $\dfrac{40 \text{ mg}}{125 \text{ mg}} \times 2 \text{ mL} = x \text{ mL}; \quad \dfrac{40 \text{ mg}}{125 \text{ mg}} = \dfrac{x \text{ mL}}{2 \text{ mL}}$

Answer: 0.6 mL. 0.64 mL is rounded to nearest tenth. The dose ordered is less than what is available. You will need less than 1 mL to administer the dose.

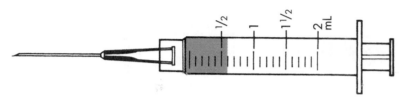

20. Conversion is required. Equivalent: 1,000 mcg = 1 mg

Therefore 200 mcg = 0.2 mg

$0.2 \text{ mg} : 1 \text{ mL} = 0.2 \text{ mg} : x \text{ mL}$ OR $\dfrac{0.2 \text{ mg}}{0.2 \text{ mg}} \times 1 \text{ mL} = x \text{ mL}; \quad \dfrac{0.2 \text{ mg}}{0.2 \text{ mg}} = \dfrac{x \text{ mL}}{1 \text{ mL}}$

Answer: 1 mL. Since 200 mcg = 0.2 mg, you will need 1 mL to administer the required dose.

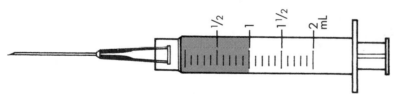

21. $5,000 \text{ U} : 1 \text{ mL} = 2,500 \text{ U} : x \text{ mL}$ OR $\dfrac{2,500 \text{ U}}{5,000 \text{ U}} \times 1 \text{ mL} = x \text{ mL}; \quad \dfrac{2,500 \text{ U}}{5,000 \text{ U}} = \dfrac{x \text{ mL}}{1 \text{ mL}}$

Answer: 0.5 mL. The dose ordered is less than what is available. You will need less than 1 mL to administer the dose.

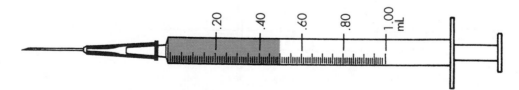

22. $50 \text{ mg} : 1 \text{ mL} = 35 \text{ mg} : x \text{ mL}$ OR $\dfrac{35 \text{ mg}}{50 \text{ mg}} \times 1 \text{ mL} = x \text{ mL}; \quad \dfrac{35 \text{ mg}}{50 \text{ mg}} = \dfrac{x \text{ mL}}{1 \text{ mL}}$

Answer: 0.7 mL. The dose ordered is less than what is available. You will need less than 1 mL to administer the required dose.

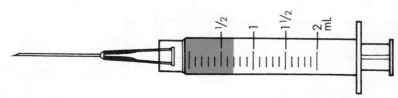

23. 75 mg : 1 mL = 60 mg : x mL   OR $\dfrac{60 \text{ mg}}{75 \text{ mg}} \times 1 \text{ mL} = x \text{ mL}$; $\dfrac{60 \text{ mg}}{75 \text{ mg}} = \dfrac{x \text{ mL}}{1 \text{ mL}}$

Answer: 0.8 mL. The dose ordered is less than what is available. You will need less than 1 mL to administer the required dose.

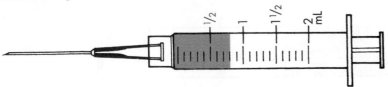

24. 300,000 U : 1 mL = 400,000 U : x mL   OR $\dfrac{400{,}000 \text{ U}}{300{,}000 \text{ U}} \times 1 \text{ mL} = x \text{ mL}$; $\dfrac{400{,}000 \text{ U}}{300{,}000 \text{ U}} = \dfrac{x \text{ mL}}{1 \text{ mL}}$

Answer: 1.3 mL. 1.33 mL is rounded to the nearest tenth. The dose ordered is more than what is available. You will need more than 1 mL to administer the required dose.

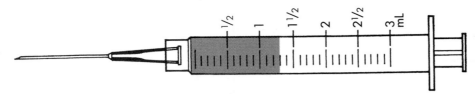

25. 0.5 mg : 2 mL = 0.4 mg : x mL   OR $\dfrac{0.4 \text{ mg}}{0.5 \text{ mg}} \times 2 \text{ mL} = x \text{ mL}$; $\dfrac{0.4 \text{ mg}}{0.5 \text{ mg}} = \dfrac{x \text{ mL}}{2 \text{ mL}}$

Answer: 1.6 mL. The dose ordered is less than what is available. You will need less than 2 mL to administer the required dose.

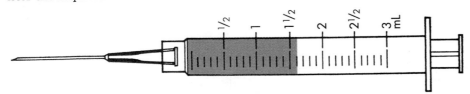

26. 500 mg : 2 mL = 100 mg : x mL   OR $\dfrac{100 \text{ mg}}{500 \text{ mg}} \times 2 \text{ mL} = x \text{ mL}$; $\dfrac{100 \text{ mg}}{500 \text{ mg}} = \dfrac{x \text{ mL}}{2 \text{ mL}}$

Answer: 0.4 mL. The dose ordered is less than what is available. You will need less than 2 mL to administer the required dose.

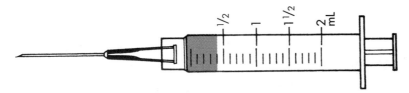

27. 80 mg : 1 mL = 60 mg : x mL   OR $\dfrac{60 \text{ mg}}{80 \text{ mg}} \times 1 \text{ mL} = x \text{ mL}$; $\dfrac{60 \text{ mg}}{80 \text{ mg}} = \dfrac{x \text{ mL}}{1 \text{ mL}}$

Answer: 0.8 mL. 0.75 mL is rounded to the nearest tenth. The dose ordered is less than what is available. You will need less than 1 mL to administer the dose.

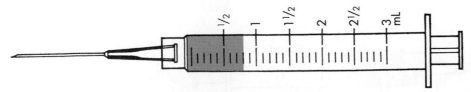

28. $4 \text{ mg} : 1 \text{ mL} = 2 \text{ mg} : x \text{ mL}$ OR $\dfrac{2 \text{ mg}}{4 \text{ mg}} \times 1 \text{ mL} = x \text{ mL}; \dfrac{2 \text{ mg}}{4 \text{ mg}} = \dfrac{x \text{ mL}}{1 \text{ mL}}$

Answer: 0.5 mL or $\dfrac{1}{2}$ mL. ($\dfrac{1}{2}$ mL is preferred for administration purposes.) The dose ordered is less than what is available. Therefore you will need less than 1 mL to administer the dose.

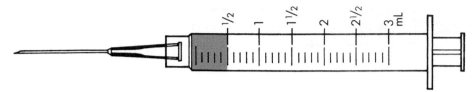

29. $25 \text{ mg} : 1 \text{ mL} = 75 \text{ mg} : x \text{ mL}$ OR $\dfrac{75 \text{ mg}}{25 \text{ mg}} \times 1 \text{ mL} = x \text{ mL}; \dfrac{75 \text{ mg}}{25 \text{ mg}} = \dfrac{x \text{ mL}}{1 \text{ mL}}$

Answer: 3 mL. The dose ordered is greater than what is available. Therefore you will need more than 1 mL to administer the dose.

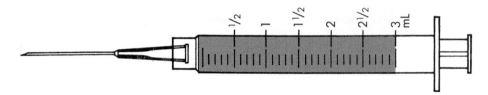

30. $50 \text{ mg} : 1 \text{ mL} = 120 \text{ mg} : x \text{ mL}$ OR $\dfrac{120 \text{ mg}}{50 \text{ mg}} \times 1 \text{ mL} = x \text{ mL}; \dfrac{120 \text{ mg}}{50 \text{ mg}} = \dfrac{x \text{ mL}}{1 \text{ mL}}$

Answer: 2.4 mL. The dose ordered is greater than what is available. Therefore you will more than 1 mL to administer the dose.

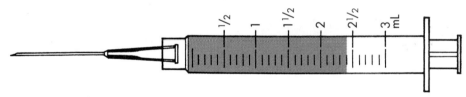

31. $2,000 \text{ U} : 1 \text{ mL} = 3,000 \text{ U} : x \text{ mL}$ OR $\dfrac{3,000 \text{ U}}{2,000 \text{ U}} \times 1 \text{ mL} = x \text{ mL}; \dfrac{3,000 \text{ U}}{2,000 \text{ U}} = \dfrac{x \text{ mL}}{1 \text{ mL}}$

Answer: 1.5 mL or $1\dfrac{1}{2}$ mL. The dose ordered is greater than what is available. Therefore you will need more than 1 mL to administer the dose. (The preferred answer is $1\dfrac{1}{2}$ mL for administration purposes.)

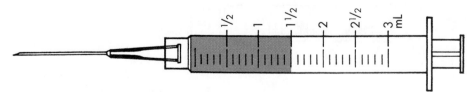

32. 25 mg : 1 mL = 50 mg : x mL   OR $\dfrac{50 \text{ mg}}{25 \text{ mg}} \times 1 \text{ mL} = x \text{ mL}; \quad \dfrac{50 \text{ mg}}{25 \text{ mg}} = \dfrac{x \text{ mL}}{1 \text{ mL}}$

Answer: 2 mL. The dose ordered is greater than what is available. Therefore you will need more than 1 mL to administer the dose.

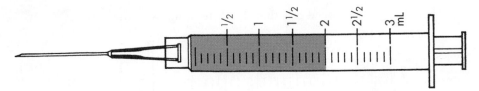

33. 30 mg : 0.3 mL = 30 mg : x mL   OR $\dfrac{30 \text{ mg}}{30 \text{ mg}} \times 0.3 \text{ mL} = x \text{ mL}; \quad \dfrac{30 \text{ mg}}{30 \text{ mg}} = \dfrac{x \text{ mL}}{0.3 \text{ mL}}$

Answer: 0.3 mL. The label indicates that the dose ordered, 30 mg, is contained in a volume of 0.3 mL.

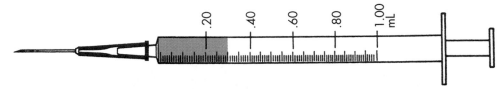

34. Conversion is required. Equivalent: 1,000 mg = 1 g

Therefore 0.3 g = 300 mg

300 mg : 2 mL = 300 mg : x mL   OR $\dfrac{300 \text{ mg}}{300 \text{ mg}} \times 2 \text{ mL} = x \text{ mL}; \quad \dfrac{300 \text{ mg}}{300 \text{ mg}} = \dfrac{x \text{ mL}}{2 \text{ mL}}$

Answer: 2 mL. The label indicates that the dose ordered, 300 mg, is contained in a volume of 2 mL.

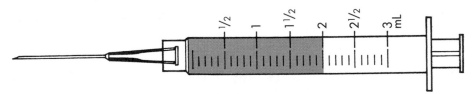

35. 5 mg : 1 mL = 7.5 mg : x mL   OR $\dfrac{7.5 \text{ mg}}{5 \text{ mg}} \times 1 \text{ mL} = x \text{ mL}; \quad \dfrac{7.5 \text{ mg}}{5 \text{ mg}} = \dfrac{x \text{ mL}}{1 \text{ mL}}$

Answer: 1.5 mL or $1\frac{1}{2}$ mL. ($1\frac{1}{2}$ mL is preferred for administration purposes.) The dose ordered is greater than what is available. Therefore you will need more than 1 mL to administer the dose.

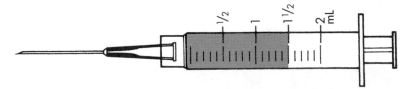

36. 1 mg : 1 mL = 1 mg : x mL   OR $\dfrac{1 \text{ mg}}{1 \text{ mg}} \times 1 \text{ mL} = x \text{ mL}; \quad \dfrac{1 \text{ mg}}{1 \text{ mg}} = \dfrac{x \text{ mL}}{1 \text{ mL}}$

Answer: 1 mL. The label indicates that the dose ordered, 1 mg, is contained in a volume of 1 mL.

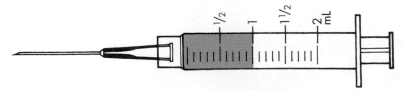

37. 20 mg : 2 mL = 30 mg : x mL   OR $\dfrac{30 \text{ mg}}{20 \text{ mg}} \times 2 \text{ mL} = x \text{ mL}; \dfrac{30 \text{ mg}}{20 \text{ mg}} = \dfrac{x \text{ mL}}{2 \text{ mL}}$

Answer: 3 mL. The dose ordered is greater than what is available. Therefore you will need more than 2 mL to administer the dose.

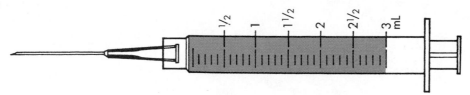

38. 4 mg : 1 mL = 12 mg : x mL   OR $\dfrac{12 \text{ mg}}{4 \text{ mg}} \times 1 \text{ mL} = x \text{ mL}; \dfrac{12 \text{ mg}}{4 \text{ mg}} = \dfrac{x \text{ mL}}{1 \text{ mL}}$

Answer: 3 mL. The dose ordered is greater than what is available. Therefore you will need more than 1 mL to administer the dose.

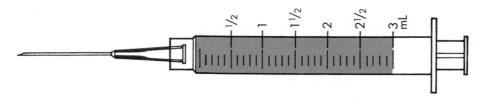

39. Conversion is required. Equivalent: 1,000 mg = 1 g

Therefore 0.25 g = 250 mg

25 mg : 1 mL = 250 mg : x mL   OR $\dfrac{250 \text{ mg}}{25 \text{ mg}} \times 1 \text{ mL} = x \text{ mL}; \dfrac{250 \text{ mg}}{25 \text{ mg}} = \dfrac{x \text{ mL}}{1 \text{ mL}}$

Answer: 10 mL. The dose ordered is greater than what is available. Therefore you will need more than 1 mL to administer the dose.

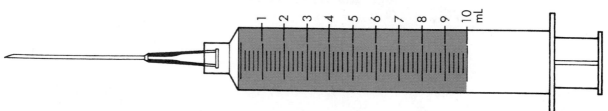

Alternate method for solving:

500 mg : 20 mL = 250 mg : x mL   OR $\dfrac{250 \text{ mg}}{500 \text{ mg}} \times 20 \text{ mL} = x \text{ mL}; \dfrac{250 \text{ mg}}{500 \text{ mg}} = \dfrac{x \text{ mL}}{20 \text{ mL}}$

40. Conversion is required. Equivalent: 1,000 mg = 1 g

Therefore 0.5 g = 500 mg

500 mg : 1 mL = 500 mg : x mL   OR $\dfrac{500 \text{ mg}}{500 \text{ mg}} \times 1 \text{ mL} = x \text{ mL}; \dfrac{500 \text{ mg}}{500 \text{ mg}} = \dfrac{x \text{ mL}}{1 \text{ mL}}$

Answer: 1 mL. The dose ordered, 500 mg, is contained in a volume of 1 mL.

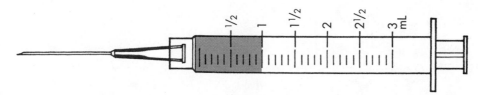

CHAPTER 18

Answers to Practice Problems

1. 1 g (1 gram)
2. 3.5 mL
3. none stated
4. 250 mg/mL
5. 1 hr
6. 2 mL

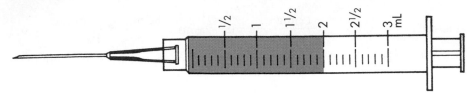

7. 1 g
8. 5.7 mL
9. sterile water for injection
10. 250 mg per 1.5 mL
11. 3 days
12. 7 days
13. 2.4 mL

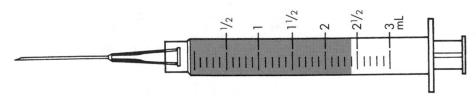

14. 1 g (1 gram)
15. sterile water for injection or 1% lidocaine solution without epinephrine
16. 2 mL
17. 1 g/2.6 mL
18. 1.3 mL

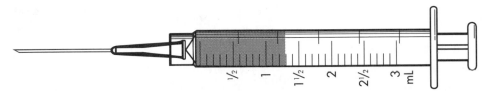

19. 10 g
20. I.V. (intravenous)
21. 95 mL
22. sterile water for injection
23. 100 mg/mL
24. 24 hrs

25. 5 days
26. 10 mL

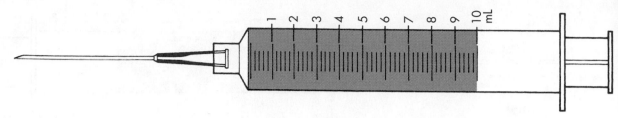

27. 5 mL; 1 tsp
28. water
29. 250 mg/5 mL
30. Refrigerate and keep tightly closed.
31. 1,000 mg (1 g)
32. 20 mL
33. sterile water for injection
34. 50 mg/mL
35. I.V.
36. 140 mL
37. 200 mL
38. 200 mg/5 mL
39. 10 days
40. 20,000,000 U
41. 500,000 U/mL

42. 1,000,000 U/mL—This strength is closest to what is ordered.
43. 2 mL
44. 7 days (1 week)
45. 5,000,000 U
46. 500,000 U/mL
47. 1.4 mL
48. refrigerator
49. 7 days
50. 250,000 U/mL
51. 7 days (1 week)
52. 3 mL
53. sterile water for injection
54. 280 mg/mL
55. 1 g (1 gram)

Answers to Chapter Review

Note:

For problems where conversion is indicated, answers are shown with order converted to what is available.

1. 250 mg : 1 mL = 400 mg : x mL   OR $\dfrac{400 \text{ mg}}{250 \text{ mg}} \times 1 \text{ mL} = x \text{ mL}; \quad \dfrac{400 \text{ mg}}{250 \text{ mg}} = \dfrac{x \text{ mL}}{1 \text{ mL}}$

   $\dfrac{250x}{250} = \dfrac{400}{250}$ $\dfrac{400}{250} = x$ $\dfrac{400}{250} = x$

   $x = 1.6$ mL

   Answer: 1.6 mL. The dose ordered is more than what is available. You will need more than 1 mL to administer the dose.

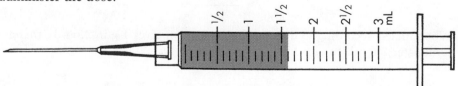

2. 1 g : 10 mL = 1 g : x mL   OR $\dfrac{1 \text{ g}}{1 \text{ g}} \times 10 \text{ mL} = x \text{ mL}; \quad \dfrac{1 \text{ g}}{1 \text{ g}} = \dfrac{x \text{ mL}}{10 \text{ mL}}$

   $\dfrac{10}{1} = x \quad x = 10$ mL $\dfrac{10}{1} = x$

a) Answer: 10 mL. The dose ordered is equal to the volume of the reconstituted solution. Large volumes of I.V. solution may be administered; therefore 10 mL I.V. is acceptable.

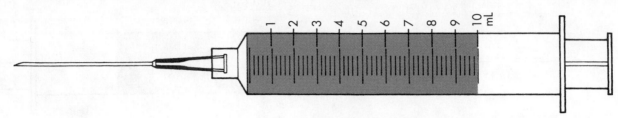

3.   250 mg : 1.5 mL = 300 mg : x mL   OR $\dfrac{300\ mg}{250\ mg} \times 1.5\ mL = x\ mL;$ $\dfrac{300\ mg}{250\ mg} = \dfrac{x\ mL}{1.5\ mL}$

$\dfrac{250x}{250} = \dfrac{450}{250}$

$\dfrac{300 \times 1.5}{250} = x$ $\dfrac{450}{250} = x$

$x = 1.8\ mL$

$\dfrac{450}{250} = x$

a) Answer: 1.8 mL. The dose ordered is greater than what is available; you will need more than 1.5 mL to administer the dose.

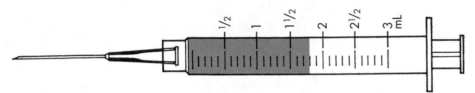

4.   3 g : 30 mL = 1.5 g : x mL   OR $\dfrac{1.5\ g}{3.0\ g} \times 30\ mL = x\ mL;$ $\dfrac{1.5\ g}{3\ g} = \dfrac{x\ mL}{30\ mL}$

$\dfrac{3x}{3} = \dfrac{45}{3}$

$\dfrac{1.5 \times 30}{3.0} = x$ $\dfrac{45}{3} = x$

$x = 15\ mL$

$\dfrac{45}{3.0} = x$

a) Answer: 15 mL. The dose ordered is less than the available dose. You will need less than 30 mL to administer the dose; 15 mL I.V. can be administered.

5.   a) 2 mL

b) sterile water or lidocaine 1% HCl without epinephrine

c) 1 g = 2.6 mL; 1 g/2.6 mL

1 g : 2.6 mL = 1 g : x mL   OR $\dfrac{1\ g}{1\ g} \times 2.6\ mL = x\ mL;$ $\dfrac{1\ g}{1\ g} = \dfrac{x\ mL}{2.6\ mL}$

$x = 2.6\ mL$

$\dfrac{1 \times 2.6}{1} = x$ $\dfrac{2.6}{1} = x$

d) Answer: 2.6 mL. When mixed according to directions, the solution gives 1 g in 2.6 mL; therefore you will need to administer 2.6 mL to give 1 g.

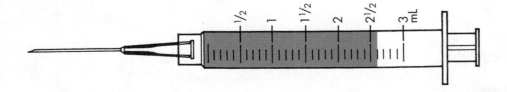

6. a) 500,000 U/mL

    b) 1.6 mL

    $500,000 \text{ U} : 1 \text{ mL} = 600,000 \text{ U} : x \text{ mL}$ OR $\dfrac{600,000 \text{ U}}{500,000 \text{ U}} \times 1 \text{ mL} = x \text{ mL}; \dfrac{600,000 \text{ U}}{500,000 \text{ U}} = \dfrac{x \text{ mL}}{1 \text{ mL}}$

    $\dfrac{500,000x}{500,000} = \dfrac{600,000}{500,000}$ $\dfrac{600,000 \times 1}{500,000} = x \qquad \dfrac{600,000}{500,000} = x$

    $\dfrac{600,000}{500,000}$ $\dfrac{600,000}{500,000} = x$

    $x = 1.2 \text{ mL}$ $x = 1.2 \text{ mL}$

    d) Answer: 1.2 mL. The dose ordered is more than what is available; therefore you will need more than 1 mL to administer the dose.

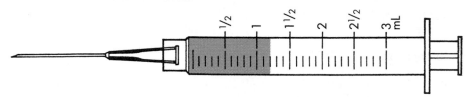

7. a) 250 mg/2 mL

    $250 \text{ mg} : 2 \text{ mL} = 200 \text{ mg} : x \text{ mL}$ OR $\dfrac{200 \text{ mg}}{250 \text{ mg}} \times 2 \text{ mL} = x \text{ mL}; \dfrac{200 \text{ mg}}{250 \text{ mg}} = \dfrac{x \text{ mL}}{2 \text{ mL}}$

    $\dfrac{250x}{250} = \dfrac{400}{250}$ $\dfrac{200 \times 2}{250} = x \qquad \dfrac{400}{250} = x$

    $x = 1.6 \text{ mL}$ $\dfrac{400}{250} = x$

    b) Answer: 1.6 mL. The dose ordered is less than what is available; therefore you will need less than 2 mL to administer the dose.

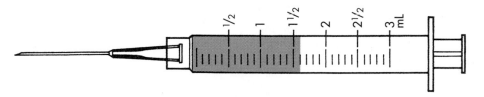

8. a) 5 g

    b) sterile water for injection

    $1 \text{ g} : 2.5 \text{ mL} = 1 \text{ g} : x \text{ mL}$ OR $\dfrac{1 \text{ g}}{1 \text{ g}} \times 2.5 \text{ mL} = x \text{ mL}; \dfrac{1 \text{ g}}{1 \text{ g}} = \dfrac{x \text{ mL}}{2.5 \text{ mL}}$

    $x = 2.5 \text{ mL} \left(2\frac{1}{2} \text{ mL}\right)$ $\dfrac{1 \times 2.5}{1} = x \qquad \dfrac{2.5}{1} = x$

    $\dfrac{2.5}{1} = x$

    c) Answer: 2 1/2 mL (for administration purposes). When mixed according to directions, 1 g will be contained in 2.5 mL. Administer 2 1/2 mL.

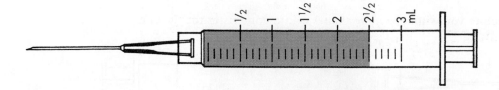

9. a) 78 mL

b) 125 mg per 5 mL

c) 20 mL

$$125 \text{ mg} : 5 \text{ mL} = 500 \text{ mg} : x \text{ mL} \qquad \text{OR} \qquad \frac{500 \text{ mg}}{125 \text{ mg}} \times 5 \text{ mL} = x \text{ mL}; \quad \frac{500 \text{ mg}}{125 \text{ mg}} = \frac{x \text{ mL}}{5 \text{ mL}}$$

$$\frac{125x}{125} = \frac{2{,}500}{125} \qquad\qquad \frac{500 \times 5}{125} = x \qquad\qquad \frac{2{,}500}{125} = x$$

$$x = 20 \text{ mL} \qquad\qquad\qquad \frac{2{,}500}{125} = x$$

Answer: 20 mL. The dose ordered is more than what is available. You will need more than 5 mL to give the dose. Since it's a p.o. liquid and sometimes large volumes are administered, 20 mL p.o. can be administered.

10. a) 2.5 mL of sterile water for injection

b) 330 mg/mL

$$330 \text{ mg} : 1 \text{ mL} = 500 \text{ mg} : x \text{ mL} \qquad \text{OR} \qquad \frac{500 \text{ mg}}{330 \text{ mg}} \times 1 \text{ mL} = x \text{ mL}; \quad \frac{500 \text{ mg}}{330 \text{ mg}} = \frac{x \text{ mL}}{1 \text{ mL}}$$

Answer: 1.5 mL ($1\frac{1}{2}$ mL for administration purposes.) The dose ordered is more than what is

available; therefore you will need more than 1 mL to administer the dose.

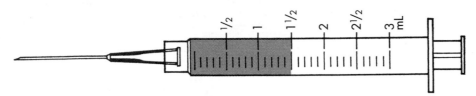

11. a) 250 mg/mL

A conversion is required.

1,000 mg = 1 g; therefore 0.5g = 500 mg

$$250 \text{ mg} : 1 \text{ mL} = 500 \text{ mg} : x \text{ mL} \qquad \text{OR} \qquad \frac{500 \text{ mg}}{250 \text{ mg}} \times 1 \text{ mL} = x \text{ mL}; \quad \frac{500 \text{ mg}}{250 \text{ mg}} = \frac{x \text{ mL}}{1 \text{ mL}}$$

b) Answer: 2 mL. The dose ordered is more than what is available; therefore you will need more than 1 mL to administer the dose.

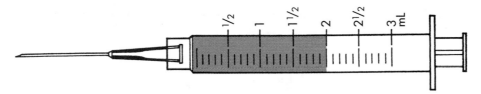

12. a) 1 g

b) 3 mL

c) 300 mg/mL

$$300 \text{ mg} : 1 \text{ mL} = 750 \text{ mg} : x \text{ mL} \qquad \text{OR} \qquad \frac{750 \text{ mg}}{300 \text{ mg}} \times 1 \text{ mL} = x \text{ mL}; \quad \frac{750 \text{ mg}}{300 \text{ mg}} = \frac{x \text{ mL}}{1 \text{ mL}}$$

d) Answer: 2.5 mL ($2\frac{1}{2}$ mL for administration purposes.) The dose ordered is more than what is

available; therefore you will need more than 1 mL to administer the dose.

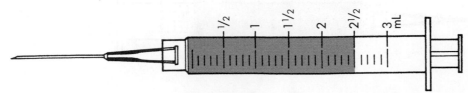

13. a) 5 g

b) 9 mL

c) 400 mg/mL

Conversion: 1,000 mg = 1 g; therefore 0.5 g = 500 mg

$$400 \text{ mg} : 1 \text{ mL} = 500 \text{ mg} : x \text{ mL} \quad \text{OR} \quad \frac{500 \text{ mg}}{400 \text{ mg}} \times 1 \text{ mL} = x \text{ mL}; \quad \frac{500 \text{ mg}}{400 \text{ mg}} = \frac{x \text{ mL}}{1 \text{ mL}}$$

d) Answer: 1.3 mL. 1.25 mL is rounded up to the nearest tenth. The dose ordered is more than what is available per mL; therefore more than 1 mL is required. The small hypodermics are marked in tenths of a mL. To round to the nearest tenth, the math is carried to the hundredth's place.

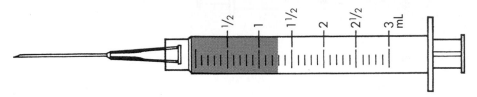

14. a) 10 mL

b) 100 mg/mL

Conversion: 1,000 mg = 1 g; therefore 0.5 g = 500 mg

$$100 \text{ mg} : 1 \text{ mL} = 500 \text{ mg} : x \text{ mL} \quad \text{OR} \quad \frac{500 \text{ mg}}{100 \text{ mg}} \times 1 \text{ mL} = x \text{ mL}; \quad \frac{500 \text{ mg}}{100 \text{ mg}} = \frac{x \text{ mL}}{5 \text{ mL}}$$

c) Answer: 5 mL. The dose ordered is more than what is available; therefore you will need more than 1 mL to administer the dose.

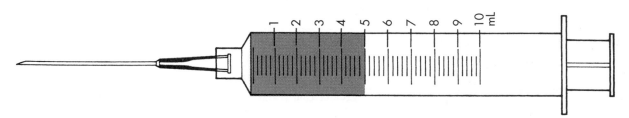

15. $$500,000 \text{ U} : 1 \text{ mL} = 400,000 \text{ U} : x \text{ mL} \quad \text{OR} \quad \frac{400,000 \text{ U}}{500,000 \text{ U}} \times 1 \text{ mL} = x \text{ mL}; \quad \frac{400,000 \text{ U}}{500,000 \text{ U}} = \frac{x \text{ mL}}{1 \text{ mL}}$$

a) Answer: 0.8 mL. The dose ordered is less than what is available; therefore you will need less than 1 mL to administer the dose.

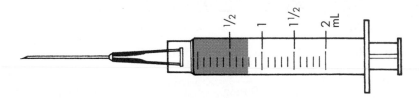

16. $$300 \text{ mg} : 1 \text{ mL} = 250 \text{ mg} : x \text{ mL} \quad \text{OR} \quad \frac{250 \text{ mg}}{300 \text{ mg}} \times 1 \text{ mL} = x \text{ mL}; \quad \frac{250 \text{ mg}}{300 \text{ mg}} = \frac{x \text{ mL}}{1 \text{ mL}}$$

a) Answer: 0.8 mL. 0.83 is rounded to the nearest tenth. The dose ordered is less than what is available; therefore you will need less than 1 mL to administer the dose.

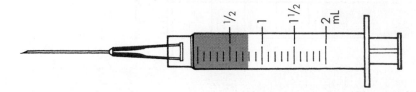

17. a) 2 mL

   b) 1 g = 2.6 mL; 1g/2.6 mL

   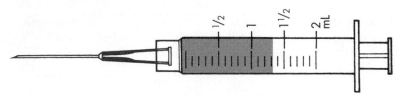

   $$1 \text{ g} : 2.6 \text{ mL} = 0.5 \text{ g} : x \text{ mL} \qquad \text{OR} \qquad \frac{0.5 \text{ g}}{1 \text{ g}} \times 2.6 \text{ mL} = x \text{ mL}; \quad \frac{0.5 \text{ g}}{1 \text{ g}} = \frac{x \text{ mL}}{2.6 \text{ mL}}$$

   c) Answer: 1.3 mL. The dose ordered is one half of the dose available; therefore you will need less than 2.6 mL to administer the dose.

   ![syringe diagram]

18. Conversion is required. Equivalent: 1,000 mg = 1 g; therefore 0.4 g = 400 mg

   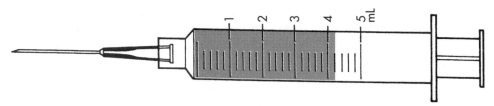

   $$95 \text{ mg} : 1 \text{ mL} = 400 \text{ mg} : x \text{ mL} \qquad \text{OR} \qquad \frac{400 \text{ mg}}{95 \text{ mg}} \times 1 \text{ mL} = x \text{ mL}; \quad \frac{400 \text{ mg}}{95 \text{ mg}} = \frac{x \text{ mL}}{1 \text{ mL}}$$

   Answer: 4.2 mL. 4.21 mL is rounded to the nearest tenth. The dose ordered is greater than what is available. Therefore you will need more than 1 mL to administer the dose. (Syringe is calibrated in 0.2 increments.)

   ![syringe diagram]

19. Conversion is required. Equivalent: 1,000 mg = 1 g; therefore 0.5 g = 500 mg

   $$50 \text{ mg} : 1 \text{ mL} = 500 \text{ mg} : x \text{ mL} \qquad \text{OR} \qquad \frac{500 \text{ mg}}{50 \text{ mg}} \times 1 \text{ mL} = x \text{ mL}; \quad \frac{500 \text{ mg}}{50 \text{ mg}} = \frac{x \text{ mL}}{1 \text{ mL}}$$

   a) Answer: 10 mL. The dose ordered is greater than what is available; therefore you will need more than 1 mL to administer the dose.

   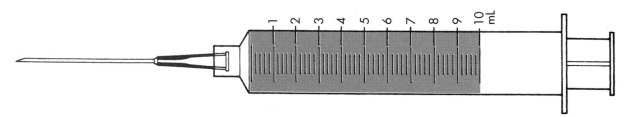

20. Conversion is required. Equivalent: 1,000 mcg = 1 mg; therefore 0.05 mg = 50 mcg

   $$200 \text{ mcg} : 5 \text{ mL} = 50 \text{ mcg} : x \text{ mL} \qquad \text{OR} \qquad \frac{50 \text{ mcg}}{200 \text{ mcg}} \times 5 \text{ mL} = x \text{ mL}; \quad \frac{50 \text{ mcg}}{200 \text{ mcg}} = \frac{x \text{ mL}}{5 \text{ mL}}$$

   a) Answer: 1.3 mL. 1.25 mL is rounded to the nearest tenth. The dose ordered is less than what is available; therefore you will need less than 5 mL to administer the dose.

   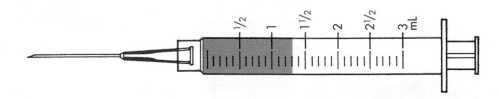

21. Conversion is required. Equivalent: 1,000 mg = 1 g; therefore 0.25 g = 250 mg

$$50 \text{ mg} : 1 \text{ mL} = 250 \text{ mg} : x \text{ mL} \qquad \text{OR} \qquad \frac{250 \text{ mg}}{50 \text{ mg}} \times 1 \text{ mL} = x \text{ mL}; \quad \frac{250 \text{ mg}}{50 \text{ mg}} = \frac{x \text{ mL}}{1 \text{ mL}}$$

a) Answer: 5 mL. The dose ordered is more than what is available; therefore you will need more than 1 mL to administer the dose.

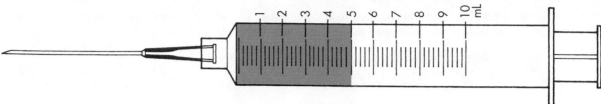

22. a) 69 mL

b) 20 mL

$$100 \text{ mg} : 5 \text{ mL} = 400 \text{ mg} : x \text{ mL} \qquad \text{OR} \qquad \frac{400 \text{ mg}}{100 \text{ mg}} = \frac{x \text{ mL}}{5 \text{ mL}}; \quad \frac{400 \text{ mg}}{100 \text{ mg}} = \frac{x \text{ mL}}{5 \text{ mL}}$$

Answer: 20 mL. The dose ordered is greater than what is available; therefore you will need more than 5 mL to administer the dose.

23. Conversion is required. Equivalent: 1000 mg = 1 g; therefore 2 g = 2,000 mg

$$200 \text{ mg} : 1 \text{ mL} = 2,000 \text{ mg} : x \text{ mL} \qquad \text{OR} \qquad \frac{2,000 \text{ mg}}{200 \text{ mg}} \times 1 \text{ mL} = x \text{ mL}$$

$$\frac{2,000 \text{ mg}}{200 \text{ mg}} = \frac{x \text{ mL}}{1 \text{ mL}}$$

a) Answer: 10 mL. The dose ordered is more than what is available; therefore you will need more than 1 mL to administer the dose.

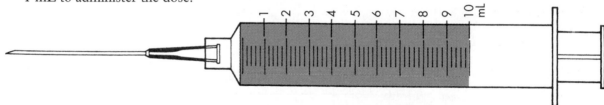

24. Conversion is required. Equivalent: 1,000 mg = 1 g; therefore 2 g = 2,000 mg

$$160 \text{ mg} : 1 \text{ mL} = 2,000 \text{ mg} : x \text{ mL} \qquad \text{OR} \qquad \frac{2,000 \text{ mg}}{160 \text{ mg}} \times 1 \text{ mL} = x \text{ mL}$$

$$\frac{2,000 \text{ mg}}{160 \text{ mg}} = \frac{x \text{ mL}}{1 \text{ mL}}$$

a) Answer: 12.5 mL. The dose ordered is more than what is available; therefore you will need more than 1 mL to administer the dose.

25. $$250 \text{ mg} : 1 \text{ mL} = 300 \text{ mg} : x \text{ mL} \qquad \text{OR} \qquad \frac{300 \text{ mg}}{250 \text{ mg}} \times 1 \text{ mL} = x \text{ mL}$$

$$\frac{300 \text{ mg}}{250 \text{ mg}} = \frac{x \text{ mL}}{1 \text{ mL}}$$

a) Answer: 1.2 mL. The dose ordered is more than what is available; therefore you will need more than 1 mL to administer the dose.

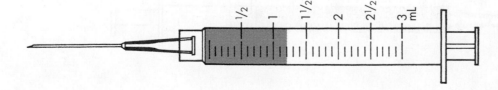

26. Conversion is required. Equivalent: 1,000 mg = 1 g; therefore 1 g = 1,000 mg

$$95 \text{ mg} : 1 \text{ mL} = 1,000 \text{ mg} : x \text{ mL} \quad \text{OR} \quad \frac{1,000 \text{ mg}}{95 \text{ mg}} \times 1 \text{ mL} = x \text{ mL}$$

$$\frac{1,000 \text{ mg}}{95 \text{ mg}} = \frac{x \text{ mL}}{1 \text{ mL}}$$

a) Answer: 10.5 mL. 10.52 is rounded to the nearest tenth. The dose ordered is more than what is available; therefore you will need more than 1 mL to administer the dose.

27. Conversion is required. Equivalent: 1,000 mg = 1 g; therefore 0.75 g = 750 mg

$$100 \text{ mg} : 1 \text{ mg} = 750 \text{ mg} : x \text{ mL} \quad \text{OR} \quad \frac{750 \text{ mg}}{100 \text{ mg}} \times 1 \text{ mL} = x \text{ mL}$$

$$\frac{750 \text{ mg}}{100 \text{ mg}} = \frac{x \text{ mL}}{1 \text{ mL}}$$

a) Answer: 7.5 mL. The dose ordered is more that what is available; therefore you will need more than 1 mL to administer the dose.

CHAPTER 19

Answers to Practice Problems

1. Lente; human
2. Regular human
3. NPH (ilentin I); beef and pork
4. Ultralente; human
5. 22 U
6. 41 U
7.

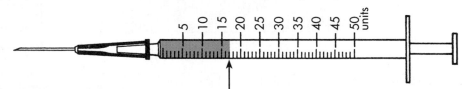

8.

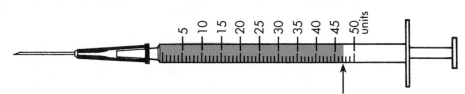

9. 40 U
10. 27 U
11. 53 U
12. 14 U
13.

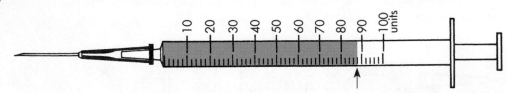

14.

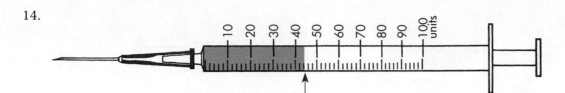

15.

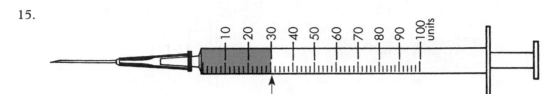

Answers to Chapter Review

1.

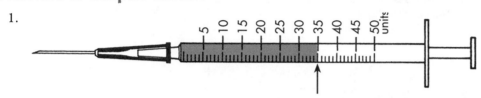

2.

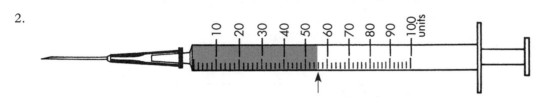

3.

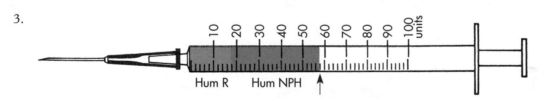

Hum R   Hum NPH

4.

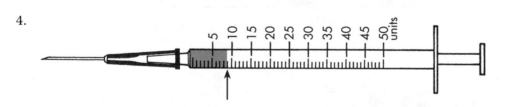

5. 15 U
6. 26 U
7. 16 U
8. 52 U
9. 38 U
10. 65 U
11. 15 U
12.

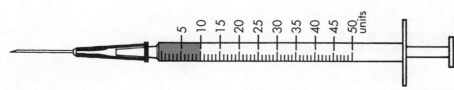

13.

14.

15.

16.

17.

18.

19.

20.

21.

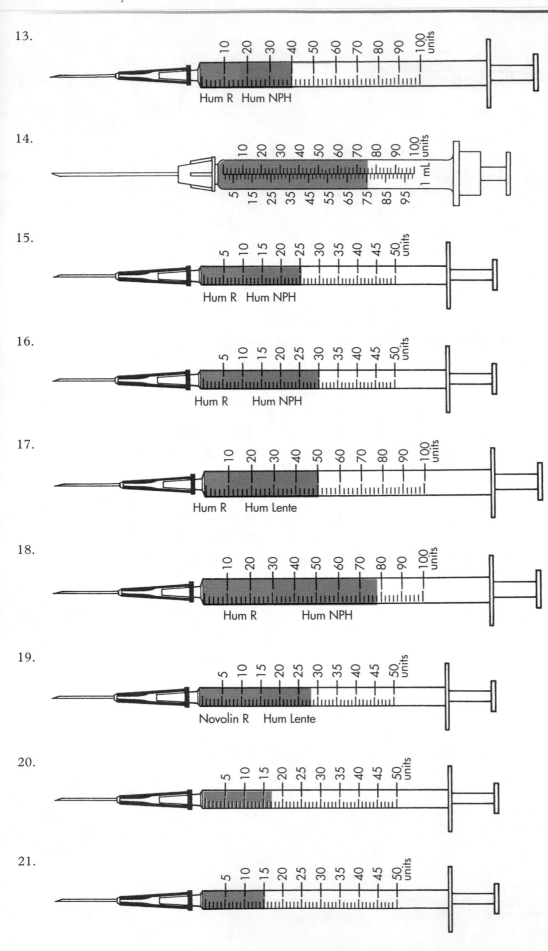

22.

23.

24.

25.

26.

27. 6 U for blood sugar level of 364

28.

29.

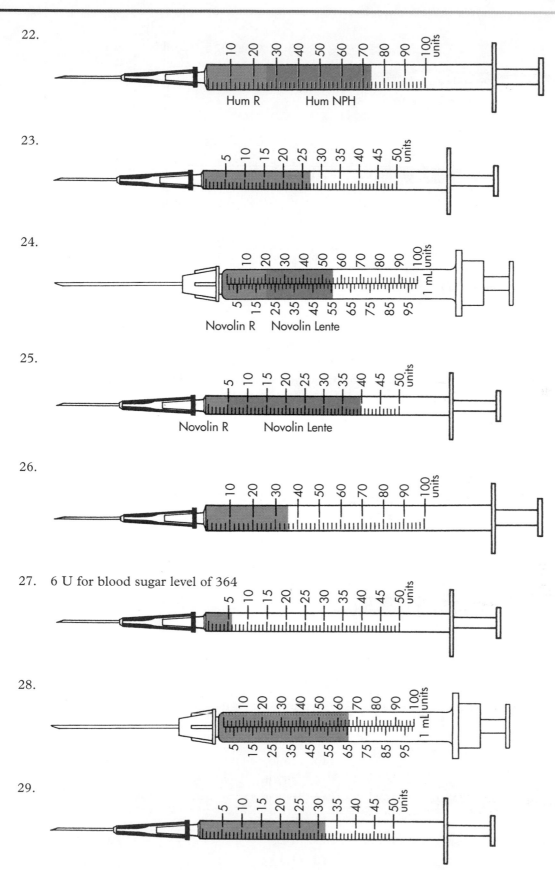

30. 35 U

31. 9 U

32. 24 U

33. 26 U total

34. 11 U total

35. 20 U total

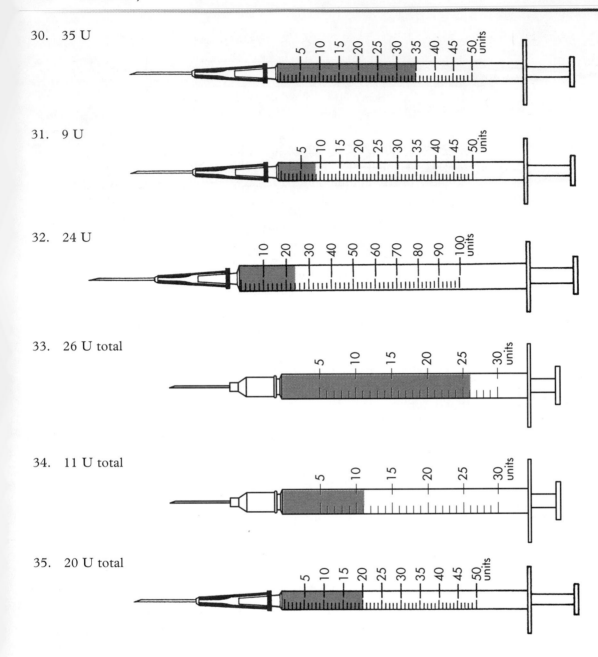

CHAPTER 20

Answers to Practice Problems

1. 6.8 kg
2. 30.9 kg
3. 14.1 kg
4. 23.6 kg
5. 32.3 kg
6. 60.5 kg
7. 3.8 kg
8. 2.5 kg
9. 47 lb
10. 39 lb
11. 48 lb

12. 33 lb
13. 75 lb
14. 157 lb
15. 161 lb
16. 216 lb
17. 4 kg
18. 1.5 kg
19. 2.9 kg
20. 3.6 kg
21. 1.9 kg

22. a) 25–50 mg/kg/day

b) Convert weight first (2.2 lb = 1 kg).
   $35 \div 2.2 = 15.9$ kg

$$\frac{25 \text{ mg}}{x \text{ mg}} = \frac{1 \text{ kg}}{15.9 \text{ kg}} \qquad x = 397.5 \text{ mg}$$

$$\frac{50 \text{ mg}}{x \text{ mg}} = \frac{1 \text{ kg}}{15.9 \text{ kg}} \qquad x = 795 \text{ mg}$$

OR

$$25 \text{ mg} \times 15.9 \text{ kg} = 397.5 \text{ mg}$$

$$50 \text{ mg} \times 15.9 \text{ kg} = 795 \text{ mg}$$

c) Dose range is 397.5-795 mg.

d) The dose ordered falls within the range that is safe.

$$(150 \text{ mg} \times 4 = 600 \text{ mg})$$

e) 125 mg : 5 mL = 150 mg : x mL

OR

$$\frac{150 \text{ mg}}{125 \text{ mg}} \times 5 \text{ mL} = x \text{ mL}; \frac{150 \text{ mg}}{125 \text{ mg}} = \frac{x \text{ mL}}{5 \text{ mL}}$$

$$x = 6 \text{ mL}$$

23. a) $\dfrac{15 \text{ mg}}{x \text{ mg}} = \dfrac{1 \text{ kg}}{35 \text{ kg}} \qquad x = 525 \text{ mg}$

525 mg—maximum dose for 24 hr

OR

$$35 \text{ kg} \times 15 \text{ mg} = 525 \text{ mg}$$

b) $\dfrac{525 \text{ mg}}{3} = 175 \text{ mg}$

c) No, not safe. 200 mg × 3 = 600 mg. This is greater than the maximum dose. Check order with the prescriber.

24. a) $\dfrac{8 \text{ mg}}{x \text{ mg}} = \dfrac{1 \text{ kg}}{40 \text{ kg}} \qquad x = 320 \text{ mg}$

OR

$$8 \text{ mg} \times 40 \text{ kg} = 320 \text{ mg}$$

$$\frac{25 \text{ mg}}{x \text{ mg}} = \frac{1 \text{ kg}}{40 \text{ kg}} \qquad x = 1,000 \text{ mg}$$

OR

$$25 \text{ mg} \times 40 \text{ kg} = 1,000 \text{ mg}$$

Answer: 1,000 mg is maximum dose.

b) four divided doses

$$320 \text{ mg} \div 4 = 80 \text{ mg}$$

$$1000 \text{ mg} \div 4 = 250 \text{ mg}$$

Answer: 80-250 mg divided dose range (250 mg is maximum divided dose)

25. a) Weight conversion (2.2 lb = 1 kg)
   $9 \div 2.2 = 4.1$ kg

b) $\dfrac{3 \text{ mg}}{x \text{ mg}} = \dfrac{1 \text{ kg}}{4.1 \text{ kg}} \qquad x = 12.3 \text{ mg}$

OR

$$3 \text{ mg} \times 4.1 \text{ kg} = 12.3 \text{ mg}$$

$$\frac{5 \text{ mg}}{x \text{ mg}} = \frac{1 \text{ kg}}{4.1 \text{ kg}} \qquad x = 20.5 \text{ mg}$$

OR

$$5 \text{ mg} \times 4.1 \text{ kg} = 20.5 \text{ mg}$$

Safety dose range for the child for a day is 12.3-20.5 mg.

c) The dose ordered is safe.

10 mg × 2 = 20 mg. The maximum dose per day is 20.5 mg.

d) 20 mg : 5 mL = 10 mg : x mL

OR

$$\frac{10 \text{ mg}}{20 \text{ mg}} \times 5 \text{ mL} = x \text{ mL}; \frac{10 \text{ mg}}{20 \text{ mg}} = \frac{x \text{ mL}}{5 \text{ mL}}$$

$$x = 2.5 \text{ mL}$$

You need to give 2.5 mL to administer the ordered dose of 10 mg. (State as 2 1/2 mL for administration purposes.)

26. a) Convert weight to kg (2.2 lb = 1 kg).
   $84 \text{ lb} \div 2.2 = 38.2$ kg

$$\frac{0.1 \text{ mg}}{x \text{ mg}} = \frac{1 \text{ kg}}{38.2 \text{ kg}} \qquad x = 3.8 \text{ mg}$$

OR

$$38.2 \text{ kg} \times 0.1 \text{ mg} = 3.82 \text{ mg} = 3.8 \text{ mg}$$

OR

$$\frac{0.2 \text{ mg}}{x \text{ mg}} = \frac{1 \text{ kg}}{38.2 \text{ kg}} = 7.6 \text{ mg}$$

b) 3.8-7.6 mg/dose

$$0.2 \text{ mg} \times 38.2 \text{ kg} = 7.64 \text{ mg} = 7.6 \text{ mg}$$

c) The dose ordered is safe. 7.5 mg is less than 7.6 mg

d) You would administer 0.5 mL.

$$15 \text{ mg} : 1 \text{ mL} = 7.5 \text{ mg} : x \text{ mL}$$

OR

$$\frac{7.5 \text{ mg}}{15 \text{ mg}} \times 1 \text{ mL} = x \text{ mL}; \quad \frac{7.5 \text{ mg}}{15 \text{ mg}} = \frac{x \text{ mL}}{1 \text{ mL}}$$

$x = 0.5$ mL (State as 1/2 mL for administration purposes.)

27. Convert weight to kg (2.2 lb = 1 kg).

a) 11 lb ÷ 2.2 = 5 kg

$$\frac{4 \text{ mg}}{x \text{ mg}} = \frac{1 \text{ kg}}{5 \text{ kg}} \qquad x = 20 \text{ mg}$$

OR

$$4 \text{ mg} \times 5 \text{ kg} = 20 \text{ mg}$$

$$\frac{8 \text{ mg}}{x \text{ mg}} = \frac{1 \text{ kg}}{5 \text{ kg}} \qquad x = 40 \text{ mg}$$

OR

$$8 \text{ mg} \times 5 \text{ kg} = 40 \text{ mg}$$

b) 20-40 mg/day

c) The dose that is ordered is safe. It falls within the safe range. 15 mg × 2 = 30 mg.

d) 30 mg : 5 mL = 15 mg : x mL

OR

$$\frac{15 \text{ mg}}{30 \text{ mg}} \times 5 \text{ mL} = x \text{ mL}; \quad \frac{15 \text{ mg}}{30 \text{ mg}} = \frac{x \text{ mL}}{5 \text{ mL}}$$

You would give 2.5 mL (2 1/2 mL for administration purposes).

28. Convert the child's weight to kg (2.2 lb = 1 kg).

a) 44 lbs ÷ 2.2 = 20 kg

$$\frac{2.5 \text{ mg}}{x \text{ mg}} = \frac{1 \text{ kg}}{20 \text{ kg}} \qquad x = 50 \text{ mg}$$

OR

$$20 \text{ kg} \times 2.5 \text{ mg} = 50 \text{ mg}$$

b) $x = 50$ mg/day

29. a) Convert weight (2.2 lb = 1 kg).

38 lb ÷ 2.2 = 17.3 kg

b) $$\frac{40 \text{ mg}}{x \text{ mg}} = \frac{1 \text{ kg}}{17.3 \text{ kg}} \qquad x = 692 \text{ mg}$$

OR

$$40 \text{ mg} \times 17.3 \text{ kg} = 692 \text{ mg}$$

$x = 692$ mg/day

c) $$\frac{692 \text{ mg}}{4} = 173 \text{ mg}$$

d) The dose ordered is not safe. 200 mg × 4 = 800 mg. 800 mg > 692 mg; check with prescriber.

30. a) 20-40 mg/kg/day

b) Convert weight (2.2 lb = 1 kg).

16 lb ÷ 2.2 = 7.27 kg, round to 7.3 kg

$$\frac{20 \text{ mg}}{x \text{ mg}} = \frac{1 \text{ kg}}{7.3 \text{ kg}} \qquad x = 146 \text{ mg}$$

OR

$$20 \text{ mg} \times 7.3 \text{ kg} = 146 \text{ mg}$$

$$\frac{40 \text{ mg}}{x \text{ mg}} = \frac{1 \text{ kg}}{7.3 \text{ kg}} \qquad x = 292 \text{ mg}$$

OR

$$40 \text{ mg} \times 7.3 \text{ kg} = 292 \text{ mg}$$

c) Safe dose range for the child is 146-292 mg/day

d) The dose ordered is not safe. 125 mg × 3 = 375 mg. 375 mg > 275 mg; check with prescriber.

31. Convert weight (2.2 lb = 1 kg).

a) 44 lb ÷ 2.2 = 20 kg

$$\frac{30 \text{ mg}}{x \text{ mg}} = \frac{1 \text{ kg}}{20 \text{ kg}} \qquad x = 600 \text{ mg}$$

OR

$$30 \text{ mg} \times 20 \text{ kg} = 600 \text{ mg}$$

$$\frac{50 \text{ mg}}{x \text{ mg}} = \frac{1 \text{ kg}}{20 \text{ kg}} = 1,000 \text{ mg}$$

OR

$$50 \text{ mg} \times 20 \text{ kg} \qquad x = 1,000 \text{ mg}$$

b) 600-1,000 mg/day

c) The dose ordered is safe. 250 mg × 4 = 1,000 mg. 1,000 mg falls within the safe range.

32. No weight conversion is required.

$$\frac{0.25 \text{ mg}}{x \text{ mg}} = \frac{1 \text{ kg}}{66.3 \text{ kg}} \qquad x = 16.57 = 16.6 \text{ mg}$$

OR

$$0.25 \text{ mg} \times 66.3 \text{ kg} = 16.57 = 16.6 \text{ mg}$$

Answer: 16.6 mg is the dose for the adult.

33. Weight conversion is required (2.2 lb = 1 kg).

a) 200 lb ÷ 2.2 = 90.9 kg

$$\frac{150 \text{ mg}}{x \text{ mg}} = \frac{1 \text{ kg}}{90.9 \text{ kg}} \qquad x = 13,635 \text{ mg}$$

OR

$$150 \text{ mg} \times 90.9 \text{ kg} = 13,635 \text{ mg}$$
$$x = 13,635 \text{ mg}$$

$$\frac{200 \text{ mg}}{x \text{ mg}} = \frac{1 \text{ kg}}{90.9 \text{ kg}} \qquad x = 18,180 \text{ mg}$$

OR

$$200 \text{ mg} \times 90.9 \text{ kg} = 18,180 \text{ mg}$$

To determine the number of g, convert the mg obtained to g (1,000 mg = 1 g).

13,635 mg ÷ 1,000 = 13.63 g

(13.6 g to nearest tenth)

18,180 mg ÷ 1,000 = 18.18 g

(18.2 g to nearest tenth)

b) The daily dose range in g is 13.6-18.2 g.

34. Convert weight (2.2. lb = 1 kg, 16 oz = 1 lb).

6 oz ÷ 16 = 0.37 lb = 0.4 lb (to nearest tenth)

Total weight in lb = 12.4 lb

a) 12.4 lb ÷ 2.2 = 5.63 kg (5.6 to nearest tenth)

$$\frac{15 \text{ mg}}{x \text{ mg}} = \frac{1 \text{ kg}}{5.6 \text{ kg}} \qquad x = 84 \text{ mg}$$

OR

$$15 \text{ mg} \times 5.6 \text{ kg} = 84 \text{ mg}$$
$$x = 84 \text{ mg}$$

$$\frac{50 \text{ mg}}{x \text{ mg}} = \frac{1 \text{ kg}}{5.6 \text{ kg}} \qquad x = 280 \text{ mg}$$

OR

$$50 \text{ mg} \times 5.6 \text{ kg} = 280 \text{ mg}$$
$$x = 280 \text{ mg}$$

b) The safe dose range is 84-280 mg/day.

35.	0.60 m²	43.	0.52 m²
36.	0.27 m²	44.	0.45 m²
37.	0.90 m²	45.	0.9 m²
38.	0.80 m²	46.	0.3 m²
39.	0.29 m²	47.	0.58 m²
40.	0.44 m²	48.	0.51 m²
41.	0.80 m²	49.	0.68 m²
42.	0.28 m²	50.	0.18 m²

Answers to Practice Problems: Determining the Dose Using the Formula

51. a) 0.52 m²

b) $\dfrac{0.52}{1.7} \times 25 = \dfrac{0.52 \times 25}{1.7} = \dfrac{13}{1.7} = 7.64$

Answer: 7.6 mg

52. a) 0.52 m²

b) $\dfrac{0.52}{1.7} \times 200 = \dfrac{0.52 \times 200}{1.7} = \dfrac{104}{1.7}$

$\dfrac{104}{1.7} = 61.17 = 61.2$ mg

$\dfrac{0.52}{1.7} \times 400 = \dfrac{208}{1.7} = 122.35$

122.35 mg = 122.4 mg

Answer: The child's dose range is 61.2-122.4 mg.

53. $\dfrac{1.5}{1.7} \times 5$ mg $= \dfrac{1.5 \times 5}{1.7} = \dfrac{7.5}{1.7}$

$\dfrac{7.5}{1.7} = 4.41$ mg $= 4.4$ mg

$\dfrac{1.5}{1.7} \times 15$ mg $= \dfrac{22.5}{1.7} = 13.23$

13.23 mg = 13.2 mg

Answer: 4.4–13.2 mg

54. $\dfrac{0.8}{1.7} \times 20$ mg $= \dfrac{0.8 \times 20}{1.7} = \dfrac{16}{1.7}$

$\dfrac{16}{1.7} = 9.41$ mg $= 9.4$ mg

Answer: The dose is incorrect. The correct dose is 9.4 mg.

55. $\dfrac{0.92}{1.7} \times 25$ mg $= \dfrac{0.92 \times 25}{1.7} = \dfrac{23}{1.7}$

$\dfrac{23}{1.7} = 13.52$ mg $= 13.5$ mg

Answer: The dose is incorrect. The correct dose is 13.5 mg.

56. $\dfrac{1.5}{1.7} \times 250$ mg $= \dfrac{1.5 \times 250}{1.7} = \dfrac{375}{1.7}$

$\dfrac{375}{1.7} = 220.58$ mg

Answer: The child's dose is 220.6 mg.

57. 0.74 × 20 = 14.8 mg

0.74 × 30 = 22.2 mg

Answer: The child's dose range is 14.8-22.2 mg.

58. $\dfrac{0.67}{1.7} \times 20$ mg $= \dfrac{13.4}{1.7} = 7.88$ mg $= 7.9$ mg.

The dose is correct.

59. $\dfrac{0.94}{1.7} \times 10 = 5.5$ mg

$\dfrac{0.94}{1.7} \times 20 = 11.1$ mg

Answer: The child's dose range is 5.5-11.1 mg.

60. a) 0.45 m²

b) $\dfrac{0.45}{1.7} \times 500$ mg $= \dfrac{225}{1.7} = 132.35$

Answer: The child's dose is 132.4 mg.

61. $\dfrac{1.3}{1.7} \times 500 = \dfrac{1.3 \times 500}{1.7} = \dfrac{650}{1.7} = 382.35$

Answer: The child's dose is 382.4 mg.

62. a) 0.55 m²

b) $\dfrac{0.55}{1.7} \times 25 = \dfrac{0.55 \times 25}{1.7} = \dfrac{13.75}{1.7}$

$\dfrac{13.75}{1.7} = 8.08$

Answer: The child's dose is 8.1 mg.

63. $\dfrac{0.52}{1.7} \times 15 = \dfrac{0.52 \times 15}{1.7} = \dfrac{7.8}{1.7} = 4.58$

Answer: The child's dose is 4.6 mg.

64. $\dfrac{1.10}{1.7} \times 150 = \dfrac{1.10 \times 150}{1.7} = \dfrac{165}{1.7} = 97.05$

Answer: The child's dose is 97.1 mg.

65. $\sqrt{\dfrac{95.5 \text{ (kg)} \times 180 \text{ (cm)}}{3{,}600}}$

$\sqrt{4.775} = 2.185 = 2.19$ m²

Answer: 2.19 m²

66. $\sqrt{\dfrac{10 \text{ (kg)} \times 70 \text{ (cm)}}{3{,}600}}$

$\sqrt{0.194} = 0.440$ m²

Answer: 0.440 m²

67. $\sqrt{\dfrac{4.8 \text{ (lb)} \times 21 \text{ (in)}}{3{,}131}}$

$\sqrt{0.032} = 0.178 = 0.18$ m²

Answer: 0.18 m²

68. $\sqrt{\dfrac{170 \text{ (lb)} \times 67 \text{ (in)}}{3{,}131}}$

$\sqrt{3.637} = 1.907 = 1.91$ m²

Answer: 1.91 m²

69. $\sqrt{\dfrac{92 \text{ (lb)} \times 35 \text{ (in)}}{3,131}}$

$\sqrt{1.028} = 1.014 = 1.01 \text{ m}^2$

Answer: 1.01 m²

Answers to Chapter Review

Note:

Alternate ways of doing problems 1-13 in the Chapter Review are possible, such as a ratio-proportion. This method is shown in the Practice Problems.

1. Convert weight (2.2 lb = 1 kg).

    22 lb = 2.2 ÷ 2.2 = 10 kg

    1 mg × 10 kg = 10 mg

    The dose ordered for this child is safe.

2. Convert weight (2.2 lb = 1 kg).

    a) 23 lb = 23 ÷ 22 = 10.5 kg

    b) 20 mg × 10.5 kg = 210 mg/day

    40 mg × 10.5 kg = 420 mg/day

    The safety range for this 10.5 kg child is 210-420 mg/day.

    c) The drug is given in divided doses q8h.

    q8h = 24 ÷ 8 = 3 doses per day

    210 mg ÷ 3 = 70 mg per dose

    420 mg ÷ 3 = 140 mg per dose

    The dose range is 70-140 mg per dose q8h.

    d) The dose ordered is not safe; 150 mg × 3 = 450 mg. 450 mg > 420 mg.

    Notify the prescriber and question the order.

3. Convert child's weight in kg to lb. The recommended dose is stated in lb.

    2.2 lb = 1 kg

    a) 17 kg = 17 × 2.2 = 37.4 lb.

    The dose range is stated as

    2.2-3.2 mg/lb/day.

    2.2 mg × 37.4 lb = 82.28 mg = 82.3 mg

    3.2 mg × 37.4 lb = 119.68 mg = 119.7 mg

    b) The dose range is 82.3-119.7 mg.

    q6h = 4 doses

    82.3 mg ÷ 4 = 20.57 mg = 20.6 mg

    119.7 mg ÷ 4 = 29.92 mg = 29.9 mg

    The divided dose range is 20.6-29.9 mg per dose.

    The dose ordered: 25 mg q6h.

    c) This dose is safe because 25 mg × 4 = 100 mg. It falls in the safe dose range.

    d) 5 mg : 1 mL = 25 mg : x mL

70. $\sqrt{\dfrac{24 \text{ (kg)} \times 92 \text{ (cm)}}{3,600}}$

$\sqrt{0.613} = 0.783 = 0.78 \text{ m}^2$

Answer: 0.78 m²

OR

$\dfrac{25 \text{ mg}}{5 \text{ mg}} \times 1 \text{ mL} = x \text{ mL}$

$x = 5 \text{ mL}$

$\dfrac{25 \text{ mg}}{5 \text{ mg}} = \dfrac{x \text{ mL}}{5 \text{ mL}}$

$x = 5 \text{ mL}$

Answer: Give 5 mL per dose. The dose ordered is greater that what is available; therefore you need more than 5 mL to administer the dose.

4. No conversion of weight is required. The child's weight is in kg, and the recommended dose is expressed in kg (12.5 mg/kg).

    12.5 mg × 35 kg = 437.5 mg/day

    q6h = 4 doses

    437.5 mg ÷ 4 =

    109.37 = 109.4 mg per dose

    Dose ordered is safe because 100 mg × 4 = 400 mg. 400 mg < 437.5 mg.

5. No conversion of weight is required. The child's weight is in lb, and the recommended dose is expressed in lb (2 mg/lb).

    2 mg × 30 lb = 60 mg/day

    q12 = 2 doses

    60 mg ÷ 2 = 30 mg per dose

    75 mg × 2 = 150 mg. This dose is too high; notify the prescriber. 150 mg > 60 mg.

6. Convert the child's weight in lb to kg. The recommended dose is expressed in kg (50 mg/kg/day).

    50 mg × 19.1 kg = 955 mg/day

    995 mg ÷ 4 = 238.8 mg per dose

    The dose ordered is not safe because 250 mg × 4 = 1,000 mg. 1,000 mg > 955 mg; notify the prescriber.

7. Convert the child's weight in lbs to kg. The recommended dose is stated in kg (10 to 25 mg/kg/24 hr).

    36 lb = 36 ÷ 2.2 = 16.4 kg

    10 mg × 16.4 kg = 164 mg/day

    25 mg × 16.4 kg = 410 mg/day

    The safe dose range is 164-410 mg/day.

The drug is given q6-8h. The dose in this problem is ordered q8h.

$$24 \div 8 = 3 \text{ doses}$$
$$164 \text{ mg} \div 3 = 54.7 \text{ mg/dose}$$
$$410 \text{ mg} \div 3 = 136.7 \text{ mg/dose}$$

The dose ordered is 150 mg q8h.

$$150 \text{ mg} \times 3 = 450 \text{ mg}$$

Notify the prescriber; the dose is high (not safe). 450 mg > the dose range 164-410 mg.

8. a) Convert the child's weight in lb to kg. The recommended dose is expressed in kg (25-50 mg/kg).

$$66 \text{ lbs} = 66 \div 2.2 = 30 \text{ kg}$$
$$25 \text{ mg} \times 30 \text{ kg} = 750 \text{ mg/day}$$
$$50 \text{ mg} \times 30 \text{ kg} = 1,500 \text{ mg/day}$$

The safety range is 750-1,500 mg/day.

The drug is given in divided doses (4).

The dosage ordered is q6h.

$$24 \div 6 = 4 \text{ doses}$$
$$750 \text{ mg} \div 4 = 187.5 \text{ mg/per dose}$$
$$1,500 \text{ mg} \div 4 = 375 \text{ mg/per dose}$$

The dose range is 187.5-375 mg per dose q6h. 250 mg $\times$ 4 = 1,000 mg. This is a safe dose since the total dose falls within the safe range for 24 hr, and the divided dose also falls within the safe range.

b) You would give 10 mL for one dose.

$$125 \text{ mg} : 5 \text{ mL} = 250 \text{ mg} : x \text{ mL}$$

OR

$$\frac{250 \text{ mg}}{125 \text{ mg}} \times 5 \text{ mL} = x \text{ mL};$$

$$\frac{250 \text{ mg}}{125 \text{ mg}} = \frac{x \text{ mL}}{5 \text{ mL}}$$

$$x = 10 \text{ mL}$$

The dose ordered is greater than what is available; you will need more than 5 mL to administer the dose.

9. a) No conversion of weight is required. The child's weight is stated in kg, and the recommended dose is (20-40 mg/kg).

$$20 \text{ mg} \times 35 \text{ kg} = 700 \text{ mg}$$
$$40 \text{ mg} \times 35 \text{ kg} = 1,400 \text{ mg}$$

The safety range is 700-1,400 mg/day.

The drug is given in divided doses q12h.

$$24 \div 12 = 2 \text{ doses}$$
$$700 \text{ mg} \div 2 = 350 \text{ mg}$$
$$1,400 \text{ mg} \div 2 = 700 \text{ mg}$$

350-700 mg per dose is safe.

The doctor ordered 400 mg I.M. q12h. This dose is safe. 400 mg $\times$ 2 = 800 mg. The total dose falls within the safe range for 24 hr.

b) Administer 1 mL.

$$400 \text{ mg} : 1 \text{ mL} = 400 \text{ mg} : x \text{ mL}$$

OR

$$\frac{400 \text{ mg}}{400 \text{ mg}} \times 1 \text{ mL} = x \text{ mL};$$

$$\frac{400 \text{ mg}}{400 \text{ mg}} = \frac{x \text{ mL}}{1 \text{ mL}}$$

$$x = 1 \text{ mL}$$

The dose ordered is contained in 1 mL.

10. Convert the child's weight in lb to kg. The recommended dose is expressed in kg (120 mg/kg).

$$46 \text{ lb} = 46 \div 2.2 = 20.9 \text{ kg}$$
$$120 \text{ mg} \times 20.9 \text{ kg} = 2,508 \text{ mg/day}$$

The drug is given in four equally divided doses.

The dose for this child is ordered q6h.

$$24 \div 6 = 4 \text{ doses.}$$
$$2,508 \text{ mg} \div 4 = 627 \text{ mg per dose}$$
$$250 \text{ mg} \times 4 = 1,000 \text{ mg}$$

The dose ordered is too low. Notify the prescriber. 250 mg each dose is less than 627 mg, and 1,000 mg < 2,508 mg. While the dose ordered may be safe, it may not be effective.

11. Convert the neonate's weight in g to kg (1,000 g = 1 kg).

a) 3,500 g = 3.5 kg

b) 30 mg $\times$ 3.5 kg = 105 mg

The safe dose for the neonate is 105 mg/day.

12. No weight conversion is required. The child's weight is in kg and the recommended dose is expressed in kg (50-100 mg/kg/day).

a) 50 mg $\times$ 14 kg = 700 mg

100 mg $\times$ 14 kg = 1,400 mg

700-1,400 mg/day

b) 24 $\div$ 6 = 4 doses

700 mg $\div$ 4 = 175 mg

1,400 mg $\div$ 4 = 350 mg

Divided dose range is 175-350 mg per dose.

c) 250 mg $\times$ 4 = 1,000 mg

The dose ordered is safe. 1,000 mg is less than 1,400; it doesn't exceed the dose allowed for the day.

13. Weight conversion is required (2.2 lb = 1 kg).

a) 190 lb $\div$ 2.2 = 86.4 kg

b) 86.4 kg × 25 mcg = 2,160 mcg

c) 86.4 kg × 30 mcg = 2,592 mcg

To determine the number of mg, convert the mcg obtained to mg (1,000 mcg = 1 mg).

2,160 mcg ÷ 1,000 = 2.16 mg (2.2 mg, to the nearest tenth)

2,592 mcg ÷ 1000 = 2.59 (2.6 mg to the nearest tenth)

The daily dosage range in mg is 2.2-2.6 mg.

14. a) 0.45 m²

b) $\dfrac{0.45}{17} \times 50 \text{ mg} = 13.23 = 13.2 \text{ mg}$

15. a) 0.54 m²

b) $\dfrac{0.54}{1.7} \times 25 \text{ mg} = 7.9 \text{ mg}$

16. a) 1.2 m²

b) $\dfrac{1.2}{1.7} \times 250 \text{ mg} = 176.5 \text{ mg}$

17. a) 1.1 m²

b) $\dfrac{1.1}{1.7} \times 30 \text{ mg} = 19.4 \text{ mg}$

18. a) 1.05 m²

b) $\dfrac{1.05}{1.7} \times 150 \text{ mg} = 92.6 \text{ mg}$

19. $\dfrac{0.70}{1.7} \times 50 \text{ mg} = 20.6 \text{ mg}$

20. $\dfrac{0.66}{1.7} \times 10 \text{ mg} = 3.9 \text{ mg}$

$\dfrac{0.66}{1.7} \times 20 \text{ mg} = 7.8 \text{ mg}$

The dose range is 3.9-7.8 mg.

21. $\dfrac{0.55}{1.7} \times 2,000 \text{ U} = 647.1 \text{ U}$

22. $\dfrac{0.55}{1.7} \times 200 \text{ mg} - 64.7 \text{ mg}$

$\dfrac{0.55}{1.7} \times 250 \text{ mg} = 80.9 \text{ mg}$

The dose range is 64.7-80.9 mg.

23. $\dfrac{0.22}{1.7} \times 150 \text{ mg} = 19.4 \text{ mg}$

24. Dose is incorrect; the child's dose is 17.3 mg.

$\dfrac{0.49}{1.7} \times 60 \text{ mg} = 17.3 \text{ mg}$

The dose of 25 mg is too high.

25. $\dfrac{0.32}{1.7} \times 10 \text{ mg} = 1.9 \text{ mg}$

The dose of 4 mg is too high.

26. Dose is correct.

$\dfrac{0.68}{1.7} \times 125 \text{ mg} = 50 \text{ mg}$

$\dfrac{0.68}{1.7} \times 150 \text{ mg} = 60 \text{ mg}$

The dose of 50 mg falls within the range of 50-60 mg.

27. Dose is incorrect.

$\dfrac{0.55}{1.7} \times 25 \text{ mg} = 8.1 \text{ mg}$

The dose of 5 mg is too low.

28. The dose is correct.

$\dfrac{1.2}{1.7} \times 75 \text{ mg} = 52.9 \text{ mg}$

$\dfrac{1.2}{1.7} \times 100 \text{ mg} = 70.6 \text{ mg}$

The dose ordered is 60 mg and falls within the dose range of 52.9-70.6 mg.

29. $\sqrt{\dfrac{100 \text{ (lb)} \times 55 \text{ (in)}}{3,131}} = \dfrac{5500}{3,131} = 1.756$

$\sqrt{1.756} = 1.325$

Answer: 1.33 m²

30. $\sqrt{\dfrac{60.9 \text{ (kg)} \times 130 \text{ (cm)}}{3,600}} = \dfrac{7,917}{3,600} = 2.199$

$\sqrt{2.199} = 1.482$

Answer: 1.48 m²

31. $\sqrt{\dfrac{55 \text{ (lb)} \times 45 \text{ (in)}}{3,131}} = \dfrac{2,475}{3,131} = 0.790$

$\sqrt{0.790} = 0.888$

Answer: 0.89 m²

32. $\sqrt{\dfrac{60 \text{ (lb)} \times 35 \text{ (in)}}{3,131}} = \dfrac{2,100}{3,131} = 0.670$

$\sqrt{0.670} = 0.818$

Answer: 0.82 m²

33. $\sqrt{\dfrac{65 \text{ (kg)} \times 132 \text{ (cm)}}{3,600}} = \dfrac{8,580}{3,600} = 2.383$

$\sqrt{2.383} = 1.543$

Answer: 1.54 m²

34. $\sqrt{\dfrac{24 \text{ (lb)} \times 28 \text{ (in)}}{3,131}} = \dfrac{672}{3,131} = 0.214$

$\sqrt{0.214} = 0.462$

Answer: 0.46 m²

35. $\sqrt{\dfrac{6 \text{ (kg)} \times 55 \text{ (cm)}}{3,600}} = \dfrac{330}{3,600} = 0.091$

$\sqrt{0.091} = 0.301$

Answer: 0.30 m²

36. $\sqrt{\dfrac{42 \text{ (lb)} \times 45 \text{ (in)}}{3,131}} = \dfrac{1,890}{3,131} = 0.603$

$\sqrt{0.603} = 0.776$

Answer: 0.78 m²

37. $\sqrt{\dfrac{8 \text{ (kg)} \times 70 \text{ (cm)}}{3,600}} = \dfrac{560}{3,600} = 0.155$

$\sqrt{0.155} = 0.393$

Answer: 0.39 m²

38. $\sqrt{\dfrac{74 \text{ (kg)} \times 160 \text{ (cm)}}{3,600}} = \dfrac{11,840}{3,600} = 3.288$

$\sqrt{3.288} = 1.813$

Answer: 1.81 m²

39. 10 mg : 1 mL = 7 mg : x mL

OR

$\dfrac{7 \text{ mg}}{10 \text{ mg}} \times 1 \text{ mL} = x \text{ mL}$

OR

$\dfrac{7 \text{ mg}}{10 \text{ mg}} = \dfrac{x \text{ mL}}{1 \text{ mL}}$

Answer: 0.7 mL. The dose ordered is less than what is available; therefore you will need less than 1 mL to administer the dose.

40. 10 mg : 1 mL = 150 mg : x mL

OR

$\dfrac{150 \text{ mg}}{10 \text{ mg}} \times 1 \text{ mL} = x \text{ mL}; \dfrac{150 \text{ mg}}{10 \text{ mg}} = \dfrac{x \text{ mL}}{1 \text{ mL}}$

Answer: 15 mL. The dose ordered is more than what is available; therefore you will need more than 1 mL to administer the dose.

41. 0.05 mg : 1 mL = 0.1 mg : x mL

OR

$\dfrac{0.1 \text{ mg}}{0.05 \text{ mg}} \times 1 \text{ mL} = x \text{ mL}; \dfrac{0.1 \text{ mg}}{0.05 \text{ mg}} = \dfrac{x \text{ mL}}{1 \text{ mL}}$

Answer: 2 mL. The dose ordered is more than what is available; therefore you will need more than 1 mL to administer the dose.

42. 50 mg : 5 mL = 80 mg : x mL

OR

$\dfrac{80 \text{ mg}}{50 \text{ mg}} \times 5 \text{ mL} = x \text{ mL}; \dfrac{80 \text{ mg}}{50 \text{ mg}} = \dfrac{x \text{ mL}}{5 \text{ mL}}$

Answer: 8 mL. The dose ordered is greater than what is available; therefore you will need more than 5 mL to administer the dose.

43. 125 mg : 5 mL = 250 mg : x mL

OR

$\dfrac{250 \text{ mg}}{125 \text{ mg}} \times 5 \text{ mL} = x \text{ mL}; \dfrac{250 \text{ mg}}{125 \text{ mg}} = \dfrac{x \text{ mL}}{5 \text{ mL}}$

Answer: 10 mL. The dose ordered is greater than what is available; therefore you will need more than 5 mL to administer the dose.

44. Conversion is required:
Equivalent: 1,000 mg = 1 g

Therefore 0.25 g = 250 mg

100 mg : 5 mL = 250 mg : x mL

OR

$\dfrac{250 \text{ mg}}{100 \text{ mg}} \times 5 \text{ mL} = x \text{ mL}; \dfrac{250 \text{ mg}}{100 \text{ mg}} = \dfrac{x \text{ mL}}{5 \text{ mL}}$

Answer: 12.5 mL. The dose ordered is greater than what is available; therefore, you would need more than 5 mL to administer the dose.

45. 250 mg : 5 mL = 100 mg : x mL

OR

$\dfrac{100 \text{ mg}}{250 \text{ mg}} \times 5 \text{ mL} = x \text{ mL}; \dfrac{100 \text{ mg}}{250 \text{ mg}} = \dfrac{x \text{ mL}}{5 \text{ mL}}$

Answer: 2 mL. The dose ordered is less than what is available; therefore you will need less than 5 mL to administer the dose.

46. 20 mg : 2 mL = 7.3 mg : x mL

OR

$\dfrac{7.3 \text{ mg}}{20 \text{ mg}} \times 2 \text{ mL} = x \text{ mL}; \dfrac{7.3 \text{ mg}}{20 \text{ mg}} = \dfrac{x \text{ mL}}{2 \text{ mL}}$

Answer: 0.73 mL. The dose ordered is less than what is available; therefore you will need less than 2 mL to administer the dose.

47. 0.4 mg : 1 mL = 0.1 mg : x mL

OR

$\dfrac{0.1 \text{ mg}}{0.4 \text{ mg}} \times 1 \text{ mL} = x \text{ mL}; \dfrac{0.1 \text{ mg}}{0.4 \text{ mg}} = \dfrac{x \text{ mL}}{1 \text{ mL}}$

Answer: 0.25 mL. The dose ordered is less than what is available; therefore you would need less than 1 mL to administer the dose.

48. 250 mg : 1 mL = 160 mg : x mL

OR

$\dfrac{160 \text{ mg}}{250 \text{ mg}} \times 1 \text{ mL} = x \text{ mL}; \quad \dfrac{160 \text{ mg}}{250 \text{ mg}} = \dfrac{x \text{ mL}}{1 \text{ mL}}$

Answer: 0.64 mL. The dose ordered is less than what is available; therefore you will need less than 1 mL to administer the dose.

49. 15 mg : 1 mL = 3.5 mg : x mL

OR

$\dfrac{3.5 \text{ mg}}{15 \text{ mg}} \times 1 \text{ mL} = x \text{ mL}; \quad \dfrac{3.5 \text{ mg}}{15 \text{ mg}} = \dfrac{x \text{ mL}}{1 \text{ mL}}$

Answer: 0.23 mL. The dose ordered is less than what is available; therefore you will need less than 1 mL to administer the dose.

50. 20 mg : 2 mL = 60 mg : x mL

OR

$\dfrac{60 \text{ mg}}{20 \text{ mg}} \times 2 \text{ mL} = x \text{ mL}; \quad \dfrac{60 \text{ mg}}{20 \text{ mg}} = \dfrac{x \text{ mL}}{2 \text{ mL}}$

Answer: 6 mL. The dose ordered is more than what is available; therefore you will need more than 2 mL to administer the dose.

51. Conversion required. Equivalent: 1,000 mg = 1 g

Therefore 0.4 g = 400 mg

160 mg : 5 mL = 400 mg : x mL

OR

$\dfrac{400 \text{ mg}}{160 \text{ mg}} \times 5 \text{ mL} = x \text{ mL}; \quad \dfrac{400 \text{ mg}}{160 \text{ mg}} = \dfrac{x \text{ mL}}{5 \text{ mL}}$

Answer: 12.5 mL. The dose ordered is more than what is available; therefore you will need more than 5 mL to administer the dose.

52. 25 mg : 1 mL = 35 mg : x mL

OR

$\dfrac{35 \text{ mg}}{25 \text{ mg}} \times 1 \text{ mL} = x \text{ mL}; \quad \dfrac{35 \text{ mg}}{25 \text{ mg}} = \dfrac{x \text{ mL}}{1 \text{ mL}}$

Answer: 1.4 mL. The dose ordered is more than what is available; therefore you will need more than 1 mL to administer the dose.

53. 150 mg : 1 mL = 100 mg : x mL

OR

$\dfrac{100 \text{ mg}}{150 \text{ mg}} \times 1 \text{ mL} = x \text{ mL}; \quad \dfrac{100 \text{ mg}}{150 \text{ mg}} = \dfrac{x \text{ mL}}{1 \text{ mL}}$

Answer: 0.66 = 0.7 mL. The dose ordered is less than what is available; therefore you will need less than 1 mL to administer the dose.

54. 300,000 U : 1 mL = 150,000 U : x mL

OR

$\dfrac{150,000 \text{ U}}{300,000 \text{ U}} \times 1 \text{ mL} = x \text{ mL}; \quad \dfrac{150,000 \text{ U}}{300,000 \text{ U}} = \dfrac{x \text{ mL}}{1 \text{ mL}}$

Answer: 0.5 mL (1/2 mL is preferred for administration purposes.) The dose ordered is less than what is available; therefore you will need less than 1 mL to administer the dose.

55. 100 mg : 2 mL = 150 mg : x mL

OR

$\dfrac{150 \text{ mg}}{100 \text{ mg}} \times 2 \text{ mL} = x \text{ mL}; \quad \dfrac{150 \text{ mg}}{100 \text{ mg}} = \dfrac{x \text{ mL}}{2 \text{ mL}}$

Answer: 3 mL. The dose ordered is more than what is available; therefore you will need more than 2 mL to administer the dose.

56. 125 mg : 5 mL = 62.5 mg : x mL

OR

$\dfrac{62.5 \text{ mg}}{125 \text{ mg}} = 5 \text{ mL} = x \text{ mL}; \quad \dfrac{62.5 \text{ mg}}{125} = \dfrac{x \text{ mL}}{5 \text{ mL}}$

Answer: 2.5 mL (for administration purposes, state as 2 1/2 mL). The dose ordered is less than what is available; therefore you would need less that 5 mL to administer the dose.

57. 25 mg : 1 mL = 20 mg : x mL

OR

$\dfrac{20 \text{ mg}}{25 \text{ mg}} \times 1 \text{ mL} = x \text{ mL}; \quad \dfrac{20 \text{ mg}}{25 \text{ mg}} = \dfrac{x \text{ mL}}{1 \text{ mL}}$

Answer: 0.8 mL. The dose ordered is less than what is available; therefore you will need less than 1 mL to administer the dose.

58. 200 mg : 5 mL = 300 mg : x mL

OR

$\dfrac{300 \text{ mg}}{200 \text{ mg}} \times 5 \text{ mL} = x \text{ mL}; \quad \dfrac{300 \text{ mg}}{200 \text{ mg}} = \dfrac{x \text{ mL}}{5 \text{ mL}}$

Answer: 7.5 mL. The dose ordered is more than what is available; therefore you will need more than 5 mL to administer the dose.

59. 2 mg : 5 mL = 3 mg : x mL

OR

$\dfrac{3 \text{ mg}}{2 \text{ mg}} \times 5 \text{ mL} = x \text{ mL}; \quad \dfrac{3 \text{ mg}}{2 \text{ mg}} = \dfrac{x \text{ mL}}{5 \text{ mL}}$

Answer: 7.5 mL. The dose ordered is more than what is available; therefore you will need more than 5 mL to administer the dose.

60. 125 mg : 5 mL = 250 mg : x mL

OR

$$\frac{250\ mg}{125\ mg} \times 5\ mL = x\ mL;\ \frac{250\ mg}{125\ mg} = \frac{x\ mL}{5\ mL}$$

Answer: 10 mL. The dose ordered is more than what is available; therefore you will need more than 5 mL to administer the dose.

61. 80 mg : 15 mL = 40 mg : x mL

OR

$$\frac{40\ mg}{80\ mg} \times 15\ mL = x\ mL;\ \frac{40\ mg}{80\ mg} = \frac{x\ mL}{15\ mL}$$

Answer: 7.5 mL. The dose ordered is less than what is available; therefore you will need less than 15 mL to administer the dose.

CHAPTER 21

Answers to Practice Problems

1. Patient-controlled analgesia
2. peripheral
3. Intravenous piggyback
4. 0.9% normal saline
5. higher
6. pressure
7. 20% dextrose in water
8. 5% dextrose in water with 10 mEq potassium chloride (KCl)
9. 50 grams
10. Dextrose : 5 g : 100 mL = x g : 750 mL

OR

$$\frac{5\ g}{100\ mL} = \frac{x\ g}{1,000\ mL};\ \frac{100x}{100} = \frac{3,750}{100}$$

x = 37.5 g dextrose

NaCl: 0.9 g : 100 mL = x g : 750 mL

OR

$$\frac{100x}{100} = \frac{675}{100}$$

x = 6.75 g NaCl

11. 10 g : 100 mL = x g : 250 mL

OR

$$\frac{10\ g}{100\ mL} = \frac{x\ g}{250\ mL};\ \frac{100x}{100} = \frac{2,500}{100}$$

x = 25 g dextrose

12. Dextrose: 5 g : 100 mL = x g : 1,000 mL

OR

$$\frac{5\ g}{100\ mL} = \frac{x\ g}{1,000\ mL};\ \frac{100x}{100} = \frac{5,000}{100}$$

x = 50 g dextrose

NaCl: 0.33 g : 100 mL = x g : 1,000 mL

OR

$$\frac{0.33g}{100\ mL} = \frac{x\ g}{1,000\ mL};\ \frac{100x}{100} = \frac{330}{100}$$

x = 3.3 g NaCl

13. Dextrose: 5 g : 100 mL = x g : 500 mL

OR

$$\frac{5\ g}{100\ mL} = \frac{x\ g}{500\ mL};\ \frac{100x}{100} = \frac{2,500}{100}$$

x = 25 g dextrose

NaCl: 0.45 g : 100 mL = x g : 500 mL

OR

$$\frac{0.45g}{100\ mL} = \frac{x\ g}{500\ mL}$$

$$\frac{100x}{100} = \frac{225}{100}$$

x = 2.25 g NaCl

Note:

Any of the problems shown can be solved by ratio-proportion. Answers will be shown using Formula "A."

14. x mL/hr = $\dfrac{1,800\ mL}{24\ hr}$, x = 75 mL/hr

15. x mL/hr = $\dfrac{2,000\ mL}{24\ hr}$; x = 83.3 = 83 mL/hr

16. x mL/hr = $\dfrac{500\ mL}{12\ hr}$; x = 41.6 = 42 mL/hr

17. *Remember:* when infusion time is less than an hour, use a ratio-proportion to determine mL/hr.

100 mL : 45 min = x mL : 60 min

$$\frac{45x}{45} = \frac{6,000}{45} = 133.3;\ x = 133\ mL/hr$$

18. x mL/hr = $\dfrac{1,500\ mL}{24\ hr}$; x = 62.5 = 63 mL/hr

19. x mL/hr = $\dfrac{750\ mL}{16\ hr}$; x = 46.8 = 47 mL/hr

20. *Remember:* when infusion time is less than an hour, use a ratio proportion to determine mL/hr.

30 mL : 20 min = x mL : 60 min

$$\frac{20x}{20} = \frac{1,800}{20} = 90; \, x = 90 \text{ mL/hr}$$

21. 10 gtt/mL, macrodrop
22. 60 gtt/mL, microdrop
23. 20 gtt/mL, macrodrop
24. 15 gtt/mL, macrodrop

25. $x \text{ gtt/min} = \dfrac{75 \text{ (mL)} \times 10 \text{ (gtt/mL)}}{60 \text{ (min)}} =$

$$\frac{75 \times 10}{60} = \frac{75 \times 1}{6} = \frac{75}{6}$$

$$x = \frac{75}{6} = 12.5 = 13 \text{ gtt/min}$$

Answer: 13 gtt/min; 13 macrogtt/min

26. $x \text{ gtt/min} = \dfrac{30 \text{ (mL)} \times 60 \text{ (gtt/mL)}}{60 \text{ (min)}} =$

$$\frac{30 \times 60}{60} = \frac{30 \times 1}{1} = \frac{30}{1}$$

$$x = \frac{30}{1} = 30 \text{ gtt/min}$$

Answer: 30 gtt/min; 30 microgtt/min

27. $x \text{ gtt/min} = \dfrac{125 \text{ (mL)} \times 15 \text{ (gtt/mL)}}{60 \text{ (min)}} =$

$$\frac{125 \times 15}{60} = \frac{125 \times 1}{4} = \frac{125}{4}$$

$$x = \frac{125}{4} = 31.2 = 31 \text{ gtt/min}$$

Answer: 31 gtt/min; 31 macrogtt/min

28. Step 1: Calculate mL/hr

$$x \text{ mL/hr} = \frac{1,000 \text{ mL}}{6 \text{ hr}}; \, x = 166.6 = 167 \text{ mL/hr}$$

Step 2: Calculate gtt/min

$$x \text{ gtt/min} = \frac{167 \text{ (mL)} \times 15 \text{ (gtt/mL)}}{60 \text{ (min)}} =$$

$$\frac{167 \times 15}{60} = \frac{167 \times 1}{4} = \frac{167}{4}$$

$$x = \frac{167}{4} = 41.7 = 42 \text{ gtt/min}$$

Answer: 42 gtt/min; 42 macrogtt/min

29. $x \text{ gtt/min} = \dfrac{60 \text{ (mL)} \times 60 \text{ (gtt/mL)}}{45 \text{ (min)}} =$

$$\frac{60 \times 60}{45} = \frac{60 \times 4}{3} = \frac{240}{3}$$

$$x = \frac{240}{3} = 80 \text{ gtt/min}$$

Answer: 80 gtt/min; 80 microgtt/min

Note:

This problem could also be done by first determining mL/min to be administered then calculating gtt/min.

30. Step 1: Calculate mL/hr.

$$x \text{ mL/hr} = \frac{1,000 \text{ mL}}{16 \text{ hr}}; \, x = 62.5 = 63 \text{ mL/hr}$$

Step 2: Calculate gtt/min.

$$x \text{ gtt/min} = \frac{63 \text{ (mL)} \times 15 \text{ (gtt/mL)}}{60 \text{ (min)}} =$$

$$\frac{63 \times 15}{60} = \frac{63 \times 1}{4} = \frac{63}{4}$$

$$x = \frac{63}{4} = 15.7 = 16 \text{ gtt/min}$$

Answer: 16 gtt/min; 16 macrogtt/min

31. Step 1: Calculate mL/hr.

$$x \text{ mL/hr} = \frac{150 \text{ mL}}{2 \text{ hr}}; \, x = 75 \text{ mL/hr}$$

Step 2: Calculate gtt/min

$$x \text{ gtt/min} = \frac{75 \text{ (mL)} \times 20 \text{ (gtt/mL)}}{60 \text{ (min)}} =$$

$$\frac{75 \times 20}{60} = \frac{75 \times 1}{3} = \frac{75}{3}$$

$$x = \frac{75}{3} = 25 \text{ gtt/min}$$

Answer: 25 gtt/min; 25 macrogtt/min

32. Step 1: Calculate mL/hr.

$$x \text{ mL/hr} = \frac{3,000 \text{ mL}}{24 \text{ hr}}; \, x = 125 \text{ mL/hr}$$

Step 2: Calculate gtt/min.

$$x \text{ gtt/min} = \frac{125 \text{ (mL)} \times 10 \text{ (gtt/mL)}}{60 \text{ (min)}} =$$

$$\frac{125 \times 10}{60} = \frac{125 \times 1}{6} = \frac{125}{6}$$

$$x = \frac{125}{6} = 20.8 = 21 \text{ gtt/min}$$

Answer: 21 gtt/min; 21 macrogtt/min

33. Step 1: Calculate mL/hr.

$$x \text{ mL/hr} = \frac{2,000 \text{ mL}}{12 \text{ hr}}; \, x = 166.6 = 167 \text{ mL/hr}$$

Step 2: Calculate gtt/min.

$$x \text{ gtt/min} = \frac{167 \text{ (mL)} \times 15 \text{ (gtt/mL)}}{60 \text{ (min)}} =$$

$$\frac{167 \times 15}{60} = \frac{167 \times 1}{4} = \frac{167}{4}$$

$$x = \frac{167}{4} = 41.7 = 42 \text{ gtt/min}$$

Answer: 42 gtt/min; 42 macrogtt/min

34. x gtt/min $= \dfrac{60 \text{ (mL)} \times 60 \text{ (gtt/mL)}}{30 \text{ (min)}} =$

$$\frac{60 \times 60}{30} = \frac{60 \times 2}{1} = \frac{120}{1}$$

$$x = \frac{120}{1} = 120 \text{ gtt/min}$$

Answer: 120 gtt/min; 120 microgtt/min

Note:

This could have also been done by first determining mL/min, then calculating gtt/min.

35. 20 gtt/mL

$$\frac{60}{20}$$

Answer: 3

36. 10 gtt/mL

$$\frac{60}{10}$$

Answer: 6

37. 60 gtt/mL

$$\frac{60}{60}$$

Answer: 1

38. Step 1: Determine the drop factor constant.
$$60 \div 10 = 6$$

Step 2: Calculate the gtt/min.

x gtt/min $= \dfrac{200 \text{ mL/hr}}{6}$; $x = 33.3 =$

33 gtt/min

Answer: 33 gtt/min; 33 macrogtt/min

39. Step 1: Determine the drop factor constant.
$$60 \div 15 = 4$$

Step 2: Calculate the gtt/min.

x gtt/min $= \dfrac{50 \text{ mL/hr}}{4}$; $x = 12.5 = 13 \text{ gtt/min}$

Answer: 13 gtt/min; 13 macrogtt/min

40. Step 1: Determine drop factor constant.
$$60 \div 60 = 1$$

Step 2: Calculate gtt/min.

x gtt/min $= \dfrac{80 \text{ mL/hr}}{1}$; $x = 80 \text{ gtt/min}$

Answer: 80 gtt/min; 80 microgtt/min

41. Step 1: Determine drop factor constant.
$$60 \div 20 = 3$$

Step 2: Calculate gtt/min.

x gtt/min $= \dfrac{140 \text{ mL/hr}}{3}$; $x = 46.6 = 47 \text{ gtt/min}$

Answer: 47 gtt/min; 47 macrogtt/min

42. Step 1: Determine mL/hr.

x mL/hr $= \dfrac{1,000 \text{ mL}}{10 \text{ hr}}$; $x = 100 \text{ mL/hr}$

Step 2: Determine the drop factor constant.
$$60 \div 10 = 6$$

Step 3: Calculate gtt/min.

x gtt/min $= \dfrac{100 \text{ mL/hr}}{6}$; $x = 16.6 = 17 \text{ gtt/min}$

Answer: 17 gtt/min; 17 macrogtt/min

43. Step 1: Determine mL/hr.

x mL/hr $= \dfrac{1,500 \text{ mL}}{12 \text{ hr}}$; $x = 125 \text{ mL/hr}$

Step 2: Determine the drop factor constant.
$$60 \div 15 = 4$$

Step 3: Calculate gtt/min.

x gtt/min $= \dfrac{125 \text{ mL/hr}}{4}$; $x = 31.2 = 31 \text{ gtt/min}$

Answer: 31 gtt/min; 31 macrogtt/min

44. Remember small volumes are multiplied and expressed in mL/hr.

Step 1: Determine mL/hr.

$$40 \text{ mL/20 min} = 40 \times 3 \ (3 \times 20 \text{ min})$$
$$= 120 \text{ mL/hr}$$

Step 2: Determine the drop factor constant.
$$60 \div 10 = 6$$

Step 3: Calculate gtt/min.

x gtt/min $= \dfrac{120 \text{ mL/hr}}{6}$; $x = 20 \text{ gtt/min}$

Answer: 20 gtt/min; 20 macrogtt/min

45. x gtt/min $= \dfrac{125 \text{ (mL)} \times 15 \text{ (gtt/mL)}}{60 \text{ (min)}} =$

$$\frac{125 \times 15}{60} = \frac{125 \times 1}{4} = \frac{125}{4}$$

$$x = \frac{125}{4} = 31.2 = 31 \text{ gtt/min}$$

Answer: 31 gtt/min; 31 macrogtt/min

46. Step 1: Determine mL/hr.

$x \text{ mL/hr} = \dfrac{2,500 \text{ mL}}{16 \text{ hr}}; x = 156.2 = 156 \text{ mL/hr}$

Step 2: Calculate gtt/min.

$x \text{ gtt/min} = \dfrac{156 \text{ (mL)} \times 10 \text{ (gtt/mL)}}{60 \text{ (min)}} =$

$\dfrac{156 \times 10}{60} = \dfrac{156 \times 1}{6} = \dfrac{156}{6}$

$x = \dfrac{156}{6} = 26 \text{ gtt/min}$

Answer: 26 gtt/min; 26 macrogtt/min

47. $x \text{ gtt/min} = \dfrac{100 \text{ (mL)} \times 60 \text{ (gtt/mL)}}{60 \text{ (min)}} =$

$\dfrac{100 \times 60}{60} = \dfrac{100 \times 1}{1} = \dfrac{100}{1}$

$x = \dfrac{100}{1} = 100 \text{ gtt/min}$

Answer: 100 gtt/min; 100 microgtt/min

48. 1 L = 1,000 mL

2 L = 2,000 mL

Step 1: Determine mL/hr.

$x \text{ mL/hr} = \dfrac{2,000 \text{ mL}}{10 \text{ hr}}; x = 200 \text{ mL/hr}$

Step 2: Calculate gtt/min.

$x \text{ gtt/min} = \dfrac{200 \text{ (mL)} \times 15 \text{ (gtt/mL)}}{60 \text{ (min)}} =$

$\dfrac{200 \times 15}{60} = \dfrac{200 \times 1}{4} = \dfrac{200}{4}$

$x = \dfrac{200}{4} = 50 \text{ gtt/min}$

Answer: 50 gtt/min; 50 macrogtt/min

Note:

Practice problems 45–48 could have also been done by using the shortcut method (determining drop factor constant, then calculating gtt/min). This method would give the same answers.

49. $x \text{ gtt/min} = \dfrac{130 \text{ (mL)} \times 15 \text{ (gtt/min)}}{60 \text{ (min)}} =$

$\dfrac{130 \times 15}{60} = \dfrac{130 \times 1}{4} = \dfrac{130}{4}$

$x = \dfrac{130}{4} = 32.5 = 33 \text{ gtt/min}$

Answer: 33 gtt/min; 33 macrogtt/min

50. $x \text{ gtt/min} = \dfrac{250 \text{ (mL)} \times 10 \text{ (gtt/min)}}{60 \text{ (min)}} =$

$\dfrac{250 \times 10}{60} = \dfrac{250 \times 1}{6} = \dfrac{250}{6}$

$x = \dfrac{250}{6} = 41.6 = 42 \text{ gtt/min}$

Answer: 42 gtt/min; 42 macrogtt/min

51. $x \text{ gtt/min} = \dfrac{50 \text{ (mL)} \times 10 \text{ (gtt/mL)}}{45 \text{ (min)}} =$

$\dfrac{50 \times 10}{45} = \dfrac{50 \times 2}{9} = \dfrac{100}{9}$

$x = \dfrac{100}{9} = 11.1 = 11 \text{ gtt/min}$

Answer: 11 gtt/min; 11 macrogtt/min

52. $x \text{ gtt/min} = \dfrac{75 \text{ (mL)} \times 10 \text{ (gtt/mL)}}{30 \text{ (min)}} =$

$\dfrac{75 \times 10}{30} = \dfrac{75 \times 1}{3} = \dfrac{75}{3}$

$x = \dfrac{75}{3} = 25 \text{ gtt/min}$

Answer: 25 gtt/min; 25 macrogtt/min

53. $x \text{ gtt/min} = \dfrac{50 \text{ (mL)} \times 10 \text{ (gtt/mL)}}{30 \text{ (min)}} =$

$\dfrac{50 \times 10}{30} = \dfrac{50 \times 1}{3} = \dfrac{50}{3}$

$x = \dfrac{50}{3} = 16.6 = 17 \text{ gtt/min}$

Answer: 17 gtt/min; 17 macrogtt/min

54. a) 50 mg : 1 mL = 500 mg : x mL

OR

$\dfrac{500 \text{ mg}}{50 \text{ mg}} \times 1 \text{ mL} = x \text{ mL}; \dfrac{500 \text{ mg}}{50 \text{ mg}} = \dfrac{x \text{ mL}}{1 \text{ mL}}$

Answer: 10 mL

b) $x \text{ gtt/min} = \dfrac{100 \text{ (mL)} \times 15 \text{ (gtt/mL)}}{60 \text{ (min)}} =$

$\dfrac{100 \times 15}{60} = \dfrac{100 \times 1}{4} = \dfrac{100}{4}$

$x = \dfrac{100}{4} = 25 \text{ macrogtt/min}$

Answer: 25 gtt/min; 25 macrogtt/min

55. a) 50 mg : 10 mL = 20 mg : x mL

OR

$\dfrac{20 \text{ mg}}{50 \text{ mg}} \times 10 \text{ mL} = x \text{ mL}; \dfrac{20 \text{ mg}}{50 \text{ mg}} = \dfrac{x \text{ mL}}{10 \text{ mL}}$

Answer: 4 mL

Step 1: Calculate mL/hr

$$x \text{ mL/hr} = \frac{300 \text{ mL}}{6 \text{ hr}}; x = 50 \text{ mL/hr}$$

Step 2: Calculate gtt/min.

b) $x \text{ gtt/min} = \dfrac{50 \text{ (mL)} \times 60 \text{ (gtt/mL)}}{60 \text{ (min)}} =$

$$\frac{50 \times 60}{60} = \frac{50 \times 1}{1} = \frac{50}{1}$$

$$x = \frac{50}{1} = 50 \text{ gtt/min}$$

Answer: 50 gtt/min; 50 microgtt/min

56. a) $16 \text{ mg} : 1 \text{ mL} = 300 \text{ mg} : x \text{ mL}$

OR

$$\frac{300 \text{ mg}}{16 \text{ mg}} \times 1 \text{ mL} = x \text{ mL}; \frac{300 \text{ mg}}{16 \text{ mg}} = \frac{x \text{ mL}}{1 \text{ mL}}$$

Answer: 18.8 mL (18.75 mL rounded to the nearest tenth)

Alternate method for calculating dose:

$320 \text{ mg} : 20 \text{ mL} = 300 \text{ mg} : x \text{ mL}$

OR

$$\frac{300 \text{ mg}}{320 \text{ mg}} \times 20 \text{ mL} = x \text{ mL}; \frac{300 \text{ mg}}{320 \text{ mg}} = \frac{x \text{ mL}}{20 \text{ mL}}$$

Answer: 18.8 mL (18.75 mL rounded to nearest tenth)

b) $x \text{ gtt/min} = \dfrac{300 \text{ (mL)} \times 10 \text{ (gtt/mL)}}{60 \text{ (min)}} =$

$$\frac{300 \times 10}{60} = \frac{300 \times 1}{6} = \frac{300}{6}$$

$$x = \frac{300}{6} = 50 \text{ gtt/min}$$

Answer: 50 gtt/min; 50 macrogtt/min

57. $x \text{ gtt/min} = \dfrac{100 \text{ (mL)} \times 10 \text{ (gtt/mL)}}{60 \text{ (min)}} =$

$$\frac{100 \times 10}{60} = \frac{100 \times 1}{6} = \frac{100}{6}$$

$$x = \frac{100}{6} = 16.6 = 17 \text{ gtt/min}$$

Answer: 17 gtt/min; 17 macrogtt/min

58. a) $15 \text{ mEq} : 1,000 \text{ mL} = 4 \text{ mEq} : x \text{ mL}$

OR

$$\frac{15 \text{ mEq}}{1,000 \text{ mL}} = \frac{4 \text{ mEq}}{x \text{ mL}}; \frac{15x}{15} = \frac{4,000}{15} = 266.6$$

$x = 267 \text{ mL/hr}$ to deliver 4 mEq of potassium chloride

b) $x \text{ gtt/min} = \dfrac{(267 \text{ mL}) \times 10 \text{ (gtt/mL)}}{60 \text{ (min)}} =$

$$\frac{267 \times 10}{60} = \frac{267 \times 1}{6} = \frac{267}{6}$$

$$x = \frac{267}{6} = 44.5 = 45 \text{ gtt/min}$$

Answer: 45 gtt/min; 45 macrogtt/min

45 gtt/min or 45 macrogtt/min would deliver 4 mEq of potassium chloride each hour.

59. a) $50 \text{ U} : 250 \text{ mL} = 10 \text{ U} : x \text{ mL}$

OR

$$\frac{50 \text{ U}}{250 \text{ mL}} = \frac{10 \text{ U}}{x \text{ mL}}; \frac{50x}{50} = \frac{2,500}{50} = 50 \text{ mL/hr}$$

50 mL/hr must be administered for the client to receive 10 U/hr.

b) $x \text{ gtt/min} = \dfrac{50 \text{ (mL)} \times 15 \text{ (gtt/mL)}}{60 \text{ (min)}} =$

$$\frac{50 \times 15}{60} = \frac{50 \times 1}{4} = \frac{50}{4}$$

$$x = \frac{50}{4} = 12.5 = 13 \text{ gtt/min}$$

Answer: 13 gtt/min; 13 macrogtt/min

13 gtt/min (13 macrogtt/min) of this solution would deliver 10 U/hr.

60. a) $40 \text{ U} : 250 \text{ mL} = 15 \text{ U} : x \text{ mL}$

OR

$$\frac{40 \text{ U}}{250 \text{ mL}} = \frac{15 \text{ U}}{x \text{ mL}}; \frac{40x}{40} = \frac{3750}{40} = 93.7 =$$

94 mL/hr

b) $x \text{ gtt/min} = \dfrac{94 \text{ (mL)} \times 60 \text{ (gtt/mL)}}{60 \text{ (min)}} =$

$$\frac{94 \times 60}{60} = \frac{94 \times 1}{1} = \frac{94}{1}$$

$$x = \frac{94}{1} = 94 \text{ gtt/min}$$

Answer: 94 gtt/min; 94 microgtt/min

94 gtt/min (94 microgtt/min) of this solution would deliver 15 U/hr.

61. $60 \text{ microgtt/min} = \dfrac{150 \text{ (mL)} \times 60 \text{ (gtt/mL)}}{x \text{ (min)}}$

$$60 = \frac{150 \times 60}{x}$$

$$60 = \frac{9,000}{x}$$

$$\frac{60x}{60} = \frac{9,000}{60}$$

$$x = 150 \text{ minutes}$$

$$60 \text{ min} = 1 \text{ hr}; 150 \text{ min} \div 60 = 2.5 \text{ hrs}$$

Answer: 2 1/2 hr

Note:

The problem asks for time in hours, so minutes are changed to hours.

62. $35 \text{ macrogtt/min} = \dfrac{x \text{ (mL)} \times 15 \text{ (gtt/mL)}}{300 \text{ (min)}}$

$$35 = x \ (\times) \ \dfrac{\cancel{15}^{\,1}}{\cancel{300}_{\,2}}$$

$$35 = \dfrac{x}{20}$$

$$x = 35 \times 20 = 700$$

$$x = 700 \text{ mL}$$

Note:

Since the formula is time in minutes, 5 hours was changed to minutes by multiplying 5×60 (60 min = 1 hr).

63. $45 \text{ macrogtt/min} = \dfrac{180 \text{ (mL)} \times 15 \text{ (gtt/mL)}}{x \text{ (min)}}$

$$45 = \dfrac{180 \times 15}{x}$$

$$45 = \dfrac{2,700}{x}$$

$$\dfrac{45x}{45} = \dfrac{2,700}{45}$$

$$x = 60 \text{ minutes}$$

$$60 \text{ min} = 1 \text{ hr}; 60 \text{ min} \div 60 = 1 \text{ hr}$$

Answer: 1 hr

64. $45 \text{ macrogtt/min} = \dfrac{x \text{ (mL)} \times 15 \text{ (gtt/mL)}}{480 \text{ (min)}}$

$$45 = x \ (\times) \ \dfrac{\cancel{15}^{\,1}}{\cancel{480}_{\,32}}$$

$$45 = \dfrac{x}{32}$$

$$x = 45 \times 32 = 1,440$$

$$x = 1,440 \text{ mL}$$

Answer: 1,440 mL

Note:

Formula is in minutes, therefore 8 hr $\times$ 60 = 480 minutes.

65. $60 \text{ microgtt/min} = \dfrac{90 \text{ (mL)} \times 60 \text{ (gtt/mL)}}{x \text{ (min)}}$

$$60 = \dfrac{90 \times 60}{x}$$

$$60 = \dfrac{5,400}{x}$$

$$\dfrac{60x}{60} = \dfrac{5,400}{60}$$

$$x = 90 \text{ minutes}$$

$$60 \text{ min} = 1 \text{ hr}; 90 \text{ min} \div 60 = 1.5 \text{ hr}$$

Answer: $1^{1}/_{2}$ hr

66. Step 1: Determine mL/hr for the remaining solution.

$$x \text{ mL/hr} = \dfrac{250 \text{ mL}}{3 \text{ hr}}; x = 83.3 \div 83 \text{ mL/hr}$$

Step 2: Calculate gtt/min.

$$x \text{ gtt/min} = \dfrac{83 \text{ (mL)} \times 15 \text{ (gtt/mL)}}{60 \text{ (min)}} =$$

$$\dfrac{83 \times 15}{60} = \dfrac{83 \times 1}{4} = \dfrac{83}{4}$$

$$x = \dfrac{83}{4} = 20.7 = 21 \text{ gtt/min}$$

Answer: a) 21 gtt/min; 21 macrogtt/min

b) Determine the percentage of change.

$$\dfrac{21 - 16}{16} = \dfrac{5}{16} = 0.31 = 31\%$$

Percentage of change is greater than 25%. Consult prescriber; order may need to be revised.

67. Step 1: Determine mL/hr for the remaining solution

$$x \text{ mL/hr} = \dfrac{200 \text{ mL}}{1.5 \text{ hr}} \ x = 133.3 = 133 \text{ mL/hr}$$

Step 2: Calculate gtt/min

$$x \text{ gtt/min} = \dfrac{133 \text{ (mL)} \times 15 \text{ (gtt/mL)}}{60 \text{ min}} =$$

$$\dfrac{133 \times 15}{60} = \dfrac{133 \times 1}{4} = \dfrac{133}{4}$$

$$x = \dfrac{133}{4} = 33.2 = 33 \text{ gtt/min}$$

Answer: a) 33 gtt/min; 33 macrogtt/min.

b) Determine the percentage of change.

$$\dfrac{33 - 21}{21} = \dfrac{12}{21} = 0.57 = 57\%$$

Percentage of change is greater than 25%. Consult prescriber; order may need to be revised.

68. Step 1: Determine mL/hr for the remaining solution.

$$x \text{ mL/hr} = \dfrac{850 \text{ mL}}{6 \text{ hr}}; x = 141.6 = 142 \text{ mL/hr}$$

Step 2: Calculate gtt/min.

$$x \text{ gtt/min} = \frac{142 \text{ (mL)} \times 20 \text{ (gtt/mL)}}{60 \text{ (min)}} =$$

$$\frac{142 \times 20}{60} = \frac{142 \times 1}{3} = \frac{142}{3}$$

$$x = \frac{142}{3} = 47.3 = 47 \text{ gtt/min}$$

Answer a) 47 gtt/min; 47 macrogtt/min

b) Determine the percentage of change.

$$\frac{47 - 42}{42} = \frac{5}{42} = 12\%$$

This is an acceptable increase. Assess if client can tolerate adjustment in rate. Check hospital policy.

69. Step 1: Determine mL/hr for the remaining solution.

$$x \text{ mL/hr} = \frac{750 \text{ mL}}{8 \text{ hr}}; x = 93.7 = 94 \text{ mL/hr}$$

Step 2: Calculate gtt/min.

$$x \text{ gtt/min} = \frac{94 \text{ (mL)} \times 20 \text{ (gtt/mL)}}{60 \text{ (min)}} =$$

$$\frac{94 \times 20}{60} = \frac{94 \times 1}{3} = \frac{94}{3}$$

$$x = \frac{94}{3} = 31.3 = 31 \text{ gtt/min}$$

Answer: a) 31 gtt/min; 31 macrogtt/min

b) Determine the percentage of change.

$$\frac{31 - 28}{28} = \frac{3}{28} = 11\%$$

The percentage of change is 11%. This is an acceptable increase. Assess if client can tolerate adjustment in rate. Check if allowed by institution policy.

70. Step 1: Determine mL/hr for remaining solution.

$$x \text{ mL/hr} = \frac{250 \text{ mL}}{3 \text{ hr}}; x = 83.3 = 83 \text{ mL/hr}$$

Step 2: Calculate gtt/min.

$$x \text{ gtt/min} = \frac{83 \text{ (mL)} \times 60 \text{ (gtt/mL)}}{60 \text{ (min)}} =$$

$$\frac{83 \times 60}{60} = \frac{83 \times 1}{1} = \frac{83}{1}$$

$$x = 83 \text{ gtt/min}$$

Answer: 83 gtt/min; 83 microgtt/min

b) Determine the percentage of change.

$$\frac{83 - 33}{33} = \frac{50}{33} = 152\%$$

The percentage of change is 152%. This is not acceptable because it is greater than 25%.

Consult prescriber; the order may need to be revised. (Do not increase IV rate.)

71. $\dfrac{500 \text{ mL}}{60 \text{ mL/hr}} = 8.33 \text{ hrs}$

$0.33 \times 60 = 19.8 = 20 \text{ minutes}$

a) Answer: 8 hr + 20 minutes = infusion time

b) Answer: 6:20 AM (10:00 PM + 8 hr + 20 minutes); military time: 0620

72. $\dfrac{250 \text{ mL}}{80 \text{ mL/hr}} = 3.12 \text{ hrs}$

$0.12 \times 60 = 7.2 = 7 \text{ minutes}$

a) Answer: 3 hr + 7 minutes = infusion time

b) Answer: 5:07 AM (2:00 AM + 3 hr + 7 minutes); military time: 0507

73. $\dfrac{1,000 \text{ mL}}{40 \text{ mL/hr}} = 25 \text{ hours}$

a) Answer: 25 hr = infusion time

b) Answer: 3:10 PM August 27 (2:10 PM on August 26 + 25 hr); military time: 1510

(Most I.V solutions are not considered sterile after 24 hrs; therefore it should be changed after 24 hrs.)

74. $\dfrac{1,000 \text{ mL}}{60 \text{ mL/hr}} = 16.66 \text{ hrs}$

$0.66 \times 60 = 39.6 = 40 \text{ minutes}$

a) Answer 16 hr + 40 minutes = infusion time

b) Answer: 10:40 PM (6:00 AM + 16 hr + 40 minutes); military time: 2240

75. $\dfrac{500 \text{ mL}}{75 \text{ mL/hr}} = 6.66 \text{ hrs}$

$0.66 \times 60 = 39.6 = 40 \text{ minutes}$

a) Answer: 6 hr + 40 minutes = infusion time

b) Answer: 8:40 PM (2:00 PM + 6 hr + 40 minutes); military time: 2040

76. Step 1: 60 gtt : 1 mL = 25 gtt : x mL

$$60x = 25$$

$$x = 25 \div 60 = 0.41 \text{ mL/min}$$

Step 2: 0.41 mL/min $\times$ 60 min = 24.6 = 25 mL/hr

Step 3: $\dfrac{1,000 \text{ mL}}{25 \text{ mL/hr}} = 40 \text{ hr}$

Answer: 40 hr = infusion time

77. Step 1: 15 gtt : 1 mL = 17 gtt : x mL

$$15x = 17$$

$$x = 17 \div 15 = 1.13 = 1.1 \text{ mL/min}$$

Step 2: 1.1 mL/min $\times$ 60 min = 66 mL/hr

Step 3: $\dfrac{250 \text{ mL}}{66 \text{ mL/hr}} = 3.78$

$60 \times 0.78 = 46.8 = 47$ minutes

Answer: 3 hr + 47 minutes = infusion time

78. Step 1: 20 gtt : 1 mL = 30 gtt : x mL

$20x = 30$

$x = 30 \div 20 = 1.5$ mL/min

Step 2: 1.5 mL/min $\times$ 60 min = 90 mL/hr

Step 3: $\dfrac{1,000 \text{ mL}}{90 \text{ mL/hr}} = 11.11$

$60 \times 0.11 = 6.6 = 7$ minutes

Answer: 11 hr + 7 minutes = infusion time

79. Step 1: 10 gtt : 1 mL = 20 gtt : x mL

$\dfrac{10x}{10} = \dfrac{20}{10}$

$x = 2$ mL/min

Step 2: 2 mL/min $\times$ 60 min = 120 mL/hr

Step 3: $\dfrac{1,000 \text{ mL}}{120 \text{ mL/hr}} = 8.33$

$60 \times 0.33 = 19.8 = 20$ minutes

Answer: 8 hrs + 20 minutes = infusion time

80. Step 1: 15 gtt : 1 mL = 10 gtt : x mL

$\dfrac{15x}{15} = \dfrac{10}{15}$

$x = 0.66 = 0.67$ mL/min

Step 2: 0.67 mL/min $\times$ 60 min = 40.2 mL/hr

Step 3: $\dfrac{100 \text{ mL}}{40 \text{ mL/hr}} = 2.5$

Answer: 2 hr + 30 minutes = infusion time

81. Step 1: 15 gtt : 1 mL = 30 gtt : x mL

$\dfrac{15x}{15} = \dfrac{30}{15}$

$x = 2$ mL/min

Step 2: 35 mL $\div$ 2 mL/min = 17.5 = 18 minutes

Answer: Infusion time is 18 minutes

82. Step 1: 60 gtt : 1 mL = 35 gtt : x mL

$\dfrac{60x}{60} = \dfrac{35}{60}$

$x = 0.58$ mL/min

Step 2: 20 mL $\div$ 0.58 mL/min = 34.4 = 34 minutes

Answer: Infusion time is 34 minutes.

83. a) Dilution volume: 27 mL

b) x gtt/min =

$\dfrac{30 \text{ mL (diluted drug)} \times 60 \text{ gtt/mL}}{50 \text{ min}}$

$x = \dfrac{30 \times 60}{50} = \dfrac{1,800}{50} = 36$ gtt/min

OR

Use a ratio-proportion to determine mL/hr first. Remember with a burette where a pump or controller is not used, mL/hr = gtt/min.

30 mL : 50 min = x mL : 60 min

$\dfrac{30 \text{ mL}}{50 \text{ min}} = \dfrac{x \text{ mL}}{60 \text{ min}}$

Answer: $x = 36$ gtt/min; 36 microgtt/min

c) 36 mL/hr

84. a) Dilution volume: 13 mL

b) x gtt/min =

$\dfrac{15 \text{ mL (diluted drug)} \times 60 \text{ gtt/mL}}{45 \text{ min}}$

$x = \dfrac{15 \times 60}{45} = \dfrac{900}{45} = 20$ gtt/min

OR

Use a ratio-proportion and determine mL/hr first.

15 mL : 45 min = x mL : 60 min

OR

$\dfrac{15 \text{ mL}}{45 \text{ min}} = \dfrac{x \text{ mL}}{60 \text{ min}}$

Answer: $x = 20$ gtt/min; 20 microgtt/min

c) 20 mL/hr

85. Step 1: Determine the dose range per hour.

10 U/kg/hr $\times$ 17 kg = 170 U/hr

25 U/kg/hr $\times$ 17 kg = 425 U/hr

Step 2: Determine dose infusing per hour.

2,500 U : 250 mL = U : 50 mL

$250x = 2,500 \times 50$

$\dfrac{250x}{250} = \dfrac{125,000}{250} = 500$

$x = 500$ U/hr

Step 3: Compare the dose ordered to see if its within normal range.

The IV is infusing at 50 mL/hr, which is 500 U/hr. The normal dosage range is 170-425 U/hr. 500 U/hr is greater than the dose range. Check with the prescriber before administering.

86. Step 1: Determine the dose range.

$0.75 \text{ m}^2 \times 100 \text{ mg} = 75 \text{ mg}$

$0.75 \text{ m}^2 \times 250 \text{ mg} = 187.5 \text{ mg}$

The dose range is 75-187.5 mg per day.

Step 2: Determine the dose the child is receiving.

84 mg q12h (2 doses)

$84 \text{ mg} \times 2 = 168 \text{ mg}$

Step 3: Determine if dose is within safe range. The 84 mg q12h (84 mg × 2 = 168 mg) is within the safe range of 75-187.5 mg, so administer the medication.

87. $\dfrac{480 \text{ mL}}{8 \text{ hr}} = 60 \text{ mL/hr}$

88. $\dfrac{1,600 \text{ mL}}{24 \text{ hr}} = 66.6 = 67 \text{ mL/hr}$

89. 300 mL qid = 300 mL × 4 = 1,200 mL

$2/3 \times 1,200 \text{ mL} = x \text{ mL}$

$\dfrac{2,400}{3} = x$

Answers to Chapter Review

Note:

Many of the IV problems involving gtt/min could also be done using the shortcut method that was presented in the chapter.

Note:

Some answers in the Chapter Review reflect the number of gtt rounded to the nearest whole number, and mL/hr.

1. a) Determine mL/hr.

$x \text{ mL/hr} = \dfrac{1,000 \text{ mL}}{8 \text{ hr}}; x = 125 \text{ mL/hr}$

b) Calculate gtt/min.

$x \text{ gtt/min} = \dfrac{125 \text{ (mL)} \times 20 \text{ (gtt/mL)}}{60 \text{ (min)}} =$

42 gtt/min; 42 macrogtt/min

2. a) Determine mL/hr.

$x \text{ mL/hr} = \dfrac{2,500 \text{ mL}}{24 \text{ hr}}; x = 104 \text{ mL/hr}$

$x = 800 \text{ mL of formula needed}$

1,200 mL − 800 mL = 400 mL (water)

Therefore you will add 400 mL of water to 800 mL of Sustacal to make 1,200 mL of 2/3-strength Sustacal.

90. 1 oz = 30 mL; therefore 16 oz = 480 mL

$3/4 \times 480 \text{ mL} = x \text{ mL OR } 3/4 \times 16 \text{ oz} = x \text{ oz}$

$\dfrac{1,440}{4} = x \qquad\qquad \dfrac{48}{4} = x$

$\qquad\qquad\qquad\qquad\qquad x = 12 \text{ oz}$

$x = 12 \text{ oz } (360 \text{ mL})$ of formula needed.

16 oz (480 mL) − 12 oz (360 mL) = 4 oz water (120 mL). You would need 360 mL of formula and 120 mL of water.

Note:

For question using ounces, give answer in ounces.

91. 1 oz = 30 mL   20 oz = 600 mL

$1/2 \times 600 \text{ mL} = x \text{ mL OR } 1/2 \times 20 \text{ oz} = x \text{ oz}$

$\dfrac{600}{2} = x \qquad\qquad \dfrac{20}{2} = x$

$\qquad\qquad\qquad\qquad\qquad x = 10 \text{ oz}$

$x = 300 \text{ mL}$; you need 10 oz of Ensure.

600 mL (20 oz) − 300 mL (10 oz) Ensure = 300 mL (10 oz of water)

Answer: 10 oz Ensure + 10 oz water = 20 oz 1/2-strength Ensure.

b) Calculate gtt/min.

$x \text{ gtt/min} = \dfrac{104 \text{ (mL)} \times 10 \text{ (gtt/mL)}}{60 \text{ (min)}} =$

17 gtt/min; 17 macrogtt/min

3. a) Determine mL/hr.

$x \text{ mL/hr} = \dfrac{500 \text{ mL}}{4 \text{ hr}}; x = 125 \text{ mL/hr}$

b) Calculate gtt/min.

$x \text{ gtt/min} = \dfrac{125 \text{ (mL)} \times 15 \text{ (gtt/mL)}}{60 \text{ (min)}} =$

31 gtt/min; 31 macrogtt/min

4. a) Determine mL/hr.

$x \text{ mL/hr} = \dfrac{300 \text{ mL}}{6 \text{ hr}}; x = 50 \text{ mL/hr}$

b) Calculate gtt/min.

$x \text{ gtt/min} = \dfrac{50 \text{ (mL)} \times 60 \text{ (gtt/mL)}}{60 \text{ (min)}} =$

50 gtt/min; 50 microgtt/min

5. a) Determine mL/hr.

$$x \text{ mL/hr} = \frac{1{,}000 \text{ mL}}{24 \text{ hr}}; x = 42 \text{ mL/hr}$$

b) Calculate gtt/min.

$$x \text{ gtt/min} = \frac{42 \text{ (mL)} \times 60 \text{ (gtt/mL)}}{60 \text{ (min)}} =$$

42 gtt/min; 42 microgtt/min

6. a) Determine mL/hr.

$$x \text{ mL/hr} = \frac{1{,}000 \text{ mL}}{12 \text{ hr}}; x = 83 \text{ mL/hr}$$

b) Calculate gtt/min.

$$x \text{ gtt/min} = \frac{83 \text{ (mL)} \times 10 \text{ (gtt/mL)}}{60 \text{ (min)}} =$$

14 gtt/min; 14 macrogtt/min

7. a) Determine mL/hr.

$$x \text{ mL/hr} = \frac{1{,}000 \text{ mL}}{10 \text{ hr}}; x = 100 \text{ mL/hr}$$

b) Calculate gtt/min.

$$x \text{ gtt/min} = \frac{100 \text{ (mL)} \times 20 \text{ (gtt/mL)}}{60 \text{ (min)}} =$$

33 gtt/min; 33 macrogtt/min

8. a) Determine mL/hr.

$$x \text{ mL/hr} = \frac{1{,}500 \text{ mL}}{12 \text{ hr}}; x = 125 \text{ mL/hr}$$

b) Calculate gtt/min.

$$x \text{ gtt/min} = \frac{125 \text{ (mL)} \times 10 \text{ (gtt/mL)}}{60 \text{ (min)}} =$$

21 gtt/min; 21 macrogtt/min

9. a) Determine mL/hr.

$$x \text{ mL/hr} = \frac{500 \text{ mL}}{4 \text{ hr}}; x = 125 \text{ mL/hr}$$

b) Calculate gtt/min.

$$x \text{ gtt/min} = \frac{125 \text{ (mL)} \times 20 \text{ (gtt/mL)}}{60 \text{ (min)}} =$$

42 gtt/min; 42 macrogtt/min

10. a) Determine mL/hr.

$$x \text{ mL/hr} = \frac{250 \text{ mL}}{4 \text{ hr}}; x = 63 \text{ mL/hr}$$

b) Calculate gtt/min.

$$x \text{ gtt/min} = \frac{63 \text{ (mL)} \times 20 \text{ (gtt/mL)}}{60 \text{ (min)}} =$$

21 gtt/min; 21 macrogtt/min

11. a) Determine mL/hr.

$$x \text{ mL/hr} = \frac{1{,}500 \text{ mL}}{8 \text{ hr}}; x = 188 \text{ mL/hr}$$

b) Calculate gtt/min.

$$x \text{ gtt/min} = \frac{188 \text{ (mL)} \times 20 \text{ (gtt/mL)}}{60 \text{ (min)}} =$$

63 gtt/min; 63 macrogtt/min

12. a) Determine mL/hr.

$$x \text{ mL/hr} = \frac{3{,}000 \text{ mL}}{24 \text{ hr}}; x = 125 \text{ mL/hr}$$

b) Calculate gtt/min.

$$x \text{ gtt/min} = \frac{125 \text{ (mL)} \times 15 \text{ (gtt/mL)}}{60 \text{ (min)}} =$$

31 gtt/min; 31 macrogtt/min

13. 1 L = 1,000 mL

2 L = 2,000 mL

a) Determine mL/hr.

$$x \text{ mL/hr} = \frac{2{,}000 \text{ mL}}{24 \text{ hr}}; x = 83 \text{ mL/hr}$$

b) Calculate gtt/min.

$$x \text{ gtt/min} = \frac{83 \text{ (mL)} \times 15 \text{ (gtt/mL)}}{60 \text{ (min)}} =$$

21 gtt/min; 21 macrogtt/min

14. a) Determine mL/hr.

$$x \text{ mL/hr} = \frac{1{,}000 \text{ mL}}{7 \text{ hr}}; x = 143 \text{ mL/hr}$$

b) Calculate gtt/min.

$$x \text{ gtt/min} = \frac{143 \text{ (mL)} \times 10 \text{ (gtt/mL)}}{60 \text{ (min)}} =$$

24 gtt/min; 24 macrogtt/min

15. a) Determine mL/hr.

$$x \text{ mL/hr} = \frac{500 \text{ mL}}{4 \text{ hr}}; x = 125 \text{ mL/hr}$$

b) Calculate gtt/min.

$$x \text{ gtt/min} = \frac{125 \text{ (mL)} \times 60 \text{ (gtt/mL)}}{60 \text{ (min)}} =$$

125 gtt/min; 125 microgtt/min

16. a) Determine mL/hr.

$$x \text{ mL/hr} = \frac{1{,}000 \text{ mL}}{6 \text{ hr}}; x = 167 \text{ mL/hr}$$

b) Calculate gtt/min.

$$x \text{ gtt/min} = \frac{167 \text{ (mL)} \times 20 \text{ (gtt/mL)}}{60 \text{ (min)}} =$$

56 gtt/min; 56 macrogtt/min

17. a) Determine mL/hr.

$$x \text{ mL/hr} = \frac{250 \text{ mL}}{8 \text{ hr}}; x = 31 \text{ mL/hr}$$

b) Calculate gtt/min.

$$x \text{ gtt/min} = \frac{31 \text{ (mL)} \times 60 \text{ (gtt/mL)}}{60 \text{ (min)}} =$$

31 gtt/min; 31 macrogtt/min

18. $x \text{ gtt/min} = \dfrac{50 \text{ (mL)} \times 60 \text{ (gtt/mL)}}{60 \text{ (min)}} =$

50 gtt/min; 50 microgtt/min

19. $x \text{ gtt/min} = \dfrac{150 \text{ (mL)} \times 15 \text{ (gtt/mL)}}{60 \text{ (min)}} =$

38 gtt/min; 38 macrogtt/min

20. a) Determine mL/hr.

$$x \text{ mL/hr} = \frac{500 \text{ mL}}{6 \text{ hr}}; x = 83 \text{ mL/hr}$$

b) Calculate gtt/min.

$$x \text{ gtt/min} = \frac{83 \text{ (mL)} \times 15 \text{ (gtt/mL)}}{60 \text{ (min)}} =$$

21 gtt/min; 21 macrogtt/min

21. a) Determine mL/hr.

$$x \text{ mL/hr} = \frac{1,500 \text{ mL}}{12 \text{ hr}}; x = 125 \text{ mL/hr}$$

b) Calculate gtt/min.

$$x \text{ gtt/min} = \frac{125 \text{ (mL)} \times 10 \text{ (gtt/mL)}}{60 \text{ (min)}} =$$

21 gtt/min; 21 macrogtt/min

22. a) Determine mL/hr.

$$x \text{ mL/hr} = \frac{1,500 \text{ mL}}{24 \text{ hr}}; x = 63 \text{ mL/hr}$$

b) Calculate gtt/min.

$$x \text{ gtt/min} = \frac{63 \text{ (mL)} \times 15 \text{ (gtt/mL)}}{60 \text{ (min)}} =$$

16 gtt/min; 16 macrogtt/min

23. a) Determine mL/hr.

$$x \text{ mL/hr} = \frac{2,000 \text{ mL}}{16 \text{ hr}}; x = 125 \text{ mL/hr}$$

b) Calculate gtt/min.

$$x \text{ gtt/min} = \frac{125 \text{ (mL)} \times 20 \text{ (gtt/mL)}}{60 \text{ (min)}} =$$

42 gtt/min; 42 macrogtt/min

24. a) Determine mL/hr.

$$x \text{ mL/hr} = \frac{500 \text{ mL}}{8 \text{ hr}}; x = 63 \text{ mL/hr}$$

b) Calculate gtt/min.

$$x \text{ gtt/min} = \frac{63 \text{ (mL)} \times 15 \text{ (gtt/mL)}}{60 \text{ (min)}} =$$

16 gtt/min; 16 macrogtt/min

25. a) Determine mL/hr.

$$x \text{ mL/hr} = \frac{250 \text{ mL}}{10 \text{ hr}}; x = 25 \text{ mL/hr}$$

b) Calculate gtt/min.

$$x \text{ gtt/min} = \frac{25 \text{ (mL)} \times 60 \text{ (gtt/mL)}}{60 \text{ (min)}} =$$

25 gtt/min; 25 microgtt/min

26. $x \text{ gtt/min} = \dfrac{75 \text{ (mL)} \times 60 \text{ (gtt/mL)}}{60 \text{ (min)}} =$

75 gtt/min; 75 microgtt/min

27. $x \text{ gtt/min} = \dfrac{125 \text{ (mL)} \times 20 \text{ (gtt/mL)}}{60 \text{ (min)}} =$

42 gtt/min; 42 macrogtt/min

28. $x \text{ gtt/min} = \dfrac{40 \text{ (mL)} \times 60 \text{ (gtt/mL)}}{60 \text{ (min)}} =$

40 gtt/min; 40 microgtt/min

29. $x \text{ gtt/min} = \dfrac{50 \text{ (mL)} \times 60 \text{ (gtt/mL)}}{45 \text{ (min)}} =$

67 gtt/min; 67 microgtt/min

30. $x \text{ gtt/min} = \dfrac{90 \text{ (mL)} \times 15 \text{ (gtt/mL)}}{60 \text{ (min)}} =$

23 gtt/min; 23 macrogtt/min

31. $x \text{ gtt/min} = \dfrac{150 \text{ (mL)} \times 10 \text{ (gtt/mL)}}{60 \text{ (min)}} =$

25 gtt/min; 25 macrogtt/min

32. a) Determine mL/hr.

$$x \text{ mL/hr} = \frac{2,500 \text{ mL}}{24 \text{ hr}}; x = 104 \text{ mL/hr}$$

b) Calculate gtt/min.

$$x \text{ gtt/min} = \frac{104 \text{ (mL)} \times 15 \text{ (gtt/mL)}}{60 \text{ (min)}} =$$

26 gtt/min; 26 macrogtt/min

33. $x \text{ gtt/min} = \dfrac{50 \text{ (mL)} \times 10 \text{ (gtt/mL)}}{40 \text{ (min)}} =$

13 gtt/min; 13 macrogtt/min

34. $x \text{ gtt/min} = \dfrac{100 \text{ (mL)} \times 20 \text{ (gtt/mL)}}{30 \text{ (min)}} =$

67 gtt/min; 67 macrogtt/min

35. a) Determine mL/hr.

$$x \text{ mL/hr} = \frac{250 \text{ mL}}{5 \text{ hr}}; x = 50 \text{ mL/hr}$$

b) Calculate gtt/min.

$$x \text{ gtt/min} = \frac{50 \text{ (mL)} \times 20 \text{ (gtt/mL)}}{60 \text{ (min)}} =$$

17 gtt/min; 17 macrogtt/min

36. x gtt/min $= \dfrac{80 \text{ (mL)} \times 20 \text{ (gtt/mL)}}{60 \text{ (min)}} =$

27 gtt/min; 27 macrogtt/min

37. x gtt/min $= \dfrac{150 \text{ (mL)} \times 10 \text{ (gtt/mL)}}{30 \text{ (min)}} =$

50 gtt/min; 50 macrogtt/min

38. x gtt/min $= \dfrac{50 \text{ (mL)} \times 60 \text{ (gtt/mL)}}{30 \text{ (min)}} =$

100 gtt/min; 100 microgtt/min

39. a) Determine mL/hr.

x mL/hr $= \dfrac{500 \text{ mL}}{3 \text{ hr}}$; $x = 167$ mL/hr

b) Calculate gtt/min.

x gtt/min $= \dfrac{167 \text{ (mL)} \times 10 \text{ (gtt/mL)}}{60 \text{ (min)}} =$

28 gtt/min; 28 macrogtt/min

40. a) Determine mL/hr.

x mL/hr $= \dfrac{250 \text{ mL}}{2 \text{ hr}}$; $x = 125$ mL/hr

b) Calculate gtt/min.

x gtt/min $= \dfrac{125 \text{ (mL)} \times 15 \text{ (gtt/mL)}}{60 \text{ (min)}} =$

31 gtt/min; 31 macrogtt/min

41. a) Determine mL/hr.

x mL/hr $= \dfrac{1{,}750 \text{ mL}}{24 \text{ hr}}$; $x = 73$ mL/hr

b) Calculate gtt/min.

x gtt/min $= \dfrac{73 \text{ (mL)} \times 10 \text{ (gtt/mL)}}{60 \text{ (min)}} =$

12 gtt/min; 12 macrogtt/min

42. a) Determine mL/hr.

x mL/hr $= \dfrac{150 \text{ mL}}{1.5 \text{ hr}}$; $x = 100$ mL/hr

b) Calculate gtt/min.

x gtt/min $= \dfrac{100 \text{ (mL)} \times 60 \text{ (gtt/mL)}}{60 \text{ (min)}} =$

100 gtt/min; 100 microgtt/min

43. 1 L $= 1{,}000$ mL

2 L $= 2{,}000$ mL

x mL/hr $= \dfrac{2{,}000 \text{ mL}}{16 \text{ hr}}$; $x = 125$ mL/hr

44. x mL/hr $= \dfrac{500 \text{ mL}}{4 \text{ hr}}$; $x = 125$ mL/hr

45. x mL/hr $= \dfrac{200 \text{ mL}}{2 \text{ hr}}$; $x = 100$ mL/hr

46. x mL/hr $= \dfrac{500 \text{ mL}}{8 \text{ hr}}$; $x = 63$ mL/hr

47. a) Determine mL/hr.

x mL/hr $= \dfrac{1{,}100 \text{ mL}}{12 \text{ hr}}$; $x = 92$ mL/hr

48. a) Determine mL/hr.

x mL/hr $= \dfrac{500 \text{ mL}}{6 \text{ hr}}$; $x = 83$ mL/hr

b) Calculate gtt/min.

x gtt/min $= \dfrac{83 \text{ (mL)} \times 10 \text{ (gtt/mL)}}{60 \text{ (min)}} =$

14 gtt/min; 14 macrogtt/min

49. a) Determine mL/hr.

x mL/hr $= \dfrac{3{,}000 \text{ mL}}{20 \text{ hr}}$; $x = 150$ mL/hr

b) Calculate gtt/min.

x gtt/min $= \dfrac{150 \text{ (mL)} \times 20 \text{ (gtt/mL)}}{60 \text{ (min)}} =$

50 gtt/min; 50 macrogtt/min

50. a) Determine mL/hr.

x mL/hr $= \dfrac{500 \text{ mL}}{6 \text{ hr}}$; $x = 83$ mL/hr

b) Calculate gtt/min.

x gtt/min $= \dfrac{83 \text{ (mL)} \times 15 \text{ (gtt/mL)}}{60 \text{ (min)}} =$

21 gtt/min; 21 macrogtt/min

51. Time remaining $= 7$ hr

Volume remaining $= 300$ mL

a) Determine mL/hr for remaining solution.

x mL/hr $= \dfrac{300 \text{ mL}}{7 \text{ hr}}$; $x = 43$ mL/hr

b) Determine gtt/min (recalculated rate).

x gtt/min $= \dfrac{43 \text{ (mL)} \times 15 \text{ (gtt/mL)}}{60 \text{ (min)}} =$

11 gtt/min

Answer: 11 macrogtt/min; 11 gtt/min

c) Determine the percentage change.

$$\dfrac{11 - 13}{13} = \dfrac{-2}{13} = -15\%$$

The -15% is within the acceptable 25% variation. Assess if client can tolerate adjustment in rate.

Negative percent of variation (-15%) indicates the adjusted rate will be decreased. Check institution policy. Assess client during rate change.

52. Time remaining = 4 hr

Volume remaining = 600 mL

a) Determine mL/hr for remaining solution.

$$x \text{ mL/hr} = \frac{600 \text{ mL}}{4 \text{ hr}}; x = 150 \text{ mL/hr}$$

b) Determine gtt/min (recalculated rate).

$$x \text{ gtt/min} = \frac{150 \text{ (mL)} \times 20 \text{ (gtt/mL)}}{60 \text{ (min)}} =$$

50 gtt/min

Answer: 50 gtt/min; 50 macrogtt/min

c) Determine the percentage change. Increase IV rate from 42 gtt/min to 50 gtt/min

$$\frac{50 - 42}{42} = \frac{8}{42} = 19\%$$

The percentage of change is 19%. This is an acceptable increase. Assess if client can tolerate the adjustment in rate. Check if allowed by institution policy. Assess client during rate change.

53. Time remaining = 4 hr

Volume remaining = 400 mL

a) Determine mL/hr for remaining solution.

$$x \text{ mL/hr} = \frac{400 \text{ mL}}{4 \text{ hr}}; x = 100 \text{ mL/hr}$$

After determining mL/hr, gtt/min is recalculated.

b) Determine gtt/min (recalculated rate).

$$x \text{ gtt/min} = \frac{100 \text{ (mL)} \times 15 \text{ (gtt/mL)}}{60 \text{ (min)}} =$$

25 gtt/min

Answer: 25 gtt/min; 25 macrogtt/min

c) The IV was ahead. The original IV order of 125 mL/hr = 31 gtt/min (31 macrogtt/min). The IV is being decreased from 31 gtt/min (31 macrogtt/min) to 25 gtt/min (25 macrogtt/min). Determine the percentage change.

$$\frac{25 - 31}{31} = \frac{-6}{31} = -19\%$$

The -19% is within acceptable 25% variation. Assess if client can tolerate the adjustment in rate. Negative percent of variation (-19%) indicates the adjusted rate will be decreased. Check institution policy. Assess client during rate change.

54. Time remaining = 5 hr

Volume remaining = 250 mL

a) Determine mL/hr for remaining solution.

$$x \text{ mL/hr} = \frac{250 \text{ mL}}{5 \text{ hr}}; x = 50 \text{ mL/hr}$$

b) Determine gtt/min (recalculated rate).

$$x \text{ gtt/min} = \frac{50 \text{ (mL)} \times 10 \text{ (gtt/mL)}}{60 \text{ (min)}} =$$

8 gtt/min

Answer: 8 gtt/min; 8 macrogtt/min

c) The IV is ahead. The IV rate must be decreased from 14 gtt/min (14 macrogtt/min) to 8 gtt/min (8 macrogtt/min). Determine the percentage change.

$$\frac{8 - 14}{14} = \frac{-6}{14} = -43\%$$

The percentage of change is greater than 25%. Check with prescriber, order may need to be revised, even though a negative variation indicates IV will be decreased. (Do not decrease.)

55. Time remaining = 4 hr

Volume remaining = 600 mL

a) Determine mL/hr for remaining solution.

$$x \text{ mL/hr} = \frac{600 \text{ mL}}{4 \text{ hr}}; x = 150 \text{ mL/hr}$$

b) Determine gtt/min (recalculated rate).

$$x \text{ gtt/min} = \frac{150 \text{ (mL)} \times 15 \text{ (gtt/mL)}}{60 \text{ (min)}} =$$

38 gtt/min

Answer: 38 gtt/min; 38 macrogtt/min

I.V. is not on schedule.

c) The IV will have to be increased from 25 gtt/min (25 macrogtt/min) to 38 gtt/min (38 macrogtt/min). Determine the percentage of increase.

$$\frac{38 - 25}{25} = \frac{13}{25} = 52\%$$

The percentage of change is greater than 25%. Check with prescriber; order may need to be revised. (Do not increase.)

56. 80 macrogtt/min (80 gtt/min) =

$$\frac{900 \text{ (mL)} \times 15 \text{ (gtt/mL)}}{x \text{ (min)}}$$

$$80 = \frac{900 \times 15}{x}$$

$$\frac{80x}{80} = \frac{13,500}{80}$$

$$x = 168.75 \text{ minutes}$$

60 min = 1 hr; $168.75 \div 60 = 2.81$ hr

Time: 2.81 hr. Since .81 represents a fraction of an additional hour, convert it to minutes—multiply by 60 minutes.

Answer: 2 hr and 49 minutes

57. $\dfrac{1,000 \text{ mL}}{100 \text{ mL/hr}} = 10 \text{ hr}$

58.
$$20 \text{ macrogtt/min (20 gtt/min)} = \dfrac{1,000 \text{ (mL)} \times 10 \text{ (gtt/mL)}}{x \text{ (min)}}$$

$$20 = \dfrac{1,000 \times 10}{x}$$

$$\dfrac{20x}{20} = \dfrac{10,000}{20}$$

$$x = 500 \text{ minutes}$$

60 min = 1 hr; 500 ÷ 60 = 8.33 hr

Time: 8.33 hr

$$0.33 \times 60 = 19.8 = 20 \text{ minutes}$$

Answer: 8 hr and 20 minutes

59.
$$25 \text{ macrogtt/min (25 gtt/min)} = \dfrac{450 \text{ (mL)} \times 20 \text{ (gtt/mL)}}{x \text{ (min)}}$$

$$25 = \dfrac{450 \times 20}{x}$$

$$\dfrac{25x}{25} = \dfrac{9,000}{25}$$

$$x = 360 \text{ minutes}$$

60 min = 1 hr; 360 ÷ 60 = 6 hr

Answer: 6 hr

60.
$$10 \text{ macrogtt/min (10 gtt/min)} = \dfrac{100 \text{ (mL)} \times 15 \text{ (gtt/mL)}}{x \text{ (min)}}$$

$$10 = \dfrac{100 \times 15}{x}$$

$$\dfrac{10x}{10} = \dfrac{1,500}{10}$$

$$x = 150 \text{ min}$$

60 min = 1 hr; 150 ÷ 60 = 2.5 = 2 1/2 hr

Answer: 2 1/2 hr

61.
$$25 \text{ macrogtt/min (25 gtt/min)} = \dfrac{x \text{ (mL)} \times 15 \text{ (gtt/mL)}}{480 \text{ (min)}}$$

$$25 = \dfrac{x \times 15}{480}$$

$$25 = \dfrac{15x}{480}$$

$$\dfrac{15x}{15} = \dfrac{25 \times 480}{15}$$

$$\dfrac{15x}{15} = \dfrac{12,000}{15}$$

$$x = 800 \text{ mL}$$

Note:

Formula, time expressed in minutes; therefore hours are expressed as minutes. 8 hr = 480 min (60 min = 1 hr).

62.
$$40 \text{ microgtt/min (40 gtt/min)} = \dfrac{x \text{ (mL)} \times 60 \text{ (gtt/mL)}}{600 \text{ (min)}}$$

$$40 = \dfrac{x \times 60}{600}$$

$$40 = \dfrac{60x}{600}$$

$$\dfrac{60x}{60} = \dfrac{40 \times 600}{60}$$

$$\dfrac{60x}{60} = \dfrac{24,000}{60}$$

$$x = 400 \text{ mL}$$

Note:

Formula, time expressed in minutes; therefore hours are expressed as minutes. 10 hr = 600 min (60 min = 1 hr)

63.
$$30 \text{ macrogtt/min (30 gtt/min)} = \dfrac{x \text{ (mL)} \times 15 \text{ (gtt/mL)}}{300 \text{ (min)}}$$

$$30 = \dfrac{x \times 15}{300}$$

$$30 = \dfrac{15x}{300}$$

$$\dfrac{15x}{15} = \dfrac{30 \times 300}{15}$$

$$\dfrac{15x}{15} = \dfrac{9,000}{5}$$

$$x = 600 \text{ mL}$$

Note:

Formula, time expressed in minutes; therefore hours are expressed as minutes. 5 hr = 300 min (60 min = 1 hr).

64. a) 10 mEq : 500 mL = 2 mEq : x mL

$$10x = 500 \times 2$$

$$\dfrac{10x}{10} = \dfrac{1,000}{10}$$

$$x = 100 \text{ mL}$$

Therefore 100 mL of fluid would be needed to administer 2 mEq of potassium chloride.

b) x gtt/min = $\dfrac{100 \text{ (mL)} \times 20 \text{ (gtt/mL)}}{60 \text{ (min)}} =$

33 gtt/min

Answer: 33 gtt/min; 33 macrogtt/min would deliver 2 mEq of potassium chloride each hour.

65. a) 30 mEq : 1,000 mL = 4 mEq : x mL

$$\frac{30x}{30} = \frac{4000}{30} = 133.3$$

133 mL would deliver 4 mEq of potassium chloride.

b) x gtt/min = $\dfrac{133 \ (\text{mL}) \times 15 \ (\text{gtt/mL})}{60 \ (\text{min})}$ =

33 gtt/min

Answer: 33 gtt/min; 33 macrogtt/min would deliver 4 mEq of potassium chloride each hour.

66. 50 U : 250 mL = 7 U : x mL

$$\frac{50x}{50} = \frac{1,750}{50} = 35 \text{ mL/hr}$$

Answer: 35 mL/hr

67. 100 U : 250 mL = 18 U : x mL

$$\frac{100x}{100} = \frac{4,500}{100} = 45 \text{ mL/hr}$$

Answer: 45 mL/hr

68. 100 U : 100 mL = 11 U : x mL

$$\frac{100x}{100} = \frac{1,100}{100} = 11 \text{ mL/hr}$$

Answer: 11 mL/hr

Note:

For problems 64–68 a ratio-proportion could be set up in different formats other than the format shown in the problems.

69. x gtt/min = $\dfrac{150 \ (\text{mL}) \times 10 \ (\text{gtt/mL})}{60 \ (\text{min})}$ =

25 gtt/min

Answer: 25 gtt/min; 25 macrogtt/min

70. x gtt/min = $\dfrac{40 \ (\text{mL}) \times 60 \ (\text{gtt/mL})}{40 \ (\text{min})}$ =

60 gtt/min

Answer: 60 gtt/min; 60 microgtt/min

71. x gtt/min = $\dfrac{35 \ (\text{mL}) \times 60 \ (\text{gtt/mL})}{30 \ (\text{min})}$ =

70 gtt/min

Answer: 70 gtt/min; 70 microgtt/min

72. x gtt/min = $\dfrac{80 \ (\text{mL}) \times 15 \ (\text{gtt/mL})}{40 \ (\text{min})}$ =

30 gtt/min

Answer: 30 gtt/min; 30 macrogtt/min

73. x gtt/min = $\dfrac{50 \ (\text{mL}) \times 10 \ (\text{gtt/mL})}{25 \ (\text{min})}$ =

20 gtt/min

Answer: 20 gtt/min; 20 macrogtt/min

74. x gtt/min = $\dfrac{65 \ (\text{mL}) \times 15 \ (\text{gtt/mL})}{60 \ (\text{min})}$ =

16 gtt/min

Answer: 16 gtt/min; 16 macrogtt/min

75. Step 1: 60 gtt : 1 mL = 50 gtt : x mL

$$60x = 50$$

$$x = 50 \div 60; \ x = 0.83 \text{ mL/min}$$

Step 2: 0.83 mL $\times$ 60 (min) = 49.8 = 50 mL/hr

Step 3: $\dfrac{50 \text{ mL}}{50 \text{ mL/hr}} = 1 \text{ hr}$

Answer: Infusion time = 1 hr

76. Step 1: $\dfrac{500 \text{ mL}}{80 \text{ mL/hr}} = 6.25$

Step 2: 60 $\times$ 0.25 = 15 minutes

Infusion time is 6 hrs and 15 minutes.

Step 3: (7 PM + 6 hrs + 15 minutes)

Answer: 1:15 AM; military time: 0115

77. $\dfrac{150 \text{ mL}}{25 \text{ mL/hr}} = 6 \text{ hr}$

a) Infusion time = 6 hr

b) (3:10 AM + 6 hrs = 9:10 AM) I.V. will be completed at 9:10 AM; military time: 0910

78. Conversion is required. Equivalent:

1 L = 1,000 mL

Therefore 2.5 L = 2,500 mL

Step 1: $\dfrac{2,500 \text{ mL}}{150 \text{ mL/hr}} = 16.66$

Step 2: 60 $\times$ 0.66 = 39.6 = 40 minutes

Infusion time is 16 hr and 40 minutes.

Note:

For problems 79–81 a ratio-proportion could be set up and mL/hr determined first, which, when a burette is used without a pump or controller, is the same as gtt/min. If gtt/min is determined first remember that is the same as mL/hr.

79. x gtt/min $= \dfrac{30\ (\text{mL}) \times 60\ (\text{gtt/mL})}{20\ (\text{min})}$ OR   mL/hr determined with ratio proportion.

$\dfrac{1,800}{20} = 90$ gtt/min

$$30\ \text{mL} : 20\ \text{min} = x\ \text{mL} : 60\ \text{min}$$
OR
$$\dfrac{30\ \text{mL}}{20\ \text{min}} = \dfrac{x\ \text{mL}}{60\ \text{min}}$$

a) 90 gtt/min; 90 microgtt/min
b) 90 mL/hr

80. x gtt/min $= \dfrac{80\ (\text{mL}) \times 60\ (\text{gtt/mL})}{60\ (\text{min})}$ OR   Determine mL/hr

$$80\ \text{mL} : 60\ \text{min} = x\ \text{mL} : 60\ \text{min}$$
$$\dfrac{80\ \text{mL}}{60\ \text{min}} = \dfrac{x\ \text{mL}}{60\ \text{min}}$$

$\dfrac{4,800}{60} = 80$ gtt/min

a) 80 gtt/min; 80 microgtt/min
b) 80 mL/hr

81. x gtt/min $= \dfrac{40\ (\text{mL}) \times 60\ (\text{gtt/mL})}{45\ (\text{min})}$ OR   Determine mL/hr.

$$40\ \text{mL} : 45\ \text{min} = x\ \text{mL} : 60\ \text{min}$$
$$\dfrac{40\ \text{mL}}{45\ \text{min}} = \dfrac{x\ \text{mL}}{60\ \text{min}}$$

$\dfrac{2,400}{45} = 53$ gtt/min

a) 53 gtt/min; 53 microgtt/min
b) 53 mL/hr

82. Step 1: Calculate the normal dose range for child.

23 kg × 40 mg/day = 920 mg
23 kg × 50 mg/day = 1,150 mg

Step 2: Calculate the dose the child receives in 24 hours.

500 mg q12hr (2 doses) 500 × 2 = 1,000 mg

Step 3: Compare dose ordered to normal range.

The dose order is 1,000 mg; it is within the normal range of 920–1,150 mg/day. Calculate the dose to give and administer.

83. Step 1: Calculate the normal dose range for the child.

20 kg × 0.05 mg/day = 1 mg

Step 2: Child receives 2 mg of medication at 10 AM.

Step 3: The dose ordered is 2 mg. 1 mg is the normal dose; consult with the prescriber before administering. (2 mg > 1 mg)

84. Step 1: Determine the normal dose range for the child.

15 kg × 6 mcg/day = 90 mcg
15 kg × 8 mcg/day = 120 mcg

Step 2: 55 mcg q12h (2 doses); 55 mcg × 2 = 110 mcg

Step 3: The dose ordered is 110 mcg; it is within the normal range of 90-120 mcg/day. Calculate the dose to give and administer.

85. $x \text{ mL/hr} = \dfrac{1{,}200 \text{ mL}}{16 \text{ hr}} = 75$

Answer: 75 mL/hr. Set the infusion pump to deliver 75 mL/hr.

86. Equivalent: 1 L = 1,000 mL

Therefore 0.5 L = 500 mL

Dextrose:

$5 \text{ g} : 100 \text{ mL} = x \text{ g} : 500 \text{ mL}$ OR $\dfrac{5 \text{ g}}{100 \text{ mL}} = \dfrac{x \text{ g}}{500 \text{ mL}}$

$\dfrac{100x}{100} = \dfrac{2{,}500}{100}$

$x = 25 \text{ g dextrose}$

NaCl:

$0.225 \text{ g} : 100 \text{ mL} = x \text{ g} : 500 \text{ mL}$ OR $\dfrac{0.225 \text{ g}}{100 \text{ mL}} = \dfrac{x \text{ g}}{500 \text{ mL}}$

$\dfrac{100x}{100} = \dfrac{112.5}{100}$

$x = 1.125 \text{ g NaCl}$

87. Dextrose:

$5 \text{ g} : 100 \text{ mL} = x \text{ g} : 750 \text{ mL}$ OR $\dfrac{5 \text{ g}}{100 \text{ mL}} = \dfrac{x \text{ g}}{750 \text{ mL}}$

$\dfrac{100x}{100} = \dfrac{3{,}750}{100}$

$x = 37.5 \text{ g of dextrose}$

NaCl:

$0.45 \text{ g} : 100 \text{ mL} = x\text{g} : 750 \text{ mL}$ OR $\dfrac{0.45 \text{ g}}{100 \text{ mL}} = \dfrac{x \text{ g}}{750 \text{ mL}}$

$\dfrac{100x}{100} = \dfrac{337.5}{100}$

$x = 3.375 \text{ g NaCl}$

88. 4 oz q4h = 6 feedings; 4 oz × 6 = 24 oz

1 oz = 30 mL; therefore 24 oz = 720 mL

$1/8 \times 720 \text{ mL} = x \text{ mL}$

$\dfrac{720}{8} = x$

$x = 90 \text{ mL of the formula}$

b) 720 mL − 90 mL = 630 mL

Answer: You would add 630 mL of water to 90 mL of Ensure to make 720 mL 1/8-strength Ensure.

CHAPTER 22

Answers to Practice Problems

1. 25,000 U : 1,000 mL = 1,000 U : x mL

   OR

   $$\frac{25,000 \text{ U}}{1,000 \text{ mL}} = \frac{1,000 \text{ U}}{x \text{ mL}}$$

   $$25,000x = 1,000 \times 1,000$$

   $$\frac{25,000x}{25,000} = \frac{1,000,000}{25,000}$$

   $$x = 40 \text{ mL/hr}$$

   Answer: 40 mL/hr. To infuse 1,000 U/hr from a solution of 25,000 U in D5 0.9% N.S., the flow rate would be 40 mL/hr.

2. First calculate mL/hr to be administered.

   30,000 U : 500 mL = 600 U : x mL

   $$\frac{30,000x}{30,000} = \frac{300,000}{30,000} = 10 \text{ mL/hr}$$

   Calculate the flow rate in gtt/min.

   $$x \text{ gtt/min} = \frac{10 \text{ mL} \times 10 \text{ gtt/mL}}{60 \text{ min}} = \frac{100}{60} = 1.6$$

   Answer: 2 gtt/min; 2 macrogtt/min

3. First convert gtt/min to mL/min.

   20 gtt : 1 mL = 40 gtt : x mL

   $$\frac{20x}{20} = \frac{40}{20}$$

   $$x = 2 \text{ mL/min}$$

   Then convert mL/min to mL/hr.

   2 mL/min × 60 min = 120 mL/hr

   Calculate U/hr.

   25,000 U : 500 mL = x U : 120 mL

   $$\frac{500x}{500} = \frac{3,000,000}{500}$$

   $$x = 6,000 \text{ U/hr}$$

4. 30,000 U : 750 mL = x U : 25 mL

   $$\frac{750x}{750} = \frac{750,000}{750}$$

   $$x = 1,000 \text{ U/hr}$$

   Answer: 1,000 U/hr

5. Calculate U/hr infusing.

   1,000 mL : 25,000 U = 100 mL : x U

   $$\frac{1,000x}{1,000} = \frac{2,500,000}{1,000}$$

   $$x = 2,500 \text{ U/hr}$$

   Answer: 2,500 U/hr

   Determine the heparinizing dose.

   2,500 U/hr × 24 = 60,000 U/24 hr

   The dose is more than the 20,000-40,000 U in 24 hr heparinizing range, so notify the prescriber.

Answers to Chapter Review

1. 10,000 U : 1 mL = 3,500 U : x mL   OR $\frac{3,500 \text{ U}}{10,000 \text{ U}} \times 1 \text{ mL} = x \text{ mL}; \quad \frac{3,500 \text{ U}}{10,000 \text{ U}} = \frac{x \text{ mL}}{1 \text{ mL}}$

   x = 0.35 mL. The dose ordered is less than what is available, therefore you will need less than 1 mL to administer the dose.

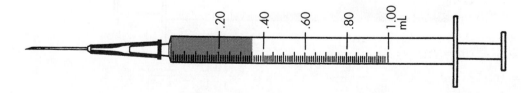

2. $20{,}000 \text{ U} : 1 \text{ mL} = 16{,}000 \text{ U} : x \text{ mL}$ OR $\dfrac{16{,}000 \text{ U}}{20{,}000 \text{ U}} \times 1 \text{ mL} = x \text{ mL}; \quad \dfrac{16{,}000 \text{ U}}{20{,}000 \text{ U}} = \dfrac{x \text{ mL}}{1 \text{ mL}}$

Answer: 0.8 mL. The dose ordered is less than what is available; therefore you will need less than 1 mL to administer the dose.

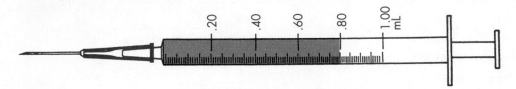

3. $2{,}500 \text{ U} : 1 \text{ mL} = 2{,}000 \text{ U} : x \text{ mL}$ OR $\dfrac{2{,}000 \text{ U}}{2{,}500 \text{ U}} \times 1 \text{ mL} = x \text{ mL}; \quad \dfrac{2{,}000 \text{ U}}{2{,}500 \text{ U}} = \dfrac{x \text{ mL}}{1 \text{ mL}}$

Answer: 0.8 mL. The dose ordered is less than what is available; therefore you will need less than 1 mL to administer the dose.

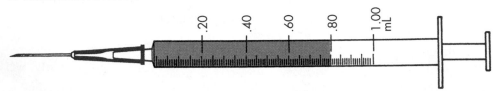

4. $5{,}000 \text{ U} : 1 \text{ mL} = 2{,}000 \text{ U} : x \text{ mL}$ OR $\dfrac{2{,}000 \text{ U}}{5{,}000 \text{ U}} \times 1 \text{ mL} = x \text{ mL}; \quad \dfrac{2{,}000 \text{ U}}{5{,}000 \text{ U}} = \dfrac{x \text{ mL}}{1 \text{ mL}}$

Answer: 0.4 mL. The dose ordered is less than what is available; therefore you will need less than 1 mL to administer the dose.

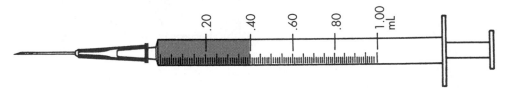

5. $1{,}000 \text{ U} : 1 \text{ mL} = 500 \text{ U} : x \text{ mL}$ OR $\dfrac{500 \text{ U}}{1{,}000 \text{ U}} \times 1 \text{ mL} = x \text{ mL}; \quad \dfrac{500 \text{ U}}{1{,}000 \text{ U}} = \dfrac{x \text{ mL}}{1 \text{ mL}}$

Answer: 0.5 mL. The dose ordered is less than what is available; therefore you will need less than 1 mL to administer the dose.

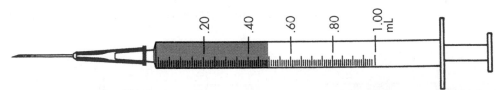

6. $10 \text{ U} : 1 \text{ mL} = 10 \text{ U} : x \text{ mL}$ OR $\dfrac{10 \text{ U}}{10 \text{ U}} \times 1 \text{ mL} = x \text{ mL}; \quad \dfrac{10 \text{ U}}{10 \text{ U}} = \dfrac{x \text{ mL}}{1 \text{ mL}}$

1 mL contains 10 U, so you will need 1 mL to administer the dose.

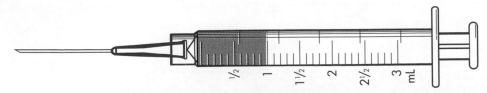

7. $10{,}000 \text{ U} : 1 \text{ mL} = 50{,}000 \text{ U} : x \text{ mL}$ $\qquad$ $\dfrac{50{,}000 \text{ U}}{10{,}000 \text{ U}} \times 1 \text{ mL} = x \text{ mL}; \quad \dfrac{50{,}000 \text{ U}}{10{,}000 \text{ U}} = \dfrac{x \text{ mL}}{1 \text{ mL}}$

Answer: 5 mL would be needed to administer the dose. The dose ordered is greater than what is available; therefore you will need more than 1 mL to administer the dose.

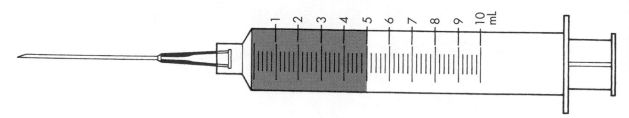

8. $20{,}000 \text{ U} : 1 \text{ mL} = 15{,}000 \text{ U} : x \text{ mL}$ $\quad$ OR $\quad$ $\dfrac{15{,}000 \text{ U}}{20{,}000 \text{ U}} \times 1 \text{ mL} = x \text{ mL}; \quad \dfrac{15{,}000 \text{ U}}{20{,}000 \text{ U}} = \dfrac{x \text{ mL}}{1 \text{ mL}}$

Answer: 0.75 mL. The dose ordered is less than what is available; therefore you will need less than 1 mL to administer the dose.

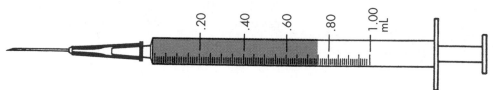

9. $2{,}500 \text{ U} : 1 \text{ mL} = 3{,}000 \text{ U} : x \text{ mL}$ $\quad$ OR $\quad$ $\dfrac{3{,}000 \text{ U}}{2{,}500 \text{ U}} \times 1 \text{ mL} = x \text{ mL}; \quad \dfrac{3{,}000 \text{ U}}{2{,}500 \text{ U}} = \dfrac{x \text{ mL}}{1 \text{ mL}}$

Answer: 1.2 mL. The dose ordered is more than what is available; therefore you will need more than 1 mL to administer the dose.

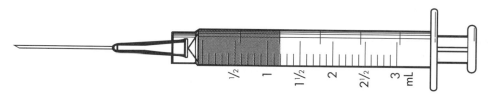

10. $20{,}000 \text{ U} : 1 \text{ mL} = 17{,}000 \text{ U} : x \text{ mL}$ $\quad$ OR $\quad$ $\dfrac{17{,}000 \text{ U}}{20{,}000 \text{ U}} \times 1 \text{ mL} = x \text{ mL}; \quad \dfrac{17{,}000 \text{ U}}{20{,}000 \text{ U}} = \dfrac{x \text{ mL}}{1 \text{ mL}}$

Answer: 0.85 mL. The dose ordered is less than what is available; therefore you will need less than 1 mL to administer the dose.

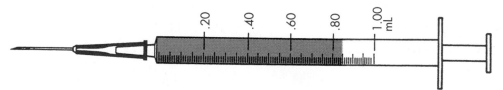

11. $10{,}000 \text{ U} : 1 \text{ mL} = 8{,}500 \text{ U} : x \text{ mL}$ $\quad$ OR $\quad$ $\dfrac{8{,}500 \text{ U}}{10{,}000 \text{ U}} \times 1 \text{ mL} = x \text{ mL}; \quad \dfrac{8{,}500 \text{ U}}{10{,}000 \text{ U}} = \dfrac{x \text{ mL}}{1 \text{ mL}}$

Answer: 0.85 mL. The dose ordered is less than what is available; therefore you will need less than 1 mL to administer the dose.

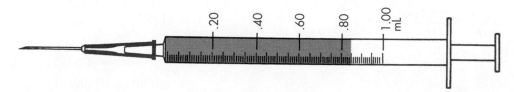

12. $10,000 \text{ U} : 1 \text{ mL} = 2,500 \text{ U} : x \text{ mL}$ OR $\dfrac{2,500 \text{ U}}{10,000 \text{ U}} \times 1 \text{ mL} = x \text{ mL};$ $\dfrac{2,500 \text{ U}}{10,000 \text{ U}} = \dfrac{x \text{ mL}}{1 \text{ mL}}$

Answer: 0.25 mL. The dose ordered is less than what is available; therefore you will need less than 1 mL to administer the dose.

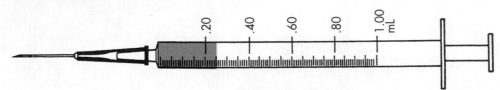

13. $25,000 \text{ U} : 1,000 \text{ mL} = 2,000 \text{ U} : x \text{ mL}$

$\dfrac{25,000x}{25,000} = \dfrac{2,000,000}{25,000}$

$x = 80 \text{ mL/hr}$. To administer 2,000 U of heparin per hour, 80 mL/hr must be given.

14. $25,000 \text{ U} : 500 \text{ mL} = 1,500 \text{ U} : x \text{ mL}$

$\dfrac{25,000x}{25,000} = \dfrac{750,000}{25,000}$

$x = \dfrac{750,000}{25,000}$

$x = 30 \text{ mL/hr}$. To administer 1,500 U of heparin per hour, 30 mL/hr must be given.

15. $25,000 \text{ U} : 250 \text{ mL} = 1,800 \text{ U} : x \text{ mL}$

$\dfrac{25,000x}{25,000} = \dfrac{450,000}{25,000}$

$x = 18 \text{ mL/hr}$. To administer 1,800 U of heparin per hour, 18 mL/hr must be given.

16. $40,000 \text{ U} : 1,000 \text{ mL} = x \text{ U} : 25 \text{ mL}$

$\dfrac{1,000x}{1,000} = \dfrac{1,000,000}{1,000}$

$x = \dfrac{1,000,000}{1,000}$

$x = 1,000 \text{ U/hr}$

17. $25,000 \text{ U} : 250 \text{ mL} = x \text{ U} : 11 \text{ mL}$

$\dfrac{250x}{250} = \dfrac{275,000}{250}$

$x = 1,100 \text{ U/hr}$

18. $40,000 \text{ U} : 500 \text{ mL} = x \text{ U} : 30 \text{ mL}$

$\dfrac{500x}{500} = \dfrac{1,200,000}{500}$

Answer: 2,400 U/hr

19. $20,000 \text{ U} : 500 \text{ mL} = x \text{ U} : 12 \text{ mL}$

$\dfrac{500x}{500} = \dfrac{240,000}{500}$

Answer: 480 U/hr

20. $25,000 \text{ U} : 500 \text{ mL} = x \text{ U} : 15 \text{ mL}$

$\dfrac{500x}{500} = \dfrac{375,000}{500}$

Answer: 750 U/hr

Note:

Problems 21b, 23b, and 27-30 could also be calculated using the shortcut method.

21. $1 \text{ L} = 1,000 \text{ mL}$

a) $\dfrac{1,000 \text{ mL}}{24 \text{ hr}} = 41.6 = 42 \text{ mL/hr}$

$40,000 \text{ U} : 1,000 \text{ mL} = x \text{ U} : 42 \text{ mL}$

$\dfrac{1,000x}{1,000} = \dfrac{1,680,000}{1000}$

$x = \dfrac{1,680,000}{1,000}$

$x = 1,680 \text{ U/hr}$

b) $x \text{ gtt/min} = \dfrac{42 \text{ mL} \times 15 \text{ gtt/mL}}{60 \text{ min}}$

$x = 11 \text{ gtt/min}; 11 \text{ macrogtt/min}$

22. $1 \text{ L} = 1,000 \text{ mL}$

a) Calculate mL/hr.

$\dfrac{1,000 \text{ mL}}{10 \text{ hr}} = 100 \text{ mL/hr}$

b) Calculate U/hr.

$15,000 \text{ U} : 1,000 \text{ mL} = x \text{ U}: 100 \text{ mL}$

$\dfrac{1,000x}{1,000} = \dfrac{1,500,000}{1,000}$

$x = \dfrac{1,500,000}{1,000}$

$x = 1,500 \text{ U/hr}$

23.   a) $35,000 \text{ U} : 1,000 \text{ mL} = x \text{ U} : 20 \text{ mL}$

$\dfrac{1,000x}{1,000} = \dfrac{700,000}{1,000}$

$x = \dfrac{700,000}{1,000}$

$x = 700 \text{ U/hr}$

b) $x \text{ gtt/min} = \dfrac{20 \text{ mL} \times 60 \text{ gtt/mL}}{60 \text{ min}}$

$x = 20 \text{ gtt/min}; 20 \text{ microgtt/min}$

24. a) Convert gtt/min to mL/min.

$$10 \text{ gtt} : 1 \text{ mL} = 20 \text{ gtt} : x \text{ mL}$$

$$\frac{10x}{10} = \frac{20}{10}$$

$$x = 2 \text{ mL/min}$$

Convert mL/min to mL/hr.

$$2 \text{ mL} \times 60 \text{ min} = 120 \text{ mL/hr}$$

b) $10{,}000 \text{ U} : 500 \text{ mL} = x \text{ U} : 120 \text{ mL}$

$$\frac{500x}{500} = \frac{1{,}200{,}000}{500}$$

$$x = \frac{1{,}200{,}000}{500}$$

$$x = 24{,}000 \text{ U/hr}$$

25. $25{,}000 \text{ U} : 500 \text{ mL} = x \text{ U} : 25 \text{ mL}$

$$\frac{500x}{500} = \frac{625{,}000}{500}$$

Answer: 1,250 U/hr

26. $20{,}000 \text{ U} : 500 \text{ mL} = x \text{ U} : 40 \text{ mL}$

$$\frac{500x}{500} = \frac{800{,}000}{500}$$

Answer: 1,600 U/hr

27. a) Calculate mL/hr to be administered.

$$40{,}000 \text{ U} : 1{,}000 \text{ mL} = 1{,}400 \text{ U} : x \text{ mL}$$

$$\frac{40{,}000x}{40{,}000} = \frac{1{,}400{,}000}{40{,}000}$$

$$x = 35 \text{ mL/hr}$$

b) Calculate gtt/min.

$$x \text{ gtt/min} = \frac{35 \text{ mL} \times 15 \text{ gtt/mL}}{60 \text{ min}}$$

$$x = 9 \text{ gtt/min}; \ 9 \text{ macrogtt/min}$$

28. a) $40{,}000 \text{ U} : 1{,}000 \text{ mL} = 1{,}000 \text{ U} : x \text{ mL}$

$$\frac{40{,}000x}{40{,}000} = \frac{1{,}000{,}000}{40{,}000}$$

$$x = \frac{1{,}000{,}000}{40{,}000}$$

$$x = 25 \text{ mL/hr}$$

b) $x \text{ gtt/min} = \dfrac{25 \text{ mL} \times 15 \text{ gtt/mL}}{60 \text{ min}}$

$$x = 6 \text{ gtt/min}; \ 6 \text{ macrogtt/min}$$

29. $25{,}000 \text{ U} : 500 \text{ mL} = 1{,}000 \text{ U} : x \text{ mL}$

$$\frac{25{,}000x}{25{,}000} = \frac{500{,}000}{25{,}000}$$

$$x = \frac{500{,}000}{25{,}000}$$

$$x = 20 \text{ mL/hr}$$

$$x \text{ gtt/min} = \frac{20 \text{ mL} \times 60 \text{ gtt/mL}}{60 \text{ min}}$$

$$x = 20 \text{ gtt/min}; \ 20 \text{ microgtt/min}$$

30. $25{,}000 \text{ U} : 1{,}000 \text{ mL} = 2{,}000 \text{ U} : x \text{ mL}$

$$\frac{25{,}000x}{25{,}000} = \frac{2{,}000{,}000}{25{,}000}$$

$$x = \frac{2{,}000{,}000}{25{,}000}$$

$$x = 80 \text{ mL/hr}$$

$$x \text{ gtt/min} = \frac{80 \text{ mL} \times 15 \text{ gtt/mL}}{60 \text{ min}}$$

$$x = 20 \text{ gtt/min}; \ 20 \text{ macrogtt/min}$$

31. Step 1: Convert gtt/min to mL/min.

$$15 \text{ gtt} : 1 \text{ mL} = 15 \text{ gtt} : x \text{ mL}$$

$$\frac{15x}{15} = \frac{15}{15}$$

$$x = 1 \text{ mL/min}$$

Step 2: Convert mL/min to mL/hr.

$$1 \text{ mL/min} \times 60 \text{ min} = 60 \text{ mL/hr}$$

Step 3: Calculate units per hour.

$$50{,}000 \text{ U} : 1{,}000 \text{ mL} = x \text{ U} : 60 \text{ mL}$$

$$\frac{1{,}000x}{1{,}000} = \frac{3{,}000{,}000}{1{,}000}$$

$$x = \frac{3{,}000{,}000}{1{,}000}$$

$$x = 3{,}000 \text{ U/hr}$$

32. Step 1: Convert gtt/min to mL/min.

$$10 \text{ gtt} : 1 \text{ mL} = 20 \text{ gtt} : x \text{ mL}$$

$$\frac{10x}{10} = \frac{20}{10}$$

$$x = 2 \text{ mL/min}$$

Step 2: Convert mL/min to mL/hr.

$$2 \text{ mL/min} \times 60 \text{ min} = 120 \text{ mL/hr}$$

Step 3: Calculate units per hour.

$$25{,}000 \text{ U} : 250 \text{ mL} = x \text{ U} : 120 \text{ mL}$$

$$\frac{250x}{250} = \frac{3{,}000{,}000}{250}$$

$$x = \frac{3{,}000{,}000}{250}$$

$$x = 12{,}000 \text{ U/hr}$$

33. Step 1: Convert gtt/min to mL/min.

$$60 \text{ gtt} : 1 \text{ mL} = 20 \text{ gtt} : x \text{ mL}$$

$$\frac{60x}{60} = \frac{20}{60}$$

$$x = 0.33 \text{ mL/min}$$

Step 2: Convert mL/min to mL/hr.

0.33 mL/min $\times$ 60 min = 19.8 mL/hr = 20 mL/hr

Step 3: Calculate units per hour.

20,000 U : 500 mL = x U : 20 mL

$$\frac{500x}{500} = \frac{400,000}{500}$$

$$x = \frac{400,000}{500}$$

$$x = 800 \text{ U/hr}$$

34. Step 1: Convert gtt/min to mL/min.

15 gtt : 1 mL = 14 gtt : x mL

$$\frac{15x}{15} = \frac{14}{15}$$

$$x = 0.93 \text{ mL/min}$$

Step 2: Convert mL/min to mL/hr.

0.93 mL/min $\times$ 60 min = 55.8 = 56 mL/hr

Step 3: Calculate units per hour.

25,000 U : 1,000 mL = x U : 56 mL

$$\frac{1,000x}{1,000} = \frac{1,400,000}{1,000}$$

$$x = \frac{1,400,000}{1,000}$$

$$x = 1,400 \text{ U/hr}$$

35. Step 1: Convert gtt/min to mL/min.

10 gtt : 1 mL = 24 gtt : x mL

$$\frac{10x}{10} = \frac{24}{10}$$

$$x = 2.4 \text{ mL/min}$$

Step 2: Convert mL/min to mL/hr.

2.4 mL/min $\times$ 60 min = 144 mL/hr

Step 3: Calculate units per hour.

20,000 U : 1,000 mL = x U : 144 mL

$$\frac{1,000x}{1,000} = \frac{2,880,000}{1,000}$$

$$x = \frac{2,800,000}{1,000}$$

$$x = 2,880 \text{ U/hr}$$

36. 30,000 U : 500 mL = x U : 25 mL

$$\frac{500x}{500} = \frac{750,000}{500}$$

$$x = \frac{750,000}{500}$$

$$x = 1,500 \text{ U/hr}$$

37. 20,000 U : 1,000 mL = x U : 40 mL

$$\frac{1,000x}{1,000} = \frac{800,000}{1,000}$$

$$x = \frac{800,000}{1,000}$$

$$x = 800 \text{ U/hr}$$

38. 40,000 U : 500 mL = x U : 25 mL

$$\frac{500x}{500} = \frac{1,000,000}{500}$$

$$x = \frac{1,000,000}{500}$$

$$x = 2,000 \text{ U/hr}$$

39. 35,000 U : 1,000 mL = x U : 20 mL

$$\frac{1,000x}{1,000} = \frac{700,000}{1,000}$$

$$x = \frac{700,000}{1,000}$$

$$x = 700 \text{ U/hr}$$

40. 25,000 U : 1,000 mL = x U: 30 mL

$$\frac{1,000x}{1,000} = \frac{750,000}{1,000}$$

$$x = \frac{750,000}{1,000}$$

$$x = 750 \text{ U/hr}$$

41. 40,000 U : 1,000 mL = x U: 30 mL

$$\frac{1,000x}{1,000} = \frac{1,200,000}{1,000}$$

$$x = 1,200 \text{ U/hr}$$

42. 20,000 U : 1,000 mL = x U : 80 mL

$$\frac{1,000x}{1,000} = \frac{1,600,000}{1,000}$$

$$x = 1,600 \text{ U/hr}$$

43. 50,000 U : 1,000 mL = x U : 70 mL

$$\frac{1,000x}{1,000} = \frac{3,500,00}{1,000}$$

$$x = 3,500 \text{ U/hr}$$

44. 20,000 U : 500 mL = x U : 30 mL

$$\frac{500x}{500} = \frac{600,000}{500}$$

$$x = 1,200 \text{ U/hr}$$

45. 30,000 U : 1,000 mL = x U : 25 mL

$$\frac{1,000x}{1,000} = \frac{750,000}{1,000}$$

$$x = 750 \text{ U/hr}$$

46. Calculate U/hr infusing.

$$1{,}000 \text{ mL} : 50{,}000 \text{ U} = 40 \text{ mL} : x \text{ U}$$

$$\frac{1{,}000\,x}{1{,}000} = \frac{2{,}000{,}000}{1{,}000}$$

$$x = 2{,}000 \text{ U/hr}$$

a) 2,000 U/hr

Determine U/24 hr.

b) 2,000 U/hr × 24 hr = 48,000 U/24 hr

c) This dose is more than the 20,000-40,000 U in 24 hr heparinizing range. Check order with prescriber.

47. Calculate U/hr infusing.

$$500 \text{ mL} : 30{,}000 \text{ U} = 15 \text{ mL} : x \text{ U}$$

$$\frac{500x}{500} = \frac{450{,}000}{500}$$

$$x = 900 \text{ U/hr}$$

a) 900 U/hr

Determine U/24 hr

b) 900 U/hr × 24 hr = 21,600 U/24 hr

c) This dose is within the 20,000-40,000 U in 24 hr heparinizing range.

CHAPTER 23

Answers to Practice Problems

1. a) Step 1: Conversion: Equivalent:
    1,000 mcg = 1 mg

    Therefore 250 mg = 250,000 mcg

    Step 2: 250,000 mcg : 500 mL =
    x mcg : 1 mL

    $$\frac{500x}{500} = \frac{250{,}000}{500} = 500 \text{ mcg/mL}$$

    Concentration of solution is 500 mcg/mL.

    Step 3: Calculate dose range.

    Lower dose:

    2.5 mcg × 50 kg = 125 mcg/min

    Upper dose:

    5 mcg × 50 kg = 250 mcg/min

    Step 4: Convert dosage range to mL/min.

    Lower dose:

    500 mcg : 1 mL = 125 mcg : x mL

    $$\frac{500x}{500} = \frac{125}{500}$$

    $$x = 0.25 \text{ mL/min}$$

    Upper dose:

    500 mcg : 1 mL = 250 mcg : x mL

    $$\frac{500x}{500} = \frac{250}{500}$$

    $$x = 0.5 \text{ mL/min}$$

    Step 5: Convert mL/min to mL/hr.

    Lower dose: 0.25 mL × 60 min =
    15 mL/hr (gtt/min)

    Upper dose: 0.5 mL × 60 min = 30 mL/hr
    (gtt/min)

    A dose range of 2.5-5 mcg/kg/min is equal
    to a flow rate of 15-30 mL/hr (gtt/min).

    b) Determine dose infusing per minute at
    25 mL/hr:

    500 mcg : 1 mL = x mcg : 25 mL

    $$x = 12{,}500 \text{ mcg/hr}$$

    12,500 mcg ÷ 60 min = 208.3 mcg/min

2. a) 2 mg : 250 mL = x mg : 30 mL

    $$\frac{250x}{250} = \frac{60}{250}$$

    $$x = 0.24 \text{ mg/hr}$$

    b) Convert mg to mcg
    (1,000 mcg = 1 mg).

    0.24 mg = 240 mcg/hr

    c) Convert mcg/hr to mcg/min.

    240 mcg/hr ÷ 60 min = 4 mcg/min

3. a) Change g to mg. (Note you were asked mg/min and mg/hr.)

    $0.25 \text{ g} = 250 \text{ mg} (1 \text{ g} = 1,000 \text{ mg})$

    Calculate mg/hr.

    $250 \text{ mg} : 8 \text{ hr} = x \text{ mg} : 1 \text{ hr}$

    $$\frac{8x}{8} = \frac{250}{8}$$

    $x = 31.25 = 31.3 \text{ mg/hr}$

    Answer: 31.3 mg/hr

    b) Convert mg/hr to mg/min:

    $31.3 \text{ mg/hr} \div 60 = 0.52 \text{ mg/min}$

4. Note: Calculate units per hour only.

    Step 1: $60 \text{ gtt} : 1 \text{ mL} = 15 \text{ gtt} : x \text{ mL}$

    $$\frac{60x}{60} = \frac{15}{60}$$

    $x = 0.25 \text{ mL/min}$

    Step 2: $0.25 \text{ mL/min} \times 60 = 15 \text{ mL/hr}$

    Step 3: $10 \text{ U} : 1,000 \text{ mL} = x \text{ U} : 15 \text{ mL}$

    $$\frac{1,000x}{1,000} = \frac{150}{1,000}$$

    $x = 0.15 \text{ U/hr}$

5. Step 1: Determine the dose per minute.

    $60 \text{ kg} \times 3 \text{ mcg/kg} = 180 \text{ mcg/min}$

    Step 2: Convert to dose per hour.

    $180 \text{ mcg/min} \times 60 = 10,800 \text{ mcg/hr}$

    Step 3: Convert to like units.

    $10,800 \text{ mcg} = 10.8 \text{ mg}$

    Calculate flow rate (mL/hr).

    $50 \text{ mg} : 250 \text{ mL} = 10.8 \text{ mg} : x \text{ mL}$

    $50x = 250 \times 10.8$

    $$\frac{50x}{50} = \frac{2,700}{50}$$

    $x = 54 \text{ mL/hr}$

6. a) $50 \text{ mg} : 250 \text{ mL} = x \text{ mg} : 3 \text{ mL}$

    $$\frac{250x}{250} = \frac{150}{250}$$

    $x = 0.6 \text{ mg/hr}$

    Convert to mcg (1,000 mcg = 1 mg).

    $0.6 \text{ mg} = 600 \text{ mcg/hr}$

    b) Convert mcg/hr to mcg/min.

    $60 \text{ mcg/hr} \div 60 \text{ min} = 10 \text{ mcg/min}$

Answers to Chapter Review

1. a) Calculate the dose per hr.

    $2 \text{ mg} : 250 \text{ mL} = x \text{ mg} : 30 \text{ mL}$

$$\frac{250x}{250} = \frac{60}{250}$$

$$x = \frac{60}{250}$$

$x = 0.24 \text{ mg/hr}$

b) Convert mg to mcg (1,000 mcg = 1 mg).

$1,000 \times 0.24 \text{ mg/hr} = 240 \text{ mcg/hr}$

c) Convert mcg/hr to mcg/min.

$240 \text{ mcg/hr} \div 60 \text{ min} = 4 \text{ mcg/min}$

2. a) Calculate dose per hr.

    $4 \text{ mg} : 500 \text{ mL} = x \text{ mg} : 40 \text{ mL}$

    $$\frac{500x}{500} = \frac{160}{500}$$

    $$x = \frac{160}{500}$$

    $x = 0.32 \text{ mg/hr}$

    b) Convert to mcg (1,000 mcg = 1 mg).

    $1,000 \times 0.32 \text{ mg/hr} = 320 \text{ mcg/hr}$

    c) Convert mcg/hr to mcg/min.

    $320 \text{ mcg/hr} \div 60 \text{ min} = 5.33 = 5.3 \text{ mcg/min}$

3. Step 1: Determine dose per hour.

    $800 \text{ mg} : 500 \text{ mL} = x \text{ mg} : 30 \text{ mL}$

    $$\frac{24,000}{500} = \frac{500x}{500}$$

    $$x = \frac{24,000}{500} = 48 \text{ mg/hr}$$

    a) Step 2: Convert mg to mcg (1,000 mcg = 1 mg).

    $48 \text{ mg/hr} \times 1,000 = 48,000 \text{ mcg/hr}$

    b) Step 3: Convert mcg/hr to mcg/min.

    $48,000 \text{ mcg/hr} \div 60 \text{ min} = 800 \text{ mcg/min}$

    c) $200 \text{ mg} : 5 \text{ mL} = 800 \text{ mg} : x \text{ mL}$

    OR

    $$\frac{800 \text{ mg}}{200 \text{ mg}} \times 5 \text{ mL} = x \text{ mL};$$

    $$\frac{800 \text{ mg}}{200 \text{ mg}} = \frac{x \text{ mL}}{5 \text{ mL}}$$

    Answer: 20 mL. The dose ordered is greater than what is available. Therefore you will need more than 5 mL to administer the dose.

4. a) Determine dose per hour.

    $50 \text{ mg} : 250 \text{ mL} = x \text{ mg} : 30 \text{ mL}$

$$\frac{1,500}{250} = \frac{250x}{250}$$

$$x = \frac{1,500}{250}$$

$$x = 6 \text{ mg/hr}$$

Convert mg to mcg
(1,000 mcg = 1 mg).

$$6 \text{ mg/hr} \times 1,000 = 6,000 \text{ mcg/hr}$$

b) Convert mcg/hr to mcg/min.

$$6,000 \text{ mcg/hr} \div 60 \text{ min} = 100 \text{ mcg/min}$$

5. a) Calculate mg/hr.

$$100 \text{ mg} : 250 \text{ mL} = x \text{ mg} : 25 \text{ mL}$$

$$\frac{250x}{250} = \frac{2,500}{250}$$

$$x = \frac{2,500}{250}$$

$$x = 10 \text{ mg/hr}$$

Convert mg to mcg
(1,000 mcg = 1 mg).

$$10 \text{ mg} = 10,000 \text{ mcg/hr}$$

b) Convert mcg/hr to mcg/min.

$$10,000 \text{ mcg/hr} \div 60 \text{ min} = 166.66 =$$
166.7 mcg/min

6. a) Convert metric weight to the same as answer request.

$$1 \text{ g} - 1,000 \text{ mg}$$

$$2,000 \text{ mg} : 250 \text{ mL} = x \text{ mg} : 60 \text{ mL}$$

$$\frac{250x}{250} = \frac{120,000x}{250}$$

$$x = \frac{120,000}{250}$$

$$x = 480 \text{ mg/hr}$$

b) Convert mg/hr to mg/min.

$$480 \text{ mg/hr} \div 60 \text{ min} = 8 \text{ mg/min}$$

7. Step 1: Convert g to mg (1000 mg = 1 g).

$$0.25 \text{ g} = 250 \text{ mg}$$

Step 2: Calculate mg/hr.

$$250 \text{ mg} : 6 \text{ hr} = x \text{ mg} : 1 \text{ hr}$$

$$\frac{250}{6} = \frac{6x}{6}$$

$$x = \frac{250}{6}$$

$$x = 41.66 = 41.7 \text{ mg/hr.}$$

8. a) Convert g to mg (1,000 mg = 1 g).

$$2 \text{ g} = 2,000 \text{ mg}$$

Calculate mg/hr.

$$2,000 \text{ mg} : 250 \text{ mL} = x \text{ mg} : 30 \text{ mL}$$

$$\frac{250x}{250} = \frac{60,000}{250}$$

$$x = \frac{60,000}{250}$$

$$x = 240 \text{ mg/hr}$$

b) Convert mg/hr to mg/min.

$$240 \text{ mg} \div 60 \text{ min} = 4 \text{ mg/min}$$

9. a) Step 1: Calculate gtt/min to mL/min.

$$60 \text{ gtt} : 1 \text{ mL} = 45 \text{ gtt} : x \text{ mL}$$

$$\frac{60x}{60} = \frac{45}{60}$$

$$x = \frac{45}{60}$$

$$x = 0.75 \text{ mL/min}$$

Step 2: Calculate U/min.

$$20 \text{ U} : 1,000 \text{ mL} = x \text{ units} : 0.75 \text{ mL}$$

$$\frac{15}{1,000} = \frac{1,000x}{1,000}$$

$$x = \frac{15}{1,000}$$

$$x = 0.015 \text{ U/min}$$

b) Calculate U/hr.

$$0.015 \text{ U/min} \times 60 \text{ min} = 0.9 \text{ U/hr}$$

10. $30 \text{ U} : 1,000 \text{ mL} = x \text{ U} : 40 \text{ mL}$

$$\frac{1,200}{1,000} = \frac{1,000x}{1,000}$$

$$x = \frac{1,200}{1,000}$$

$$x = 1.2 \text{ U/hr}$$

11. $30 \text{ U} : 500 \text{ mL} = x \text{ U} : 45 \text{ mL}$

$$\frac{1,350}{500} = \frac{500x}{500}$$

$$x = \frac{1,350}{500}$$

$$x = 2.7 \text{ U/hr}$$

12. a) Change metric measures to same as question. 1 g = 1,000 mg; therefore 2 g = 2,000 mg

Calculate mg/hr.

$$2,000 \text{ mg} : 500 \text{ mL} = x \text{ mg} : 30 \text{ mL}$$

$$\frac{600,000}{500} = \frac{500x}{500}$$

$$x = \frac{60,000}{500}$$

$$x = 120 \text{ mg/hr}$$

b) Change mg/hr to mg/min.

$$120 \text{ mg/hr} \div 60 \text{ min} = 2 \text{ mg/min}$$

13. a) Change metric measures to same as question.

$$2 \text{ g} = 2,000 \text{ mg} \ (1 \text{ g} = 1,000 \text{ mg})$$

Calculate mg/hr:

$$2,000 \text{ mg} : 500 \text{ mL} = x \text{ mg} : 45 \text{ mL}$$

$$\frac{90,000}{500} = \frac{500x}{500}$$

$$x = \frac{90,000}{500}$$

$$x = 180 \text{ mg/hr}$$

b) Change mg/hr to mg/min

$$180 \text{ mg/hr} \div 60 \text{ min} = 3 \text{ mg/min}$$

14. Determine dose per hour:

$$500 \text{ mcg/min} \times 60 \text{ min} = 30,000 \text{ mcg/hr}$$

Convert mcg to mg.

$$1,000 \text{ mcg} = 1 \text{ mg}$$

$$30,000 \text{ mcg/hr} = 30 \text{ mg/hr}$$

Calculate flow rate in mL/hr.

$$50 \text{ mg} : 250 \text{ mL} = 30 \text{ mg} : x \text{ mL}$$

$$\frac{50x}{50} = \frac{7,500}{50}$$

$$x = 150 \text{ mL/hr}$$

Set at 150 mL/hr to deliver 30 mg/hr.

15. $400 \text{ mg} : 500 \text{ mL} = x \text{ mg} : 35 \text{ mL}$

$$\frac{500x}{500} = \frac{14,000x}{500}$$

$$x = 28 \text{ mg/hr}$$

16. a) Calculate mg/hr.

$$2 \text{ mg} : 250 \text{ mL} = x \text{ mg} : 30 \text{ mL}$$

$$\frac{60}{250} = \frac{250x}{250}$$

$$x = \frac{60}{250}$$

$$x = 0.24 \text{ mg/hr}$$

b) Convert mg to mcg.

$$(1,000 \text{ mcg} = 1 \text{ mg})$$

$$0.24 \text{ mg} \times 1,000 = 240 \text{ mcg/hr}$$

c) Convert mcg/hr to mcg/min.

$$240 \text{ mcg} \div 60 \text{ min} = 4 \text{ mcg/min}$$

17. Convert metric weight to same as question.

$$1,000 \text{ mg} = 1 \text{ g}$$

Calculate mg/hr.

$$1,000 \text{ mg} : 10 \text{ hr} = x \text{ mg} : 1 \text{ hr}$$

$$\frac{10x}{10} = \frac{1,000}{10}$$

$$x = 100 \text{ mg/hr}$$

18. $150 \text{ mg} : 500 \text{ mL} = x \text{ mg} : 30 \text{ mL}$

$$\frac{500x}{500} = \frac{4,500}{500}$$

$$x = \frac{4,500}{500}$$

$$x = 9 \text{ mg/hr}$$

19. a) Convert metric weights g to mg.

$$2 \text{ g} = 2,000 \text{ mg} \ (1,000 \text{ mg} = 1 \text{ g})$$

$$2,000 \text{ mg} : 250 \text{ mL} = x \text{ mg} : 22 \text{ mL}$$

$$\frac{250x}{250} = \frac{44,000x}{250}$$

$$x = \frac{44,000}{250}$$

$$x = 176 \text{ mg/hr}$$

b) Change mg/hr to mg/min.

$$176 \text{ mg/hr} \div 60 \text{ min} = 2.93 = 2.9 \text{ mg/min}$$

20. Calculate dose per hour

$$4 \text{ mg} : 250 \text{ mL} = x \text{ mg} : 8 \text{ mL}$$

$$\frac{250x}{250} = \frac{32}{250}$$

$$x = \frac{32}{250}$$

$$x = 0.128 \text{ mg/hr}$$

Convert mg to mcg. $(1,000 \text{ mcg} = 1 \text{ mg})$

$$0.128 \text{ mg} \times 1,000 = 128 \text{ mcg/hr}$$

21. a) $500 \text{ mg} : 250 \text{ mL} = x \text{ mg} : 30 \text{ mL}$

$$\frac{250x}{250} = \frac{15,000}{250}$$

$$x = \frac{15,000}{250}$$

$$x = 60 \text{ mg/hr}$$

b) Convert mg/hr to mg/min.

$$60 \text{ mg/hr} \div 60 \text{ min} = 1 \text{ mg/min}$$

22. a) Calculate mg/hr.

500 mg : 500 mL = x mg : 30 mL

$$\frac{500x}{500} = \frac{15,000}{500}$$

$$x = \frac{15,000}{500}$$

$$x = 30 \text{ mg/hr}$$

Convert mg to mcg (1,000 mcg = 1 mg).

30 mg = 30,000 mcg/hr

b) Convert mcg/hr to mcg/min.

30,000 mcg/hr ÷ 60 min = 500 mcg/min

23. 25 g : 300 mL = 2 g : x mL

$$\frac{25x}{25} = \frac{600}{25}$$

$$x = \frac{600}{25}$$

$$x = 24 \text{ mL/hr to administer 2 g}$$

24. Determine dose per hour.

200 mcg/min × 60 min = 12,000 mcg/hr

Convert mcg to mg

(1,000 mcg = 1 mg)

12,000 mcg ÷ 1,000 = 12 mg/hr

Calculate the mL/hr.

400 mg : 500 mL = 12 mg : x mL

$$\frac{400x}{400} = \frac{6,000}{400}$$

$$x = 15 \text{ mL/hr}$$

25. 25 g : 300 mL = 3 g : x mL

$$\frac{25x}{25} = \frac{900}{25}$$

$$x = \frac{900}{25}$$

$$x = 36 \text{ mL/hr to admin-ister 3 g}$$

26. Convert dose per min to dose per hour.

10 mcg/min × 60 = 600 mcg/hr

Convert measures to like units (mcg to mg)
1,000 mcg = 1 mg

600 mcg = 600 ÷ 1,000 = 0.6 mg

c) Calculate mL/hr.

50 mg : 250 mL = 0.6 mg : x mL

$$\frac{50x}{50} = \frac{150}{50}$$

$$x = 3 \text{ mL/hr}$$

Calculate the flow rate in gtt/min.

$$x \text{ gtt/min} = \frac{3 \text{ mL} \times 60 \text{ gtt/mL}}{60 \text{ min}}$$

x = gtt/min; 3 microgtt/min

To deliver 10 mcg/min, the I.V. is to infuse at 3 gtt/min (3 microgtt/min).

27. Convert weight in lb to kg.

120 lb = 54.54 = 54.5 kg

Calculate dose per minute.

54.5 kg × 2 mcg = 109 mcg/min

28. No conversion of weight is required.

80 kg × 3 mcg = 240 mcg/minute

29. No conversion of weight is required.

73.5 kg × 0.7 mg = 51.45 mg/hr

30. a) Convert weight in lb to kg.

110 lb ÷ 2.2 = 50 kg

Calculate the dose per hour.

50 kg × 0.7 mg = 35 mg/hr

b) Calculate the dose per minute.

35 mg/hr ÷ 60 min = 0.58 mg/min = 0.6 mg/min

c) The dose is safe, it falls within the safe range.

31. Step 1: Convert to like units.

Equivalent: 1,000 mcg = 1 mg

Therefore 2 mg = 2,000 mcg

Step 2: Calculate the concentration of solution in mcg/mL.

2,000 mcg : 500 mL = x mcg : 1 mL

$$\frac{500x}{500} = \frac{2,000}{500}$$

$$x = 4 \text{ mcg/mL}$$

Lower dose: 4 mcg : 1 mL = 2 mcg : x mL

$$\frac{4x}{4} = \frac{2}{4}$$

$$x = 0.5 \text{ mL/min}$$

Upper dose: 4 mcg : 1 mL = 6 mcg : x mL

$$\frac{4x}{4} = \frac{6}{4}$$

$$x = 1.5 \text{ mL/min}$$

Step 3: Convert mL/min to mL/hr.

Lower dose: 0.5 mL × 60 min = 30 mL/hr (gtt/min)

Upper dose: 1.5 mL × 60 min = 90 mL/hr (gtt/min)

A dose range of 2-6 mcg/min is equal to a flow rate of 30-90 mL/hr (gtt/min).

32. Determine the doe per hour.

0.15 mg/min × 60 min = 9 mg/hr

Calculate the flow rate (mL/hr, gtt/min).

$$150 \text{ mg} : 500 \text{ mL} = 9 \text{ mg} : x \text{ mL}$$

$$\frac{150x}{150} = \frac{4,500}{150} = 30 \text{ mL/hr}$$

To infuse 0.15 mg/min set the flow rate at 30 mL/hr (gtt/min).

33. Step 1: Convert to like units.

   Equivalent: 1,000 mcg = 1 mg

   Therefore 5,000 mg = 5,000,000 mcg

   Step 2: Calculate the concentration of solution in mcg/mL.

   $$5,000,000 \text{ mcg} : 500 \text{ mL} = x \text{ mcg} : 1 \text{ mL}$$

   $$\frac{500x}{500} = \frac{5,000,000}{500}$$

   $$x = 10,000 \text{ mcg/mL}$$

   The concentration of solution is 10,000 mcg/mL.

   Step 3: Calculate the dose range.

   Lower dose: 50 mcg × 60 kg = 3,000 mcg/min

   Upper dose: 75 mcg × 60 kg = 4,500 mcg/min

   Step 4: Convert the dose range to mL/min.

   Lower dose: 10,000 mcg : 1 mL = 3,000 mcg : x mL

   $$\frac{10,000x}{10,000} = \frac{3,000}{10,000}$$

   $$x = 0.3 \text{ mL/min}$$

   Upper dose: 10,000 mcg : 1 mL = 4,500 mcg : x mL

   $$\frac{10,000x}{10,000} = \frac{4,500}{10,000}$$

   $$x = 0.45 \text{ mL/min}$$

   Step 5: Convert mL/min to mL/hr.

   Lower dose: 0.3 mL × 60 min = 18 mL/hr (gtt/min)

   Upper dose: 0.45 mL × 60 min = 27 mL/hr (gtt/min)

   a) A dose range of 50-75 mcg is equal to a flow rate of 18-27 mL/hr (gtt/min).

   b) Determine the dose per minute infusing at 30 mL/hr.

   $$10,000 \text{ mcg} : 1 \text{ mL} = x \text{ mcg} : 30 \text{ mL}$$

   $$x = 10,000 \times 30 = 300,000 \text{ mcg/hr}$$

   300,000 mcg/hr ÷ 60 min = 5,000 mcg/min

34. Calculate the dose per minute for client.

   65 kg × 10 mcg = 650 mcg/min

   Determine the dose per hour.

   650 mcg/min × 60 min = 39,000 mcg/hr

   Convert to like units.

   1,000 mcg = 1 mg

   39,000 mcg = 39 mg/hr

   Calculate mL/hr flow rate:

   $$500 \text{ mg} : 250 \text{ mL} = 39 \text{ mg} : x \text{ mL}$$

   $$x = 19.5 = 20 \text{ mL/hr}$$

   Answer: To deliver a dose of 10 mcg/kg set the flow rate at 20 mL/hr (gtt/min).

35. Convert g to mg.

   1,000 mg = 1 g

   0.25 g = 250 mg

   Calculate mg/hr.

   250 mg ÷ 6 = 41.6 = 42 mg/hr

   Answer: The client is receiving 42 mg/hr of aminophylline.

36. a) Convert g to mg.

   1 g = 1,000 mg

   Calculate mg/hr.

   $$1,000 \text{ mg} : 500 \text{ mL} = x \text{ mg} : 20 \text{ mL}$$

   $$x = 40 \text{ mg/hr}$$

   b) Convert mg/hr to mg/min.

   40 mg/hr ÷ 60 min = 0.66 mg/min = 0.7 mg

   Answer: At the rate of 20 mL/hr, the client is receiving a dose of 40 mg/hr or 0.7 mg/min.

37. a) Convert gtt/min to mL/min.

   $$60 \text{ gtt} : 1 \text{ mL} = 15 \text{ gtt} : x \text{ mL}$$

   $$x = 0.25 = 0.3 \text{ mL/min}$$

   Determine mg/min.

   $$300 \text{ mg} : 500 \text{ mL} = x \text{ mg} : 0.3 \text{ mL}$$

   $$x = 0.18 = 0.2 \text{ mg/min}$$

   b) Calculate mg/hr.

   0.2 mg/min × 60 min = 12 mg/hr

   Answer: At 15 gtt/min, the client is receiving a dose of 0.2 mg/min and 12 mg/hr.

38. a) 10,240 mcg/min

   b) 102 mL/hr

   Calculate the dosage per min.

   100 mcg/kg/min × 102.4 kg = 10,240 mcg/min

   Convert mcg/min to mg/min.

   10,240 mcg ÷ 1,000 = 10.24 = 10.2 mg/min

Convert mg/min to mg/hr.

$$10.2 \text{ mg/min} \times 60 \text{ min} = 612 \text{ mg/hr}$$

Calculate flow rate.

$$1 \text{ g} = 1,000 \text{ mg}; 1.5 \text{ g} = 1,500 \text{ mg}$$

$$1,500 \text{ mg} : 250 \text{ mL} = 612 \text{ mg} : x \text{ mL}$$

$$1,500 \ x = 250 \times 612$$

$$\frac{1,500x}{1,500} = \frac{153,000}{1,500}$$

$$x = 102 \text{ mL/hr}$$

OR

$$\frac{1,500 \text{ mg}}{250 \text{ mL}} = \frac{612 \text{ mg}}{x \text{ mL}}$$

39. a) 0.27 mg/min

    b) 270 mcg/min

    Calculate mg/hr infusing.

    $$500 \text{ mL} : 400 \text{ mg} = 20 \text{ mL} : x \text{ mg}$$

    OR

    $$\frac{500 \text{ mL}}{400 \text{ mg}} = \frac{20 \text{ mL}}{x \text{ mg}}$$

    $$500x = 400 \times 20$$

    $$\frac{500x}{500} = \frac{8,000}{500}$$

    $$x = 16 \text{ mg/hr}$$

    Calculate the mg/min infusing.

    $$16 \text{ mg/hr} \div 60 \text{ min} = 0.266 = 0.27 \text{ mg/min}$$

    $$0.27 \text{ mg} = 270 \text{ mcg/min}$$

40. 11 mL/hr

    Calculate dose per minute.

    $$3 \text{ mcg/kg/min} \times 59.1 \text{ kg} = 177.3 \text{ mcg/min}$$

    Convert mcg/min to mcg/hr.

    $$177.3 \text{ mcg/min} \times 60 = 10,638 \text{ mcg/hr}$$

Convert mcg/hr to mg/hr.

$$10,638 \text{ mcg/hr} = 10.63 = 10.6 \text{ mg/hr}$$

Calculate the flow rate.

$$250 \text{ mg} : 250 \text{ mL} = 10.6 \text{ mg} : x \text{ mL}$$

OR

$$\frac{250 \text{ mg}}{250 \text{ mL}} = \frac{10.6 \text{ mg}}{x \text{ mL}}$$

$$250x = 250 \times 10.6$$

$$\frac{250x}{250} = \frac{2,650}{250}$$

$$x = 10.6 = 11 \text{ mL/hr}$$

41. a) 375 mcg/min

    b) 22,500 mcg/hr

    c) 23 mL/hr

    Convert client's weight to kg (2.2 lb = 1 kg).

    $$165 \text{ lb} \div 2.2 = 75 \text{ kg}$$

    Calculate dosage per minute.

    $$5 \text{ mcg/kg/min} \times 75 \text{ kg} = 375 \text{ mcg/min}$$

    Convert mcg/min to mcg/hr.

    $$375 \text{ mcg/min} \times 60 = 22,500 \text{ mcg/hr}$$

    Convert mcg/hr to mg/hr.

    $$22,500 \text{ mcg/hr} = 22.5 \text{ mg/hr}$$

    Calculate flow rate.

    $$250 \text{ mg} : 250 \text{ mL} = 22.5 \text{ mg} : x \text{ mL}$$

    OR

    $$\frac{250 \text{ mg}}{250 \text{ mL}} = \frac{22.5 \text{ mg}}{x \text{ mL}}$$

    $$250x = 250 \times 22.5$$

    $$\frac{250x}{250} = \frac{5,625}{250}$$

    $$x = 22.5 = 23 \text{ mL/hr}$$

CHAPTER 24

Answers to Practice Problems

Note:

The following problems could be set up without placing 1 under a value; however placing a 1 under the value as shown in the set-up for problems 1-20 doesn't alter the value of the number.

1. $\text{gr } x = \dfrac{\text{gr } 1}{60 \text{ mg}} \times \dfrac{15 \text{ mg}}{1}$

2. $x \text{ mg} = \dfrac{60 \text{ mg}}{\text{gr } 1} \times \dfrac{\text{gr v}}{1}$

3. $x \text{ mg} = \dfrac{1 \text{ mg}}{1,000 \text{ mcg}} \times \dfrac{400 \text{ mcg}}{1}$

4. $x \text{ mL} = \dfrac{15 \text{ mL}}{1 \text{ tbs}} \times \dfrac{2 \text{ tbs}}{1}$

5. $x \text{ mg} = \dfrac{1,000 \text{ mg}}{1 \text{ g}} \times \dfrac{0.007 \text{ g}}{1}$

6. $x \text{ mL} = \dfrac{1,000 \text{ mL}}{1 \text{ L}} \times \dfrac{0.5 \text{ L}}{1}$

7. $x \text{ g} = \dfrac{1 \text{ g}}{1,000 \text{ mg}} \times \dfrac{529 \text{ mg}}{1}$

8. $x \text{ L} = \dfrac{1 \text{ L}}{1,000 \text{ mL}} \times \dfrac{1,600 \text{ mL}}{1}$

9. $x \text{ lb} = \dfrac{1 \text{ lb}}{2.2 \text{ kg}} \times \dfrac{46.4 \text{ kg}}{1}$

10. $x \text{ inch} = \dfrac{1 \text{ inch}}{2.5 \text{ cm}} \times \dfrac{5 \text{ cm}}{1}$

11. $x \text{ mL} = \dfrac{1.5 \text{ mL}}{0.4 \text{ g}} \times \dfrac{0.3 \text{ g}}{1}$

12. $x \text{ mL} = \dfrac{1 \text{ mL}}{15 \text{ mg}} \times \dfrac{60 \text{ mg}}{\text{gr } 1} \times \dfrac{\text{gr } 1/4}{1}$

13. $x \text{ cap} = \dfrac{1 \text{ cap}}{500 \text{ mg}} \times \dfrac{1,000 \text{ mg}}{1 \text{ g}} \times \dfrac{1 \text{ g}}{1}$

14. $x \text{ mL} = \dfrac{5 \text{ mL}}{400 \text{ mg}} \times \dfrac{400 \text{ mg}}{1}$

15. $x \text{ mL} = \dfrac{1 \text{ mL}}{25 \text{ mg}} \times \dfrac{150 \text{ mg}}{1}$

16. $x \text{ tab} = \dfrac{1 \text{ tab}}{125 \text{ mg}} \times \dfrac{250 \text{ mg}}{1}$

17. $x \text{ tab} = \dfrac{1 \text{ tab}}{0.25 \text{ mg}} \times \dfrac{0.125 \text{ mg}}{1}$

18. $x \text{ mL} = \dfrac{5 \text{ mL}}{125 \text{ mg}} \times \dfrac{300 \text{ mg}}{1}$

19. $x \text{ mL} = \dfrac{5 \text{ mL}}{125 \text{ mg}} \times \dfrac{1,000 \text{ mg}}{1 \text{ g}} \times \dfrac{1 \text{ g}}{1}$

20. $x \text{ mL} = \dfrac{1 \text{ mL}}{150 \text{ mg}} \times \dfrac{1,000 \text{ mg}}{1 \text{ g}} \times \dfrac{0.3 \text{ g}}{1}$

21. $\dfrac{x \text{ gtt}}{\text{min}} = \dfrac{15 \text{ gtt}}{1 \text{ mL}} \times \dfrac{100 \text{ mL}}{40 \text{ min}}$

$x = \dfrac{15 \times 100}{40} = 37.5 = 38 \text{ gtt/min}$

$x = 38 \text{ gtt/min; } 38 \text{ macrogtt/min}$

Note:

Placing a 1 under the value doesn't alter the value of the number.

Answers to Chapter Review

1. $x \text{ tab} = \dfrac{1 \text{ tab}}{12.5 \text{ mg}} \times \dfrac{25 \text{ mg}}{1}$

$x = \dfrac{25}{12.5}$

$x = 2 \text{ tabs}$

2. $x \text{ mL} = \dfrac{15 \text{ mL}}{30 \text{ mEq}} \times \dfrac{20 \text{ mEq}}{1}$

$x = \dfrac{15 \times 20}{30}$

$x = \dfrac{300}{30}$

$x = 10 \text{ mL}$

22. $\dfrac{x \text{ gtt}}{\text{min}} = \dfrac{60 \text{ gtt}}{1 \text{ mL}} \times \dfrac{40 \text{ mL}}{30 \text{ min}}$

$x = \dfrac{60 \times 40}{30} = \dfrac{2,400}{30} = 80 \text{ gtt/min}$

$x = 80 \text{ gtt/min; } 80 \text{ microgtt/min}$

23. $\dfrac{x \text{ gtt}}{\text{min}} = \dfrac{60 \text{ gtt}}{1 \text{ mL}} \times \dfrac{20 \text{ mL}}{60 \text{ min}}$

$x = \dfrac{60 \times 20}{60} = 20 \text{ gtt/min}$

$x = 20 \text{ gtt/min; } 20 \text{ microgtt/min}$

24. $\dfrac{x \text{ gtt}}{\text{min}} = \dfrac{15 \text{ gtt}}{1 \text{ mL}} \times \dfrac{150 \text{ mL}}{60 \text{ min}}$

$x = \dfrac{15 \times 150}{60} = 37.5 = 38 \text{ gtt/min}$

$x = 38 \text{ gtt/min; } 38 \text{ macrogtt/min}$

25. $\dfrac{x \text{ gtt}}{\text{min}} = \dfrac{10 \text{ gtt}}{1 \text{ mL}} \times \dfrac{125 \text{ mL}}{60 \text{ min}}$

(Note that mL/hr was determined first.

$\dfrac{1,500 \text{ mL}}{12 \text{ hr}} = 125 \text{ mL/hr, expressed}$

as $\dfrac{125 \text{ mL}}{60 \text{ min}}$)

$x = \dfrac{10 \times 125}{60} = 20.8 = 21 \text{ gtt/min}$

$x = 21 \text{ gtt/min; } 21 \text{ macrogtt/min}$

Note:

The I.V. problems have been done expressing 1 hr as 60 minutes (1 hr = 60 minutes). Time has been expressed in minutes. This relates to rates to infuse within 1 hour. Problems could have been done using 1 hr in the equation; however, remember then you must add the conversion factor to the equation: 1 hr = 60 minutes.

3. $x \text{ mL} = \dfrac{1 \text{ mL}}{15 \text{ mg}} \times \dfrac{20 \text{ mg}}{1}$

$x = \dfrac{20}{15}$

$x = 1.3 \text{ mL}$

4. $x \text{ mL} = \dfrac{1 \text{ mL}}{225 \text{ mg}} \times \dfrac{1,000 \text{ mg}}{1 \text{ g}} \times \dfrac{0.5 \text{ g}}{1}$

$x = \dfrac{1 \times 1,000}{225} \times 0.5 = \dfrac{500}{225}$

$x = 2.2 \text{ mL}$

5. $x \text{ tab} = \dfrac{1 \text{ tab}}{25 \text{ mg}} \times \dfrac{18.75 \text{ mg}}{1}$

    $x = \dfrac{18.75}{25}$

    $x = 0.75 = 3/4$ tab (state as 3/4 tab; tablets scored in fourths)

6. $x \text{ mL} = \dfrac{1 \text{ mL}}{100 \text{ mg}} \times \dfrac{80 \text{ mg}}{1}$

    $x = \dfrac{80}{100}$

    $x = 0.8 \text{ mL}$

7. $x \text{ mL} = \dfrac{1 \text{ mL}}{10,000 \text{ U}} \times \dfrac{6,500 \text{ U}}{1}$

    $x = \dfrac{6,500}{10,000}$

    $x = 0.65 \text{ mL}$

8. $x \text{ mL} = \dfrac{4 \text{ mL}}{0.6 \text{ g}} \times \dfrac{1 \text{ g}}{1,000 \text{ mg}} \times \dfrac{300 \text{ mg}}{1}$

    $x = \dfrac{4 \times 300}{0.6 \times 1,000} = \dfrac{1,200}{600}$

    $x = 2 \text{ mL}$

9. $x \text{ tab} = \dfrac{1 \text{ tab}}{150 \text{ mg}} \times \dfrac{300 \text{ mg}}{1}$

    $x = \dfrac{300}{150}$

    $x = 2 \text{ tabs}$

10. $x \text{ mL} = \dfrac{1 \text{ mL}}{62.5 \text{ mg}} \times \dfrac{175 \text{ mg}}{1}$

    $x = \dfrac{175}{62.5}$

    $x = 2.8 \text{ mL}$

11. $x \text{ mL} = \dfrac{1,000 \text{ mL}}{1 \text{ qt}} \times \dfrac{3 \text{ qt}}{1}$

    $x = \dfrac{1,000 \times 3}{1}$

    $x = \dfrac{3,000}{1}$

    $x = 3,000 \text{ mL}$

12. $x \text{ kg} = \dfrac{1 \text{ kg}}{2.2 \text{ lb}} \times \dfrac{79 \text{ lb}}{1}$

    $x = \dfrac{79}{2.2}$

    $x = 35.9 \text{ kg}$ (to the nearest tenth)

13. $x \text{ mg} = \dfrac{1 \text{ mg}}{1,000 \text{ mcg}} \times \dfrac{5 \text{ mcg}}{1}$

    $x = \dfrac{5}{1,000}$

    $x = 0.005 \text{ mg}$

14. $x \text{ L} = \dfrac{1 \text{ L}}{1,000 \text{ mL}} \times \dfrac{2,400 \text{ mL}}{1}$

    $x = \dfrac{2,400}{1,000}$

    $x = 2.4 \text{ L}$

15. $x \text{ cm} = \dfrac{2.5 \text{ cm}}{1 \text{ in}} \times \dfrac{8 \text{ in}}{1}$

    $x = \dfrac{2.5 \times 8}{1}$

    $x = 20 \text{ inches}$

16. $\dfrac{x \text{ gtt}}{\text{min}} = \dfrac{10 \text{ gtt}}{1 \text{ mL}} \times \dfrac{75 \text{ mL}}{60 \text{ min}}$

    $x = \dfrac{10 \times 75}{60} = 12.5 = 13 \text{ gtt/min}$

    $x = 13 \text{ gtt/min}; 13 \text{ macrogtt/min}$

17. $\dfrac{x \text{ gtt}}{\text{min}} = \dfrac{15 \text{ gtt}}{1 \text{ mL}} \times \dfrac{150 \text{ mL}}{60 \text{ min}}$

    $x = \dfrac{15 \times 150}{60} = 37.5 = 38 \text{ gtt/min}$

    $x = 38 \text{ gtt/min}; 38 \text{ macrogtt/min}$

18. $\dfrac{x \text{ gtt}}{\text{min}} = \dfrac{60 \text{ gtt}}{1 \text{ mL}} \times \dfrac{100 \text{ mL}}{60 \text{ min}}$

    $x = \dfrac{60 \times 100}{60} = 100 \text{ gtt/min}$

    $x = 100 \text{ gtt/min}; 100 \text{ microgtt/min}$

           OR

    $\dfrac{x \text{ gtt}}{\text{min}} = \dfrac{60 \text{ gtt}}{1 \text{ mL}} \times \dfrac{100 \text{ mL}}{1 \text{ hr}} \times \dfrac{1 \text{ hr}}{60 \text{ min}}$

19. $\dfrac{x \text{ gtt}}{\text{min}} = \dfrac{60 \text{ gtt}}{1 \text{ mL}} \times \dfrac{17 \text{ mL}}{60 \text{ min}}$

$$x = \frac{60 \times 17}{60} = 17 = 17 \text{ gtt/min}$$

$x = 17$ gtt/min; 17 microgtt/min

OR

$$\frac{x \text{ gtt}}{\text{min}} = \frac{60 \text{ gtt}}{1 \text{ mL}} \times \frac{17 \text{ mL}}{1 \text{ hr}} \times \frac{1 \text{ hr}}{60 \text{ min}}$$

20. $$\frac{x \text{ gtt}}{\text{min}} = \frac{15 \text{ gtt}}{1 \text{ mL}} \times \frac{63 \text{ mL}}{60 \text{ min}}$$

$$x = \frac{15 \times 63}{60} = 15.7 = 16 \text{ gtt/min}$$

$x = 16$ gtt/min; 16 macrogtt/min

OR

$$\frac{x \text{ gtt}}{\text{min}} = \frac{15 \text{ gtt}}{1 \text{ mL}} \times \frac{63 \text{ mL}}{1 \text{ hr}} \times \frac{1 \text{ hr}}{60 \text{ min}}$$

Note:

Note for I.V. rates to infuse in 1 hr: if the rate is not stated in minutes (60 min) then the conversion factor (1 hr = 60 min) must be included as part of the dimensional analysis equation (see illustration of this in problems 18–20). Larger volumes with time periods greater than an hour have been calculated by determining mL/hr first before proceeding with the calculation to make numbers smaller.

ANSWERS TO COMPREHENSIVE POSTTEST

1. 200 mg : 5 mL = 300 mg : x mL

   OR

   $$\frac{300 \text{ mg}}{200 \text{ mg}} \times 5 \text{ mL} = x \text{ mL}; \quad \frac{300 \text{ mg}}{200 \text{ mg}} = \frac{x \text{ mL}}{5 \text{ mL}}$$

   Answer: 7.5 mL or $7\frac{1}{2}$ mL

2. Conversion is required.

   Equivalent: 1,000 mg = 1 g

   500 mg : 1 tab = 1,000 mg : x tab

   OR

   $$\frac{1,000 \text{ mg}}{500 \text{ mg}} \times 1 \text{ tab} = x \text{ tab}; \quad \frac{1,000 \text{ mg}}{500 \text{ mg}} = \frac{x \text{ tab}}{1 \text{ tab}}$$

   Answer: 2 tabs

3. 0.1 mg : 1 cap = 0.2 mg : x cap

   OR

   $$\frac{0.2 \text{ mg}}{0.1 \text{ mg}} \times 1 \text{ cap} = x \text{ cap}; \quad \frac{0.2 \text{ mg}}{0.1 \text{ mg}} = \frac{x \text{ cap}}{1 \text{ cap}}$$

   Answer: 2 caps

4. Tablets B Septra DS. The doctor's order indicates DS, which means double strength; therefore the client should be given the tabs that are labeled DS.

5. 0.1 mg : 1 mL = 1 mg : x mL

   OR

   $$\frac{1 \text{ mg}}{0.1 \text{ mg}} \times 1 \text{ mL} - x \text{ mL}; \quad \frac{1 \text{ mg}}{0.1 \text{ mg}} = \frac{x \text{ mL}}{1 \text{ mL}}$$

   Answer: 10 mL

6. 10,000 U : 1 mL = 6,500 U : x mL

    OR

    $$\frac{6{,}500 \text{ U}}{10{,}000 \text{ U}} \times 1 \text{ mL} = x \text{ mL}; \quad \frac{6{,}500 \text{ U}}{10{,}000 \text{ U}} = \frac{x \text{ mL}}{1 \text{ mL}}$$

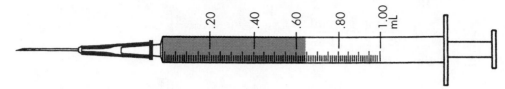

    Answer: 0.65 mL

7. Conversion is required. Equivalent: 1,000 mg = 1 g

    Therefore 0.75 g = 750 mg

    1,200 mg : 120 mL = 750 mg : x mL

    OR

    $$\frac{750 \text{ mg}}{1{,}200 \text{ mg}} \times 120 \text{ mL} = x \text{ mL}; \quad \frac{750 \text{ mg}}{1{,}200 \text{ mg}} = \frac{x \text{ mL}}{120 \text{ mL}}$$

    Answer: 75 mL

8. a) 50 mg : 10 mL = 75 mg : x mL

    OR

    $$\frac{75 \text{ mg}}{50 \text{ mg}} \times 10 \text{ mL} = x \text{ mL}; \quad \frac{75 \text{ mg}}{50 \text{ mg}} = \frac{x \text{ mL}}{10 \text{ mL}}$$

    Answer: 15 mL

    b) 1. Determine mL/hr.

    $$x \text{ mL/hr} = \frac{1{,}000 \text{ mL}}{6}; \quad x = 166.6 = 167 \text{ mL/hr}$$

    2. Use formula and determine gtt/min.

    $$x \text{ gtt/min} = \frac{167 \text{ (mL)} \times 10 \text{ (gtt/mL)}}{60 \text{ (min)}} = 27.8 = 28 \text{ gtt/min}$$

    Answer: 28 macrogtt/min; 28 gtt/min

Note:

Problem 8 could also be done using the shortcut method illustrated in Chapter 21.

9. Convert weight in lb to kg. Equivalent: 2.2 lb = 1 kg

    Therefore 110 ÷ 2.2 = 50 kg

    50 kg × 1 mg = 50 mg

    Answer: 50 mg

10. Conversion is required. Equivalent: 1,000 mg = 1 g

    Therefore 0.3 g = 300 mg

    150 mg : 1 tab = 300 mg : x tab

    OR

    $$\frac{300 \text{ mg}}{150 \text{ mg}} \times 1 \text{ tab} = x \text{ tab}; \quad \frac{300 \text{ mg}}{150 \text{ mg}} = \frac{x \text{ tab}}{1 \text{ tab}}$$

    Answer: 2 tabs

11. a) 95 mg/mL (Vial is 1 g.)

    b) Conversion is required. 1,000 mg = 1 g

    Therefore 0.25 g = 250 mg

    95 mg : 1 mL = 250 mg : x mL

    OR

    $\dfrac{250 \text{ mg}}{95 \text{ mg}} \times 1 \text{ mL} = x \text{ mL}; \dfrac{250 \text{ mg}}{95 \text{ mg}} = \dfrac{x \text{ mL}}{1 \text{ mL}}$

    Answer: 2.63 mL = 2.6 mL to nearest tenth

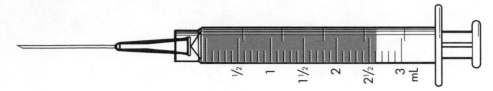

12. Answer: 2 tabs (one 50-mg tab and one 25-mg tab)

    Total = 75 mg (one 50-mg tab and one 25-mg tab)

    Administer the least number of tablets to client.

13. Step 1: Determine mL/hr.

    $x \text{ mL/hr} = \dfrac{250 \text{ mL}}{3 \text{ hr}}; x = 83.3 =$

    83 mL/hr

    Step 2: Calculate gtt/min.

    $x \text{ gtt/min} = \dfrac{83 \text{ (mL)} \times 20 \text{ (gtt/mL)}}{60 \text{ (min)}}$

    $x = 27.6 = 28 \text{ gtt/min}$

    Answer: 28 macrogtt/min; 28 gtt/min

    The shortcut method could also have been used to do the problem.

14. $x \text{ gtt/min} = \dfrac{80 \text{ (mL)} \times 15 \text{ (gtt/mL)}}{60 \text{ (min)}}$

    $x = 20 \text{ gtt/min}$

    Answer: 20 macrogtt/min; 20 gtt/min

15. $x \text{ gtt/min} = \dfrac{100 \text{ (mL)} \times 10 \text{ (gtt/mL)}}{45 \text{ (min)}}$

    $x = 22.2 = 22 \text{ gtt/min}$

    Answer: 22 macrogtt/min; 22 gtt/min

16. $\dfrac{1,000 \text{ mL}}{60 \text{ mL/hr}} = 16.66$

    $60 \times 0.66 = 39.6 = 40 \text{ minutes}$

    Answer: 16 hr + 40 minutes

17. 6 mg TMP × 12 kg = 72 mg/day

    12 mg TMP × 12 kg = 144 mg/day

    Divided dose: 72 mg/day ÷ 2 = 36 mg q12h

    144 mg/day ÷ 2 = 72 mg q12h

    The safe dose range is 72-144 mg/day

    The divided dose is 36-72 mg q12h

    Answer: The doctor ordered 60 mg q12h. The dose is safe (60 mg × 2 = 120 mg); it falls within the safe dose range.

18. $\dfrac{100 \text{ mL}}{50 \text{ mL/hr}} = 2 \text{ hr}$

    a) 2 hr

    b) 12 noon or 12 PM (10:00 AM and 2 hours); military time: 1200

19. Determine the dose per hour.

    10 mcg/min × 60 min = 600 mcg/hr

    Convert to like units:

    1,000 mcg = 1 mg, therefore

    600 mcg = 0.6 mg

    Calculate mL/hr.

    50 mg : 250 mL = 0.6 mg : x mL

    OR

    $\dfrac{50 \text{ mg}}{250 \text{ mL}} = \dfrac{0.6 \text{ mg}}{x \text{ mL}}$

    $x = 3 \text{ mL/hr}$

    Answer: To deliver 10 mcg/min, set the flow rate at 3 mL/hr (gtt/min).

20. a) 22 units

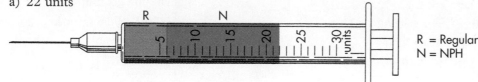

R = Regular
N = NPH

21. a) 52 mL

b) $x \text{ gtt/min} = \dfrac{55 \text{ (mL)} \times 60 \text{ (gtt/mL)}}{50 \text{ (min)}}$

$x = 66 \text{ gtt/min}$

Answer: 66 microgtt/min; 66 gtt/min. The shortcut method could also have been used to do this problem.

c) 66 mL/hr (gtt/min with a microdrip = mL/hr)

22. Administer 2 20-mg tablets. The client should receive the least number of tabs. If 10 mg tabs are used, the client would require 4 tabs. The maximum number of tablets that should be administered is 3. Remember: question any order requiring more than this.

   1 20-mg tab
 + 1 20-mg tab
   40 mg

23. $\sqrt{\dfrac{102 \text{ (lb)} \times 51 \text{ (in)}}{3,131}} = \sqrt{1.66} = 1.288 = 1.29 \text{ m}^2$

Answer: 1.29 m²

24. a) $\sqrt{\dfrac{13.6 \text{ (kg)} \times 60 \text{ cm}}{3,600}} = \sqrt{0.226} = 0.475 = 0.48 \text{ m}^2$

   Answer: 0.48 m². The amount required is greater than what is available. Therefore you would need more than 1 mL to administer the dose.

b) 0.48 m² × 500 mg/m² = 240 mg

   Answer: 240 mg

c) 50 mg : 1 mL = 240 mg : x mL

   OR

   $\dfrac{240 \text{ mg}}{50 \text{ mg}} \times 1 \text{ mL} = x \text{ mL}; \dfrac{240 \text{ mg}}{50 \text{ mg}} = \dfrac{x \text{ mL}}{1 \text{ mL}}$

   Answer: 4.8 mL

25. a) 25 mg : 1 tab = 50 mg : x tab

   OR

   $\dfrac{50 \text{ mg}}{25 \text{ mg}} \times 1 \text{ tab} = x \text{ tab}; \dfrac{50 \text{ mg}}{25 \text{ mg}} = \dfrac{x \text{ tab}}{1 \text{ tab}}$

   Answer: 2 tabs

b) Hold the medication since the systolic b/p (top number) is less than 100 and notify the prescriber.

26. $\dfrac{2}{5} \times 250 \text{ mL} = x \text{ mL}$

   $\dfrac{500}{5} = x$

   $x = 100 \text{ mL of Ensure Plus}$

   250 mL − 100 mL = 150 mL (water)

   Therefore you would add 150 mL water to 100 mL Ensure Plus to make 250 mL 2/5-strength Ensure Plus.

27. $x \text{ mL/hr} = \dfrac{400 \text{ mL}}{6 \text{ hr}}$

   $x = 66.6 = 67 \text{ mL/hr}$

   Answer: 67 mL/hr

28. $x \text{ gtt/min} = \dfrac{70 \text{ (mL)} \times 60 \text{ (gtt/mL)}}{50 \text{ (min)}}$

   $x = 84 \text{ gtt/min}$

   a) 84 microgtt/min; 84 gtt/min. The shortcut method could also have been used to do this problem.

   b) 84 mL/hr

29. Step 1: Calculate the normal daily dosage range.

   40 mg/day × 21.4 kg = 856 mg
   50 mg/day × 21.4 kg = 1,070 mg

   The normal dosage range is 856-1,070 mg/day.

   Step 2: Calculate the dose infusing in 24 hr.

   500 mg q12h = (2 doses)
   500 mg × 2 = 1,000 mg in 24/hr

   Step 3: Assess the accuracy of dose ordered.

   500 mg q12hr (1,000 mg) falls within the 856-1,070 mg/day dosage range. Administer the medication as ordered.

30. 1 L = 1,000 mL; therefore 2 L = 2,000 mL

Dextrose: 5 g : 100 mL = x g : 2,000 mL

$$\frac{100x}{100} = \frac{10,000}{100}$$

OR

$$\frac{5\ g}{100\ mL} = \frac{x\ g}{2,000\ mL}$$

x = 100 g dextrose

NaCl: 0.225 g : 100 mL = x g : 2,000 mL

$$\frac{100x}{100} = \frac{450}{100}$$

OR

$$\frac{0.225\ g}{100\ mL} = \frac{x\ g}{2,000\ mL}$$

x = 4.5 g NaCl

Note:

Remember 1/4 NS is written as 0.225.

31. Time remaining: 3 hr − 1.5 hr = 1.5 hr (1 1/2)

Volume remaining: 500 mL − 175 mL = 325 mL

Step 1: Calculate mL/hr

325 mL ÷ 1.5 hr = 216.6 = 217 mL/hr

Step 2: Calculate the gtt/min

$$x\ gtt/min = \frac{217\ mL \times 10\ gtt/mL}{60\ min}$$

$$x = \frac{217 \times 1}{6} = \frac{217}{6}$$

x = 36 gtt/min; 36 macrogtt/min

The I.V. rate would have to be changed to 36 gtt/min (36 macrogtt/min).

Step 3: Determine the percentage of change

$$\frac{36 - 28}{28} = \frac{8}{28} = 0.285 = 29\%$$

Course of action: Assess the client, and notify the prescriber. This increase is greater than 25%.

32. Time remaining: 8 hr − 4hr = 4 hr

Volume remaining: 1,000 mL − 600 mL = 400 mL

Step 1: Calculate mL/hr

400 mL ÷ 4 hr = 100 mL/hr

Step 2: Calculate the gtt/min

$$x\ gtt/min = \frac{100\ mL \times 15\ gtt/mL}{60\ min}$$

$$x = \frac{100 \times 1}{4} = \frac{100}{4}$$

x = 25 gtt/min; 25 macrogtt/min

The I.V. rate would have to be changed to 25 gtt/min (25 macrogtt/min).

Step 3: Determine the percentage of change

$$\frac{25 - 31}{31} = \frac{-6}{31} = -0.193 = -19\%$$

Course of action: Assess the client and lower the I.V. rate to 25 gtt/min (25 macrogtt/min). This is an acceptable decrease (−19%); it's within the acceptable 25% variation. Also check the institution's policy and continue observation of the client.

Note:

In problems 31 and 32, in addition to determining mL/hr, another shortcut method could be used to determine the drop factor constant.

33. Step 1: Calculate the U/hr infusing

500 mL : 20,000 U = 25 mL : x U

$$\frac{500x}{500} = \frac{500,000}{500}$$

$$x = 1,000\ U/hr$$

An I.V. of 500 mL containing 20,000 U of heparin infusing at 25 mL/hr is administering 1,000 U /hr.

Step 2: Determine the heparinizing dose

1,000 U/hr × 24 hr = 24,000 U/24 hr

The dose is safe. It is within the 20,000 to 40,000 U in 24 hr heparinizing range.

Index

A

Abbreviations
  for common intravenous solutions, 388
  for scheduling medications, 139
  medication, 121
  metric, 62
Absorbed fluids, 86
Access devices, I.V. therapy and, 382
Acetaminophen, 225
Acetaminophen elixir, 238
Acetic acid solution, 74
Acquired immunodeficiency syndrome
    (AIDS), 110
Addition
  of decimals, 26-27
  of fractions, 16-17
Add-Vantage System, 381-382
Administration
  and calculation, methods of, 101-204
    calculating doses using ratio-
      proportion, 165-186
    dose calculation using the formula
      method, 187-204
    medication administration, 103-117
    medication administration records,
      131-146
    reading medication labels, 147-164
    understanding medication orders,
      119-130
  of medication. *See* Medication adminis-
    tration.
Administration sets, drip factor and, 397
Afronad, 463
Aging, special considerations and, 105
AIDS. *See* Acquired immunodeficiency
    syndrome (AIDS).
Aldomet, 142, 223, 473
Amikacin, 197, 371
Amikin, 285
Aminophylline, 182, 199, 262, 290, 459,
    462, 463, 465
Amoxicillin, 180, 197, 236, 244, 308-309,
    355, 365, 371
Amoxil, 266
Amphotericin B, 481
Ampicillin, 128, 129, 171, 209, 213-214,
    221, 294, 305, 371, 409, 472-473

Ampule, 247-248
Amrinone, 466
Analysis, dimensional. *See* Dimensional
    analysis.
Ancef, 309
Antiarrhythmic drugs, 455
Antivert, 245, 477
AOT. *See* Assisted outpatient treatment
    (AOT).
Apothecaries' system, 7, 69-72
  converting within and between other sys-
    tems of measurement and, 77-92
  equivalents among household and metric
    systems and, 77, 78
  fractions and, 215
Apresoline. *See* Hydralazine (Apresoline).
Aquamephyton, 275
Arabic system, 7, 8, 70
Aramine, 455, 461
Ascorbic acid, 235
Aspirin, 69, 128, 194, 228
Assisted outpatient treatment (AOT), 108
Atacand, 243
Ativan, 164, 180, 199, 243, 286
Atropine, 69, 128, 147, 148, 180, 199,
    278, 371, 373
Atropine sulfate, 271-272
Augmentin, 156, 174, 182, 201, 228, 240,
    297, 370, 473, 479
Azathioprine (Imuran), 122
Azidothymidine (AZT), 369
AZT, 122, 369

B

Baclofen, 172, 222
Bacteriostatic water, powdered drugs
    and, 292
Bactrim, 153
Barrel of syringe, 251
Baxer Mini-Bag Plus, 380, 382
Benadryl, 129, 178, 203
Betamethasone, 290
Bicillin, 284
Body surface area (BSA), 41, 367-369
  pediatric dose calculation and, 356-364
Body weight, 99
  pediatric dose calculation and, 343,
    344, 348

Boiling point of water, 94
Bolus, I.V., 382-383
Brand name, 122
Bretylium, 462, 463
BSA. *See* Body surface area (BSA).
Buccal route of administration of
    medications, 110
Buretrol, 380
    pediatric intravenous administra-
        tion and, 420
Burette, 421
    calculating I.V. medications by,
        420-424
    calibrated, pediatric intravenous
        administration and, 420

C

Calcium carbonate, 222
Calcium gluconate, 264
Calculation
    administration and. *See* Adminis-
        tration and calculation,
        methods of.
    critical care. *See* Critical care
        calculations.
    dose. *See* Dose calculation.
    heparin. *See* Heparin calculations.
    intravenous. *See* Intravenous (I.V.)
        calculations.
    of oral liquids, 230
    of oral medications. *See* Oral med-
        ications, calculation of.
Calculators in calculation of critical
    care doses, 361-362
Calibrated burettes, pediatric
    intravenous administration
    and, 420
Calibrated dropper, 111, 112, 230
Caplets, 207
Capoten, 23, 208, 220, 227, 228,
    477, 486
Capsules, 41, 208-209, 210-230
Carafate, 129, 175
Carbenicillin, 308
Carbidopa, 153, 154
Cardizem, 163, 164, 175
Carpuject, 250, 251
Cartridge, 251
Ceclor, 186
Cefadyl, 316
Cefepime hydrochloride (Maxipime),
    315-316
Cefobid, 296
Cefotaxime, 310-311
Ceftazidime (Tazidime), 312,
    351-352, 367
Celsius and Fahrenheit, converting
    between, 93-96
Centigrade, 93-95
Centimeter (cm), 96
    cubic, 251-254

Centimeter (cm)—cont'd
    formula for calculating body
        surface area from, 362
Central line, I.V. therapy and, 378
Cephradine, 196
Charting of I.V. therapy, 418-419
Chemical compound of drug, 122
Children. *See* pediatric entries.
Chloromycetin, 311-312
Cimetidine, 289
Cipro, 161, 184, 203, 481
Cisplatin, 363
Cleocin, 366, 371, 477
Client
    education of, medication adminis-
        tration and, 108-109
    full name of, on medication
        order, 121
    right, medication administration
        and, 106
Clindamycin, 203, 278, 353,
    409, 474
Clonazepam, 228
Clonidine, 110, 245
Clozaril, 203
Codeine, 195, 281
Cogentin, 174, 196, 225, 263, 275
Colace, 124, 209, 235
Combined drugs, medication labels
    for, 153-158
Compazine, 129, 185, 274
Complex fraction, 12-15
Comprehensive posttest, 479-487
Computer controlled dispensing sys-
    tem, 137, 138
Computerized infusion pumps, 386
Computerized medication records,
    137, 138
Computer time, 139-140
Continu-Flo Solution Set, 397
Conversion clock, 71
Conversion factors, dimensional
    analysis and, 467-468
Conversions
    between Celsius and Fahrenheit,
        93-96
    between metric units, 63-64
    between systems of measurement,
        77-81, 83-84
    calculating intake and output and,
        84-89
    from military to traditional time,
        140-141
    from traditional to military time,
        139-140
    methods of, 78-81
    metric measures relating to length
        and, 96-97, 99
    of mg to g, 167
    performing, using dimensional
        analysis, 468-469

Conversions—cont'd
    relating to length, 96, 99
    relating to weight, 97-99
    useful in health care setting,
        93-100
    within and between systems, 77-92
    within same system of measure-
        ment, 81-83
Corvert, 163, 262-263, 480
Coumadin, 157, 221
Coverage orders for insulin, 326,
    327-328
Critical care calculations, 455-466
    calculating doses based on
        mcg/kg/min, 457-458
    calculating mL/hr rate, 456
    drugs ordered in milligrams per
        minute, 457
    per hour, 456-457
    per minute, 456-457
    titration of infusions, 458-459
Critical thinking
    and medication administration, 104
    drug calculation errors and, 98,
        112, 120, 152, 155, 216
    errors in administration and, 149
CSII pump, 321
Cubic centimeter (cc), 61, 63,
    251-254
Cubic millimeter, 60
Cyanocobalamin, 152

D

D5, 417, 418
Dakins solution, 74
Dalteparin. *See* Fragmin (Dal-
    teparin).
Daraprim. *See* Pyrimethamine
    (Daraprim).
Date
    on medication order, 121-122
    on medication record, 132
Decadron, 159, 224
Deciliter, 60
Decimal place values, 24
Decimal point, movement of, conver-
    sion and, 78-79
Decimals, 23-35
    addition and subtraction of, 26-27
    changing, to fractions, 32-33
    changing, to percentages, 48-49
    changing fractions to, 32
    changing percentages to, 47-48
    comparing value of, 25-26
    division of, 29-30
        by decimal, 30
        by decimal movement, 30
        by whole number, 30
    multiplying, 27-29
    reading and writing, 24-25
    rounding off, 31-32, 41

Demerol. *See* Meperidine (Demerol).
Denominator
    of fraction, 11
    of ratio, 37
Depakote, 243
Depo-Medrol, 198, 286
Depo-Provera, 161, 185, 202
Dexamethasone, 172, 226
Dextrose, 390, 392, 487
    powdered drugs and, 292
5% Dextrose, 388
    in normal saline, 389
Diabetes mellitus, insulin for, 317
Diabinese, 172
Dicloxacillin, 130, 223, 365
Dicloxacillin sodium, 237, 350-351
Digoxin, 23, 128, 142, 173, 194,
    212-213, 236, 244, 278,
    370, 473
Dilantin, 128, 129, 157, 178, 196,
    222, 229, 233, 235, 242, 245,
    348-349, 354, 474
Dilaudid, 152, 279, 281
Diluent, powdered drugs and, 291
Dimensional analysis, 82, 467-478
    basics of, 467-470
    dosage calculation using, 470-474
    performing conversions using,
        468-469
    using, to calculate I.V. flow rates,
        474-477
Diphenhydramine HCl, 236
Displacement, reconstitution of,
    292-293
Displacement factor, reconstitution
    of powdered drugs and,
    292-293
Dividend, division of decimals
    and, 29
Division
    of decimals, 29-30
    of fractions, 19-20
Division factor in calculation of I.V.
    flow rates, 404
Divisor, division of decimals and, 29
D5 0.9% N.S., 453
Dobutamine, 457, 458, 464, 465
Dobutrex, 459, 465
Doctor's orders. *See* Medication
    orders.
Doctor's order sheet, 120
Documentation
    of medications administered on
        medication record, 132,
        133-135
    right, medication administration
        and, 106
Dopamine, 456-457, 461, 463,
    464, 466
Dosage strength, 149
Dosage volume (DV), 188

Dosage weight (DW), 188
Dose
    factors influencing, 104-105
    on medication order, 122
    parenteral, calculation of, 267
    right, medication administration
        and, 107
Dose calculation
    applying ratio-proportion to,
        41-43
    equipment used for, 111-112
    for medications in units, 272-277
    pediatric. *See* Pediatric dose calcu-
        lation.
    reconstitution of powdered drugs
        and, 302-304
    using dimensional analysis,
        470-474
    using formula method, 187-204
    using ratio-proportion, 165-186
Double-scale 1-mL syringe, 324
dr. *See* Dram (dr).
Dram (dr), 69, 71, 72
Drip factor, administration sets
    and, 397
D5 R/L, 416
Drop (gtt), 73
Dropper
    calibrated, 111, 112, 230
    medicine, 112, 231
Drug doses. *See* Dose.
Drugs. *See also* Medications;
    Powdered drugs.
DTNS, 484
Dual-channel infusion pump, I.V.
    therapy and, 385
DV. *See* Dosage volume (DV).
D5W, 391, 395, 401-403, 405, 406,
    416, 417-418, 450, 451, 452,
    453, 456, 460, 464, 465, 476,
    477, 478, 487
DW. *See* Dosage weight (DW).

E

Effexor, 178
Elderly, special considerations for,
    105-106
Electronic dispensing system,
    137, 138
Electronic infusion devices, I.V.
    therapy and, 383-387
Electronic rate controllers, I.V.
    therapy and, 383-384
Electronic volumetric pumps, I.V.
    therapy and, 384-385
Elixir, 230
    of phenobarbital, 197, 233-234
Elixophyllin elixir, 245
Emulsions, lipid, 392-393
Enoxaprin. *See* Lovenox
    (Enoxaprin).

Ensure Plus, 486
Enteral feedings, 424-430
Enteric-coated tablets, 208, 209
Epinephrine, 455, 459, 460, 463
Epivir, 160, 184, 238, 369, 482
Epivir Oral Solution, 149
Epogen, 287
Equipment
    for administering oral medications
        to children, 112-115
    for dose calculation, 111-112
Equivalents, dimensional analysis
    and, 467-468
Erythromycin, 235, 245, 298,
    373, 409
Esmolol, 465, 466
Ethambutol, 220
Expiration date (EXP) on
    medication administration
    record, 151
Extended release tablets, 208, 209
Extenders for inhalers, 110
Extremes, proportions and, 38

F

Factor-label method, dimensional
    analysis and, 467
Fahrenheit and Celsius, converting
    between, 93-96
Fast-acting insulin, 317, 319
Fixed combination insulins, 320, 321
Flagyl, 177
Flagyl IVPB, 484
Fleming, Doris R., 320, 329-330
Flow rates
    I.V. *See* Intravenous flow rates.
    of heparin, 442-443
Fluids
    absorbed, 86
    infused, 86
    I.V. *See* Intravenous fluids.
Folic acid, 128
Form of medication, 150
Formula
    calculation of doses using, 165
    in calculation of critical care doses,
        362
    solution using, 441
Formula method
    dose calculation using, 187-204
    for calculating I.V. flow rate,
        400-406
    solution using, 212-213, 214-216,
        217-218, 233, 234, 237,
        269-270, 271-272, 273-274,
        302-304
Fractions, 11-22
    adding, 16-17
    Apothecaries' system and, 215
    changing, to decimals, 32
    changing, to percentages, 48-49

Fractions—cont'd
changing decimals to, 32-33
changing percentages to, 47-48
complex, 12-15
dividing, 19-20
fundamental rules of, 14
improper, 12-15
multiplying, 18
proper, 12-15
reducing, 15-16
rules for comparing size of, 13
subtracting, 17-18
types of, 12-15
Fragmin (Dalteparin), 440
Freezing point of water, 94
Frequency of administration on
medication order, 123-124
Fungizone, 161, 355-356, 410
Furadantin, 365
Furosemide (Lasix), 128, 142, 178,
226, 277, 290, 365, 471

G

Gantrisin, 193, 367
Gelatin-coated liquid capsule, 209
Generic name, 122, 147-148
Gentamicin, 178, 179, 198, 269,
349-350
Gentamycin, 371, 471-472
Gentamycin Sulfate, 126
Glucephage, 243
Glucophage, 204
Glyburide, 226
Grain (gr), 71, 77
Gram (g), 59, 62-63
Gravity flow intravenous
piggyback, 379
gtt. *See* Drop (gtt).

H

Haldol, 237, 282
Heparin, 129, 180, 180, 198, 258,
264, 266, 272-273, 276, 280,
283, 382, 446, 447, 448,
449, 450, 451, 452, 453,
477, 480
Heparin calculations, 439-453
calculation of I.V. heparin solutions, 441-443
calculation of S.C. doses, 440-441
determining if dose is within safe
heparinizing range, 443-444
Heparin labels, 440
Heparin sodium, 163, 439
Hep-Lock flush solution, 440
Heplocks, I.V. therapy and, 382
Home care
infusion devices for, 387, 388
medication administration and, 109
Hourly urine output, 86

Household system, 72-75
converting within and between
other systems of measurement
and, 77-92
equivalents among Apothecaries'
and metric systems and,
77, 78
Humalog insulin, 317
Humalog U-100, 338
Humulin, 318
Humulin Lente U-100, 336, 337,
339, 340
Humulin NPH, 332
Humulin NPH U-100, 329, 337,
339, 340, 341
Humulin R, 317
Humulin Regular, 122
Humulin Regular U-100, 326, 329,
330, 331, 334, 336, 338, 339,
340, 341
Humulin 70/30 U-100, 338, 341
Humulin U U-100, 340
Hydralazine (Apresoline), 148
Hydrochlorothiazide, 194, 244
Hydromorphone HCl, 152
Hydroxyzine (Vistaril), 148, 156,
182, 198, 262, 284
Hyperalimentation, 393
Hypodermic, 251-258
large, 257
small, 253

I

Ilosone, 355
I.M. route of administration,
concentration of medication
and, 299
Improper fraction, 12-15
Imuran. *See* Azathioprine (Imuran).
Inches, formula for calculating body
surface area from, 362-363
Inderal LA, 230
Indocin, 151, 193, 227
Indomethacin, 151
Indwelling infusion ports, I.V. ther-
apy and, 382
Infused fluids, 86
Infusion
methods of, intravenous, 378-387
titration of, 458-459
Infusion devices
electronic, I.V. therapy and,
383-387
for home care setting, 387, 388
Infusion ports, I.V. therapy and, 382
Infusion pump
computerized, 386
I.V. therapy and, 384-385
Infusion times
and volumes, calculation of,
412-413

Infusion times—cont'd
calculation of, when mL/hr is not
indicated, 419-421
total, calculation of, 417-418
Inhalation route of administration of
medications, 110
Initials on medication record, 132
Injectable medications, calculation
of, according to syringe,
267-272
Inocar, 466
Instillation of medications into body
cavity, 110
Insulin, 264, 266, 317-343, 412
appearance of, 320
fixed combination, 320, 321
insulin orders, 326, 327-328
MAR for administration of,
327-328
measuring two types of, in same
syringe, 329-332
mixing, 330
preparing single dose of, in insulin
syringe, 329
types of, 258-259, 317-320
U-100 syringe, 321-325
Insulin orders, 326
Insulin syringes, 258-261, 267, 322
preparing single dose of insulin
in, 329
same, measuring two types of insulin in, 329-332
Intake
liquid, 84
oral, 84
and output (I&O), calculation of,
84-89
and output (I&O) sheet, 84, 85,
87, 88, 391
InterLink System, 397
Intermediate-acting insulin, 317,
319-320
International System of Units (SI),
59
Intravenous (I.V.) bolus, 382-383
Intravenous (I.V.) calculations,
377-438
calculating infusion time when
ml/hr is not indicated,
419-421
calculating I.V. medications by
burette, 420-424
charting, 418-419
determining amount of drug in
specific amount of solution,
410-412
determining infusion times and
volumes, 412-413
determining total infusion times,
417-418
enteral feedings, 424-430

Intravenous (I.V.) calculations—cont'd
  for I.V. therapy for children, 420
  I.V. fluids, 387-394
  I.V. medications, 408-410
  I.V. tubing, 396-398
  labeling solution bags, 421
  methods of infusion, 378-387, 388
  of flow rates. *See* Intravenous flow
    rates.
  steps to calculating problem with
    an unknown, 413-414
Intravenous (I.V.) flow rates
  calculation of, 394-395
    formula method for, 400-406
    in gtt/min, 399-400
    using dimensional analysis,
      474-477
    using formula method, 400-406
    using shortcut method, 404-406
    when several solutions are
      ordered, 407-408
  recalculation of, 414-417
Intravenous (I.V.) fluids, 387-394.
    See also Intravenous calcula-
    tions.
  calculating gtt/min using large
    volumes of, 475-477
  calculating percentage in, 390-394
  calculating small volumes of, in
    gtt/min, 474-475
  charting, on I&O record, 391
Intravenous (I.V.) heparin solutions,
    calculation of, 441-443
Intravenous (I.V.) infusion set, 379
Intravenous (I.V.) medications,
    408-410. *See also* Intravenous
    calculations.
  calculation of, by burette, 420-424
  determining amount of, in specific
    amount of solution, 410-412
  protocols for, 393
Intravenous piggyback (IVPB),
    378-380, 408
Intravenous (I.V.) push, 382-383
Intravenous (I.V.) route of adminis-
    tration, concentration of med-
    ication and, 299
Intravenous solutions
  common, abbreviations for, 388.
    See also Intravenous (I.V.) cal-
    culations
  percentage strengths of, 46
Intravenous (I.V.) therapy. *See* Intra-
    venous (I.V.) calculations.
Intravenous (I.V.) tubing, 396-398
I&O. *See* Intake and output (I&O).
Isoniazid, 229
Isosorbide dinitrate, 172
Isuprel, 456, 463
I.V. *See* Intravenous entries.
IVPB. *See* Intravenous piggyback.

K
Kanamycin (Kantrex), 199, 245,
    270, 353
Kangaroo pump, 425
Kantrex. *See* Kanamycin (Kantrex).
Kaon-Cl, 180, 235
Kardex, 131
Keflex, 174, 195, 236, 237, 366, 474
Keflin, 408-409
Kefzol, 477
Kendra's law, 107-108
Kilo, 60
Kilogram (kg), 60, 63
  converting lb to, 97-98
    pediatric dose calculation and,
      344-345
  converting, to lb, 98-99
    pediatric dose calculation and,
      346
  formula for calculating body
    surface area from, 362
Kiloliter, 60

L
Labeling. *See also* Medication labels.
  for combined drugs, 153-158
  for multiple-strength solution, 299
  of solution bags, 421
  parenteral, reading, 261-263
Labetalol. *See* Trandate (Labetalol).
Lactated Ringer's solution, 389, 484
Lactulose, 185, 233, 245
Lanoxicaps, 177, 209, 479
Lanoxin, 159, 208, 221, 285
Lasix. *See* Furosemide (Lasix).
lb
  converting kg to, 98-99
    pediatric dose calculation and,
      346
  converting, to kg, 97-98
    pediatric dose calculation and,
      344-345
  formula for calculating body sur-
    face area from, 362-363
Length
  conversions relating to, 99
  metric measures relating to, 96-97
  of stay (LOS), 122
Lente, 317
Levodopa, 153, 154
Levophed. *See* Norepinephrine
    (Levophed).
Levothyroxine sodium, 314
Librium, 128
Lidocaine, 263, 457, 461, 463, 466
Like units, 458
Lipid emulsions, 392-393
Liquid intake, 84
Liquids, oral. *See* Oral liquids.
Lispro, 317
Liter (l), 59, 62, 63

Lithium carbonate, 237
Lithium citrate, 199
Lo-Dose syringe, 259, 260, 321,
    322, 323
  double-scale 1-mL, 321, 322, 324
  single-scale 1-mL, 321, 322, 324
Long-acting insulin, 317, 320
Lopid, 200
Lopressor, 177, 242, 243
LOS. *See* Length of stay (LOS).
Lovenox (Enoxaprin), 288, 440
Lowest terms, fractions and, 41
Lozenges, 209
Luer-Lok syringe, 251

M
Macrodantin, 173
Macrodrip chamber, 398
Macrodrop, 398
Macrodrop tubing, 396
Magnesium sulfate, 464
MAR. *See* Medication administration
    record (MAR).
Math review, 1-55
  decimals, 23-35
  fractions, 11-22
  percentages, 45-51
  ratio and proportion, 37-44
  Roman numerals, 7-9
Maxipime. *See* Cefepime hydro-
    chloride (Maxipime).
MDI. *See* Metered dose inhaler
    (MDI).
Means, proportions and, 38
Measurement, systems of. *See*
    Systems of measurement.
Measuring cup, 73, 230
Medication abbreviations, 121
Medication administration, 103-117
  critical thinking and, 104
  equipment for administering oral
    medications to children,
    112-115
  equipment used for dose calcula-
    tion, 111-112, 113, 114
  factors influencing drug doses and
    action in, 104-105
  home care considerations an, 109
  patient education and, 108-109
  routes of, 109-110
  six rights of, 106-108
  special considerations for elderly,
    105-106
  symbols and abbreviations for
    units of measure used in, 120
Medication administration record
    (MAR), 119, 125, 131-146
  computerized, 137, 138
  documentation of medications ad-
    ministered and, 132, 133-135

Medication administration record—cont'd
  essential information on, 132, 136
  explanation of, 135-137
  for insulin administration, 327-328
  medication administration and, 106
  military time and, 139-141
  scheduling medication times, 138-139
  unit dose system and, 137-138
Medication information on medication record, 132
Medication labels, 147-164. *See also* Labeling.
  directions for mixing or reconstituting a medication, 151
  dosage strength, 149
  for combined drugs, 153-158
  form of, 150
  generic name, 147-148
  precautions on, 151-153, 154
  route of administration, 150, 151
  total volume, 150-151
  trade name, 148-149, 150
Medication orders, 119-130
  components of, 120-124
  interpreting of, 124-126
  writing of, 120
Medications, 7
  calculation of, when final concentration is not stated, 298
  calculation of doses for, in units, 272-277
  combined, medication labels for, 153-158
  daily, container for, 106
  documentation of administration of, on medication record, 132, 133-135
  injectable, calculation of, according to syringe, 267-272
  I.V. *See* Intravenous medications.
  labeled in percentage strengths, 263-264
  name of, on medication order, 122
  oral. *See* Oral medications.
  parenteral. *See* Parenteral medications.
  reading measured amount of, in syringe, 255
  right, medication administration and, 106
  right to refuse, 106
  solid, forms of, 207-209
  titrated, 455
  week's, container for, 106
  weight of, in volume of solution, ratio and, 41
Medication ticket, medication administration and, 106

Medicine cup, 61, 73, 111, 231
Medicine dropper, 112, 231
Medlocks, I.V. therapy and, 382
Mellaril, 185, 236, 241
Meniscus, 231
Meperidine (Demerol), 128, 147-148, 276, 284, 373
Meperidine hydrochloride, 179, 196
Mercaptopurine, 354
Mestonin. *See* Pyridostigmine bromide (Mestonin).
Meter, 59
Metered dose inhaler (MDI), 110
Methergine, 127, 280
Methotrexate, 371
Metric abbreviations, 62
Metric measures relating to length, 96-97
Metric system, 59-67, 69
  conversions between metric units, 63-64
  converting within and between other systems of measurement and, 77-92
  equivalents among Apothecaries' and household systems and, 77, 78
  particulars of, 59-62
  rules of, 62
  units of measure of, 62-63
Mevacor, 178, 245
Mezlocillin, 306, 409
Microdrip, 455
Microdrip chamber, 398
Microdrop, 398
Microdrop sets, 420
Microdrop tubing, 396-398
Microgram (mcg), 61, 62
Military time, medication administration records and, 139-141
Milk of magnesia, 129
Milliequivalents (mEq), parenteral medications in, 265-266
Milligram (mg), 61, 62, 63
Milliliter (mL), 60, 61, 62, 63, 251-254
Millimeter (mm), 96
  cubic, 60
Mini-Bag Plus, 380, 382
Minim (m), 69, 71, 254, 269
Minipress, 128, 158, 195
Mistaken identity of name of medication, 122
Mithracin, 367
Mix-O-Vial, 249, 250
Morphine, 69, 147, 179, 180, 371
Morphine sulfate, 129, 198, 270-271, 277, 280, 354, 477
Motrin, 178, 195, 229
Multiple-strength solution, label for, 299

Multiplication
  by decimal movement, 28-29
  of decimals, 27-29
  of fractions, 18
Mycostatin suspension, 239
Mylanta, 126
Mylicon, 128

N

NaCl. *See* Sodium chloride (NaCl).
Nafcillin, 310, 316
Name
  brand, 122
  generic, 122, 147-148
  proprietary, 148-149, 150
  trade, 122, 148-149, 150
Nasogastric (NG), 424
National Drug Code (NDC) number on medication administration record, 151
National Formulary (N.F.), 148
NDC number. *See* National Drug Code (NDC) number.
Nebcin. *See* Tobramycin sulfate (Nebcin).
Needleless infusion system, I.V. therapy and, 384
Needle sticks, needle with plastic guard in prevention of, 253
Needle with plastic guard to prevent needle sticks, 253
Nembutal, 128, 202, 216-217, 287
Neomycin ophthalmic ointment, 129
Nepro, 425
N.F. *See* National Formulary (N.F.).
NG. *See* Nasogastric (NG).
Nicoderm, 110
Nicotine patch, 110
Nipride. *See* Sodium nitroprusside (Nipride).
Nitrofurantoin, 130
Nitroglycerin (Nitrostat), 69, 70, 208, 214-216, 225, 245, 459, 463, 464, 484
Nitroglycerin patch, 110
Nitroprusside, 455
Nitrostat. *See* Nitroglycerin (Nitrostat).
Nomogram, West, pediatric dose calculation and, 359
Non-Luer-Lok syringe, 251
Norepinephrine (Levophed), 455, 465
Normal saline (NS), 74, 387, 388, 395, 401, 403, 405, 416, 450, 451, 476, 478
  5% dextrose in, 389
  I.V. therapy and, 382
Norvasc, 243
Novolin R, 318

Novolin Regular U-100, 337, 338, 339
Novolin R U-100, 334
NPH insulin, 317
NS. *See* Normal saline (NS).
Numerals, Roman, 7-9
Numerator
    of fraction, 11
    of ratio, 37
Numorphan, 289
Nutrition
    parenteral, 392. See also Parenteral medications.
    total parenteral, 393
Nystatin, 180

O

Oral intake, 84
Oral liquids
    calculation of, 230
    measurement of, 230-241
Oral medications
    calculation of, 207-245
        capsules, 208-209, 210-230
        forms of solid medications, 207-209
        oral liquids, 230-241
        tablets, 207-208, 210-230
    equipment for administering, to children, 112-115
    pediatric, 364
Oral route of administration of medications, 110
Oral syringes, 111, 113, 231
Ounce (oz), 71, 72
Oxacillin, 294-295, 306, 366
Oxacillin sodium, reconstitution of, 292, 293
Oxytocin (Pitocin), 264, 459, 462

P

Packaging of parenteral medications, 247-251
Parenteral dosages, calculation of, 267
Parenteral labels, reading, 261-263
Parenteral medications, 247-290
    calculating dosages of, 267
    calculating doses for medications in units, 272-277
    calculating injectable medications according to syringe, 267-272
    drugs labeled in percentage strengths and, 263-264
    in milliequivalents, 265-266
    measured in units, 264
    packaging of, 247-251, 252
    pediatric, 364
    reading, 261-263
    solutions expressed in ratio strength and, 264

syringes, 251-261
Parenteral nutrition, 392
Parenteral route of administration of medications, 110
Parenteral syringe, 112, 113, 114
Patch, topical medications and, 110
Patient-controlled analgesia (PCA), 385-387
Patient education, medication administration and, 108-109
PCA. *See* Patient-controlled analgesia (PCA).
PDR. *See* Physician's Desk Reference (PDR).
Pediatric dose calculation, 343-373
    calculation of doses based on body weight, 343, 344
    converting kg to lb, 346-356
    converting lb to kg, 344-345
    I.V. therapy and, 420
    oral medications, 364
    parenteral medications, 364
    principles relating to basic calculations, 344
    using body surface area, 356-357, 359-364
    West nomogram chart, 357-358
Pediatric intravenous administration, 420
Pediatric oral medications, 364
Pediatric parenteral medications, 364
PEG. *See* Percutaneous endoscopic gastrostomy (PEG).
Penicillin, 264, 298, 299
Penicillin G, 279, 307
Penicillin G potassium, 300-301, 312
Penicillin G procaine, 273-274
Pentamidine, 110
Percentages, 45-51
    calculating, in I.V. fluids, 390-394
    changing, to fractions, decimals, and ratios, 47-48
    changing fractions, decimals, and ratios to, 48-49
    determining percent of quantity, 50
    determining what percent one number is of another, 50-51
Percentage solution, 46
Percent of quantity, determining, 50
Percocet, 142
Percutaneous endoscopic gastrostomy (PEG), 424
Percutaneous route of administration of medications, 110
Peripheral line, I.V. therapy and, 378
Phenergan, 281
Phenobarbital, 147, 171, 172, 173, 182, 193, 223, 236, 353
Phenobarbital elixir, 197, 233-234

Physician's Desk Reference (PDR), 292, 343
Piggyback
    intravenous. *See* Intravenous piggyback.
    tandem, 380
Pint, 72
Pitocin. *See* Oxytocin (Pitocin).
Plunger of syringe, 251
Pneumocystis carinii pneumonia, 110
Posttest, 53-55
    comprehensive, 479-487
Potassium, 265, 410-411
Potassium chloride, 128, 142, 159, 178, 198, 201, 265, 411, 412, 477, 487
Pound. *See* lb.
Powdered drugs, 291-316
    basic principles for reconstitution of, 291-298
    calculation of doses and, 302-304
    reconstituting from package insert directions, 301-302
    reconstituting medications with more than one direction for mixing, 298-301
Pravachol, 243
Prazosin hydrochloride, 225
Precautions on medication administration record, 151-153
Prednisone, 129
Prefixes used in health care, 60
Prepackaged syringe, 251
Pretest, 3-5
Prilosec, 126
Primidone, 203
Procaine penicillin, 198, 371
Procaine penicillin G, 126
Procan SR, 245, 479
Procardia XL, 229
Product, decimals and, 27
Pronestyl, 290, 457, 462
Proper fraction, 12-15
Proper name of drug, 122
Proportion, 38-39. *See also* Ratio-proportion.
Proprietary name, 148-149, 150
Proventil, 373
Prozac, 184, 200, 241
Pulmo Care, 425, 486
Pump
    computerized infusion, 386
    CSII, 321
    electronic volumetric, I.V. therapy and, 384-385
    kangaroo, 425
    syringe, 385, 386
    volumetric. *See* Volumetric pumps.
Push, I.V., 382-383
Pyridium, 226

Pyridostigmine bromide (Mestonin), 122
Pyrimethamine (Daraprim), 122
Pyxis system, 138, 153

Q

Quart, 72
Quotient, division of decimals and, 29

R

Rapid-acting insulin, 317
Ratio, 37
  and proportion, 37-44. *See also* Ratio-proportion.
  changing percentages to, 47-48
  changing, to percentages, 48-49
Ratio-proportion, 456-457
  applying, to dosage calculation, 41-43
  calculation of doses using, 165-186
  in calculation of U/hr of heparin, 441
  in converting within and between systems, 80, 81-84
  rules for, 80-81
  solution using, 212, 213, 214, 215, 216, 218, 233, 234, 237, 269, 270, 271, 272, 273, 302, 303, 441
  solving for *x* in, 39-41
Ratio strength, solutions expressed in, 264
Reading decimals, 24-25
Reading medication labels. *See* Medication labels.
Reconstitution
  directions for, 151
  of powdered drugs, 291-316
    basic principles for, 291-298
    from package insert directions, 301-302
    with more than one direction for mixing, 298-301
Reducing fractions, 15-16
Registration symbol, 122, 149
Reglan, 221, 276
Regular-acting insulin, 317, 319
Regular Humulin insulin, 126, 128
Regular Humulin insulin U-100, 326, 329, 330, 331, 333
Respectively, medication label and, 299
Restoril, 126, 142, 173
Retrovir. *See* Zidovudine (Retrovir).
Rifampin, 175
Right
  to be educated regarding medications, 108
  to refuse medications, 106
Right client, medication administration and, 106

Right documentation, medication administration and, 106
Right dose, medication administration and, 107
Right drug, medication administration and, 106
Right route, medication administration and, 106
Right time, medication administration and, 106
Risperdal, 177
Ritodrine (Yutopar), 463, 465
R/L, 406, 416, 476, 478
Robinul, 199, 283
Roman numerals, 7-9, 70
Rounding off decimals, 31-32, 41
Route(s) of medication administration, 109-110, 150, 151
  on medication order, 122-123
  right, 106
Rule of Nines, 46

S

Safe heparinizing range, determining if dose of heparin is within, 443-444
Saline, normal. *See* Normal saline (NS).
Saline locks, I.V. therapy and, 382
Sandostatin, 275
S.C. heparin, 440-441
Schedule of medication times, 138-139
Scopolamine, 282
Scored tablets, 207-208, 209
Seconal, 195
Secondary lines, I.V. therapy and, 378
Semilente insulin, 317
Septra, 129, 153, 154-155, 410, 466, 484
Septra DS, 155, 176, 480
Set calibration and flow rate of heparin, 442-443
SI. *See* International System of Units (SI).
Signature of person writing medication order, 124
Sinemet, 153, 176, 200
Single infusion pump, I.V. therapy and, 385
Single-scale 1-mL syringe, 324
Six rights of medication administration, 106-108
Sliding scale, coverage orders for insulin and, 326, 327-328
Small hypodermic, 253
Sodium bicarbonate, 265
Sodium chloride (NaCl), 387, 391, 392
Sodium nitroprusside (Nipride), 455, 457, 458-459, 461, 464

Solid medications, forms of, 207-209
Solu-Cortef, 130, 249, 282, 307
Solu-Medrol, 180, 197, 249, 279, 283
Solumendrol, 478
Soluset, 380
  pediatric intravenous administration and, 420
Solute, definition of, 426
Solution(s)
  acetic acid, 74
  Dakins, 74
  expressed in ratio strength, 264
  intravenous, percentage strengths of, 46
  percentage, 46
  using formula method, 237
  using ratio-proportion method, 237
  volume of, weight of drug in, ratio and, 41
Solution bags, labeling, 421
Solvent
  definition of, 426
  powdered drugs and, 291
Soufflé cup, 111
Spacers for inhalers, 110
Spansules, 208
Special instructions on medication record, 132
Stadol, 199, 281
Stock volume (SV), 188
Stock weight (SW), 188
Strength of drug in volume of solution, ratio and, 41
Streptomycin, 311, 366-367
Streptomycin sulfate, 160
Sublingual route of administration of medications, 110
Sublingual tablets, 208
Subtraction
  of decimals, 26-27
  of fractions, 17-18
Sulfamethoxazole, 153
Sulfasalazine, 227
Suppositories, 110
Suprax, 315
Surfak, 160
Suspension, 230
Sustained release capsules, 208
SV. *See* Stock volume (SV).
SW. *See* Stock weight (SW).
Synthroid, 126, 130, 159, 173, 220, 222, 227, 228
Syringe(s), 251-261
  calculating injectable medications according to, 267-272
  Carpuject, 250
  filling directly from medicine cup, 231
  for measuring oral liquids, 230-231, 231

Syringe(s)—cont'd
  hypodermic, 251-258
  insulin. *See* Insulin syringes.
  Lo-Dose, 259, 260, 321, 322, 323
  Luer-Lok, 251
  Non-Luer-Lok, 251
  oral, 111, 113, 231
  parenteral, 112, 113, 114
  parts of, 113, 252
  prepackaged, 251
  reading measured amount
      of medications in, 255
  tuberculin, 258, 259, 267
  types of, 114, 251-261
  U-100, 321-325
Syringe pumps, 385, 386
Syrup, 230
Système International d'Unités, 59
Systems of measurement, 57-100
  Apothecaries' system, 69-76
  conversions useful in health care
      setting, 93-100
  converting within and between sys-
      tems, 77-92
  household system, 69-76
  metric system, 59-67

T
Tablespoon, 73
Tablets, 41, 207-208, 209, 218-229
  calculating doses involving,
      210-230
  enteric-coated, 208, 209
  extended release, 208, 209
  scored, 207-208, 209
  sublingual, 208
  timed release, 208
  unscored, breaking of, 208
Tagamet, 202, 226, 238, 409
Tandem/piggyback setup, 380
Tazicef, 301, 313, 316, 483
Tazidime. *See* Ceftazidime
      (Tazidime).
Teaspoon, 73
Tegretol, 222, 371
Tetracycline, 209, 373
Theophylline, 235, 373, 465
Thiamine, 477
Thinking, critical. *See* Critical
      thinking.
Thorazine, 183, 185, 196, 218, 224,
      239, 263, 287, 483
Ticar, 295, 306, 313
Ticket, medication, medication
      administration and, 106
Time
  computer, 139-140
  military, medication administration
      records and, 139-141

Time—cont'd
  of administration, 138-139
    on medication order, 121-122,
        123-124
    on medication record, 132
    right, medication administration
        and, 106
    traditional, conversion from
        military time to, 140-141
Timed-release capsules, 208, 209
Timed-release tablets, 208
Timentin, 315
Tip of syringe, 251
Titrated medications, 455
Titration, 455, 458-459
Tobramycin sulfate (Nebcin), 371
Tofranil, 126
Topical route of administration of
      medications, 110
Total infusion times, calculation of,
      417-418
Total parenteral nutrition
      (TPN), 393
Total volume on medication admin-
      istration record, 150-151
TPN. *See* Total parenteral nutrition
      (TPN).
Trade name, 122, 148-149, 150
Trandate (Labetalol), 456, 478
Transdermal route of administration
      of medications, 110
Trilafon, 238
Trimethoprim, 153, 155
Troches, 209
Tuberculin syringes, 258, 259, 267
Tubex, 251, 252
Tubing
  I.V., 396-398
  macrodrop, 396
  microdrop, 396-398
Tylenol, 128, 142, 242, 245, 371

U
U Humulin NPH, 485
U Humulin R, 332
U Humulin Regular, 485
U-100 insulin, 258-259, 319
Ultra Lente, 317
Understanding medication orders.
      See Medication orders.
Unit dose, 137-138
Unit dose packages, 154
Unit dose system, 137-138
United States Pharmacopoeia
      (USP), 148
Unit factor method, dimensional
      analysis and, 467
Units
  calculation of doses for medica-
      tions in, 272-277

Units—conti'd
  in metric system, 62-63
  parenteral medications measured
      in, 264
Unknown, steps to calculating prob-
      lems with, 413-414
Unscored tablets, breaking of, 208
Urine output, hourly, 86
USP. *See* United States Pharma-
      copoeia (USP).
U-100 syringe, 321-325

V
Valium, 218-219, 251, 275, 289
Vancocin HCl, 152, 153
Vancomycin, 314, 354, 409
Vancomycin hydrochloride, 152
Vasodilator drugs, 455
Vasopressor drugs, 455
Vasotec, 157, 203
V-Cillin, 356
V-Cillin K suspension, 237
Velosef, 367
Verapamil, 224
Vial, 248-249
Vibramycin, 179, 366
Vistaril. *See* Hydroxyzine (Vistaril).
Vitamin B$_{12}$, 126, 129, 179
Vitamin K, 280
Vita-Plus B-12, 152
Volume
  in Apothecaries' system, 71-72, 74
  of solution, weight of drug in, ratio
      and, 41
  total, on medication administration
      record, 150-151
  units of measure of, in metric
      system, 63
Volume-controlled devices, 380, 421
Volume control set, parts of, 383
Volumetric pumps
  calculating flow rates for, in mL/hr,
      394-395
  electronic, I.V. therapy and, 384-
      385
Volutrol, 380
  pediatric intravenous administra-
      tion and, 420

W
Water
  bacteriostatic, powdered drugs
      and, 292
  boiling point of, 94
  enteral feedings and, 425
  freezing point of, 94
Weight
  body, 99
  conversions relating to, 97-99, 99
  in Apothecaries' system, 71-72, 74

Weight—cont'd
  of drug in volume of solution,
    ratio and, 41
  pediatric dose calculation and,
    343, 344, 348
  units of measure of, in metric
    system, 62-63
West nomogram, pediatric dose cal-
    culation and, 356-364
Whole numbers, 12-15, 26
  division of, by decimal, 30
  division of decimal by, 30
Writing decimals, 24-25

X

x, solving for, in ratio-proportion,
    39-41
Xanax, 175, 245

Y

Yutopar. *See* Ritodrine (Yutopar).

Z

Zantac, 161, 182, 241, 288, 473
Zidovudine (Retrovir), 122, 126,
    176, 183, 239, 370, 410, 482
Zocor, 149, 151, 164, 485

Zovirax, 161, 174, 240, 297,
    314-315
Zovirax I.V., 486